Blackwell's Five-Minute Veterinary Consult

Clinical Companion

Small Animal Toxicology

Second Edition

Blackwell's Five-Minute Veterinary Consult

Clinical Companion

Small Animal Toxicology

Second Edition

Lynn R. Hovda, RPh, DVM, MS, DACVIM
Ahna G. Brutlag, DVM, MS, DABT, DABVT
Robert H. Poppenga, DVM, PhD, DABVT
Katherine L. Peterson, DVM, DACVECC

First Edition Editors

Lynn R. Hovda, RPh, DVM, MS, DACVIM
Ahna G. Brutlag, DVM, MS, DABT, DABVT
Gary D. Osweiler, DVM, PhD, DABVT
Justine A. Lee, DVM, DACVECC, DABT

WILEY Blackwell

Editorial offices: 1606 Golden Aspen Drive, Suites 103 and 104, Ames, Iowa 50010, USA
The Atrium, Southern Gate, Chichester, West Sussex, PO19 8SQ, UK
9600 Garsington Road, Oxford, OX4 2DQ, UK

For details of our global editorial offices, for customer services and for information about how to apply for permission to reuse the copyright material in this book please see our website at www.wiley.com/wiley-blackwell.

ISBN: 9781119036548

A catalogue record for this book is available from the Library of Congress and the British Library.

Wiley also publishes its books in a variety of electronic formats. Some content that appears in print may not be available in electronic books.

Cover image (middle): Getty Images/© perkmeup

Set in 10.5/13pt ITC Berkeley Oldstyle Std by Aptara Inc., New Delhi, India
Printed and bound in Singapore by Markono Print Media Pte Ltd

1 2016

Dedications

The second edition of this textbook in small animal toxicology is an extension of *Blackwell's Five-Minute Veterinary Consult: Canine and Feline* by Drs Larry Tilley and Frank Smith. We are grateful for their vision and foresight that fostered this textbook as well as others in the series. The editors of this edition would like to acknowledge the efforts of two prior editors, Drs. Gary Osweiler and Justine Lee, as well as the many associated authors who contributed to the original textbook. We are indebted to the current authors whose depth and width of knowledge make the second edition more thorough and complete. Deserving of recognition as well are the wonderful veterinary students who challenge us to become better teachers, clinicians, and toxicologists.

A special thank you to Dr Gretchen Gerber – no one could ask for a better friend or colleague. In remembrance of old friends, many gone but forever present in my heart, and to Bob and Tyne, the cornerstones of my world.

Lynn R. Hovda

To my colleagues and mentors at Pet Poison Helpline, I remain grateful for your continued support and our thought-provoking conversations. And to my husband, Nathan, who keeps my heart filled with joy, my head with humor, and my stomach with deliciousness.

Ahna G. Brutlag

Thanks to my family (Amy, Mia, and Zoe) for all of their support and love. And a shout-out to all of the veterinary students who have discovered (and will continue to discover) how fascinating veterinary toxicology is!

Robert H. Poppenga

To my resident-mates, Jennifer Hall, Elise Craft and Sarah Gray, for your friendship and support in my career. And to Dan for your love and support in the rest of my life.

Katherine L. Peterson

Contents

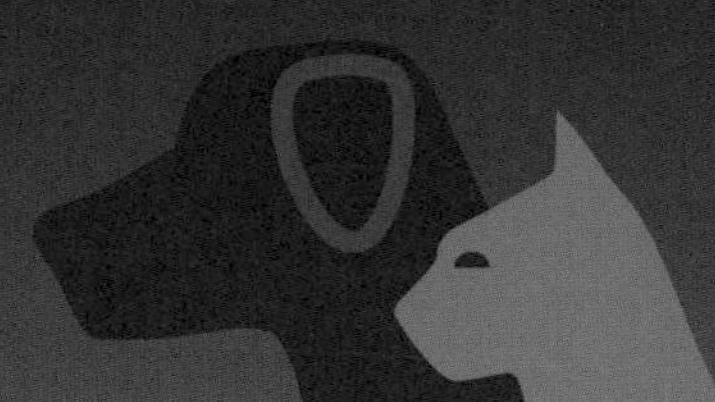

Contributor List

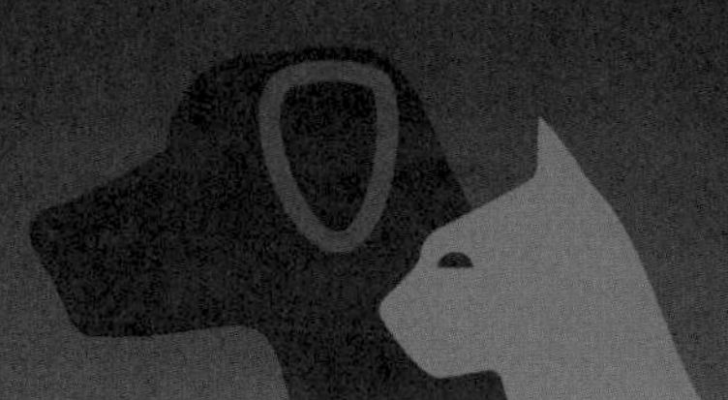

Catherine M. Adams, DVM
Veterinarian Emeritus
Pet Poison Helpline & SafetyCall International, PLLC
Bloomington, Minnesota, USA

Colleen M. Almgren, DVM, PhD, DABT, DABVT
Veterinary Toxicologist
Pet Poison Helpline & SafetyCall International, PLLC
Bloomington, Minnesota, USA

Sarah Alpert, DVM
Associate Veterinarian, Clinical Toxicology
Pet Poison Helpline & SafetyCall International, PLLC
Bloomington, Minnesota, USA

Catherine Angle, DVM, MPH
Associate Veterinarian
Rum River Veterinary Clinic
Anoka, Minnesota, USA
&
Consulting Veterinarian, Clinical Toxicology
Pet Poison Helpline & SafetyCall International, PLLC
Bloomington, Minnesota, USA
&
Chief Veterinary Officer
Vetta Health
Minnetonka, Minnesota, USA

Adrienne Bautista, DVM, PhD, DABVT
Associate Toxicologist
Pesticide and Environmental Toxicology Branch
Office of Environmental Health Hazard Assessment
California Environmental Protection Agency
Sacramento, California, USA

Karyn Bischoff, DVM, MS, DABVT
Diplomate American Board of Veterinary Toxicology
Diagnostic Toxicologist/Senior Extension Associate
New York State Animal Health Diagnostic Center/Cornell University
Ithaca, New York, USA

David R. Brown, PhD
Professor of Pharmacology and Vice Chair
Department of Veterinary and Biomedical Sciences
University of Minnesota College of Veterinary Medicine
St Paul, Minnesota, USA

Ahna G. Brutlag, DVM, MS, DABT, DABVT
Associate Director of Veterinary Services & Senior Veterinary Toxicologist
Pet Poison Helpline & SafetyCall International, PLLC
Bloomington, Minnesota, USA
&
Adjunct Assistant Professor
Department of Veterinary and Biomedical Sciences

College of Veterinary Medicine, University of Minnesota
St Paul, Minnesota, USA

Jacinda Christie, DVM
Associate Veterinarian, Clinical Toxicology
Pet Poison Helpline & SafetyCall International, PLLC
Bloomington, Minnesota, USA
&
Affiliated Emergency Veterinary Service
Blaine, Minnesota, USA

Dana L. Clarke, VMD, DACVECC
Assistant Professor, Interventional Radiology & Critical Care
University of Pennsylvania School of Veterinary Medicine
Philadelphia, Pennsylvania, USA

Seth L. Cohen, DVM
Staff Veterinarian
Trooper Veterinary Hospital
Philadelphia, Pennsylvania, USA

Camille DeClementi, VMD, DABT, DABVT
Senior Director
Animal Poison Control Center, Animal Health Services
ASPCA
Urbana, Illinois, USA

David C. Dorman, DVM, PhD, DABVT, DABT
Professor of Toxicology
College of Veterinary Medicine
North Carolina State University
Raleigh, North Carolina, USA

Eric Dunayer, MS, VMD, DABT, DABVT
Associate Professor of Veterinary Clinical Sciences
St Matthew's University School of Veterinary Medicine
Grand Cayman, Cayman Islands

James N. Eucher, DVM, DHSc, MS, MPH
Associate Veterinarian, Clinical Toxicology
Pet Poison Helpline & SafetyCall International, PLLC
Bloomington, Minnesota, USA

Kate S. Farrell, DVM
Small Animal Emergency and Critical Care Resident
University of California-Davis
Davis, California, USA

Charlotte Flint, DVM
Senior Consulting Veterinarian, Clinical Toxicology
Pet Poison Helpline & SafetyCall International, PLLC
Bloomington, Minnesota, USA

Christina Fourré
DVM Candidate, Class of 2017
North Carolina State University College of Veterinary Medicine
Raleigh, North Carolina, USA

Sarah L. Gray, DVM, DACVECC
Emergency and Critical Care Specialist
Pet Poison Helpline & SafetyCall International, PLLC
Bloomington, Minnesota, USA
&
Critical Care Specialist
Veterinary Medical and Surgical Group
Ventura, California, USA

Sharon Gwaltney-Brant, DVM, PhD, DABVT, DABT
Consultant
Veterinary Information Network
Mahomet, Illinois, USA

Jennifer M. Hall, DVM, DACVECC
Staff Criticalist
VCA West Los Angeles Animal Hospital
Los Angeles, California, USA

Jeffery O. Hall, DVM, PhD, DABVT
Professor and Head, Diagnostic Toxicology
Utah Veterinary Diagnostic Laboratory
Department of Animal, Dairy, and Veterinary Sciences
Utah State University
Logan, Utah, USA

Kelly M. Hall, DVM, MS, DACVECC
Stillwater, Minnesota, USA

Jayme E. Hoffberg, DVM, DACVECC
Clinical Instructor, Emergency and Critical Care
University of Wisconsin School of Veterinary Medicine
Madison, Wisconsin, USA

Holly Hommerding, DVM
Associate Veterinarian, Clinical Toxicology
Pet Poison Helpline & SafetyCall International, PLLC
Bloomington, Minnesota, USA

Lynn R. Hovda, RPh, DVM, MS, DACVIM
Director of Veterinary Services
Pet Poison Helpline & SafetyCall International, PLLC
Bloomington, Minnesota, USA
&
Adjunct Professor
Department of Veterinary and Biomedical Sciences
College of Veterinary Medicine
University of Minnesota
St Paul, Minnesota, USA

Tyne K. Hovda, DVM
Hospital Intern
Rood & Riddle Equine Hospital
Lexington, Kentucky, USA

Jean Ihnen, DVM
Relief Veterinarian
Princeton, Minnesota, USA

Karl E. Jandrey, DVM, MAS, DACVECC
Associate Professor of Clinical Small Animal Emergency and Critical Care
Director, Center for Continuing Professional Education
University of California-Davis
School of Veterinary Medicine
Davis, California, USA

Sarah K. Jarosinski, BS, DVM elect 2016.
Veterinary Medicine Class of 2016
Texas A&M University
College Station, Texas, USA

Tracy Julius, DVM, DACVECC
BluePearl Veterinary Partners
Eden Prairie, Minnesota, USA

Hwan-Goo Kang, DVM, PhD
Senior Researcher
Animal and Plant Quarantine Agency
Anyang, Gyeong-gi Province, Republic of Korea

Megan Kaplan, DVM, DACVECC
Emergency and Critical Care specialist
Blue Pearl Veterinary Partners
Chicago, Illinois, USA

Daniel E. Keyler, RPh, BS, Pharm D, FAACT
Senior Clinical Toxicologist
Pet Poison Helpline & SafetyCall International, PLLC
Bloomington, Minnesota, USA
&
Adjunct Professor
Department of Experimental & Clinical Pharmacology
University of Minnesota
Minneapolis, Minnesota, USA

Christy A. Klatt, DVM
Assistant Commission Veterinarian
Minnesota Racing Commission
Shakopee, Minnesota, USA

Stephanie Kleine, DVM, DACVVA
Veterinary Education Specialist II
University of Georgia College of Veterinary Medicine
Athens, Georgia, USA

Justine A. Lee, DVM, DACVECC, DABT
CEO, VETgirl
Consultant, ASPCA Animal Poison Control Center
St Paul, Minnesota, USA

Christopher M. McLaughlin, DVM
Resident, Emergency and Critical Care
North Carolina State University
Raleigh, North Carolina, USA

Katrina L. Mealey, DVM, PhD, DACVIM, DACVCP
Professor and Ott Endowed Chair of Medicine
College of Veterinary Medicine
Washington State University
Pullman, Washington, USA

Charlotte Means, DVM, MLIS, DABVT, DABT
Director of Toxicology
ASPCA Animal Poison Control Center
Urbana, Illinois, USA

Donna Mensching, DVM, MS, DABVT, DABT
High Peaks Animal Hospital
Ray Brook, New York, USA

Michael Murphy, DVM, JD, PhD, DABVT, DABT, RAC
Veterinary Medical Officer
Food and Drug Administration, Center for Veterinary Medicine
Rockville, Maryland, USA

Gary D. Osweiler, DVM, PhD, DABVT
Professor Emeritus
Veterinary Diagnostic and Production Animal Medicine
College of Veterinary Medicine
Iowa State University
Ames, Iowa, USA

Katherine L. Peterson, DVM, DACVECC
Emergency Critical Care Specialist
Pet Poison Helpline & SafetyCall International, PLLC
Bloomington, Minnesota, USA
&
Veterinary Criticalist
BluePearl Veterinary Partners
Eden Prairie, Minnesota, USA

Michael E. Peterson, DVM, MS
Staff Veterinarian
Reid Veterinary Hospital
Albany, Oregon, USA

Konnie H. Plumlee, DVM, MS, DABVT, DACVIM
Veterinary Medical Officer
USDA-APHIS-Animal Care
Ozark, Missouri, USA

Amanda L. Poldoski, DVM
Senior Consulting Veterinarian in Clinical Toxicology
Pet Poison Helpline & SafetyCall International, PLLC
Bloomington, Minnesota, USA

Robert H. Poppenga, DVM, PhD, DABVT
Professor of Clinical and Diagnostic Veterinary Toxicology
California Animal Health and Food Safety Laboratory System
School of Veterinary Medicine
University of California-Davis
Davis, California, USA

Birgit Puschner, DVM, PhD, DABVT
Professor and Chair
School of Veterinary Medicine
Department of Molecular Biosciences
University of California-Davis
Davis, California, USA

Jane Quandt, DVM, MS, DACVAA, DACVECC
Associate Professor of Comparative Anesthesia
Small Animal Medicine & Surgery
College of Veterinary Medicine
University of Georgia
Athens, Georgia, USA

Julie Schildt, DVM, DACVECC
Assistant Professor, Emergency Medicine and Critical Care
University of Minnesota, Veterinary Medical Center
St Paul, Minnesota, USA

Renee D. Schmid, DVM
Associate Veterinarian, Clinical Toxicology
Pet Poison Helpline & SafetyCall International, PLLC
Bloomington, Minnesota, USA

Kelly Sioris, PharmD, CSPI
Senior Clinical Toxicologist
Project Manager of Drug Safety & Medical Affairs
Pet Poison Helpline & SafetyCall International, PLLC
Bloomington, Minnesota, USA

Leo J. Sioris, PharmD
Senior Clinical Toxicologist
Chief Executive Officer
Pet Poison Helpline & SafetyCall International, PLLC
Bloomington, Minnesota, USA
&
Professor
Department of Experimental and Clinical Pharmacology
College of Pharmacy, University of Minnesota
Minneapolis, Minnesota, USA

Kristin Smith, DVM
Resident, Emergency and Critical Care
University of Minnesota
Veterinary Medical Center
St Paul, Minnesota, USA

Laura Stern, DVM
Consulting Veterinarian in Clinical Toxicology
ASPCA Animal Poison Control Center
Urbana, Illinois, USA

Patricia A. Talcott, MS, DVM, PhD, DABVT
Professor, Veterinary Diagnostic Toxicologist
Director of Admissions
College of Veterinary Medicine
Washington State University
Pullman, Washington, USA

Dominic Tauer, DVM
Associate Veterinarian, Clinical Toxicology
Pet Poison Helpline & SafetyCall International, PLLC
Bloomington, Minnesota, USA

John H. Tegzes, MA, VMD, DABVT
Professor of Toxicology
Western University of Health Sciences
Pomona, California, USA

Rebecca A. L. Walton, DVM
Emergency and Critical Care Resident
North Carolina State University
Raleigh, North Carolina, USA

Kirsten E. Waratuke, DVM
Consulting Veterinarian in Clinical Toxicology
ASPCA Animal Poison Control Center
Urbana, Illinois, USA

Sharon Welch, DVM, DABVT, DABT
Veterinary Toxicologist
Pet Poison Helpline & SafetyCall International, PLLC
Bloomington, Minnesota, USA

Tina Wismer, DVM, DABVT, DABT, MS
Medical Director
ASPCA Animal Poison Control Center
Urbana, Illinois, USA

Preface

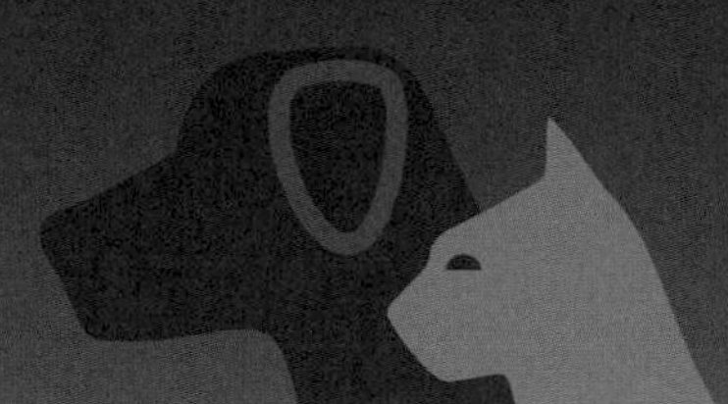

The second edition of *Blackwell's Five-Minute Veterinary Consult Clinical Companion: Small Animal Toxicology* improves on the first edition yet still follows the lead of the successful *Five-Minute Veterinary Consult: Canine and Feline*, 6th edition. The Five-Minute concept of providing essential and relevant information in an organized and easy-to-access format continues in this textbook. In addition, the format of the focused and relevant information can provide excellent support for teaching veterinary toxicology in a professional curriculum. *Blackwell's Five-Minute Veterinary Consult Clinical Companion: Small Animal Toxicology* provides selected details and expanded coverage of toxicology that meet the needs of contemporary small animal toxicology care. The coverage is organized by traditional categories of overview, etiology/pathophysiology (including mechanism of action, pharmacokinetics or toxicokinetics, toxicology, and systems affected), signalment/history, clinical features, key differential diagnoses, diagnostics and therapeutics. Incorporated is information essential to toxicology evaluation such as dosage, absorption, distribution, metabolism, excretion, toxic doses, prevention, and public health issues.

Blackwell's Five-Minute Veterinary Consult Clinical Companion: Small Animal Toxicology is designed to aid in the identification of dangerous exposures from many natural, synthetic, and consumer products, while subsequently providing the reader with necessary information to identify and confirm clinical poisoning. In addition, further information discussing prompt detoxification and supportive therapy, as well as specific antidotes or drug therapies, are reviewed. This book provides a logical, consistent, and sufficiently detailed resource to reach appropriate clinical decision making while accessing specific information quickly and efficiently.

ORGANIZATION AND FORMAT

The first section of the book, Clinical Toxicology, provides organized and detailed information on the determination of effective detoxification and effective life support measures which are often responsible for saving animals' lives even before a diagnosis can be confirmed. A separate chapter on antidotes provides rapid and useful information for known toxicants while a new chapter aids the clinician in dealing with unknown poisons.

The second section of this book, Specific Toxins & Toxicants, is organized around broad categories of toxicants generally familiar to clients and the veterinarian alike. This section details 113 individual topics representing current toxins or toxicants in small animal toxicology. The selection of these topics is based on evidence from published literature, animal poison control center databases, and advice from colleagues and professionals at veterinary colleges in North America. The multiple author format and use of four distinct editors provides a broad range of experiences by those whose professional careers are in the clinical specialties of emergency and critical care, internal medicine, and toxicology.

Section 3, Reference Information, provides useful information, including abbreviations, important resources for toxicology, and tables summarizing common metals, plants, and topical toxins.

KEY FEATURES

Within each major category of toxins or toxicants, individual chapters are arranged alphabetically to provide consistent access to the topics. Specific headings within each chapter are similar to common clinical organization of information and augmented by essential toxicological categories. These sections include Definition/Overview, Etiology/Pathophysiology, Signalment/History, Clinical Features, Differential Diagnosis, Diagnostics, Therapeutics, and Comments (including client education, patient monitoring, and expected course and prognosis). Each chapter provides up to five pertinent and clinically relevant references for additional direction to the clinician or student.

Lynn R. Hovda, Ahna G. Brutlag,
Robert H. Poppenga, Katherine L. Peterson

About the Companion Website

This book is accompanied by a companion website:

www.fiveminutevet.com/toxicology

The website includes:

- Case studies
- Client education handouts

section I

Clinical Toxicology

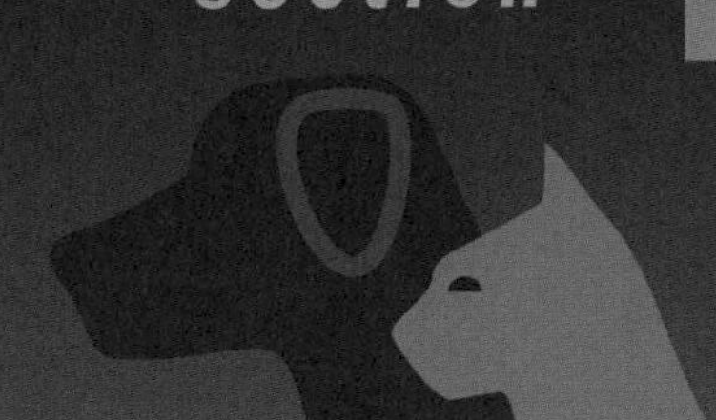

chapter 1

Decontamination and Detoxification of the Poisoned Patient

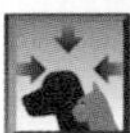

DEFINITION/OVERVIEW

- In veterinary medicine, the primary treatment for toxicant exposure should be decontamination and detoxification of the patient, along with symptomatic and supportive care.
- The goal of decontamination is to inhibit or minimize further toxicant absorption and to promote excretion or elimination of the toxicant from the body.
- When treating the poisoned patient, the clinician should have an understanding of the underlying mechanism of action of the toxicant, the pharmacokinetics (including absorption, distribution, metabolism, and excretion), and the toxic dose (if available). This will help determine appropriate decontamination and therapy for the patient.
- As decontamination can only be performed within a narrow window of time for most substances, it is important to obtain a thorough history and time since exposure.
- Emesis induction, which is the most common route of GI decontamination, is contraindicated in symptomatic patients.
- While the GI route is the most common type of decontamination in veterinary medicine, other categories may include ocular, dermal, inhalation, injection, forced diuresis, or surgical removal of the toxicant.

Ocular Decontamination

- If ocular exposure to a toxicant has occurred, thorough evaluation and appropriate medical care of the eye may be necessary.
- Ocular decontamination is often difficult for the pet owner, as it requires restraint of the animal.
- If the product is corrosive or caustic, owners should flush the eye at home with physiological saline (e.g., contact lens solution *without* any cleaners, soaps, etc.) or tepid water for 15–20 minutes prior to transportation to a veterinarian. This will help maximize decontamination and reduce secondary injury to the cornea. Immediate veterinary care is imperative. Owners should be advised to prevent injury or rubbing of the eye until veterinary attention is sought. An Elizabethan collar should be used, if available.

Blackwell's Five-Minute Veterinary Consult Clinical Companion: Small Animal Toxicology, Second Edition.
Lynn R. Hovda, Ahna G. Brutlag, Robert H. Poppenga, and Katherine L. Peterson.

Companion website: www.fiveminutevet.com/toxicology

- If the product is considered a *non*corrosive irritant, owners should flush the eye at home with physiological saline (e.g., contact lens solution *without* any cleaners, soaps, etc.) or tepid water for 10–15 minutes, if possible. Ophthalmic ointments or medications should *not* be used, and the pet should be monitored carefully for an extended period of time to prevent iatrogenic corneal abrasion or ulceration from rubbing the eyes. Owners should be advised to prevent injury or rubbing of the eye. An Elizabethan collar should be used, if available. Any change in condition (e.g., blepharospasm, pupil size change, pruritus, ocular discharge) should prompt immediate medical attention.

Dermal Decontamination

- The use of dermal decontamination is important to prevent transdermal absorption of the toxicant, but also to prevent oral reexposure secondary to grooming (particularly in cats).
- Owners should be advised to prevent the pet from grooming, and cautioned to protect themselves from exposure to the toxicant while transporting the pet to the veterinary clinic.
- When decontaminating a patient, it is important that pet owners and veterinary staff be protected from the toxic agent (e.g., pyrethrins, blue-green algae, organophosphates, corrosive or caustic chemicals, etc.). Appropriate protection should be used (e.g., rubber gloves, waterproof apron, face shield, etc.) as needed.
- Oil-based toxicities (e.g., high concentration pyrethrins) should be bathed off with tepid water and a liquid dish degreasing soap (e.g., Dawn™, Joy™, etc.). Pet owners should be specifically told not to use dish detergent from an automatic dishwasher; rather, they should be instructed to use liquid dish soap designated to wash dishes in the sink. The patient should be bathed and rinsed multiple times as soon after exposure as possible. Pet or human shampoos are typically insufficient to remove the oil-based product, as a follicular flushing shampoo or degreasing soap is necessary.
- Appropriate dermal decontamination is warranted to prevent continued absorption of the toxicant; this will also help minimize persistent clinical signs due to continued absorption. Avoid the use of shampoos containing insecticides (e.g., flea or tick shampoos), coal tar, antibiotics, or antifungals.
- The most common toxicant requiring dermal decontamination in veterinary medicine is high-concentration pyrethrins (e.g., used inappropriately in cats). In symptomatic cats exposed to pyrethrins, sedation with IV methocarbamol first may be beneficial prior to dermal decontamination (see chapter 94, Pyrethrins and Pyrethroids).
- Gentle clipping of the hair may also help remove the toxin, particularly in long-haired pets or patients that cannot be bathed.
- If caustic, acidic, or alkaline exposure has occurred to the skin, careful, gentle decontamination must occur. The skin should be thoroughly flushed with copious amounts of tepid water for 15–20 minutes, making sure not to traumatize the area with abrasive scrubbing or high-pressure water sprays.

- Avoid the use of "neutralizing" agents on the skin (e.g., an acid for an alkaline exposure), as this may cause a chemical or thermal reaction that results in more serious dermal injury.
- After dermal decontamination, the patient's temperature should be appropriately monitored. Due to cooling from the bathing process, patients may become hypothermic and may require appropriate heat support.

Inhalant Decontamination

- With exposure of an inhaled toxicant (e.g., zinc phosphide rodenticides, carbon monoxide, etc.), the patient should be removed from the environment and evaluated. Often, simple removal is all that is necessary.
- Further treatment may include administration of a humidified oxygen source, monitoring of oxygenation and ventilation (e.g., via arterial blood gas analysis, pulse oximetry, co-oximetry, etc.) and rarely, mechanical ventilation. Please see chapters 117 and 118 on toxic gases for more information.
- The nares and upper airway help filter particulate matter, helping prevent lower airway exposure. The use of bronchoscopy is typically unnecessary.
- The area where the inhalant exposure occurred should be adequately ventilated to prevent reexposure by persistent toxic fumes.

Injection Decontamination

- Injection decontamination is typically necessary when an animal has been exposed to an insect stinger or venom sac. If embedded in the patient's skin, gentle manipulation (e.g., tweezers) to remove the stinger or venom sac should be performed, after careful examination of the affected area. Typically, this does not require sedation.
- Snake bites should not be decontaminated via incision and "sucking" of the venom from the bite wound, nor should hot or cold compressions or tourniquet application be used. Please see chapters 53–60 for more information on envenomations.

Gastrointestinal Decontamination

- "At-home" decontamination (e.g., emesis induction) can be performed by pet owners to prevent or treat toxicosis; however, the medical recommendation to decontaminate a pet at home must be thoroughly evaluated by the veterinarian, veterinary staff, or an Animal Poison Control Center first.
- A complete history should be obtained from the pet owner *prior* to emesis induction (for home emesis or veterinary emesis induction).
- It is important to understand the contraindications for emesis induction to prevent secondary complications such as aspiration pneumonia, protracted emesis, hematemesis, or caustic or corrosive injury to the esophagus, oropharynx, and GIT.

- Prior to inducing emesis, several factors must be considered.
  - Time frame – A thorough history and time frame since ingestion must be obtained prior to recommendations for emesis induction. If several hours have passed, toxic contents may have moved out of the stomach. Emesis induction is indicated for most toxins ingested within 1–2 hours, provided the patient is asymptomatic.
  - Underlying medical problems – Dogs with brachycephalic syndrome (e.g., stenotic nares, everted saccules, hypoplastic trachea, and elongated soft palate) may be at higher risk for aspiration, and emesis induction at a veterinary facility may be safer. Dogs with a prior history of laryngeal paralysis, megaesophagus, aspiration pneumonia, upper airway disease, etc., should not have emesis induction performed due to the risk of aspiration pneumonia.
  - Symptomatic patients – Patients that are already symptomatic should *not* undergo emesis induction. Symptomatic patients that are excessively sedate may have a decreased gag reflex or a lowered seizure threshold and may be unable to protect their airway, resulting in aspiration pneumonia.
  - Corrosive or caustic agent – Emesis induction may cause additional injury to the esophagus, oropharynx, and GIT when these agents are expelled.
  - Hydrocarbons – Low-viscosity liquids (e.g., gasoline, kerosene, motor oil, transmission fluid, etc.) can be easily aspirated into the respiratory system, resulting in severe aspiration pneumonia. See chapter 10 on hydrocarbons for more information.

Effectiveness of Emesis Induction

- The effectiveness of emesis induction is based on several factors, including:
  - emetic agent used
  - time elapsed since ingestion
  - physical characteristics of the toxicant ingested
  - toxicant's effect on gastric emptying
  - presence of gastric contents.
- The more rapidly emesis is induced post ingestion, the greater yield of recovery of gastric contents. Studies have shown that gastric recovery within 1 hour after toxin ingestion was approximately 17–62%. When emesis was induced within an even shorter time span (within 30 minutes), mean recovery of gastric contents was approximately 49% (range 9–75%).
- While delayed emesis after 1–2 hours may still be successful, the amount of gastric recovery significantly decreases as time passes.
- Emesis induction performed after 4 hours is likely of no benefit, with the exception of delayed gastric emptying or ingestions of large bezoars or concretions of toxic agents (if still present in the stomach). Examples include:
  - large wads of xylitol gum
  - large amounts of chocolate
  - grapes and raisins

- massive ingestions that can form a concretion or bezoar (e.g., fish oil capsules, prenatal iron vitamins, etc.)
- ingestions that can form a bezoar or foreign body (e.g., blood or bone meal, fire starter logs, etc.)
- drugs that delay gastric emptying (e.g., opioids, anticholinergics, salicylates, TCA antidepressants).

Recommendations for Home Emesis

- The decision to recommend emesis induction at home is based on the clinical judgment of the veterinary facility.
- Numerous "antidotes" and "emetics" exist on the internet, and pet owners may find and use inappropriate information. Vegetable oil, milk, bread, and physical gagging with a finger have all been reportedly used by pet owners as antidotes or emetics.
- In addition, pet owners may use an inappropriate dose based on an estimated weight of the patient, resulting in side effects (e.g., protracted vomiting, hematemesis). Appropriate counseling by the veterinary staff or an Animal Poison Control Center is imperative (on which emetic to use, how much to use, if home emesis induction is warranted, etc.).
- As time is of the essence with emesis induction, it is often more effective to seek veterinary attention immediately rather than attempt emesis induction at home. This depends on the comfort and ability of the pet owner and availability of appropriate emetics (e.g., hydrogen peroxide) at home. Rather than send a pet owner to a local store to purchase hydrogen peroxide and wait 10 minutes for the effect of the emetic (which may or may not be productive), it may be more efficient to seek veterinary care for prompt emesis induction.
- As certain human medications have a rapid onset of action (e.g., SSRI antidepressants, amphetamines, etc.) and clinical signs can be seen as early as 15–30 minutes, the use of emesis induction at home is generally not recommended with certain toxicants. In these situations, emesis induction is best done under the supervision of a veterinarian; the patient should be assessed to confirm that it is asymptomatic prior to emesis induction. Other examples of toxicants with a rapid onset of action include baclofen and benzodiazepine or nonbenzodiazepine agents (e.g., sleep aids).
- There are no safe emetic agents for cats that pet owners can use at home.

Emetic Agents

- Currently the only recommended at-home, oral emetic agent is 3% hydrogen peroxide. Other emetic agents that have been previously recommended include table salt (sodium chloride), liquid dishwashing detergent, or 7% syrup of ipecac.
- Common veterinary emetics available at a veterinary clinic include apomorphine for dogs and alpha$_2$-adrenergic agonist agents (e.g. xylazine, dexmedetomidine) for cats. Hydrogen peroxide is also commonly used by veterinarians as an emetic, and is equally effective to apomorphine.

3% Hydrogen Peroxide

- Hydrogen peroxide is thought to act as an emetic by direct gastric irritation.
- Hydrogen peroxide is the *current* recommendation for at-home emesis induction in dogs. Only the 3% concentration should be used, as higher concentrations can result in severe gastritis.
- In cats, the use of hydrogen peroxide as an emetic is *not* recommended. It is not as effective in cats compared to dogs, and can result in significant adverse effects (e.g., hypersalivation, hemorrhagic gastritis, protracted hematemesis, etc.). Any toxic ingestion in a cat should be sent directly to the veterinarian for emesis induction under veterinary supervision.
- When using hydrogen peroxide, make sure the product is first aid grade (e.g., 3%) and nonexpired (e.g., fresh, bubbly, not exposed to light) to be most effective. Dose: 1–2 mL/kg orally, not to exceed 50 mL in dogs.
- It should be acknowledged that this dose has been exceeded by many veterinarians without ill effect; however, persistent emesis and hematemesis may result.
- Emesis induction typically occurs within 5–10 minutes. If the first dose is ineffective as an emetic, a second dose can be repeated and potentially doubled.
- Hydrogen peroxide is generally safe, but more than two doses should not be administered at home before seeking veterinary attention.
- Pet owners should be informed that they must carefully syringe hydrogen peroxide (via turkey baster, oral syringe, etc.), as most dogs will not electively drink this on their own, delaying emesis even further. Owners should be careful to prevent aspiration during administration.
- Anecdotally, hydrogen peroxide works best if a small amount of food is present in the stomach. When advising pet owners on how to perform emesis induction at home, the pet owner should be informed to feed a few dog treats or small amount of kibble prior to emesis induction.
- Another option is to soak a small amount of food or bread with the prescribed amount of hydrogen peroxide.

Table Salt (Sodium Chloride)

- Salt acts as an emetic by direct gastric irritation.
- The use of salt as an emetic is *no longer recommended* due to the risks of hypernatremia, persistent emesis, and hematemesis.
- Dose of salt in dogs and cats: 1–3 teaspoons orally, depending on the size of the patient.
- Emesis induction typically occurs within 10–15 minutes.
- In children treated with salt as an emetic, hypernatremia, secondary cerebral edema, and neurological complications have been seen. Rarely, death has been reported (see chapter 70 on salt toxicity).

Liquid Dish Detergent (e.g., Dawn, Palmolive, Joy)

- Liquid dish detergent acts as an emetic due to direct gastric irritation.
- The use of liquid dish detergent is not typically recommended, although it may be considered more benign than table salt or syrup of ipecac.

- Detergents containing phosphate are most effective (thus excluding eco-friendly products).
- Dose: 10 mL/kg of a mixture of 3 tablespoons of detergent to 8 ounces of water.
- Emesis induction typically occurs within 20 minutes.
- It is imperative that pet owners and veterinary staff ensure that the appropriate product is used, rather than products designed for use in automatic dishwashers (which can be corrosive). These types of detergents should *never* be used due to their alkaline nature, which may cause severe injury to the GIT.

7% Syrup of Ipecac

- Syrup of ipecac acts as an emetic due to direct gastric irritation and stimulation of the CTZ. This is likely due to the active alkaloid compounds emetine and cephaeline.
- Syrup of ipecac is derived from *Cephaelis ipecacuanha*, which is a dried root indigenous to South America.
- Syrup of ipecac is *no longer recommended* as an emetic in both human and veterinary medicine.
- Syrup of ipecac is not to be confused with ipecac fluid extract, which is estimated to be 14 times more potent.
- Dose: dogs, 1–2 mL/kg PO; cats, 3.3 mL/kg; cumulative dose in either species is not to exceed 15 mL; dose may be repeated once.
- Emesis induction typically occurs within 10–30 minutes but may take up to 1 hour.
- Potential complications from syrup of ipecac administration include:
  - delayed effect
  - lack of effectiveness in approximately 50% of small animals
  - distaste (particularly to cats)
  - protracted emesis, severe hematemesis, lethargy, diarrhea, depression
  - potential cardiotoxic arrhythmogenic action.

VETERINARY EMETIC AGENTS

Apomorphine

- Apomorphine acts directly on the CTZ.
- Apomorphine is an effective emetic agent for dogs that is commonly used by veterinarians.
- Dose: dogs, 0.02–0.04 mg/kg IV or IM; or direct application of the tablet form into the subconjunctival sac. The injectable apomorphine can also be administered SQ; however, this is not currently the recommended route due to delayed onset of action and a prolonged duration of effect. If subconjunctival apomorphine is used, thorough flushing of the subconjunctival sac must be performed after emesis induction, or protracted vomition may occur.
- Emesis occurs within 4–6 minutes.
- If emesis does not occur, a second titrated dose can be used. If emesis does not occur after a second dose, an additional oral dose of hydrogen peroxide may be beneficial.
- Apomorphine is not recommended for cats, as it is an ineffective emetic and may result in CNS stimulation.

- The use of apomorphine as an emetic should be carefully considered with opioid or sedative toxicosis, due to the potential for severe sedation.
- If a patient exhibits excessive CNS sedation or respiratory depression after apomorphine administration, naloxone can be used as a reversal (dose: 0.01–0.04 mg/kg, IV, IM, or SQ). However, naloxone will not reverse the emetic effect of apomorphine due to different receptor effects.
- Apomorphine tablets can be purchased through veterinary pharmaceutical companies.
- The emetic effects of apomorphine are counteracted by potent antiemetic agents such as maropitant, ondansetron, or dolasetron.

Xylazine

- Xylazine is a centrally mediated alpha$_2$-adrenergic agonist.
- Xylazine is an emetic used by veterinarians for emesis induction in cats. Occasionally, it can effective in dogs, but is generally not recommended due to more effective emetic agents being available (e.g., hydrogen peroxide, apomorphine).
- Dose: cats, 0.44 mg/kg, IM or SQ.
- Emesis induction typically occurs within 10–20 minutes but is not always effective.
- The use of xylazine often results in profound CNS and respiratory depression, and cats should be carefully monitored for excessive side effects (e.g., sedation, hypotension, etc.).
- Xylazine can be reversed with alpha$_2$-adrenergic antagonists.
  - Yohimbine: 0.1 mg/kg IM, SQ, or IV slowly.
  - Atipamezole (Antisedan): 0.2 mg/kg IM, IV.

Gastric Lavage (Fig. 1.1)

- The goal of gastric lavage is to remove gastric contents when emesis induction is unproductive or contraindicated.
- Human studies have shown that if gastric lavage was performed within 15–20 minutes after toxicant ingestion, gastric lavage recoveries were minimal (38% and 29%, respectively). If lavage was performed at 60 minutes post ingestion, only 8.6–13% was recovered.
- As most poisoned patients present to the veterinary clinic after 1 hour, the clinical usefulness of gastric lavage is debated.
- Despite low gastric recovery and labor intensiveness, the use of gastric lavage is indicated in certain circumstances.
  - A symptomatic patient that is already excessively sedate, unconscious, tremoring, or seizing that still needs controlled decontamination (e.g., metaldehyde, marijuana, organophosphates).
  - Material that is large in size or has formed a bezoar or concretion (e.g., bone meal, iron tablets, large amounts of chocolate, etc.).
  - Large toxic ingestions of capsules or tablets approaching the LD_{50} or toxicants with a narrow margin of safety (e.g., calcium channel blockers, beta-blockers, baclofen, ivermectin, organophosphate and carbamate insecticides).

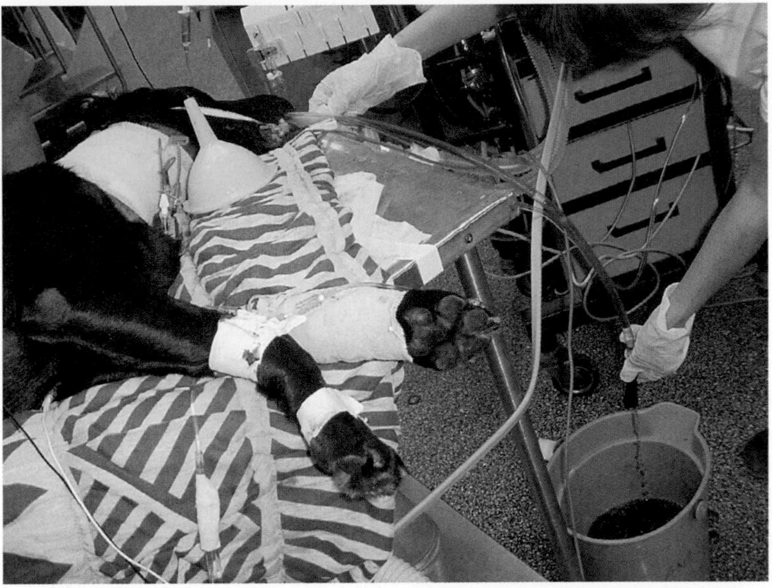

■ **Fig. 1.1.** Patient undergoing gastric lavage. Photo courtesy of Justine A. Lee, DVM, DACVECC, DABT.

- A newer modality is to administer AC via orogastric tube prior to lavage to prevent further absorption of the toxin, and then to lavage out the charcoal-toxin complex. Following copious lavage, AC is then readministered. There is lack of data evaluating this technique, and this modality still needs to be evaluated. Currently, the author does not recommend this technique without further evidence.
- Complications of gastric lavage include:
    - risks of sedation
    - aspiration pneumonia
    - hypoxemia secondary to aspiration pneumonia or hypoventilation from sedation
    - mechanical injury to the mouth, oropharynx, esophagus, or stomach.
- Contraindications for gastric lavage include:
    - a corrosive agent, where esophageal or gastric perforation can occur with orogastric tube placement
    - a hydrocarbon agent, which may be easily aspirated due to its low viscosity
    - sharp objects ingested (e.g., sewing needles, etc.).
- Many veterinarians may not feel comfortable performing gastric lavage, but it can be easily accomplished when organized with the appropriate supplies in a team-oriented approach.
    - Begin by preparing all materials in an organized fashion.
        - □ White tape
        - □ Mouth gag
        - □ Sterile lubrication
        - □ Gauze
        - □ Warm lavage fluid in a bucket

- ☐ Bilge or stomach pump
- ☐ Funnel
- ☐ Step stool
- ☐ Sedatives predrawn and labeled
- ☐ Sterile ETT, ideally with a high-volume, low-pressure cuff
- ☐ Empty syringe to inflate the cuff
- ☐ Material to secure and tie in the ETT
- ☐ IV catheter supplies
- ☐ Activated charcoal predrawn in the appropriate dose in 60 mL syringes ready for administration
- ☐ Sedation reversal agents if necessary

- Place an IV catheter.
- Sedate and intubate with ETT; secure ETT in place and connect to oxygen ± inhalant anesthesia source. Inflate cuff to prevent aspiration of gastric contents or lavage fluid. Place the patient in sternal recumbency.
- Premeasure an appropriately sized orogastric tube to the last rib and mark this line with white tape. This will be the maximum distance to pass the tube.
- Lubricate the orogastric tube, and pass the tube into the stomach using gentle, twisting motions. Blowing into the other end of the tube to inflate the esophagus with air may assist with passing of the tube into the stomach.
- Confirm orogastric tube placement by:
  - ☐ palpation of the orogastric tube on abdominal palpation
  - ☐ blowing into the orogastric tube and simultaneously ausculting for "bubbles" in the stomach
  - ☐ palpation of the neck for two tube-like structures (trachea, esophagus with tube placement).
- Infuse tepid or warm water by gravity flow via funnel, bilge, or stomach pump. The volume of the stomach is estimated to be approximately 60 mL/kg; therefore, copious amounts of fluid can be used to gavage. Fluid recovery (by gravity) should be emptied into an empty bucket.
- The stomach should be frequently palpated to monitor overdistension of the stomach and massaged/agitated to help break up contents within the stomach; this will hopefully allow small material to be removed via gastric lavage.
- Several lavage cycles (>5–20) should be performed to maximize decontamination of the stomach. All of the gavage fluid, if possible, should be removed prior to AC administration.
- The gastric lavage fluid should be examined for the presence of toxicants (e.g., plant material, mushrooms, rodenticides, medications, etc.), and can be saved for toxicological testing at a veterinary diagnostic laboratory if needed.
- Prior to removal of the orogastric tube, the appropriate amount of activated charcoal (with a cathartic for the first dose) should be instilled.
- The AC contents can then be flushed further into the orogastric tube with water or by blowing forcefully into the tube.

- Prior to removal of the orogastric tube, it is imperative that the tube be kinked off to prevent lavage fluid from being aspirated. Once kinked, the tube should be removed quickly in one sweeping movement.
- The patient should continue to be intubated until gag reflex is present. Positioning the patient in sternal recumbency with the head elevated may help prevent aspiration.
- Administration of a potent antiemetic (e.g., maropitant, dolasetron, ondansetron) should be considered.
- A video example of gastric lavage can be found here: http://vetgirlontherun.com/veterinary-continuing-education-how-perform-gastric-lavage-dog-vetgirl-video/

Whole Bowel Irrigation (WBI)

- The goal of WBI is to clean the GIT by removing toxins and normal intraluminal GI contents.
- This is done by enteral administration of large amounts of polyethylene glycol electrolyte solution (PEG-ES or PEG; e.g., Golytely™) until effluent (e.g., stool) is clear.
- WBI is frequently done in human medicine, but is rarely necessary for treatment of the poisoned veterinary patient. Rather, WBI is more commonly used for bowel preparation (e.g., for endoscopy, colonoscopy, etc.).
- WBI may be necessary in the poisoned patient if the toxicant is suspected to be present within the small intestinal tract. Examples of toxicants may include life-threatening ingestions of prenatal iron tablets, large ingestions of sustained-release medicines, etc.
- Due to the massive amount of PEG-ES that needs to be ingested, administration must typically occur via a temporary feeding tube (e.g., nasoesophageal, nasogastric, orogastric, etc.).
- Dose of PEG-ES: 25–40 mL/kg, followed by continuous oral infusion of 0.5 mL/kg/hour. Alternatively, 30–40 mL/kg can be gavaged every 2 hours.
- Stool typically appears within 2–4 hours, and WBI should be continued for approximately 8–12 hours until the effluent is clear.
- The use of antiemetics may be necessary. Metoclopramide (0.2–0.5 mg/kg, SQ or 1–2 mg/kg/day, IV CRI) would be an appropriate choice due to its antiemetic, prokinetic, and gastric-emptying effects.
- Complications of WBI include nausea, vomiting, bloating, abdominal discomfort, and aspiration pneumonia.
- Contraindications for WBI include a foreign body obstruction, ileus, perforated bowel, shock, refractory emesis, and significant GI hemorrhage.

Activated Charcoal (AC)

- The goal of AC is to act as an adsorbent and to prevent systemic absorption of the toxicant.
- While less commonly used in human medicine, AC still remains the primary treatment of choice for detoxification of the veterinary poisoned patient.

- AC is produced by heating wood pulp to extreme temperatures (900°C), washing it with inorganic acids, and drying it. This results in "activated" charcoal particles with a large surface area that promotes absorption. One gram of AC has approximately 1000 m^2 of surface area.
- AC contains carbon moieties that adsorb compounds with varying affinity.
  - Nonpolar compounds bind to AC well.
  - Heavy metals (e.g., zinc, iron, etc.) and alcohols (e.g., ethylene glycol, methanol, isopropyl alcohol, ethanol) typically are not absorbed by AC.
  - Xylitol binds poorly to AC.
- The interaction between the bound toxin and AC could potentially undergo desorption (where the toxicant unbinds from the AC over time); hence, the addition of a cathartic is often used to help promote fecal expulsion and increase GIT transit time.
- Administration of AC with a cathartic as long as 6 hours out may still be beneficial with toxicosis, particularly if the product has delayed release (e.g., extended or sustained release) or undergoes enterohepatic recirculation.
  - The use of AC with a magnesium-containing cathartic should be undertaken judiciously in cats.
- Dose: 1–5 g of AC per kg of body weight orally; in general, the higher the dosage used, the more effective the adsorption.
- Certain situations or toxicities warrant multidose administration of AC. Drugs undergoing enterohepatic recirculation (e.g., ibuprofen, carprofen, etc.), with a long half-life (naproxen), or delayed-release products will require multidose administration of AC.
- Dose: for multidose charcoal (1–2 g/kg, PO q 6 hours for 24 hours).
  - Additional doses of AC should ideally not contain a cathartic, due to increased risks for dehydration via fluid losses from the GIT. If AC without a cathartic is not available, then appropriate and aggressive hydration of the patient is imperative to prevent rare complications of hypernatremia.
- There are several types of AC commercially available, and the labeled directions should be followed appropriately for each specific type. Note that not all brands are labeled correctly; when in doubt, the appropriate dose (1–5 g/kg) should be calculated and administered.
- Many types of AC contain a cathartic already present (e.g., typically 70% sorbitol).
- At-home AC tablets and capsules (typically used by humans for colonic cleansing purposes) are not as effective as veterinary AC liquid slurries.
- The use of AC granules can also be considered (e.g., Toxiban™ granules), and mixed with a small amount of food to increase palatability for dogs.
- Few animals will ingest AC voluntarily, and administration may need to occur via forced but careful syringe feeding or orogastric tube administration.
- Based on an in vitro study assessing the administration of AC with a palatable veterinary prescription canned food (Hills™ a/d), the administration of AC with food can decrease the absorptive capacity of AC; however, this was thought to be clinically insignificant. That said, when administering AC with food, ideally the smallest amount of food should be used.

- Due to the thick viscosity of AC, it is often difficult to administer via NE or NG tube administration. Oral tubing in an awake patient (e.g., with a mouth gag and careful restraint) has been successfully used to administer AC.
- Rarely, reports of hypernatremia have been clinically seen with AC administration. This is likely due to the sorbitol effect (see "Cathartics"). The patient should be assessed for hydration status.
- To prevent dehydration and hypernatremia, the patient should be appropriately hydrated with either IV or SQ fluids.
- A potent antiemetic should be administered to prevent secondary vomition or aspiration pneumonia, and to allow for rapid return to oral water (to help maintain hydration of the patient).
    - Maropitant 1 mg/kg, SQ q 24 hours; administration to cats or by intravenous administration is considered extra-label but has been used by this author successfully.
    - Ondansetron 0.1–0.3 mg/kg, SQ, IM, IV q 6–12 hours.
    - Dolasetron 0.6–1 mg/kg, SQ, IM, IV q 24 hours.
    - Metoclopramide 0.2–0.5 mg/kg, SQ, IM q 6–12 hours; or CRI at 1–2 mg/kg/day IV; generally less effective as an antiemetic than maropitant or ondansetron, but provides gastric emptying and a prokinetic effect.
- Contraindications for AC include dehydration, hypernatremia, vomiting, late-stage presentation with clinical signs already present, a compromised airway (risk for aspiration pneumonia), endoscopy, abdominal surgery of the GIT, gastric or intestinal obstruction, perforation of the GIT, lack of borborgymi, ileus, hypovolemic shock, caustic substance ingestion, and hydrocarbon toxicosis (due to increased risk for aspiration pneumonia).

Cholestyramine

- Cholestyramine, a chloride salt of a basic anion exchange resin, is recommended by the ASPCA Animal Poison Control Center over the use of charcoal.
- Cholestyramine binds with bile acids within the intestines, producing an insoluble complex and preventing bile acids from being reabsorbed (and instead, excreted through the feces).
- Cholestyramine can be dosed at 0.3–1 g/kg every 6–8 hours with toxicants that undergo enterohepatic recirculation or biliary elimination.
- Little is known about the success of cholestyramine in veterinary medicine; anecdotally, the ASPCA Animal Poison Control Center has had success with its use instead of AC for the poisoned patient.
- Cholestyramine, like AC, has fallen out of favor in human medicine.

Cathartics

- Cathartics are designed to increase the speed and transit time of the GIT, promoting fecal excretion of the toxicant; more importantly, cathartics decrease the time allowed for toxicant absorption through the GIT.

- Two of the most common types of cathartics used in the poisoned patient are:
  - saccharide cathartics (e.g., sorbitol)
  - saline cathartics (e.g., magnesium citrate, magnesium sulfate, sodium sulfate).
- Dose: sorbitol (70% solution, 1–2 mL/kg, PO, given within 60 minutes of toxin ingestion).
- Side effects of sorbitol administration: vomiting, dehydration, secondary hypernatremia, abdominal cramping or pain, and possible hypotension.
- Contraindications for cathartics are similar to those for AC listed above.
- Mineral oil is *no longer recommended* as a cathartic due to the high risks of aspiration.
- The use of cathartics alone is no longer recommended or beneficial.
- Cathartics should not be used in a dehydrated patient, due to the risks of voluminous fluid losses through the GIT and secondary hypernatremia. For patients receiving either multidoses of AC with or without cathartics, serum sodium levels and hydration status should be carefully monitored.

Fluid Therapy

- Fluid therapy is one of the cornerstone therapies of emergency management of the poisoned patient to:
  - correct dehydration
  - maintain perfusion at a cellular level
  - vasodilate the renal vessels, flush the renal tubules, and diurese the patient. This is particularly important with nephrotoxicants such as grapes, raisins, NSAIDs, ethylene glycol, lilies, etc.
  - treat hypotension (particularly with drugs like beta-blockers, calcium channel blockers, ACE-inhibitors, etc.).
- Fluid therapy can also be used to aid in detoxification of the patient by increasing renal excretion of toxicants by forced diuresis, provided the toxicants undergo renal excretion (e.g., amphetamines, etc.).
- Dose: the dose of IV fluids to administer is dependent on the clinical state and physical examination findings of the patient.
  - In a healthy patient, fluid rates of 4–10 mL/kg/hour can be used to force renal clearance of the toxicant.
  - Neonates have a higher maintenance fluid rate (80–180 mL/kg/day), and fluid rates should be adjusted accordingly.
  - Patients with cardiac disease or respiratory disease, or those who have ingested toxicants that may increase the patient's risk of pulmonary edema (e.g., phosphide rodenticide) should have judicious fluid administration.
  - Careful assessment of hydration should be made based on PCV/TS, weight gain, CVP, and physical examination findings.
- The additional use of diuretics can be undertaken in hydrated patients to increase forced diuresis. This should be *less commonly considered*, as diuretics can result in dehydration or nephrotoxicity.
  - Furosemide 1–4 mg/kg, IV, SQ, IM q 6–8 hours.
  - Mannitol 0.5–2 g/kg, IV slow over 20–30 minutes q 6–8 hours.

- Highly protein-bound toxins are not cleared efficiently by diuresis (e.g., NSAIDs).
- Drugs that respond well to forced diuresis include:
  - phenobarbital
  - amphetamines
  - salicylate
  - lithium
  - bromide.

Surgical Decontamination

- Surgical removal of toxic agents may occasionally need to be performed, particularly if the toxicant is caustic or corrosive (e.g., batteries), results in a bezoar that cannot be removed by gastric lavage (e.g., iron tablets, bone meal), results in foreign body obstruction (e.g., Gorilla Glue), or continues to leach its toxic effect (e.g., Amitraz collars, zinc pennies, fentanyl or nicotine patches, etc.). Please see chapter 72, Foreign Objects, for more information.
- Prior to surgery, patients should have radiographs done to verify presence of the agent and presence of an obstructive pattern. Keep in mind that not all foreign bodies are radiopaque. Patients should be properly volume resuscitated with IV fluid therapy and antiemetic therapy, and have their electrolyte, glucose, and acid–base imbalances corrected prior to anesthesia.

CONCLUSIONS

- Aggressive decontamination and detoxification of the poisoned patient are imperative and still considered the mainstay therapy in veterinary medicine.
- The clinician should feel well versed in appropriate decontamination methods to treat poisoned patients.

Abbreviations

See Appendix 1 for a complete list.

PEG-ES = polyethylene glycol electrolyte solution
WBI = whole bowel irrigation

Suggested Reading

Abdallah AH, Tye A. A comparison of the efficacy of emetic drugs and stomach lavage. Am J Dis Child 1967; 113:571–575.

American Academy of Clinical Toxicology and European Association of Poisons Centres and Clinical Toxicologists. Position paper: Gastric lavage. J Toxicology 2004; 42(7):933–943.

American Academy of Clinical Toxicology and European Association of Poisons Centres and Clinical Toxicologists. Position paper: Single-dose activated charcoal. Clin Toxicol 2005; 43:61–87.

Arnold FJ, Hodges JB Jr, Barta RA Jr. Evaluation of the efficacy of lavage and induced emesis in treatment of salicylate poisoning. Pediatrics 1959; 23:286–301.

Cope RB. A screening study of xylitol binding in vitro to activated charcoal. Vet Human Tox 2004; 46:336–337.

Corby DG, Lisciandro RC, Lehman RW, et al. The efficacy of methods used to evacuate the stomach after acute ingestions. Pediatrics 1967; 40:871–874.

Khan SA, McLean MK, Slater M, et al. Effectiveness and adverse effects of the use of apomorphine and 3% hydrogen peroxide solution to induce emesis in dogs. J Am Vet Med Assoc 2012; 241(9):1179–1184.

Peterson ME. Toxicological decontamination. In: Peterson ME, Talcott PA, eds. Small Animal Toxicology, 3rd edn. St Louis, MO: Elsevier Saunders, 2013; pp. 73–85.

Plumb DC. Veterinary Drug Handbook, 7th edn. Ames, IA: Blackwell Publishing Professional, 2011.

Teshima D, Suzuki A, Otsubo K, et al. Efficacy of emetic and United States Pharmacopoeia ipecac syrup in prevention of drug absorption. Chem Pharm Bull 1990; 38:2242–2245.

Türk EE, Schulz F, Koops E, et al. Fatal hypernatremia after using salt as an emetic – report of three autopsy cases. Leg Med (Tokyo) 2005; 7(1):47–50.

Wilson HE, Humm KR. In vitro study of the effect of dog food on the adsorptive capacity of activated charcoal. J Vet Emerg Crit Care 2013; 23(3):263–267.

Author: Justine A. Lee, DVM, DACVECC, DABT
Consulting Editor: Lynn R. Hovda, RPh, DVM, MS, DACVIM

chapter 2

Emergency Management of the Poisoned Patient

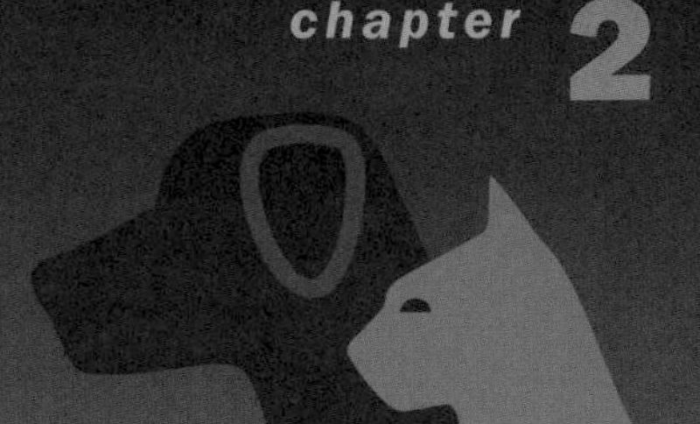

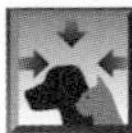

DEFINITION/OVERVIEW

- Management of the acutely poisoned patient includes initial telephone triage, appropriate communication and history gathering from the pet owner, thorough physical examination, and initial stabilization.
- It is imperative to understand the toxicant's mechanism of action, the pharmacokinetics (e.g., absorption, distribution, metabolism, and excretion), and the toxic dose to understand how to treat the poisoned patient appropriately.
- Prompt decontamination and detoxification of the patient should be performed, when appropriate. Please see chapter 1, Decontamination and Detoxification of the Poisoned Patient, for more information.
- Initial stabilization of the emergent patient should include the ABCDs.
    - Airway
    - Breathing
    - Circulation
    - Dysfunction
- Appropriate diagnostic testing (e.g., CBC, chemistry, venous blood gas analysis, electrolytes, UA) should be performed, as this may help guide or titrate therapy. Additional diagnostics include radiographs and more specific toxicant testing (e.g., prothrombin time (PT), activated partial thromboplastin time (aPTT), urine drug screening, ethylene glycol (EG), etc.). Please refer to the specific toxicant's chapter for further information.
- Appropriate monitoring of the critically ill, poisoned patient should include the following.
    - Continuous ECG (cECG)
    - Blood pressure monitoring (BP)
    - Urine output (UOP)
    - Pulse oximetry
    - End-tidal carbon dioxide ($ETCO_2$)
    - Blood gas analysis
    - Central venous pressure (CVP)
- If an antidote (e.g., fomepizole, 2-PAM, atropine, vitamin K_1) or reversal agent (e.g., naloxone, flumazenil, yohimbine, atipamezole) is available, it should be initiated promptly

Blackwell's Five-Minute Veterinary Consult Clinical Companion: Small Animal Toxicology, Second Edition.
Lynn R. Hovda, Ahna G. Brutlag, Robert H. Poppenga, and Katherine L. Peterson.

Companion website: www.fiveminutevet.com/toxicology

for the specific toxicant. Please see chapter 3, Antidotes and Other Useful Drugs, for further information specific to antidotes.

- With fat-soluble toxicants (e.g., ivermectin, moxidectin, baclofen, calcium channel blockers, etc.), the use of intravenous lipid emulsion (ILE) can be considered as a potentially life-saving antidote. Please see "Miscellaneous Treatment" later in this chapter.
- Note, the majority of toxicants do *not* have a readily available antidote; therefore the use of decontamination and symptomatic supportive care is warranted.

ABCDs of the Poisoned Patient

Airway

- Any patient presenting comatose, unconscious, neurologically impaired (e.g., decreased or absent gag reflex), or with severe respiratory distress or dyspnea should be intubated with an endotracheal tube (ETT), connected to an oxygen source, and treated with positive pressure ventilation (PPV) or manual delivery of breaths (see Breathing).
- Pulse oximetry and $ETCO_2$ monitoring should be used appropriately to monitor the patient; likewise, the use of arterial blood gas (ABG) analysis should be considered as the gold standard for measuring oxygenation and ventilation.

Breathing

- Altered breathing may be due to various toxicants, which result in hypoxemia or hypoventilation.
    - Hydrocarbons, anticoagulant rodenticides (ACR), acetaminophen, carbon monoxide, smoke inhalation, macrocyclic lactones (e.g., ivermectin, moxidectin), baclofen, barbiturates, anticonvulsants, opioids, benzodiazepines, and others.
    - Secondary causes of hypoxemia may be due to aspiration pneumonia, atelectasis, pulmonary edema, pleural effusion, or altered hemoglobin (e.g. preventing hemoglobin from carrying oxygen normally), etc.
- If the patient is not breathing, immediate intubation and PPV are indicated at 10–20 bpm, with a tidal volume of approximately 6–15 mL/kg.
- If clinical signs of tachypnea or dyspnea are present, the patient should be treated immediately with oxygen supplementation.
- The severity of the patient's tachypnea or dyspnea should be assessed based on response to oxygen supplementation, improvement in clinical signs, and measurable parameters (such as pulse oximetry, $ETCO_2$, or ABG).
- Hypoxemia is defined as an arterial partial pressure of oxygen (PaO_2) ≤80 mmHg. Hypoventilation is defined as a partial pressure of carbon dioxide (PCO_2) ≥45 mmHg.
- In general, a "50:50 rule" (PaO_2 ≤50 mmHg and a PCO_2 ≥50 mmHg) – even with oxygen supplementation – is an indication for PPV.
- First, determine why the patient is hypoxemic or hypoventilating.
    - Was it due to excessive sedation from a toxicant? If the toxicant has a reversal agent (e.g., toxicant/reversal agent: fentanyl patch/naloxone; benzodiazepine/flumazenil; imidazoline decongestants/yohimbine), prompt reversal should occur. If a reversal

agent is not available, supportive PPV until the patient is able to ventilate appropriately is indicated.
  - Why is the patient hypoxemic? Is there evidence of abnormal lung sounds or the presence of a fever or cough? Chest radiographs should be performed to rule out disease in the following anatomical locations: airway (upper and lower), pulmonary parenchyma, pleural space, and thoracic wall. Rule-outs including aspiration pneumonia, atelectasis, pulmonary edema, pleural effusion, or multilobular hemorrhage (often seen secondary to ACR) should be considered. Other rule-outs include hypemic hypoxia, where hemoglobin is unable to carry oxygen adequately (e.g., carboxyhemoglobin secondary to carbon monoxide, methemoglobin secondary to acetaminophen, etc.).
- Mechanical ventilation is indicated until the patient meets the following criteria.
  - Able to ventilate and oxygenate without assistance.
  - Spontaneous respirations.
  - Resolution of severe dyspnea.
  - Return of neurological status (e.g., palpebral or gag reflex).
  - PCO_2 ≤50 mmHg.
  - PaO_2 ≥60 mmHg with oxygen supplementation. (Note: Oxygen supplementation can then be administered via less invasive modalities such as an oxygen cage or nasal oxygen.)
- Readers are referred to the references on mechanical ventilation for more information.

Circulation

- Altered circulation secondary to inadequate perfusion (e.g., secondary to hemorrhagic shock, hypovolemic shock, profound hypotension, etc.) may be due to various toxicants: ACR, beta-blockers, calcium channel blockers, others.
- The patient should be assessed for effective circulation based on the following physical examination parameters: mentation, mucous membrane color, CRT, heart rate, pulse quality and pressure, and body temperature.
- Appropriate therapy should be initiated promptly. This may include the following:
  - Fluid therapy (including crystalloids, colloids, blood products) to maintain blood pressure and perfusion or to treat dehydration, decreased colloid osmotic pressure, coagulopathy or anemia.
  - Oxygen therapy if hypoxemic.
  - Please see Fluid Therapy later in this chapter for more specific information.

Dysfunction

- Mental dysfunction may be due to various toxicants.
  - Excessive sedation – marijuana, baclofen, opioids, benzodiazepines, sedatives, hypnotics, barbiturates, others.
  - Agitation – SSRIs, amphetamines, nonbenzodiazepine hypnotics, caffeine, theobromine, tremorgenic mycotoxins, others.

- Hypoglycemia – xylitol, volatile alcohols, hepatotoxicants (e.g., blue-green algae, xylitol, acetaminophen, *Amanita* mushrooms, NSAIDs, etc.), prolonged tremoring or seizure activity from neurotoxins, sepsis, others.
- Neurological – 5-FU, SSRIs, amphetamines, baclofen, ivermectin, bromethalin, benzodiazepines, lamotrigine, pyrethrins, organophosphates, metaldehyde, cocaine, amphetamines, mushrooms, salt, isoniazid, blue-green algae, marijuana, others.

■ On initial presentation, the poisoned patient should be evaluated for gross neurological disability. Initial neurological examination should include the following:
  - Mentation
  - Pupillary light reflex (PLR) and assessment to determine if pupils are equal and responsive to light
  - Ambulation
  - Spinal reflexes

■ Assessing neurological function prior to treatment, if possible, is imperative as patients with severe toxicosis (e.g., organophosphate, metaldehyde, pyrethrins, caffeine, bromethalin) may have suffered severe hypoxemia or even cardiopulmonary arrest. Assessing neurological function allows better prognostic guidance to pet owners.

■ Appropriate therapy should be initiated promptly. This may include the following:
  - Dextrose administration – if patient is hypoglycemic <60 mg/dL (normal 70–110 mg/dL), administer 0.5–1.5 mL/kg of 50% dextrose IV, diluted 1:3 with a crystalloid, over 1–2 minutes, followed by a CRI in IV fluids (2.5–5% dextrose supplementation).

■ Treatment for the neurologically impaired poisoned patient includes decreasing intracranial pressure, increasing perfusion to the brain, and treatment of seizure activity.

■ For more information on treatment for neurological disorders, please see Neurological Support later in this chapter.

SUPPORTIVE CARE AND TREATMENT

■ As stated previously, very few toxicities have antidotes, and treatment is often symptomatic and supportive, including the following:
  - Monitoring and supportive care
  - Fluid therapy
  - Cardiovascular support
  - Gastrointestinal support
  - Neurological support
  - Analgesia/sedation
  - Miscellaneous treatment

Monitoring and Supportive Care

■ Monitoring of the poisoned patient may include any of the following:
  - cECG
  - BP

- UOP
- Pulse oximetry
- $ETCO_2$
- Blood gas analysis
- CVP

Continuous ECG

- In general, patients with underlying heart disease, cardiac dysrhythmias, myocardial hypoxia, pain/stress, splenic disease, or severe acid–base/electrolyte disturbances may be more at risk of arrhythmias and should be monitored with a cECG.
- Likewise, poisoned patients may be at increased risk for the development of arrhythmias (e.g., tachyarrhythmias, bradyarrhythmias) or severe electrolyte or acid–base abnormalities.
- Specific toxicants that may require the use of cECG monitoring include cardiac medications (e.g., beta-blockers, calcium channel blockers, digoxin), albuterol, SSRIs, amphetamines, caffeine, lamotrigine, cardiac glycoside-containing plants, *Bufo* toads, and amitraz. This list is not exclusive.
- The ECG should be used to look for the presence of dysrhythmias, bradycardia, or tachycardia.
- In general, the following parameters should warrant treatment if detected on an ECG:
  - Dog: HR <50 bpm or >180 bpm.
  - Cat: HR <120 bpm or >240 bpm.
  - Presence of severe VPCs.
  - R on T phenomenon (often predisposing to serious ventricular arrhythmias like ventricular fibrillation).
  - VPCs >180 bpm.
  - Pulse deficits.
  - Hypotension.
  - Clinical signs of poor perfusion (e.g., prolonged CRT, poor pulse quality, pulse deficits, dull mentation, etc.).
- For more information on general treatment for arrhythmias, please see Cardiovascular Support later in this chapter. Readers are also directed to a veterinary cardiology or critical care book for more details due to the large scope of information.

Blood Pressure (BP)

- Blood pressure should be monitored frequently in hypotensive patients, as it is a reflection of cardiac output, blood volume, and vascular tone.
- Blood pressure can be monitored by direct arterial blood pressure, Doppler, or oscillometric measurement. These are listed in order of accuracy.
  - Direct arterial blood pressure is advantageous because it is continuous and very accurate, but it is invasive, requires specialized equipment, requires a high level of skill to maintain and place an arterial line, and if disconnected (and unobserved), can lead to catastrophic bleeding.

- Indirect blood pressure monitoring can be performed with oscillometric or Doppler monitoring and is often more economical.
  - The HR should match on the oscillometric device or the results are not considered accurate.
  - Appropriate cuff selection is imperative, with the cuff being approximately 40% of the limb circumference.
- Causes for hypotension include hypovolemia (low preload), peripheral vasodilation, decreased systemic vascular resistance, decreased cardiac output, and poor cardiac contractility.
- In the poisoned patient, hypotension may be seen from the following toxicants.
  - Cardiac medications (e.g., beta-blockers, calcium channel blockers, cardiac glycoside-containing plants, *Bufo* toads, others), resulting in arrhythmias or severe bradycardia, which results in poor cardiac contractility, decreased afterload, and decreased systemic vascular resistance.
  - Beta-agonists (e.g., albuterol, salmeterol, clenbuterol), resulting in severe tachycardia, which prevents adequate ventricular filling and secondary hypotension.
  - Sedatives (e.g., baclofen, opioids, others), resulting in severe sedation and CNS depression.
  - Anticoagulant rodenticides (e.g., bromadiolone, brodifacoum, etc.), which can result in hemorrhagic shock secondary to coagulopathy and secondary bleeding.
- If the patient is hypotensive (MAP <60 mmHg or systolic <90 mmHg), appropriate volume resuscitation should occur with IV fluid therapy, provided cardiogenic shock (e.g., congestive heart failure) has been ruled out.
- These treatment recommendations should be modified for patients that may potentially volume overload, such as those with a heart murmur, known cardiac disease (e.g., dilated or hypertrophic cardiomyopathy) or pulmonary disease.
- When treating hypotension, make sure the patient is adequately volume resuscitated first before reaching for a vasopressor.
- The goal of fluid therapy is to achieve the following endpoints of resuscitation:
  - Mean arterial pressure (MAP) ≥65 mmHg.
  - CVP ≥8–12 mmHg.
  - UOP ≥0.5 mL/kg/hour.
  - Normal lactate 1–2 mmol/L.
  - Normal base excess (BE) –5 to +5 mmol/L.
- When volume resuscitating a patient, the following IV fluids can be used:
  - Any balanced, isotonic crystalloid (e.g., Normosol-R, LRS): 20–30 mL/kg IV aliquots over 15–20 minutes; repeat 2–3× as needed, monitoring frequently for response to therapy.
  - If no improvement, consider colloid bolus (e.g., Hetastarch, VetStarch): 5 mL/kg IV aliquots over 20–30 minutes; repeat 2–3× as needed.
  - If no improvement, consider the following:
    - If coagulopathic (PT/aPTT prolongation as seen with ACR): fresh frozen plasma or frozen plasma 10–20 mL/kg IV over 1–4 hours.
    - If anemic: blood products (e.g., whole blood, pRBC) 10–20 mL/kg IV to effect over 1–4 hours.

- Causes for hypertension in veterinary medicine include pain, fear, renal disease, toxicosis, cardiac disease, endocrine disease (e.g., hyperadrenocorticism, hyperthyroidism), immune-mediated hemolytic anemia, pheochromocytoma, etc.
- In the poisoned patient, hypertension may be seen from the following toxicants: SSRIs, amphetamines, caffeine, theobromine, decongestants, phenylpropanolamine, others.
- Patients with a blood pressure higher than a MAP >160 mmHg or systolic >180–200 mmHg should be promptly treated.
    - The use of judicious sedation/analgesia, anxiolytics, anticonvulsants, vasodilators, or ACE inhibitors may be necessary.
    - If the hypertension is toxicant related and concurrent agitation is simultaneously observed, the use of aggressive sedation is recommended for patients with stable cardiovascular systems.
        - Acepromazine
            - Dog: 0.05–0.1 mg/kg, IV, IM, SQ PRN to effect. Rarely, higher doses may be necessary in *severe* cases, but in general no more than 3 mg total per dog is recommended.
            - Cat: 0.05–0.1 mg/kg IV, IM, SQ PRN. It is generally not recommended to give more than 1 mg total per cat.
        - Chlorpromazine
            - Dog: 0.5–1 mg/kg, IV, IM, SQ PRN to effect
            - Cat: 0.5 mg/kg, IV, IM, SQ PRN to effect
        - Butorphanol 0.1–0.8 mg/kg, IV, IM, SQ PRN to effect
        - Diazepam 0.1–0.5 mg/kg, IV only, PRN to effect
            - Diazepam is contraindicated with benzodiazepine or nonbenzodiazepine toxicosis (e.g., sleep aids). See chapters 17 and 26 for further information.
    - In the poisoned patient, persistent hypertension typically responds well to aggressive, frequent sedation of the patient. However, if the patient is persistently hypertensive despite multiple doses of sedation, the additional use of antihypertensives may be necessary to prevent vascular injury, retinal detachment, or ischemic injury. Antihypertensives include:
        - Amlodipine (calcium channel blocker)
            - Dog: 0.1–0.25 mg/kg, PO q 12–24 hours PRN to effect
            - Cat: 0.625 mg *total* per cat, PO q 12–24 PRN to effect
            - Use cautiously in patients with cardiac or hepatic disease. Do not use in hypotensive patients or those with toxicants that may result in hypotension (e.g., calcium channel blockers, beta-blockers, etc.)
        - Hydralazine (vasodilator)
            - Dog: 0.5–3 mg/kg, PO q 8–12 hours to effect
            - Cat: 2.5 mg *total* per cat, PO q 12–24 hours to effect
        - Nitroprusside (vasodilator)
            - Dog: 1.0 µg/kg/minute, IV to effect
            - Cat: 0.5 µg/kg/minute, IV to effect

Urine Output (UOP)

- Normal urine output is 1–2 mL/kg/hour.
- UOP should be monitored and fluid therapy directed toward achieving normal UOP, particularly with nephrotoxicants (e.g., NSAIDs, grapes/raisins, ethylene glycol, lilies, etc.). The need for placement of a urinary catheter is typically limited to patients that are azotemic and have abnormal UOP (e.g., excessive polyuric, oliguria, etc.).
- Ideally, a urine specific gravity (USG) should be collected *prior* to initiation of fluid therapy to adequately assess renal function. USG can be used to evaluate the following:
  - Dehydration: the presence of hypersthenuria may suggest ongoing dehydration (dog >1.025; cat >1.040), and aggressive fluid resuscitation or rehydration is warranted.
  - Appropriate hydration: one of the goals of fluid therapy is to achieve isosthenuria (e.g., 1.015–1.018) while on IV fluids. That said, certain medical conditions such as diabetes mellitus, hyperthyroidism, hyperadrenocorticism, diabetes insipidus, psychogenic polydipsia, and renal disease preclude this.
  - If UOP is decreased (particularly in azotemic patients), fluid therapy and vasopressor support (to increase renal blood flow) should be initiated to prevent oliguria or anuria. Ensure adequate hydration prior to instituting medications to increase UOP (e.g., furosemide, mannitol); otherwise, these products will result in increased UOP at the expense of dehydrating the patient.
- Increasing renal blood flow
  - Ideally, IV fluids should be the first line of defense in treatment of the poisoned patient. This will help increase renal blood flow and promote diuresis. If the patient is adequately hydrated and develops oliguria or anuria, consider the following:
    - Dopamine: 1–5 μg/kg/min IV CRI (dose for dopaminergic effect).
    - Dobutamine: 5–10 μg/kg/min IV CRI (for dogs).
    - Furosemide (if patient becoming oliguric): 0.1–1 mg/kg/hour IV CRI or intermittent 2 mg/kg IV boluses q 4–6 hours PRN.
  - Due to the complexity of this topic, readers are referred to a critical care book (see Suggested Reading) for further information.

Pulse Oximetry

- Pulse oximeters are noninvasive, easy-to-use bedside monitors that measure SpO_2 rather than SaO_2 (oxygen saturation). A pulsatile tissue bed is required for an accurate reading. Measurements can be taken on the lip, tongue, pinnae, base of tail, toe web, vulva, prepuce, or rectum (with a rectal probe).
- Reliable pulse oximetry readings are affected by ambient light, hypotension, poor perfusion, pigmentation, icterus, and nail polish.
- An accurate HR and strong signal *must* correlate with the pulse oximeter before a reliable reading can be taken.
- Normal pulse oximetry (without oxygen supplementation) is ≥95–100%. A pulse oximetry reading of 90% correlates with a PaO_2 of 60 mmHg (normal 80–100 mmHg), consistent with *severe* hypoxemia.

- While the gold standard for assessing oxygenation and ventilation is ABG analysis, a pulse oximeter reading (with the aid of the oxygen dissociation curve) and venous blood gas (VBG) can be assessed together to help identify the severity of hypoxemia and hypoventilation.
- Pulse oximetry is useful in the poisoned patient when dyspnea, tachypnea, abnormal lung sounds, or respiratory distress is evident.

End-Tidal CO_2 ($ETCO_2$)

- Capnography is a noninvasive way of continuously measuring $PaCO_2$. $ETCO_2$ is an effective way of measuring the ability to adequately ventilate. In veterinary medicine, the use of $ETCO_2$ is typically limited to sedated, intubated patients.
- With the poisoned patient, the use of $ETCO_2$ may be beneficial to assess the severity of hypercapnia (or hypoventilation).
- Patients who are excessively sedate benefit from $ETCO_2$ monitoring to determine if PPV needs to be implemented.
- When in doubt, the gold standard to confirm a PCO_2 level is the ABG (see Breathing earlier in this chapter).
- In patients with an $ETCO_2$ >40–50 mmHg, appropriate PPV may be warranted or respiratory arrest may be imminent.

Blood Gas Analysis

- Venous (VBG) or arterial (ABG) blood gas analysis is the determination of the pH, paO_2 (arterial), pCO_2 (venous or arterial), base excess (BE), and bicarbonate (HCO_3) of blood. Blood gases allow clinicians to evaluate the overall acid–base status of the blood, the respiratory and metabolic contributions, and the pulmonary function.
- HCO_3 is a measure of the metabolic component, while pCO_2 is a measure of ventilation and is the respiratory component of a patient's acid–base status.
- The reader is referred to an acid–base source for more information.
- In general, the steps for interpretation of blood gas analysis should be the following:
  1. **pH.** Is the pH acidemic or alkalemic?
  2. **BE.** As this is the truest assessment of the metabolic component, a more negative number (e.g., −15) represents a severe metabolic acidosis, while a positive number (e.g., +15) represents a severe metabolic alkalosis.
  3. **pCO_2.** This evaluates the respiratory component. As pCO_2 is an acid, a high pCO_2 indicates a respiratory acidosis. A lower pCO_2 indicates a respiratory alkalosis.
  4. **Compensation**. Is compensation occurring? For example, an animal with a severe metabolic acidosis should be hyperventilating and blowing off its extra acid (pCO_2). Keep in mind that an animal will never overcompensate. If it appears that "overcompensation" is occurring, an additional acid–base disturbance is typically present (e.g., mixed acid–base).
  5. **Hypoxia**. Evaluate if the paO_2 is <80 mmHg to rule out hypoxemia. This can only be assessed on an ABG.
  6. Do these changes correspond to the clinical picture?

- VBG analysis with pulse oximetry interpretation can be used together and is often as beneficial as ABG results. For the evaluation of acid–base parameters, a VBG is an attractive alternative as it does not require arterial sampling. Venous samples can be interpreted as previously described for an arterial sample, with three known exceptions.
    - □ The partial pressure of venous carbon dioxide ($PvCO_2$) is approximately 5–10 mmHg higher than in the arterial system. Normal $PaCO_2$ is approximately 35 mmHg.
    - □ One cannot assess PO_2 on a VBG. Only an arterial PO_2 can provide information regarding the oxygenation function of the lungs. With pulse oximetry, SpO_2 can be correlated with an oxygen-hemoglobin dissociation curve and the pO_2 can then be deduced. Pulse oximeter + VBG = ABG.
    - □ When peripheral vasoconstriction, severe shock, hypovolemia, or low flow states (e.g., saddle thrombus, tourniquet application) occur, a peripheral venous sample may not accurately reflect the patient's acid–base status. Ideally, a jugular sample may be a more accurate reflection compared to a peripheral sample.
- VBG analysis is beneficial in the poisoned patient to evaluate the severity of acid–base imbalances. There are four main causes of metabolic acidosis.
    - Lactic acidosis.
    - Uremic acidosis (e.g., acute kidney injury [AKI]).
    - Diabetic ketoacidosis.
    - Toxicants (e.g., ethylene glycol, salicylates, methanol, etc.).
- VBG analysis can be used in conjunction with other diagnostic testing (e.g., EG testing) to confirm ingestion. For example, a dog presenting to a clinic 3 hours after possibly ingesting EG should have an EG blood test and VBG done simultaneously if possible. The absence of a metabolic acidosis in the face of a weak (or false) positive result makes it unlikely that true exposure occurred, as the presence of a metabolic acidosis would be expected.
- VBG analysis may help the clinician titrate appropriate therapy; for example, if a severe metabolic acidosis (pH <7.0, BE −18, HCO_3 11 mmHg) is present, the use of sodium bicarbonate therapy may be indicated.

Central Venous Pressure (CVP)

- CVP is the hydrostatic pressure in the cranial vena cava and approximates right atrial pressure.
- CVP monitoring can be performed to estimate right ventricular end-diastolic volume and the relationship between blood volume capacity and blood volume. It indirectly correlates to intravascular volume, right heart function, and venous compliance, correlating with preload.
- Setup for CVP monitoring includes a central line, a water manometer ($10), and IV tubing.
- Normal CVP is 0–5 cmH_2O or 0–4 mm Hg.

- CVP monitoring will allow the veterinarian to titrate fluid therapy appropriately.
- A low CVP may reflect a hypovolemic state, while a high CVP may indicate fluid overload, right-sided heart failure, increased right atrial filling pressure, pericardial disease, or the presence of a cranial mediastinal mass.
- CVPs can be falsely elevated with pleural space disease (such as pneumothorax) or with positive end-expiratory pressure, and should be evaluated subjectively based on trends.
- Evaluation of perfusion and hydration status should include a global evaluation of the patient and may include HR, BP, CVP, UOP, PCV/TS, and physical exam findings.
- CVP monitoring is useful in the poisoned patient that is in AKI from nephrotoxins such as ethylene glycol, lilies, grapes/raisins, NSAIDs, etc.

Fluid Therapy

- Fluid therapy, a cornerstone therapy of emergency management of the poisoned patient:
  - corrects dehydration
  - maintains perfusion at a cellular level
  - vasodilates the renal vessels (particularly with nephrotoxic toxins like NSAIDs, lilies, etc.)
  - treats hypotension (particularly with toxicants such as beta-blockers, calcium channel blockers, others).
- Fluid therapy can also be used to aid in detoxification of the patient by increasing renal excretion of toxicants by forced diuresis.
- Patients should be evaluated for dehydration based on skin turgor, tacky mucous membrane, and the presence of sunken eyes. Depending on the severity of dehydration and illness, patients should be treated with IV fluid replacement.
- Hydration status should be appropriately monitored by assessing weight gain (or loss), PCV/TS (as evidence of hemoconcentration or hemodilution), and BUN (which gives a gross estimate of decreased renal perfusion and glomerular filtration rate, resulting in a prerenal azotemia).
  - Evidence of hypersthenuria (cat >1.040; dog >1.025) is consistent with dehydration.
- Crystalloids
  - Any balanced, isotonic buffered solution can be used (e.g., Normosol-R, LRS).
  - Dose: the dose of IV fluids to administer is dependent on the clinical state and physical examination findings of the patient.
  - In a healthy patient, fluid rates of 4–10 mL/kg/hour can be used to force renal clearance of the toxicant.
  - Neonates have a higher maintenance fluid rate (80–180 mL/kg/day), and fluid rates should be adjusted accordingly.
  - Patients with cardiac disease or respiratory disease, or those who have ingested toxins that may increase the patient's risk toward pulmonary edema (e.g., TCA antidepressants, phosphide rodenticides) should have judicious fluid administration.
  - Careful assessment of hydration should be made based on PCV/TS, weight gain, CVP, and physical examination findings.

- Colloids
  - Colloids are large molecules that stay in the intravascular space for a longer duration of time.
  - The use of colloids (e.g., Hetastarch, VetStarch) should be considered for those patients with a low colloid osmotic pressure (normal reference range 18–20 mmHg). In general, hypoproteinemic (TS <5 g/dL) or persistently hypotensive patients may benefit from the added effect of a colloid.

Cardiovascular Support

- Please see Circulation, Fluid Therapy, and Continuous ECG for more information.
- In patients with cardiac arrhythmias, the use of antiarrhythmic therapy is recommended if it is directly affecting perfusion parameters (e.g., CRT, blood pressure, pulse deficits, etc.).
  - Bradyarrhythmias (dog: HR <50 bpm; cat: HR <120 bpm)
    - Atropine: 0.02–0.04 mg/kg IV, IM, SQ PRN bradycardia.
    - Glycopyrrolate: 0.01 mg/kg IV, IM, SQ PRN bradycardia.
    - If nonresponsive, more aggressive therapy such as intravenous lipid emulsion (ILE), temporary pacemaker placement, or high-dose insulin therapy may be necessary, depending on the underlying toxicant.
  - Supraventricular tachyarrhythmias (SVTs) (dog: HR >180 bpm; cat: HR >240 bpm)
    - SVTs are differentiated from VPCs by ECG appearance. SVTs typically retain a normal-appearing QRS.
    - Esmolol: 250–500 μg/kg IV slow over 2 minutes, then 10–200 μg/kg/min CRI.
    - Verapamil: 0.025–0.15 mg/kg IV q 5 minutes, up to total dose of 0.15–0.2 mg/kg.
    - Digoxin:
      - Dogs: 3–7 μg/kg PO q 12 hours
      - Cats: 10 μg/kg PO q 24–48 hours
    - Diltiazem: 0.05–0.25 mg/kg IV slowly, repeat q 15 minutes to maximum dose of 0.75 mg/kg.
    - Amiodarone: 10–20 mg/kg PO q 12–24 hours.
  - Ventricular arrhythmias
    - VPCs have a QRS on ECG that is 90% abnormal, wide, and bizarre.
    - Lidocaine:
      - Dogs: 2–4 mg/kg IV bolus, then 25–100 μg/kg/min IV CRI
      - Cats: 0.25–0.5 mg/kg IV bolus, then 10–20 μg/kg/min IV CRI (use with caution in cats due to the risk of neurotoxicity)
    - Procainamide:
      - Dogs: 2 mg/kg IV bolus, repeated to maximum cumulative dosage of 20 mg/kg, then 25–50 μg/kg/min IV CRI (dogs only)
      - Cats: 1–2 mg/kg IV slowly, then 10–20 μg/kg/min IV CRI (use with caution in cats due to the risk of neurotoxicity)
    - Amiodarone: 10–20 mg/kg PO q 12–24 hours
    - Magnesium sulfate: 0.75–1 mEq/kg/day IV CRI

- In patients with cardiovascular collapse (e.g., hypotension, tachycardia, bradycardia, etc.), the appropriate use of IV fluids and/or antiarrhythmic therapy is warranted. In persistently hypotensive patients not responding to boluses of crystalloids, colloids, or blood products, the use of positive inotropes may be necessary to increase cardiac contractility or blood pressure. Due to the complexity of this topic, readers are directed toward the Suggested Reading at the end of this chapter.
  - Dopamine
    - 2–10 µg/kg/min IV CRI to effect (dose for beta effect).
    - >10 µg/kg/min IV CRI to effect (dose for alpha effect).
  - Dobutamine (not to be used for more than 24 hours, ideally)
    - Dogs: 5–20 µg/kg/min IV CRI.
    - Cats: 1–10 µg/kg/min IV CRI (observe closely for CNS complications such as seizures).
  - Norepinephrine: 0.1–1.0 µg/kg/min IV CRI.
  - Epinephrine: 0.05–0.4 µg/kg/min IV CRI.
  - Vasopressin: start with 0.8 U/kg IV bolus, then 0.01–0.04 units/kg/hour IV, CRI *or* 0.5–1 mU/kg/min IV CRI.

Gastrointestinal Support

- Certain toxins result in severe gastrointestinal ulceration (corrosive or caustic agents, human NSAIDs, e.g., naproxen, ibuprofen, aspirin, diclofenac, veterinary NSAIDS, e.g., carprofen, deracoxib, firocoxib, etc.).
- Patients should be monitored closely for signs of gastrointestinal ulceration, including the presence of vomiting, hematemesis, coffee-ground appearance to vomitus, diarrhea, bloody diarrhea, or melena. Dogs should have a rectal exam performed daily while hospitalized, if possible.
- As the shock organ in the dog is the GIT, appropriate fluid resuscitation is necessary to aid in perfusion of the gut.
- Treatment should be initiated promptly and includes use of the following antiulcer drugs.
  - H_2 antagonists
    - Famotidine 0.5–1.0 mg/kg, PO, SQ, IM, or IV q 12–24 hours.
    - Ranitidine 1–2 mg/kg, PO, IV, SQ q 8–12 hours.
    - Cimetidine 5–10 mg/kg, PO, IM, IV q 6–8 hours.
  - Proton pump inhibitors
    - Omeprazole 0.5–1.0 mg/kg, PO q 24 hours in dogs; 0.7 mg/kg, PO q 12–24 hours in cats.
    - Pantoprazole 0.5–1 mg/kg, IV q 24 hours.
  - Sucralfate 0.25–1 g, PO q 24 hours.
  - Antiemetic therapy
    - Maropitant 1 mg/kg, SQ q 24 hours (extra-label use for cats or via IV route of administration).
    - Ondansetron 0.1–0.3 mg/kg, SQ, IV q 8–12 hours.

- ◻ Metoclopramide 0.2–0.5 mg/kg, PO, IM, SQ q 6–8 hours or 1–2 mg/kg/day, CRI IV.
- ◻ Dolasetron mesylate 0.6–1 mg/kg, IV q 12–24 hours.

- Adequate nutritional support should be provided to critically ill patients whose calories have been restricted for more than 3–4 days, provided risks of aspiration pneumonia have resolved.
- If patients are vomiting despite antiemetic therapy, alternative nutrition such as TPN or PPN should be initiated.
- Nutrition is important to help reduce intestinal villous atrophy or bacterial translocation, prevent gastric ulceration, increase gastric or intestinal blood flow, increase GI mucous production, and preserve normal GI flora, all of which speed recovery and decrease risk for sepsis and morbidity.
- Patients should not be force fed, as this is stressful to the patient and increases the risk of aspiration pneumonia.

Neurological Support

- Certain toxicants may result in signs of agitation, CNS depression, or refractory seizures. Examples include 5-FU, amphetamines, SSRIs, baclofen, ivermectin, bromethalin, benzodiazepines, lamotrigine, pyrethrins, organophosphates, metaldehyde, cocaine, mushrooms, salt, blue-green algae, and others.
- In the poisoned patient, it is imperative that appropriate drug therapy be used to stop tremors and seizures immediately. Persistent tremoring and seizuring can result in rhabdomyolysis with secondary AKI, lowering of the seizure threshold, secondary hyperthermia, and secondary DIC. The use of muscle relaxants and anticonvulsant therapy is imperative.
  - Methocarbamol 55–220 mg/kg, IV or PO, PRN to effect.
  - Diazepam 0.25–0.5 mg/kg, IV, PRN to effect, followed by CRI if indicated.
  - Midazolam 0.1–0.5 mg/kg, IV, PRN to effect, followed by CRI if indicated.
  - Levetiracetam 20–60 mg/kg, IV, PRN to effect.
  - Phenobarbital 4–20 mg/kg, IV q 4 hours × 4 doses to load; additional doses may be necessary.
  - Pentobarbital 2–15 mg/kg, IV, PRN to effect.
  - Propofol 1–4 mg/kg, IV slow, PRN to effect, followed by CRI if indicated
  - General anesthesia (inhalant therapy).
- Severely neurologically impaired poisoned patients should be monitored and treated for cerebral ischemia or edema with the following supportive care, if needed.
  - 15–30° head elevation.
  - Oxygen therapy.
  - Fluid therapy to maintain perfusion, blood pressure, UOP.
  - ECG, pulse oximetry, or $ETCO_2$ monitoring.
  - Frequent neurological examination (PLR, mentation, etc.).
  - Treatment for cerebral edema: mannitol 0.5–2 g/kg, IV slowly over 20–30 minutes PRN.

- Patients should be monitored for increased intracranial pressure (ICP), which may be evident by Cushing's reflex (different from Cushing's disease). Cushing's reflex is seen secondary to increased ICP and clinical signs include progressive lethargy, nonresponsiveness, acute bradycardia (HR <60 bpm dog, <140 bpm cat), and concurrent hypertension (>190–200 mmHg systolic). This reflex is indicative of *severe cerebral edema* and imminent herniation; mannitol should be administered immediately.
- The use of steroids is no longer advocated for treatment for elevated ICP.

Analgesics/Sedatives

- Certain toxicities may result in severe agitation, where sedation may be necessary. Common toxicities include beta-agonist toxicity (e.g., albuterol), methylxanthines (e.g., chocolate, caffeine), SSRIs, TCAs, benzodiazepines, nonbenzodiazepines, amphetamines, methamphetamines, metaldehyde, tremorgenic toxins, and others.
- Sedatives and analgesics should be used when appropriate. For agitation and hypertension, higher doses of sedatives may be required. See treatment for "hypertension" earlier for appropriate drugs and doses.
- For patients with oral corrosive injury (e.g., ultra-bleach cleaning products, essential oils/liquid potpourri), the use of topical analgesics should be avoided in the mouth. While analgesic therapy is important, further self-mutilation or trauma may occur with the use of products such as lidocaine gels or numbing oral rinses. Rather, the use of analgesics should be considered.
  - Buprenorphine 11–22 μg/kg sublingual, IV, IM, SQ q 6 hours as needed.
  - Butorphanol 0.2–0.8 mg/kg, IV, SQ, IM, PRN to effect.
  - Tramadol 1–5 mg/kg, PO q 6–8 hours to effect.

Miscellaneous Treatment

- Vitamin K_1 should be used for ACR toxicosis. Typically, for the acutely poisoned patient, the use of oral versus injectable vitamin K_1 is sufficient, as it is absorbed rapidly when given with a fatty meal. The use of IV or IM vitamin K_1 is generally not recommended due to the risk of anaphylaxis or intramuscular hemorrhage, respectively.
  - Dose: 2.5–5 mg/kg PO, SQ q 12–24 hours PO as needed.
- Cyproheptadine, a serotonin antagonist, can be given for toxicants that result in serotonin syndrome (e.g., SSRI, TCAs, amphetamines, etc.).
  - Cats: 2–4 mg total dose q 4–6 hours PO as needed until resolution of clinical signs.
  - Dogs: 1.1 mg/kg q 4–6 hours PO as needed.
- N-acetylcysteine (NAC), a glutathione source, can be used to limit formation of toxic metabolites (e.g., NAPQI with acetaminophen toxicity) by maintaining glutathione and sulfate concentrations. NAC is most commonly used for acetaminophen toxicosis, but can also be used with other hepatotoxicants (e.g., blue-green algae, *Amanita* spp., xylitol).
  - 10–20% solutions should be diluted to a 5% solution prior to IV administration.

- Initial loading doses of 140 mg/kg, followed by 70 mg/kg PO or IV every 4–6 hours for 7–17 doses (typically, NAC is administered for 48 hours, but may be continued for longer if there is evidence of hepatic insult).
- The sterile "for inhalation only" formulation of NAC may be given IV (off-label) slowly over 15–20 minutes through a 0.22 micron bacteriostatic filter.

- S-adenosyl-methionine (SAMe), a glutathione precursor and methyl donor, can be used as a hepatoprotectant and antioxidant, and may help with glutathione production and maintenance.
  - 18 mg/kg/day PO (without food) may reduce oxidative damage × 7–30 days.
- Intravenous lipid emulsion, or IV fat, is thought to act as an antidote for fat-soluble toxicants such as macrocyclic lactones (e.g., ivermectin, moxidectin), baclofen, calcium channel blockers, cholecalciferol, pyrethrins, etc. ILE is thought to create a lipid sink, resulting in decreased volume of distribution of toxicants. It can be administered via a sterile peripheral catheter at the recommended dose (based on a 20% solution):
  - 1.5 mL/kg IV once over 1–2 minutes, followed by a CRI of 0.25–0.5 mL/kg/minute for 30–60 minutes. Multiple additional doses can be considered. The reader is referred to chapter 3 (Antidotes and Other Useful Drugs) for more information.
- Ascorbic acid (vitamin C) can be used as an antioxidant and to help reduce methemoglobinemia to hemoglobin (as seen with acetaminophen toxicosis).
  - 30 mg/kg PO, SQ, IV q 6 hours.

CONCLUSIONS

With toxicosis, the majority of toxins do not have a readily available antidote. Symptomatic and supportive care remains the primary goal of emergency management of the poisoned patient.

Abbreviations

See Appendix 1 for a complete list.

ACR = anticoagulant rodenticide
ALI = acute lung injury
AKI = acute kidney injury
cECG = continuous electrocardiography
$ETCO_2$ = end-tidal CO_2
HCM = hypertrophic cardiomyopathy
ICP = intracranial pressure
MetHb = methemoglobin
NAPQI = *N*-acetyl-*p*-benzoquinone imine
PaO_2 = partial pressure of arterial oxygen
p_aCO_2 = partial pressure of arterial carbon dioxide

pCO_2 = partial pressure of carbon dioxide
p_vCO_2 = partial pressure of venous carbon dioxide
PPN = partial parenteral nutrition
SaO_2 = arterial oxygen saturation
SpO_2 = saturation of arterial blood with oxygen as measured by pulse oximetry
SVT = supraventricular tachyarrhythmia
TPN = total parenteral nutrition
UOP = urine output
VPC = ventricular premature complex

Suggested Reading

Braswell C, Mensack S. Supportive care of the poisoned patient. In: Peterson ME, Talcott PA, eds. Small Animal Toxicology, 3rd edn. St Louis, MO: Elsevier Saunders, 2013; pp. 85–124.

Fernandez A, Lee J, Rahilly L, et al. The use of intravenous lipid emulsions as an antidote in veterinary toxicology: a review. J Vet Emerg Crit Care 2011; 21(4):309–320.

Hopper K. Basic mechanical ventilation. In: Silverstein DC, Hopper K, eds. Small Animal Critical Care Medicine, 2nd edn. St Louis, MO: Elsevier Saunders, 2015; pp. 161–165.

Hopper K. Advanced mechanical ventilation. In: Silverstein DC, Hopper K, eds. Small Animal Critical Care Medicine, 2nd edn. St Louis, MO: Elsevier Saunders, 2015; pp. 166–171.

Pypendop BH. Capnography. In: SilversteinDC, HopperK, eds. Small Animal Critical Care Medicine, 2nd edn. St Louis, MO: Elsevier Saunders, 2015; pp. 994–997.

Sorell-Raschi L. Blood gas and oximetry monitoring. In: Silverstein DC, Hopper K, eds. Small Animal Critical Care Medicine, 2nd edn. St Louis, MO: Elsevier Saunders, 2015; pp. 970–977.

Waddell LS, Brown AJ. Hemodynamic monitoring. In: Silverstein DC, Hopper K, eds. Small Animal Critical Care Medicine, 2nd edn. St Louis, MO: Elsevier Saunders, 2015; pp. 957–961.

Author: Justine A. Lee, DVM, DACVECC, DABT
Consulting Editor: Lynn R. Hovda, RPh, DVM, MS, DACVIM

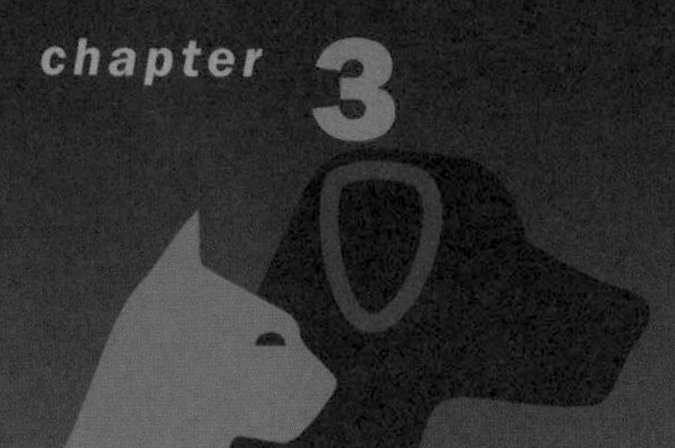

chapter 3

Antidotes and Other Useful Drugs

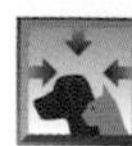

DEFINITION/OVERVIEW

- Antidotes are remedies used to counteract poisons. Specifically, antidotes are defined as any substance used to relieve or prevent the effects associated with a toxicant.
- Very few antidotes exist in medicine, and those that do are generally not approved for veterinary use. Any use associated with nonveterinary-approved antidotes is considered extra-label. The doses used are often extrapolated from human literature with very little scientific animal data available. Veterinarians are allowed to legally use medications in an extra-label manner but when doing so assume all the responsibility associated with their use.
- Little effort has been made by manufacturers to produce antidotes approved for use in veterinary medicine. There is little financial incentive for them to do this as the use of antidotes is limited, making research and manufacturing cost prohibitive.
- Antidotes can be divided into three broad categories:
  - *Chemical or causal antidotes* are those that work directly on the toxicant. They bind with the toxicant to yield an innocuous compound that is excreted from the body.
  - *Functional antidotes* have no chemical or physical interaction with toxicants but work to lessen the clinical signs associated with intoxication.
  - *Pharmacological or physiological antidotes* work in the body by several different mechanisms. Most commonly, they work directly at the receptor site, generally counteracting toxicosis by producing opposing clinical signs. They may also prevent the formation of toxic metabolites, facilitate a more rapid elimination of a toxicant, or aid in the restoration of normal body function.

Chemical Antidotes

Antivenom

- IV antivenom can be used in dogs and cats to prevent paralysis, coagulopathies, and thrombocytopenia from snake, black widow spider, or scorpion bites. They have no effect on tissue necrosis. Early administration is preferred as it not only lessens the severity of signs but attenuates the need for a large number of doses at a later date.

Blackwell's Five-Minute Veterinary Consult Clinical Companion: Small Animal Toxicology, Second Edition.
Lynn R. Hovda, Ahna G. Brutlag, Robert H. Poppenga, and Katherine L. Peterson.

Companion website: www.fiveminutevet.com/toxicology

- Anaphylactoid, anaphylactic, and serum sickness reactions can occur, especially if the animal has received antivenom at a prior time.
- Elapid antivenin (coral snakes).
  - Specific *M. fulvius* antivenin is no longer readily available in the USA and the remaining supply is primarily restricted for human use.
    - North American coral snake antivenin (Wyeth, Antivenin *Micrurus fulvius*; IgG, equine origin).
  - Alternative coral snake antivenoms produced in other countries may sometimes be obtained from local zoos.
  - The manufacturer's guidelines for dilution and administration should be followed closely.
  - Protective cross-reactivity occurs with the following antivenins:
    - Coralmyn Fab_2 (equine derived); Instituto Bioclon, Mexico.
    - Costa Rican coral snake antivenin; Instituto Clodomiro Picado, Costa Rica.
    - Australian tiger snake (*Notechis scutatus*) antivenin; CSL Limited, Parkville, Victoria, Australia.
- Crotalid antivenin (pit vipers).
  - Veterinary antivenoms – specific USDA-approved products available in USA.
    - Antivenin (Crotalidae, IgG equine derived); polyvalent (veterinary antivenin):
      - Boehringer-Ingelheim, Ridgefield, CT
      - Dose varies from 1 to 5 vials IV depending on severity of symptoms
      - 95% of cases controlled with a single vial
    - Venom Vet (Crotalidae, Fab_2 equine origin; polyvalent (injectable antivenin solution):
      - MT Venom, LLC, Canoga Park, CA
      - Ready to use, no reconstitution necessary
      - Reasonably priced and available
  - Alternative antivenoms (human) – doses not precisely determined for veterinary use.
    - CroFab (Crotalidae, Fab. ovine) – polyvalent:
      - BTG International Inc., West Conshohocken, PA
      - Supplied as a carton of two vials
    - Antivipmyn (Fab_2, equine origin) – polyvalent antiviper serum:
      - Instituto Bioclon, Mexico
      - Maintained by multiple zoos in United States
      - Currently in veterinary trials
    - Costa Rican (IgG, equine) – polyvalent pit viper antivenin:
      - Instituto Clodomiro Picado, Costa Rica
      - Maintained by multiple zoos in United States
- Black widow spider antivenin.
  - Reserved for high-risk patients (e.g., pediatric, geriatric, or metabolically compromised).

- Lycovac antivenin black widow spider (human antivenin, equine origin), Merck, West Point, PA.
  - ☐ 1 vial mixed with 100 mL crystalloid solution; administer IV slowly with monitoring of the ventral ear pinna for evidence of hyperemia (an indicator of allergic response):
    - ◦ May no longer be available for veterinary use
    - ◦ One dose is usually sufficient with response evident within 30 minutes
- Alacracmyn, Instituto Bioclon, Mexico, has completed human trials but has not yet been approved by the FDA for use in the USA. This is an equine-origin Fab_2 antivenin product and may be less likely to trigger an allergic reaction.
  - ☐ Marketed in Mexico but not the USA.
- Analatro antivenin, Instituto Bioclon, Mexico, has completed more thorough clinical trials but the data have not yet been reviewed as of April 2015.
  - ☐ Currently not on the market in the USA.

■ Scorpion antivenin.
- Anascorp (*Centruroides* Fab_2; equine origin) antivenin; Instituto Bioclon, Mexico.

Chelating agents

■ These antidotes are generally used to remove heavy metals from the body. The chelating agent combines with a metal ion to form a complex that is then excreted.

■ Calcium disodium ethylenediaminetetraacetic acid or $CaNa_2EDTA$ (Calcium Disodium Versenate, Medicis).
- Labeled for use in pediatric and adult human beings with acute and chronic lead poisoning. The use has declined over the years due to side effects and decreased incidence of lead toxicosis in human beings.
- Still widely used in veterinary medicine to chelate lead, zinc, inorganic mercury, and perhaps cadmium, particularly in birds.
- Calcium disodium EDTA (Calcium EDTA) and *not* Disodium EDTA (Sodium EDTA or Edetate Disodium) must be used. These two should not be confused.
- Should not be used while lead remains in the GIT as it may enhance the systemic absorption of lead.
- Should be used in conjunction with dimercaprol to increase lead excretion and prevent acute neurological signs.
- Dose (dogs and cats):
  - ☐ Dilute product in 5% dextrose to a final concentration of 2–4 mg/mL prior to use.
  - ☐ 25 mg/kg IV or SQ every 6 hours.
  - ☐ Maximum recommended daily dose of 2 g/day.
  - ☐ Treat for 5 days; rest for 5–7 days, and repeat if needed.
- IM injection is painful and not recommended.
- Causes GI signs and is very nephrotoxic so caution needs to be exercised to ensure hydration; should not be used in animals with chronic renal failure.

■ D-penicillamine (Cuprimine, Merck; Depen, Wallace).
- Labeled for use in human beings for copper, lead, iron, and mercury poisoning.

  - Used in veterinary medicine for acute cadmium, inorganic mercury, lead, and zinc toxicosis, and with chronic copper toxicosis in dogs with inherited copper storage disease.
  - Often difficult to obtain and may be expensive, depending on source.
  - Dose (dogs) for at-home therapy after $CaNa_2EDTA$ lead treatment: 110 mg/kg/day divided, PO q 6–8 hours for 1–2 weeks.
  - Dose (cats) for at-home therapy after $CaNa_2EDTA$ lead treatment and in the presence of elevated blood levels: 125 mg per cat, PO q 12 hours for 5 days.
- Deferoxamine (Desferal, Novartis Pharmaceutical Corporation).
  - Labeled in human beings for the treatment of acute iron intoxication and chronic iron overload due to transfusion-dependent anemia.
  - Contraindicated in patients with severe renal disease or anuria and those with high circulating levels of aluminum.
  - Complexes with iron; deferoxamine chelated complex is water soluble and excreted primarily in urine.
  - Dose (dogs and cats): 40 mg/kg IM q 4–8 hours. In critical situations, an IV infusion of 15 mg/kg/hour can be used, but the cardiovascular system must be monitored closely during this time. The excreted complex turns the urine pink or salmon colored and is sometimes referred to as the "vin rosé" of iron poisoning. Continue treatment until the urine is clear or serum iron levels are within normal limits.
  - Deferoxamine is most effective if used within the first 24 hours while iron is still in circulation and has not been distributed to tissues.
  - Ascorbic acid: 10–15 mg/kg IM, IV, SQ, PO q 4–6 hours can be used in acute situations *after* all iron has been removed from the GIT to increase the efficacy of deferoxamine, but should be used cautiously in chronic iron poisoning as it can cause adverse cardiac effects.
- Dimercaprol (BAL in oil, Taylor).
  - Labeled in human beings for use in the treatment of arsenic, gold, and mercury poisoning. Can also be used in acute lead poisoning concomitantly with $CaNa_2EDTA$ and for treatment of high copper levels in those animals with copper storage disease.
  - Complex is water soluble and excreted in urine.
  - Dose (dogs and cats):
    - For arsenic toxicosis: 5 mg/kg IM × one dose followed by 2.5 mg/kg IM q 4 hours for 2 days, q 8 hours for 1 day, and q 12 hours until recovered.
    - For lead toxicosis: 2.5–5 mg/kg IM as 10% solution q 4 hours on days 1 and 2, then q 6 hours on day 3.
  - IM injections are painful (peanut oil carrier) and should only be given deep IM.
  - Dimercaprol is nephrotoxic so limit use and monitor BUN and creatinine. Be sure patients are adequately hydrated while product is used.
- Dimercaptosuccinic acid (also referred to as DMSA or Succimer; Chemet, Schwartz).
  - Labeled for use in pediatric human beings for lead poisoning when the blood levels are >45 μg/mL. Unlabeled use includes mercury and arsenic toxicosis. It has not been shown to be effective for iron poisoning.

- Used in veterinary medicine for lead or zinc toxicosis.
- Advantages over other chelators:
  - □ Can be given PO or rectally if GI signs are severe.
  - □ Incidence of adverse GI signs is much lower.
  - □ Can be used while lead is still present in the GIT.
  - □ Has less of an effect on systemic zinc concentrations.
- Disadvantages:
  - □ Cost – expensive.
  - □ Availability – often difficult to find.
  - □ Postchelation lead level rebound can occur.
  - □ May have a transient increase in AST and ALT.
  - □ Anecdotal reports of renal failure in cats.
- Dose (dogs and cats): 10 mg/kg PO or rectal q 8 hours × 10 days; retreat only if clinical signs are present.

■ Trientine (also known as TETA or 2,2,2 tetramine; Syprine, Aton Pharma).
- Used in veterinary medicine as an oral copper chelator in the treatment of copper-associated hepatopathies in dogs.
- Advantages: fewer adverse reactions, especially vomiting.
- Disadvantages:
  - □ Limited veterinary experience.
  - □ More expensive than d-penicillamine.
  - □ Not readily available; need to compound smaller doses.
  - □ Cannot use opened capsules as oral sprinkles because exposure results in dermatitis.
  - □ Chelates zinc, iron, and other minerals so may need to supplement.
  - □ Possibility of acute kidney injury.
- Dose (dogs).
  - □ 10–15 mg/kg PO 1–2 hours before meals.
  - □ 5–7 mg/kg PO BID 1–2 hours before meals (used in dogs with very high copper levels; helps avoid acute kidney injury).

Others

■ Digoxin immune Fab fragments – ovine (Digibind, Glaxo Smith Kline).
- Specific antidote used for digoxin toxicosis. It may also protect from poisoning associated with *Rhinella (Bufo)* toads and many cardiac glycoside-containing plants. See chapters 55 and 102.
- Fab fragments should be reserved for the treatment of life-threatening cardiac arrhythmias that do not respond to conventional antiarrhythmic therapy.
- They are expensive and will likely have to be obtained from a human hospital.
- Dose depends on the amount ingested and serum digoxin level:
  - □ Serum digoxin level available.
    - ◦ Number of vials = serum digoxin level (ng/mL) × BW (kg)/100
  - □ If serum digoxin levels are not available or if treating a *Rhinella (Bufo)* toad or cardiac-containing plant toxicosis, start therapy with 1–2 vials and reassess as needed.

- Protamine sulfate (generic, various).
  - Complexes with heparin to form an inactive salt.
  - Useful in heparin overdoses when life-threatening bleeding occurs.
  - Rapid onset of action – binding begins 5 minutes after IV administration.
  - Dose (dogs and cats):
    - 1 mg protamine sulfate IV per 100 units heparin to be inactivated. Give slowly, no faster than 50 mg over 10 minutes.
    - Decrease amount of protamine sulfate by 50% for every 30–60 minutes that has passed since heparin overdose given.

Functional Antidotes

- Bisphosphonates (Pamidronate; Aredia, Novartis).
  - Used as the current and specific antidote for vitamin D_3 (cholecalciferol) toxicosis, including cholecalciferol rodenticides and calcipotriene, a human prescription medication for psoriasis.
  - Bisphosphonates are a group of compounds that lower serum calcium levels by binding to hydroxyapatite crystals in the bone.
  - Expensive and generally must be obtained from a human hospital or drug warehouse.
  - Due to the poor prognosis with hypercalcemia and secondary mineralization, the use of pamidronate, despite the cost, is highly recommended early in the treatment of hypercalcemia.
  - Aredia dose (dogs and cats):
    - 1.3–2 mg/kg diluted in 250–500 mL 0.9% NaCl, IV slowly over several hours.
    - Monitor serum calcium levels every 12–24 hours and adjust ancillary treatment as needed. If hypercalcemia is still present, a repeated dose of pamidronate may be necessary 5–7 days after the initial dose.
    - Very large overdoses of cholecalciferol may require a second dose in 3–4 days.
- Calcitonin (Micalcin, Sandoz).
  - Infrequently used to treat hypercalcemia associated with cholecalciferol toxicosis. Has largely been replaced by pamidronate.
  - Salmon calcitonin has a number of physiological effects that result in a lowering of serum calcium. Calcitonin is used less often since pamidronate became commercially available, but may be effective when pamidronate is unavailable or in cases where the serum calcium is resistant to conventional treatment. The rapid development of resistance may limit its use.
  - In general, it should not be used in conjunction with a bisphosphonate as there is some evidence that it may increase the risk of soft tissue mineralization.
  - Dose: 4–6 IU/kg, SQ q 8–12 hours.
- Cyproheptadine (various manufacturers).
  - Used for the treatment of serotonin syndrome (e.g., excitation or depression, vocalization, ataxia, hyperthermia, seizures, tremors, vomiting, diarrhea) associated with ingestions of baclofen, SSRIs, and other medications.

- Antihistamine with serotonin antagonistic properties:
    - Dose (dogs): 1.1 mg/kg PO or rectally q 4–8 hours PRN.
    - Dose (cats): 2–4 mg per cat PO or rectally q 4–8 hours PRN.

- Intravenous lipid emulsion (ILE-Intralipid, Baxter; Liposyn, Hospira; Medialipid, Braun).
  - Composed of medium to long chain triglycerides derived from plant oils (safflower oil, soybean oil), egg phosphatides, and glycerin.
    - Clinolipid (Baxter)is somewhat different as it contains olive oil and soybean oil in addition to egg phosphatides.
  - ILE was initially used in human medicine to resuscitate patients undergoing cardiac arrest from severe local anesthetic drug toxicosis.
  - It has been used successfully in veterinary medicine to treat toxicosis associated with lipid-soluble drugs such as baclofen, beta-receptor antagonists, calcium channel blockers, ivermectin, and moxidectin.
  - It has the potential to be effective for many other lipid-soluble drugs and substances including lidocaine, cholecalciferol and vitamin D_3 analogs, parasiticides (permethrin), herbicides, and antidepressant and antipsychotic drugs.
  - The exact mechanism of how ILE works is unknown, but possible mechanisms include the following:
    - ILE may create a "pharmacological sink" for fat-soluble drugs. In this widely accepted mechanism, ILE forms a lipid phase into which free drug passes, thereby lowering the tissue drug concentration.
    - ILE may increase intracellular calcium via direct activation of voltage-gated calcium channels. This may restore myocyte function in the drug-depressed myocardium.
    - ILE may also provide an additional fatty acid supply to improve cardiac performance.
  - Adverse effects of ILE are infrequent in veterinary medicine; Reported effects in humans include hyperlipidemia, hepatosplenomegaly, jaundice, seizures, hemolytic anemia, prolonged clotting time, thrombocytopenia, and fat embolism.
  - ILE dosing information is based on human dosing using a 20% solution.
  - Several different treatment suggestions exist.
    - "Standard" protocol:
      - 1.5 mL/kg IV bolus of 20% ILE over 5–15 minutes, followed immediately with CRI of 0.25mL/kg/min over 1–2 hours.
      - May repeat dose in several hours if signs of toxicity return. Examine serum for lipemia prior to repeating dose and do not use is serum is lipemic.
    - Suggested protocol:
      - 1.5–4 mL/kg IV bolus of 20% ILE over 1 minute, followed by CRI of 0.25 mL/kg/minute over 30–60 minutes
      - Individual boluses may be repeated as needed up to 7 mL/kg IV. Examine serum for lipemia prior to repeating dose and do not use if serum is lipemic.

- Phytonadione (generic, various manufacturers).
  - Used for the treatment of anticoagulant rodenticide toxicity.
  - Analog of systemic vitamin K_1, which is required for the synthesis of clotting factors II, VII, IX, and X.

- Dosing information:
    - 2–5 mg/kg PO every 24 hours or divided twice a day.
    - SQ or IM dosing can be used if need be; IM injection may cause injection site bleeding, especially early in therapy. IV administration is not recommended due to incidence of anaphylactoid reactions.

Skeletal Muscle Relaxants

- Methocarbamol (generic, various manufacturers).
    - Used for the treatment of tremors associated with pyrethrins and pyrethroids, tremorgenic mycotoxins, strychnine, and CNS stimulant toxicosis.
    - Centrally acting skeletal muscle relaxant.
    - Dose:
        - Dogs: 55–220 mg/kg slow IV. Labeled not to exceed 330 mg/kg/day but higher doses may be used in severe poisonings as long as the dog is monitored for CNS and respiratory depression.
        - Cats: 44 mg/kg slow IV, up to 330 mg/kg/day. Labeled not to exceed 330 mg/kg/day but higher doses may be needed in severe poisonings. Monitor for CNS and respiratory depression when using high doses.
- Dantrolene (Dantrium, JHP Pharmaceuticals).
    - Used for the treatment of malignant hyperthermia reactions associated with hops (*Humulus lupulus*) or as an adjunct therapy for black widow spider bites.
    - Direct-acting skeletal muscle relaxant.
    - Dose (dogs):
        - Black widow spider bites: 1 mg/kg IV followed by 1 mg/kg PO q 4 hours as needed.
        - Hops toxicosis: 2–3 mg/kg IV or 3.5 mg/kg PO.

Pharmacological or Physiological Antidotes

- Atipamezole, yohimbine, tolazoline.
    - Atipamezole (Antisedan, Pfizer) is an alpha$_2$-adrenergic antagonist labeled for reversal of medetomidine and dexmedetomidine. It is used off-label to reverse other alpha$_2$-adrenergic agonists, including amitraz, clonidine, and xylazine. The half-life is short (2–3 hours) and the drug may need to be repeated if used to reverse longer acting agonists.
        - Dose (dogs): 50–100 μg/kg IM.
        - Dose (cats): 25–50 μg/kg IM or IV (slow).
    - Tolazoline (Tolazine, Lloyd) is an alpha-adrenergic antagonist. It is used off-label primarily to reverse xylazine. The effects may be partial and transient and it is rarely used in small animal medicine.
        - Dose (dogs and cats): 4 mg/kg IV (slow).
    - Yohimbine (Yobine, Lloyd) is an alpha$_2$-adrenergic antagonist indicated to reverse the effects of xylazine. The half-life is short (1.5–2 hours) and the drug will likely

need to be repeated if used to reverse longer acting agonists. Yohimbine has more side effects at lower doses than atipamezole, including CNS excitation, tremors, and hypersalivation.

- ☐ Dose (dogs and cats): 0.11 mg/kg IV slowly.

- ■ Atropine (various manufacturers).
  - Antimuscarinic agent used for treatment of SLUDGE (salivation, lacrimation, urination, defecation, and gastroenteritis) that accompanies organophosphate (OP) and carbamate insecticide toxicity.
  - Competes with acetylcholine at the postganglionic parasympathetic sites.
  - Dose (dogs and cats): 0.2–2 mg/kg. One quarter of the dose should be given IV and the remainder IM or SQ. The dose will likely need to be repeated; heart rate and secretions should be used to guide redosing.
  - It is important that enough atropine be provided, especially in large overdoses of OP or carbamates. Atropine should be given despite initial tachycardia, in order to adequately compete with acetylcholine. Without adequate therapy for OP toxicosis, patients may drown in their own secretions.
- ■ Ethanol (various manufacturers).
  - Used as a second-line treatment for ethylene glycol toxicosis. Fomepazole is the preferred treatment.
  - The mechanism of action is similar to fomepizole (inhibits alcohol dehydrogenase), but side effects including CNS depression, metabolic acidosis, and hyperosmolality limit the use.
  - Many different IV treatment recommendations have been recommended.
    - ☐ Preferred method: using 7% ethanol (70 mg/mL), load with 8.6 mL/kg (600 mg/kg) slow IV × 1 dose and follow with 1.43 mL/kg/hour (100 mg/kg/hour) IV CRI for 24–36 hours or until ethylene glycol (EG) test is negative.
    - ☐ Other methods can be used depending on source and concentration of ethanol source:
      - 5.5 mL/kg IV of a 20% ethanol solution every 4 hours × 5 doses; follow with 5.5 mL/kg every 6 hours for 4 more doses *OR*
      - CRI 5.5 mL/kg/hour of 5% ethanol solution until EG test is negative *OR*
      - 12 mL/kg IV of 5% ethanol solution slow IV followed by 2 mL/kg/hour as CRI until EG test is negative
- ■ Fomepizole or 4-MP (currently not commercially available).
  - Indicated as the specific antidote for EG toxicosis.
  - 4-MP is a competitive inhibitor of alcohol dehydrogenase. The mechanism of action is similar to ethanol, as it prevents the conversion of EG to toxic metabolites. Unlike ethanol, fomepizole does not result in CNS depression, metabolic acidosis, or hyperosmolality.
  - Labeled for use in dogs; extra-label in cats.
    - ☐ Dogs: may be treated as late as 8 hours after ingestion and still survive.
    - ☐ Cats: must be treated within 3 hours after ingestion. Cats treated more than 4 hours after ingestion have a reported mortality rate of 100%.

- Dose (dogs):
  - □ 20 mg/kg IV over 15–20 minutes as loading dose.
  - □ 15 mg/kg IV at 12 and 24 hours.
  - □ 5 mg/kg IV at 36 hours. Repeat EG test.
  - □ If positive, continue 5 mg/kg IV every 12 hours until negative.
- Dose (cats):
  - □ 125 mg/kg slow IV as a loading dose.
  - □ 31.25 mg/kg IV at 12, 24, and 36 hours.

■ Flumazenil (Romazicon, Anexate, others).
- Reversal agent for benzodiazepine (diazepam, etc.) overdoses with marked CNS and respiratory depression that are nonresponsive to conventional therapy.
- Competitive antagonist at the benzodiazepine receptor site.
- Use needs to be carefully balanced against the side effects – lowering of seizure threshold, vomiting, and ataxia.
- The duration of action is very short (1–2 hours) and the dose often needs to be repeated, especially when longer acting benzodiazepines have been ingested.
- Dose (dog and cat): 0.01 mg/kg IV. Doses 10–20× labeled dose have been used in some animals but there are currently no scientific data to support them.

■ Leucovorin (generic, various manufacturers).
- Calcium salt of folinic acid used for toxicity associated with folic acid antagonists (methotrexate, pyrimethamine, trimethoprim, ormetoprim).
- Reduced form of folic acid – does not require conversion by dihydrofolate reductase to become biologically active.
- Dose (dogs and cats):
  - □ Pyrimethamine, trimethoprim, ormetoprim: 0.1–0.3 mg/kg PO every 24 hours.
  - □ Methotrexate: varies depending on methotrexate serum concentrations (25–200 mg/m^2 IV, IM every 6 hours for up to 8 doses).

■ Methylene blue (generic, various).
- Infrequently used to treat methemoglobinemia formed secondary to oxidative agents such as hydroxyurea, nitrates, phenols, naphthalene (moth balls), and phenazopyridine.
- Use with extreme caution or not at all in cats.
- Dog dose: 1–1.5 mg/kg as 1% solution IV over several minutes; may be repeated but use with caution as it may cause Heinz body anemia.

■ N-acetylcysteine (Acetadote, Cumberland).
- Acetylcysteine (NAC) is used to prevent hepatic necrosis that occurs secondary to acetaminophen toxicosis. It is most effective when used within 8 hours of exposure and should be used within 24 hours to be of value.
- It has also been used successfully as a liver protectant for other hepatotoxins, including *Amanita* mushroom, xylitol, and sago palm toxicosis.
- It is a sulfhydryl compound that acts to increase glutathione synthesis in the liver, providing an alternative substrate for conjugation of acetaminophen metabolites and restoring glutathione levels.

- Specifics of use:
  - Dose (dog and cat): 140 mg/kg IV or PO × 1 dose, then 70 mg/kg IV or PO q 6 hours for 7 doses. The product should be diluted to a 5% solution prior to use.
  - IV administration preferred in cats due to low oral bioavailability (20%).
  - Variety of other doses have been suggested, most based on extrapolation from human literature. Some recommend higher doses (280 mg/kg) and others additional doses (up to 17 doses) for massive ingestions.
  - Emesis frequently occurs with oral dosing, especially after the initial dose, and an antiemetic may be required prior to starting NAC therapy.

- Naloxone (Narcan, DuPont Pharmaceuticals).
  - Used for the reversal of CNS and respiratory depression associated with opiate and opioid intoxication.
  - Pure opioid antagonist with no analgesic activity.
  - Will not reverse respiratory depression associated with buprenorphine and likely butorphanol, pentazocine, and nalbuphine.
  - Rapid onset of action (1–5 minutes) and short duration of action (approximately 90 minutes). The dose will likely have to be repeated, especially with longer acting opioids.
  - Dose (dogs and cats): 0.01–0.04 mg/kg, IV, IM, SQ; may need to use 0.04 mg/kg with larger overdoses. IM and SQ routes result in slower onset of action (5 minutes). No veterinary dose available for human oral "gel" product.
- Pralidoxime (2-PAM; Protopam Chloride, Wyeth).
  - Pralidoxime is used in OP toxicosis to reactivate cholinesterase enzymes inactivated by the insecticide. It binds to the enzyme, attaches to the OP, and forms a pralidoxime-OP complex that detaches (reactivating the enzyme) and is excreted.
  - Helps prevent nicotinic signs and should be used in conjunction with atropine.
  - Limited benefits with carbamate toxicosis.
  - Generally, pralidoxime should be used within 24 hours of exposure, but may still be effective when given at 36–48 hours. There is some evidence that it is also effective when used for treatment of the intermediate syndrome of OP toxicosis.
  - Dose (dogs and cats): 20 mg/kg IM or slow IV (over 30 minutes) for first dose. Repeat dose q 8–12 hours, IM or SQ.
  - Rapid IV administration has resulted in tachycardia, neuromuscular blockade, laryngospasm, muscle rigidity, and death.
- Pyridostigmine (Mestinon, Valeant).
  - Anticholinesterase that directly competes with acetylcholine for attachment.
  - Longer t ½ (half-life) than other similar drugs.
  - Used to treat a variety of poisonings or overdoses: anticholinergic plants (*Cestrum* spp., *Datura* spp., *Solanum* spp, etc.), atropine, avermectin and ivermectin, botulism, some Elapid snake bites, and nondepolarizing neuromuscular blocking agents (curare, pancuronium, etc.).
  - Dose: 0.01–0.03 mg/kg/hour CRI.

- Pyridoxine (generic, various manufacturers).
  - Infrequently used for isoniazid toxicosis in dogs (extra-label use).
  - May have to obtain from human hospital.
  - Converted in RBCs to pyridoxal phosphate and pyridoxamine.
  - Enhances excretion.
  - Dose: 71 mg/kg as 5–10% infusion over 30–60 minutes; if total amount of isoniazid consumed is known, can give on a mg per mg (1:1) ratio.

COMMENTS

- Antidotes, in and of themselves, are not free of side effects and should never be used indiscriminately. Each case needs to be evaluated on an individual basis and the antidote used with knowledge and forethought.
- Many toxicants lack a true antidote and symptomatic and supportive care is imperative for survival of the poisoned patient. Refer to the previous chapter, Emergency Management of the Poisoned Patient, for more information on specific supportive care and treatment.
- Many other useful drugs are not mentioned in this chapter, and the reader is directed to the Suggested Reading below for further information.

Abbreviations

See Appendix 1 for a complete list.

4-MP = 4-methylpyrazole
BAL = British anti-Lewisite
Fab = fragment antigen binding
IU = international units
SLUDGE = salivation, lacrimation, urination, defecation, gastroenteritis

Suggested Reading

Bates N, Rawson-Harris P, Edwards N. Common questions in veterinary toxicology. J Sm Anim Prac 2015; 56:298–306.

Bruno M, Borron SW, Baud FJ, et al. Anti-digitalis fab fragments. In: Brent J, Wallace KL, Burkhart KK, et al, eds. Critical Care Toxicology: Diagnosis of the Critically Poisoned Patient. Philadelphia, PA: Mosby, 2005; pp. 1575–1579.

Cave G, Harvey M, Graudins A. Review article: intravenous lipid emulsion as antidote: a summary of published human experience. Emerg Med Australasia 2011; 23(2): 123–141.

Cevik SE, Tasyurek T, Guneysel O. Intralipid emulsion treatment as an antidote in lipophilic drug intoxications. Am J Emerg Med 2014; 32(9):1103–1108.

Dalefield RR, Oehme F. Antidotes for specific poisons. In: Peterson ME, Talcott PA, eds. Small Animal Toxicology, 2nd edn. St Louis, MO: Elsevier, 2006; pp. 459–474.

Fernandez AL, Lee JA, Rahilly L, et al. The use of intravenous lipid emulsion as an antidote in veterinary toxicology. J Vet Emerg Crit Care 2011; 21(4):309–320.

Gwaltney-Brant S, Meadows I. Use of intravenous lipid emulsions for treating certain poisoning cases in small animals. Vet Clin NA- SA Prac 2012; 42:251–262.

Gwaltney-Brant S, Rumbeiha W. Newer antidotal therapies. Vet Clin NA- SA Prac 2002; 32(2):323–339.

Khan SA, Common reversal agents/antidotes in small animal poisoning. Vet Clin NA- SA Prac 2012; 42:403–406.

Peterson ME, Matz M, Seibold K, et al. A randomized multicenter trial of Crotalidae polvlent immune Fab antivenom for the treatment of rattlesnake envenomation in dogs. J Vet Emerg Crit Care 2011; 21:335–345.

Plumb DC. Plumb's Veterinary Drug Handbook, 8th edn. Ames, IA: Blackwell, 2015.

Wismer T. Antidotes. In: Poppenga RH, Gwaltney-Brant S, eds. Small Animal Toxicology Essentials. Chichester, Sussex: Wiley-Blackwell, 2011; pp. 57–70.

Author: Lynn R. Hovda, RPh, DVM, MS, DACVIM
Consulting Editor: Lynn R. Hovda, RPh, DVM, MS, DACVIM

Identification and Management of the Unknown Toxicant

chapter 4

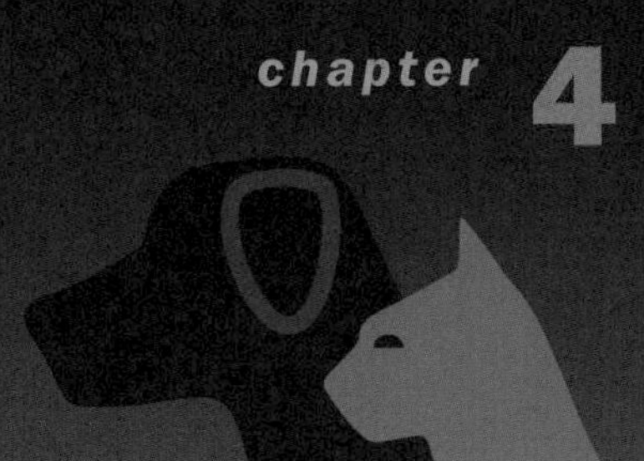

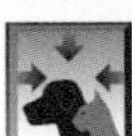

DEFINITION/OVERVIEW

- Animals are often presented to the veterinarian with a variety of clinical signs and a complaint by the owner that the animal was "poisoned."
- In reality, the incidence of true poisoning in animals is low. Other processes such as infectious or metabolic diseases, neoplasia, and trauma need to be considered when working through these cases.
- The age-old adage "treat the patient and not the toxicant" is still the basis of sound veterinary medicine in these cases.
  - Obtaining an accurate and complete history is a diagnostic cornerstone and should not be overlooked, even if the animal has life-threatening signs.
  - Stabilizing the animal and providing emergency care (see chapter 2) should be undertaken immediately. If possible, a history should be taken simultaneously by an assistant.
  - This, coupled with the physical examination findings, may help determine if a poisoning has occurred as well as suggesting what specific toxicant may have been involved.

PERTINENT INFORMATION

History

- Well-planned written protocols should be used to ensure that no details are omitted.
- These should contain, at the very least, client information (i.e. owner, address, contact information; patient information, i.e., animal species, breed, age, and weight plus any known medical conditions and medications and/or supplements taken), and a brief history of known or potential exposures.
  - Most animal owners are forthcoming with this information; however, this may not always be the case when illicit drugs are involved.
- Many owners do not know or do not remember their animal's history and only with careful questioning will this information come to light.

Blackwell's Five-Minute Veterinary Consult Clinical Companion: Small Animal Toxicology, Second Edition.
Lynn R. Hovda, Ahna G. Brutlag, Robert H. Poppenga, and Katherine L. Peterson.

Companion website: www.fiveminutevet.com/toxicology

- When questioning owners about known or potential toxicant exposures, it is often helpful to be as specific with the questioning as possible since owners might not be aware of the toxicity of many chemicals, foods, plants, or other natural products.
  - Specific questioning can be facilitated if major target organs can be identified and species sensitivities considered. For example, if an animal presents with acute renal failure, the owners can be asked specifically about possible exposure to ethylene glycol (dogs and cats), grapes/raisins (dogs), or lilies (cats).
- In addition to baseline information, other animal specific information should be obtained.
  - This may include reproductive status, vaccination history, housing (indoors or outdoors, garage or basement, etc.), environment (city, lake, farm, free roaming, or fenced in yard), and exposure to other animals.
  - A history of clinical signs should be established, including the estimated time the animal was last observed as "normal," when the clinical signs were first noted, and the progression of signs (worse, better, same).
- Any first aid provided by the owner, such as inducing emesis or bathing the animal, should also be noted as this may have complicated the situation. For example, some pet owners may have administered "home remedies" such as milk, egg whites, table salt, hydrogen peroxide, or charcoal capsules if they think their pet has been poisoned.

Physical Exam

- A complete physical examination should be performed, paying particular attention to the cardiovascular, neurological, and respiratory systems.
- Any animal with life-threatening signs should receive immediate emergency care (see chapter 2) and the physical examination should be completed when the animal is stabilized.
- Superficial physical assessment for toxicant-induced changes should include the color of the skin and mucous membranes, presence of petechiation or ecchymoses, distinctive odors or substances on the breath or body (e.g., garlic or rotten fish smell is suggestive of zinc phosphide), evidence of foreign substances on hair coat (i.e. blue-green algae, solvents, essential oils, ticks, etc.), and evidence of bites or stings.
- The animal should be examined for any signs of trauma, whether incidental such as hit by a car, or self-inflicted due to a neurological or dermal problem.
- The respiratory, gastrointestinal, cardiovascular, and neurological systems should be examined in detail for any abnormalities.
- Ocular examination may also be important. Pupil size and response should be noted, as well as irritation to the cornea or conjunctiva.

Diagnostics

- Baseline labs should include blood glucose concentration, a CBC, serum chemistries, and a urinalysis.

- If possible, stomach contents (from spontaneous or induced emesis or initial gastric lavage fluid), whole blood, serum, and urine should be saved for further testing.
    - In general, obtaining as much sample as possible for testing is desirable since the degree of testing required might be unknown.
    - All samples for toxicological testing can be refrigerated initially and frozen if to be stored for more than a few days.
- A coagulation panel should be added if hemorrhage occurs easily or if petechiae or ecchymoses were present on physical examination.
- Blood gas analysis and pulse oximetry are required for compromised respiratory systems.
- Urinalysis may include a spot check for ethylene glycol, common illicit drugs, or crystalluria.
- Other laboratory diagnostics should be ordered as needed and could include specifics such as carboxyhemoglobin concentration (carbon monoxide poisoning), cholinesterase activity (organophosphate or carbamate poisoning) or individual drug/chemical concentrations (e.g., aspirin, acetaminophen, ethanol, ethylene glycol, iron, etc.).
- Further diagnostics are performed based on the history and physical examination findings.
    - Evaluation of the body temperature is part of a routine physical examination but should be repeated often as some toxicants cause severe hyperthermia.
    - Abnormalities noted on cardiac auscultation should be evaluated with an ECG.
    - Radiographic imaging is useful to rule out radiopaque foreign objects or material.

TOXIDROMES

- Toxidromes are recognizable syndromes resulting from particular toxicants or classes of toxicants.
- They consist of a group of clinical signs or characteristic effects which can aid a practitioner or toxicologist with diagnosis. Toxidromes are analogous to a group of clinical signs associated with certain medical conditions.
    - For example, a dog suffering from bloat or GDV typically exhibits a distended, tympanic abdomen, retching, unproductive vomiting, and hypersalivation.
    - Likewise, a dog presenting with hot, dry, flushed skin, mydriasis, tacky mucous membranes, tachycardia, urinary retention, and lethargy or disorientation might suggest exposure to a toxicant with anticholinergic effects (e.g., Jimson weed or atropine).
- Common toxidromes noted in veterinary toxicology include cholinergic, anticholinergic, sympathomimetic, and serotonin toxidromes.
- The opioid toxidrome is well described in people but, due to significant interspecies variability, the signs are not as reliably similar in veterinary species.

Cholinergic Toxidrome

- The cholinergic toxidrome is produced by an overstimulation of muscarinic and nicotinic receptors by acetylcholine in the CNS, at neuromuscular junctions, and in the sympathetic and parasympathetic nervous systems. This typically occurs following the inhibition of acetylcholinesterase, the enzyme responsible for breaking down acetylcholine.

- Acute muscarinic signs include excessive salivation, lacrimation, urination (dribbling), defecation (i.e., SLUD), miosis, and coughing or dyspnea (excessive pulmonary excretions).
- Acute nicotinic signs include muscle tremors (often starting with the head and progressing toward the tail), generalized muscle stiffness/tetany, weakness with potential paresis or paralysis.

- Agents resulting in this toxidrome include organophosphate and carbamate insecticides; muscarinic mushrooms (e.g., *Inocybe* spp., *Clitocybe* spp.); pharmaceuticals used to treat glaucoma, dry mouth, or increase bladder contractility (e.g., carbachol, pilocarpine, bethenachol); and cholinergic plants.
- Atropine is the antidote for muscarinic signs and extremely large doses may be required, especially in cases of severe poisoning (0.1–2.0 mg/kg, give ¼ dose IV, remainder SQ or IM, repeat every 1–2 hours until animal is stable and secretions are controlled).
- Nicotinic signs can be treated with pralidoxime chloride or "2-PAM" (20 mg/kg IV over 15–30 minutes or SQ q 12 hours). Pralidoxime usually needs to be administered within the first 24 hours to effectively treat acute signs. For more information on the treatment of the cholinergic toxidrome, see chapter 93.

Anticholinergic Toxidrome

- The anticholinergic toxidrome is produced by the inhibition of cholinergic neurotransmission at muscarinic receptor sites in the parasympathetic nervous system.
- The common mnemonic used to describe the clinical signs associated with this toxidrome is:
  - **Mad as a hatter** (bizarre behavioral signs)
  - **Blind as a bat** (severe mydriasis which impairs visual focus)
  - **Dry as a bone** (blockade of cholinergic tone to salivary glands results in dry mouth, intense thirst, and difficulty swallowing)
  - **Red as a beet** (erythema)
  - **Hot as a pistol** (hyperthermia).
- Additional acute clinical signs may include reduced GI motility, constipation, urinary retention, restlessness, and muscular twitching. These signs may progress to incoordination, paralysis, delirium, and respiratory paralysis.
- Atropine and glycopyrolate are prototype anticholinergic agents.
  - Other agents resulting in this toxidrome include prescription and OTC anti-motion sickness agents (e.g., scopolamine patches, Dramamine® [dimenhydrinate], meclizine), drugs for overactive bladder syndrome (e.g., Detrol® [tolterodine]), antipsychotics, and many antihistamines (e.g., Benadryl® [diphenhydramine]).
  - There are also many plants with anticholinergic properties including *Datura* spp. (Jimson weed, angel's trumpet), *Atropa belladonna* (deadly nightshade), and *Convolvulus* spp. (bindweed).

- Unlike treatment for the cholinergic toxidrome, treatment for the anticholinergic toxidrome is more focused on supportive care such as IV fluids, diazepam, cooling measures, etc.
    - Physostigmine (canine dose: 1 mg total dose per dog q 12 hours IV or SQ), a parasympathomimetic drug which stimulates the parasympathetic nervous system, is available but should be reserved for cases where the patient exhibits either extreme agitation and is at risk of injuring itself or others, or where supraventricular tachycardia and sinus tachycardia are nonresponsive to traditional therapy.

Sympathomimetic Toxidrome

- Sympathomimetic agents are stimulant compounds which mimic the effects of the neurotransmitters in the sympathetic nervous system (i.e., epinephrine, norepinephrine, dopamine, etc.).
    - These agents may have a direct effect on alpha- and beta-adrenergic receptors, or may act indirectly by causing the release of norepinephrine from presynaptic nerve endings and/or by preventing the metabolism of norepinephrine by inhibiting norepinephrine transporter (NET) activity.
    - Furthermore, these agents may inhibit monoamine oxidase, an enzyme involved in the breakdown of catecholamines.
- Clinical signs associated with the sympathomimetic toxidrome include hypertension, restlessness/hyperactivity/agitation, tachycardia, and mydriasis.
    - Severe cases may display head bobbing, nausea/vomiting, tachydysrhythmias including supraventricular tachycardia and ventricular tachycardia.
    - Severe hypertension may also result in intracranial hemorrhage or renal insufficiency.
    - Reflex bradycardia due to significant hypertension is possible.
    - Prolonged agitation can lead to rhabdomyolysis and hyperthermia.
    - The $beta_2$-agonists (e.g., albuterol, clenbuterol) can cause significant electrolyte abnormalities, including severe hypokalemia.
- Unintentional pet exposure to sympathomimetic agents is frequently reported to Pet Poison Helpline, a 24/7 animal poison control center, because these drugs are commonly found in human OTC nasal decongestants (e.g., Bendaryl-D® and Clartin-D® contain pseudoephedrine), weight loss agents, anabolic bodybuilding agents, aphrodisiacs, mood stimulants, and other "energy" supplements designed to promote wakefulness. They are also present in a variety of human and veterinary prescription products such as ADD/ADHD medications (e.g., amphetamines), bronchodilators, and phenylpropanolamine.
- There is no antidote for sympathomimetic agents although helpful baseline treatments include acepromazine or chlorpromazine for sedation and to treat hypertension, injectable beta-blockers (i.e. esmolol) to treat tachycardia (if not resolved with acepromazine), and intravenous fluids to maintain perfusion.
    - Diazepam is known to produce paradoxical excitation in these patients and is usually best avoided or used with caution until the clinician is comfortable with the patient's response.

- Vital signs, including blood pressure, must be monitored closely and an ECG should be used if arrhythmias are noted.
    - If hyperthermia develops, cooling measures are recommended but should be stopped once the body reaches 103.5°F to avoid hypothermia.
- Electrolytes should be monitored closely for hypokalemia if the patient was exposed to a beta-agonist (e.g., dog biting into albuterol inhaler). For more information on specific toxicants and treatment, see chapters 13, 18, 32, 35, 43, 50, and 78.

Serotonin Toxidrome

- The serotonin toxidrome, often called serotonin syndrome or hyperactivity syndrome, is caused by overstimulation of postsynaptic serotonin receptors in the CNS.
- The main receptors responsible for serotonin syndrome are thought to be the 5-HT1A type, associated with hyperactivity, hyperreflexia, and anxiety, and the 5-HT2A type, associated with hyperthermia, incoordination, and neuromuscular excitement.
- There are at least four mechanisms by which excessive serotonin concentrations are likely to occur.
    - Decreasing serotonin breakdown (e.g., MAOIs).
    - Decreasing serotonin reuptake at presynaptic sites (e.g., SSRIs, SNRIs, TCAs, tramadol, fentanyl, cocaine, methadone, meperidine, St John's wort, amphetamines, dextromethorphan) .
    - Increasing serotonin precursors or agonists (e.g., L-tryptophan, select antimigraine medications, LSD, buspirone).
    - Increasing serotonin release (e.g., amphetamines, cocaine, buspirone, lithium).
- Acute clinical signs associated with the serotonin toxidrome include agitation, vocalization, tremors, muscle rigidity, tachycardia, hypertension, and severe hyperthermia.
    - Other reported signs include abdominal pain, diarrhea, hypersalivation, increased reflexes, ataxia, myoclonus, shivering, increased respiratory rate, transient blindness, seizures, coma, and death.
- Treatment is primarily symptomatic and supportive.
    - Cyproheptadine, a serotonin antagonist, has been used with good results in animals displaying milder signs, especially vocalization (1.1 mg/kg for dog or 2–4 mg total dose per cat given orally or rectally q 4–6 hours until signs resolve).
    - Barbiturates may be more effective for treating seizures than diazepam but either can be used.
    - As with the treatment of sympathomimetics, diazepam may cause paradoxical excitation so should be used cautiously until the practitioner can gauge the patient's response.
    - Acepromazine and chlorpromazine can used for sedation; high doses may be needed.
    - Other treatments include fluid therapy, blood pressure monitoring, ECG monitoring, and thermoregulation. For more information, see chapters 15, 28, 31, and 33.

TREATMENT PLAN

Consultation with Animal Poison Control Center

- Consultation with a specialist at an animal poison control center should be undertaken as soon as possible. Their experts have a vast amount of knowledge and experience in sorting out clinical and historic findings, providing a rule-out list and treatment advice.
- It is possible that the history and physical exam findings coupled with laboratory values may suggest a specific toxicant or toxidrome (see Toxidrome section).
    - For instance, metabolic acidosis, an increased serum osmolality, and subsequent elevations in BUN and creatinine are associated with ethylene glycol intoxication, while early and severe hypoglycemia and subsequent elevations in liver enzymes are consistent with xylitol (dogs) or alpha-lipoic acid intoxication (cats or dogs).

Decontamination

- The primary goal of decontamination, whether it is ophthalmic, dermatological, respiratory, or gastrointestinal, is to slow or prevent further absorption of a toxicant (see chapter 1).
- Care should be taken to protect workers during decontamination as some toxicants such as blue-green algae, cholinesterase-inhibiting insecticides, or zinc phosphide (which creates phosphine gas) are harmful to humans.
- Ophthalmic decontamination includes immediate lavage of the affected eye(s) for 15–20 minutes followed by a slit lamp examination to evaluate for damage.
- Moving animals to fresh air or providing oxygen assists with respiratory decontamination.
- Multiple baths with a mild, degreasing shampoo or liquid hand dishwashing detergent and tepid water followed by thorough rinsing is used to remove and prevent absorption of many dermal toxins.
- Several factors should be considered prior to undertaking gastrointestinal decontamination.
    - Important historical information includes the time since exposure, if emesis was induced at home, and whether there is any underlying medical condition that precludes decontamination (e.g., megaesophagus, seizure disorder, cardiac disease, etc.).
    - Induction of emesis is generally not an appropriate form of decontamination to use with an unknown toxicant.
        - It is contraindicated in most symptomatic patients, especially if sedate or seizing, and those with a hydrocarbon odor (e.g., gasoline, kerosene, pesticides), or lesions in mouth or oropharynx (indicative of corrosive injury).
        - Prior spontaneous vomiting is also a relative contraindication.
            - Gastric lavage is an effective form of GI decontamination, especially if the practitioner is skilled at doing so, but must be performed quickly following exposure. It allows for gastric emptying in sedate patients and the placement of activated charcoal with or without a cathartic directly

in the stomach prior to removal of the tube.The use of activated charcoal with or without a cathartic is an additional option. It is effective for most toxicants, provides rapid adsorption, and quickly moves into the small intestine where most toxicants are systemically absorbed.
    - The clinician always needs to balance the use of gastric evacuation procedures (emetics or gastric lavage) with the consequent delay in administering activated charcoal.

Case Management

- Case management depends on the history and physical exam but even stable animals should have IV catheter placement for emergency access if needed and a TPR repeated frequently.
- Very few antidotes are available and they are generally useful only for specific toxicants, although intravenous lipid emulsions have a broader range (see chapter 3).
- If a specific toxicant or toxidrome is identified during the history and physical exam, by diagnostics, or in consultation with an animal poison control center, then an appropriate antidote may be effective.
    - Even if an antidote is indicated for a particular case, it might be prohibitively expensive, not readily available, or beyond the point of clinical utility. For example, fomepizole, the preferred antidote for ethylene glycol toxicosis, is most effective if administered within 3 hours of ingestion in cats or 3–8 hours of ingestion in dogs.

Neurological Signs

- If the animal appears heavily sedated or is comatose, a stat blood glucose concentration should be obtained and dextrose administered as needed.
- If there is a potential history of opiate or opioid ingestion, as is indicated by co-existing respiratory and cardiovascular depression, response to a test dose of naloxone can be determined.
- Ingestion of benzodiazepines generally does not cause severe sedation, but if suspected, then flumazenil may be used to reverse the signs and help with the diagnosis.
- Any animal with CNS depression undergoing decontamination via bathing should be monitored closely as hypothermia may spontaneously occur.
- Neurological stimulation in the form of tremors or seizures is typical of toxicants such as pyrethrins (cats), amphetamines (see Sympathomimetic Toxidrome), caffeine/theobromine, 5-fluorouracil, ivermectin, metaldehyde, and many more.
- If the toxicant is unidentified, it is typically safe to attempt to stabilize the tremoring or seizing patient with injectable methocarbamol, diazepam, or barbiturates while simultaneously evaluating a blood glucose concentration and a serum chemistry panel.

Gastrointestinal Signs

- These signs are common, nonspecific, and may be due to a variety of toxicants or other etiologies.

- Mild gastroenteritis may require only supportive care but severe signs such as projectile vomiting, melena, HGE, cholinergic signs, etc. require urgent care coupled with IV fluids, appropriate pharmacological treatment, laboratory diagnostics, imaging, etc.
  - A test dose of atropine may be useful in animals with typical organophosphate (OP) signs (excessive salivation, lacrimation, urination, diarrhea, gastroenteritis).

Respiratory Signs

- Relatively few toxicants result in respiratory signs, with the notable offenders being OPs/carbamates (increased pulmonary secretions), or toxicants interfering with oxygen transport or hemoglobin binding such as carbon monoxide, cyanide, and hydrogen sulfide.
- Upon presentation, immediate actions should include supplemental oxygen, assessment with pulse oximetry, laboratory diagnostics including gross examination of the blood for methemoglobinemia, blood gas analysis, and thoracic radiographs (once stable).
- Additional treatments such as bronchodilators, atropine, cyanide antidotes, etc. may be warranted based on presentation and diagnostic results.

Cardiovascular Signs

- Cardiovascular signs are often relatively nonspecific and need to be contextualized with other clinical signs (see Toxidromes).
- Regardless of the cause, the first approach to treatment should be aimed at basic stabilization via IV fluid therapy and potential supplemental oxygen.
- In general, if related to intoxication, cardiovascular depression or stimulation will be apparent.
- Bradycardia, hypotension, and other signs associated with cardiac depression may be due to toxicants such as alpha$_2$-adrenergic agonists, amitraz, beta- or calcium channel blockers, cardiac glycosides, opioids, and OPs/carbamates.
  - Based on other clinical signs, agents such as atipamezole, atropine, naloxone, and calcium gluconate should be considered.
  - Reflex bradycardia (i.e., concurrent hypertension) is often due to sympathomimetic agents so treatment should be focused on decreasing the blood pressure instead of raising the heart rate.
- Cardiovascular stimulation including tachycardia and hypertension may be due to toxicants such as albuterol, amphetamines, caffeine/theobromine, metaldehyde, phenylpropanolamine, and many more (see Sympathomimetic Toxidrome).
  - If CV stimulation is coupled with hyperactivity/agitation, focus initial treatment on sedation (i.e., acepromazine for amphetamine intoxication) as this may simultaneously decrease the heart rate and blood pressure.
  - If sedation is not required or CV stimulation is refractory to sedatives, then additional agents such as injectable beta-blockers or vasodilators may be used.
  - As with all potential toxicants, treatment should be coupled with pointed historical exposure questions and diagnostics.

- As antidotes are not often available for many toxins, further care is symptomatic, supportive, and varies depending on systems affected and clinical signs. If appropriate and thorough, such treatments can still result in favorable outcomes.

Toxicological Testing

- While it is helpful to narrow down a list of possible toxicant exposures in order to select the most appropriate testing to be done, it is possible to rule out exposure to a large number of toxicants through screening approaches for unknown compounds.
- The use of powerful screening tools for both organic and inorganic toxicants is a viable option in many cases of suspected exposure to an unknown chemical.
- Depending on the specifics of a case, testing either gastric contents or urine can be useful.
    - Stomach content is often the testing sample of choice in cases of acute onset of clinical signs while urine can be a useful sample if clinical signs have been present for from several hours up to one or two days.
    - It is often recommended to test more than one sample in order to be as thorough as possible, although costs associated with testing might restrict analysis to one sample. In such a situation, a toxicologist can assist with making the most appropriate sample selection.
- In many cases, toxicological testing takes some time and therefore should not be counted on to help direct early case management.
    - Despite this limitation, test results can sometimes be available within 24 hours.
    - More delayed results are still useful to many pet owners or veterinarians in order to confirm exposure to a toxicant and to prevent further exposure risks to pets and people.
    - In addition, many suspected intoxications might result in later litigation, in which case appropriate testing can be essential.

CONCLUSIONS

- Managing an animal with a potential unknown toxicant exposure is challenging and difficult.
- Obtaining a complete and accurate history, performing a thorough physical examination followed by the appropriate laboratory diagnostics, and consultation with an animal poison control center should help the practitioner make a diagnosis and formulate an appropriate treatment plan.

Suggested Reading

Brutlag AG, Puschner B. Approach to diagnosis for the toxicology case. In: PetersonME, TalcottPA, eds. Small Animal Toxicology, 3rd edn. St Louis, MO: Elsevier, 2013; pp. 45–52.

Khan SA. Investigating fatal suspected poisonings. In: Poppenga RH, Gwaltney-Brant SM, eds. Small Animal Toxicology Essentials. Ames, IA: Wiley-Blackwell, 2011; pp. 71–76.

Khan SA. Differential diagnosis of common acute toxicologic versus nontoxicologic illness. Vet Clin Small Anim 2012; 42:389–402

Authors: Ahna G. Brutlag, DVM, MS, DABT, DABVT; Lynn R. Hovda, RPh, DVM, MS, DACVIM; Robert H. Poppenga, DVM, PhD, DABVT

Consulting Editor: Lynn R. Hovda, RPh, DVM, MS, DACVIM

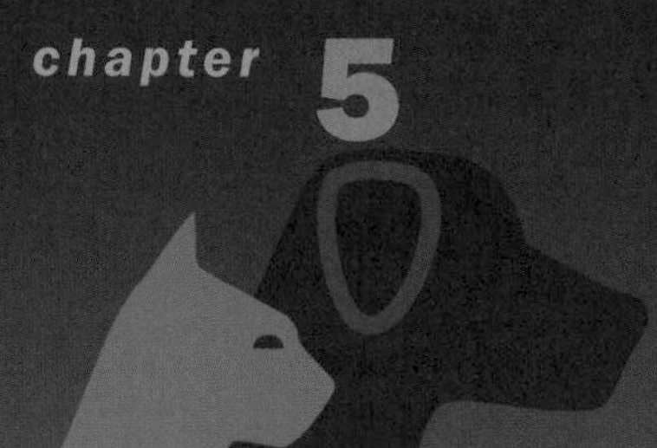

chapter 5

Laboratory Diagnostics for Toxicology

INTRODUCTION

- Diagnosis of poisoning generally depends on fulfilling five major diagnostic criteria.
  - History
  - Clinical signs
  - Clinical laboratory evaluation
  - Necropsy lesions
  - Chemical analysis
- Used properly, they are an effective combination for detecting and understanding clinical poisoning.

Historical Information

- Knowledge of a known exposure to toxicants and the circumstances surrounding an exposure are often essential to an effective toxicological diagnosis.
- One must refrain from basing a diagnosis exclusively on history of exposure. The post hoc fallacy (*Post hoc ergo propter hoc*), as translated from the original Latin, admonishes, "After the fact, therefore because of the fact."
- To avoid this, history is used only as a starting point in the diagnostic process.
- The presence of poisons such as rodenticides, insecticides, drugs, paints, household products, over-the-counter and prescription drugs, drugs of abuse, fertilizers, feed additives, and poisonous plants on the premises or a history of their availability or use should be determined when possible.
- Concurrent with this, the adage "Dosage makes the poison" means exposure alone without knowing the amount or dosage encountered is not sufficient for a diagnosis. An attempt should be made to estimate the amount or degree of exposure.
- The food and water supply along with the animal's environment should be examined carefully for algae, fungi, toxic plants, and foreign matter (e.g., baits or chemical spills) as well as odors or physical changes that suggest contamination. Detection of evidence of chewing on product containers is helpful in confirming exposures to toxicants.

Blackwell's Five-Minute Veterinary Consult Clinical Companion: Small Animal Toxicology, Second Edition.
Lynn R. Hovda, Ahna G. Brutlag, Robert H. Poppenga, and Katherine L. Peterson.

Companion website: www.fiveminutevet.com/toxicology

- A thorough history will lead to a more informed clinical examination and choice of diagnostic tests. Fundamental information should include patient identification and characteristics, important demographic factors about the environment, and group or individual issues for affected animals.
- Table 5.1 provides a guide for systematic evaluation of history, environment, and clinical effects.

TABLE 5.1. Checklist for information collection in suspect poisoning of small animals.

Owner Data:
Date: ______
Owner: ______
Manager: ______
Address: ______
Phone: ______
FAX: ______
E-mail: ______

Health History:
- Illness past 6 months:
- Exposure to other animals last 30 days:
- Vaccination history:
- Medications: sprays, dips, hormones, minerals, wormers past 6 months – administered by owner or veterinarian?
- Last exam by a veterinarian:

Environmental Data:
- Location: pasture, woods, near river or pond, confined indoors; recent location changes
- Housing: indoors, outdoors, or combination
- Approximate age of home or kennel
- Type of construction (wood frame, metal, concrete)
- Recent changes in access to trash or garbage; pesticides, flower garden, treated wood, old construction materials; recent burning of materials?
- Confined to fenced yard?
- Allowed to roam free?
- If yes, is animal always supervised?
- Businesses or commercial structures accessible?
- Other (describe): ______

Patient Data:
Species: ______
Breed: ______
Sex: ______
Pregnancy: ______
Weight: ______
Age: ______

Current Clinical and Environmental History:
- Housing: indoors/outdoors/with other animals
- Are other similar groups on the same premises?
- Common feed or water among groups?
- If a group, what is:
  - morbidity ___ mortality ___
- When first observed sick?
- How long has problem existed in this animal?
- If dead, when last seen alive and healthy?
- Any recent malicious threats; if yes, describe.
- Recent losses at home or in neighborhood?
- Pesticide use (insecticides, rodenticides, herbicides) and specific types or names if available (ask for tags or bags to ID)
- Materials used for construction/renovation
- Services: e.g., lawn care, seeding, tree planting, fertilization, pest control
- Access to automotive products, cleaning agents, hobby materials, flower gardens, ornamental trees?
- OTC and prescription medications in the home?
- Interactions with wildlife?

Dietary Data:
- Diet components: dry food only, canned food only, combination? Access to snacks or table foods? Lot number or manufacturing date
- Recent changes in total diet or specific diet component(s): list any OTC or prescribed supplements
- Method of feeding: hand feeding, free choice? Is feeding supervised? Food bowl outside?
- Access to molded or spoiled food, mushrooms, bulbs, flower garden plants, indoor plants?
- Recent changes in home/yard: painting, remodeling, pest control, weed sprays, burning trash?
- Any evidence of digging in yard or garden, evidence of damage to plants?
- Water source (flowing stream, pond, well, county or city water)

(*Continued*)

TABLE 5.1. *Continued*

Clinical Signs (check all that apply):	**GI Signs**	**Cardiovascular**	**Blood**
Nervous System	Anorexia	Arrhythmia	Anemia
Ataxia	Colic	Bradycardia	Hemorrhage
Salivation	Vomiting	Hypotension	Icterus
Blindness/vision impaired/ pupil response	Diarrhea	Tachycardia	Hemoglobinuria
Depression	Melena	Other	Methemoglobinemia
Excitement	Constipation		
Seizures	Polyphagia	**Pulmonary**	**Other**
Cerebellar signs		Cyanosis	Straining
Paraparesis or tetraparesis	**Urinary – Renal**	Dyspnea	Fever
Dysphonia	Polydipsia	Hyperpnea	Weakness
Syncope	Polyuria	Rales	
Other (describe):	Hematuria		

Clinical Signs

- Clinical signs are of prime importance to the clinician and toxicologist.
  - Both the nature of the signs and sequence of occurrence are important.
    - Did the signs begin explosively and taper off, or did they begin as mild events and worsen with time?
    - Is one body system primarily affected, or are major signs present in several systems?
- Details are often important.
  - For example, a wide range of CNS signs exists and a general description of “seizures” or “tremors” is less useful than an explicit description.
    - Are the signs a typical cranial-to-caudal epileptiform seizure?
    - Is the animal ataxic with cerebellar, vestibular, or peripheral nerve signs?
    - Are there parasympathetic signs such as vomiting, salivation, urination, diarrhea, and dyspnea?
    - Are there parasympatholytic signs such as bloat, dry mouth, mydriasis, hallucinations, or bradycardia?
  - Careful attention to changes in heart rate and rhythm can help define several cardiotoxins.
  - The attending veterinarian may see only one phase of a toxicological response, so the owner or caretaker should be queried for more information.
  - There are dangers in making a toxicological diagnosis based solely on clinical signs as there are thousands of toxic agents but only a limited range of clinical responses that can be expressed by an animal.
  - Unfortunately, in many cases an animal is found dead without any clinical signs being noted. Sudden death in an animal otherwise noted to be healthy might be a tip-off for exposure to a toxicant.

Clinical Laboratory Evaluation

- Evaluation of clinical laboratory changes can help refine associations with specific toxicants or toxicant groups, as well as suggest potential mechanisms of action and alterations in homeostasis that need correction to save the animal.
- Some changes are very characteristic of certain toxicants, while the absence of ogan damage is typical of other toxicants.
- CBC and serum chemistries are useful tools for evaluating clinical signs and formlating a treatment plan.
- Table 5.2 provides some typical clinical chemistry and hematological changes that help define various poisons.

Necropsy Lesions

- Loss of one or more animals in a group or a single animal at risk provides an invaluable opportunity to increase diagnostic information by conducting a thorough postmortem examination.
    - Necropsy may help improve diagnosis and therapy for other affected animals.
    - It can also provide guidance to the owner/manager in planning ahead and eliminating risks to other animals or people.
- Necropsy and microscopic lesions may be invaluable in supporting insurance claims or actions where liability or litigation is involved.
    - Lesions are typically absent in certain toxicoses, while the presence of lesions may correlate with other toxicoses.
    - Many insecticides and drugs, strychnine, and lead, among others, often cause few or very subtle lesions.
    - Ethylene glycol, microcystins, amanitin-containing mushrooms, bromethalin, anticoagulant rodenticides, and many other toxicants provide defined lesions helpful for making a diagnosis or narrowing a differential list.
    - Necropsy should include the brain (and a rabies exam) if neurological signs are present.
    - A thorough selection of samples collected at necropsy is easier and more inclusive if consistently performed.
    - Should legal or insurance claims be likely, a necropsy is usually essential. In this instance, photographs and detailed notes regarding the necropsy and premise examination should be taken and preserved.
    - Table 5.3 summarizes recommended necropsy specimens.
    - Specimens collected for possible toxicology testing can be stored refrigerated or frozen pending results from histopathological examination of formalin-fixed tissue samples or other postmortem testing.

Chemical Analysis

- Chemical analysis is an indispensable aid in forming a toxicological diagnosis. When used properly, and in the right context, chemical analysis may be the single best diagnostic criterion.

TABLE 5.2. Selected clinical laboratory tests supporting toxicological diagnosis.

Clinical Laboratory Assay	Example Toxicants
Ammonia (serum)	Hepatic encephalopathy secondary to a number of hepatotoxic chemicals
Aplastic anemia	Phenylbutazone, chloramphenicol, gasoline, petroleum solvents, trichothecene mycotoxins
AST, ALT, LDH increase	Aflatoxin, blue-green algae, fumonisins, pyrrolizidine alkaloids, *Lantana* spp., *Amanita* mushrooms, sago palm, xylitol
Azotemia (BUN, creatinine)	Arsenic, cadmium, antifreeze, oak, oxalate plants (e.g., lilies), NSAIDs, grapes, raisins, ACE inhibitors, beta-blockers, calcium channel antagonists, mercury
Basophilic stippling	Lead, zinc
Bile acids	Aflatoxin, other hepatotoxicants (e.g., blue-green algae, *Amanita* mushrooms, xylitol)
Bilirubin	Aflatoxin, fumonisins, zinc toxicosis, other hepatotoxicants (e.g., blue-green algae, *Amanita* mushrooms, xylitol)
Carboxyhemoglobin	Carbon monoxide (buildings, trailers), smoke inhalation
Cholinesterase	Organophosphates, blue-green algae, *Solanum* plants
CK increase	Ionophores (monensin, lasalocid), white snake root, *Cassia* spp., toxicants resulting in tremoring or seizuring (causing secondary increased CK) such as metaldehyde, tremorgenic mycotoxins, pyrethrin/pyrethroid insecticides, illicit drugs
Coagulopathy (PT, PTT)	Anticoagulant rodenticides, hepatotoxicants, DIC secondary to toxicants resulting in hyperthermia (e.g., hops, amphetamines, SSRIs)
Crystalluria	Antifreeze, oxalate plants
GGT increase	Aflatoxin, fumonisins, pyrrolizidine alkaloids; glucocorticoids, other hepatotoxicants
Hemolysis	Copper, garlic, onion, red maple, phenothiazine wormers, zinc
Hypercalcemia	Vitamin D_3, day-blooming jessamine, calcium supplements, calcipotriene
Hyperkalemia	Digitalis glycosides, oleander, nephrotoxicants (e.g., ethylene glycol, NSAIDs, grapes, raisins, calcium oxalate-containing plants, etc.).
Hyperosmolarity	Antifreeze, aspirin, ethanol, propylene glycol
Hypocalcemia	Antifreeze, oxalate poisoning, nephrotoxicants resulting in renal secondary hyperparathyroidism
Hypoproteinemia	Aflatoxins, chemotherapy, blood loss (e.g., secondary to anticoagulant rodenticides, DIC, NSAID-induced gastric ulceration, etc.)
Iron (serum) and TIBC	Iron toxicosis
Methemoglobin	Acetaminophen, copper, nitrites, chlorates, methylene blue, smoke inhalation, red maple
Urinary casts	Nephrotoxicants (e.g., aminoglycosides, NSAIDs, ethylene glycol, grapes, lilies, beta-blockers, ACE inhibitors, etc.), arsenic, cadmium, mercury, oak

TABLE 5.3. Necropsy specimen collection recommended for toxicology.
Brain ½ frozen, ½ formalin. *Leave midline in formalin for pathologist orientation.*
Ocular fluid (2–4 mL) chilled
Injection site (100 g) frozen
Stomach and intestinal contents (1 kg or as much as possible) frozen
Colon contents (1 kg) frozen
Liver (200 g) frozen
Kidney (200 g) frozen
Urine if present (100 mL or as much as possible) ½ chilled, ½ frozen

- Limitations to chemical analysis include the following.
  - Chemical tests should not be relied upon without supporting historical and/or clinical data.
  - Time course of the intoxication, changes since death, or limitations on testing methodology can render a chemical analysis less useful or ineffective for diagnostic confirmation.
  - Chemical tests for all possible poisons are rarely available.
  - Broad-spectrum screens using gas chromatography and/or high-performance liquid chromatography coupled with mass spectrometry provide more latitude for analysis but often are not quantitative and may be less sensitive than more focused assays.
  - More generalized tests that include ELISA or other immunological technology can be very sensitive but sometimes suffer from cross-reactions or low specificity.
  - Identify a laboratory in advance and be familiar with its reputation and performance prior to the time when rapid or critical testing is needed.
- Most laboratories welcome inquiries about appropriate sampling and test limitations.
- A good laboratory will inform you when a received sample is inadequate or the test requested is not part of their routine and approved offerings.
- For some toxicoses, chemical analysis may not be developed, or a toxic principle may be unknown, so reliance must be on clinical and pathological confirmation of your diagnosis.
- Depending on the circumstances of a particular case, detection of any amount of toxicant is sufficient to confirm exposure and/or intoxication. In other cases, quantification of a toxicant in a fluid or tissue sample is necessary to make a diagnosis of intoxication.

GETTING THE MOST FROM YOUR DIAGNOSTIC EFFORT

- The principles and approaches described here give your clients a combination of your best efforts, their best management and information, and the best value you can obtain from laboratory assistance. Not all acute or chronic poisonings become a positive diagnosis.

- In some cases, the poisoning suspect is actually something else that may never be identified.
- The approach outlined is widely accepted and provides a standard of diagnosis that should be supportable and acceptable in veterinary practice.

Abbreviations

See Appendix 1 for a complete list.

ACE = angiotensin-converting enzyme
NPN = nonprotein nitrogen
NSAIDs = nonsteroidal antiinflammatory drugs
SSRI = selective serotonin reuptake inhibitors

Suggested Reading

Lohmeyer C. Taking a toxicologic history. In: Poppenga RH, Gwaltney-Brant SM, eds. Small Animal Toxicology Essentials, Ames, IA: Wiley-Blackwell, 2011.

Puschner B, Brutlag AG. Approach to diagnosis for the toxicology case. In: Peterson ME, Talcott, eds. Small Animal Toxicology, 3rd edn. St Louis, MO: Elsevier, 2013; pp. 45–52.

Talcott PA. Effective use of a diagnostic laboratory. In: Peterson ME, Talcott, eds. Small Animal Toxicology, 3rd edn. St Louis, MO: Elsevier, 2013; pp. 125–132.

Authors: Gary D. Osweiler, DVM, PhD, DABVT; Robert H. Poppenga, DVM, PhD, DABVT
Consulting Editor: Robert H. Poppenga, DVM, PhD, DABVT

section II

Specific Toxins & Toxicants

Alcohols and Glycol Ethers

chapter 6

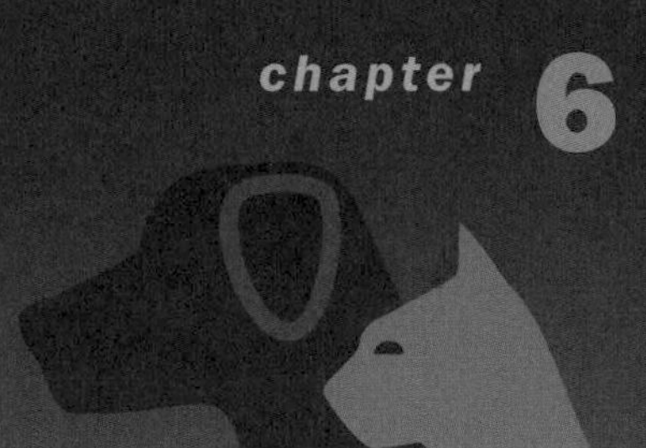

Alcohols

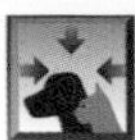

DEFINITION/OVERVIEW

- Alcohols are hydrocarbons with a hydroxyl (-OH) group.
- Methanol (wood alcohol; CH_3OH), ethanol (ethyl alcohol; CH_3CH_2OH), and isopropanol (rubbing alcohol; $(CH_3)_2CHOH$) are commonly encountered examples.
- Short carbon chain alcohols are commonly found in medicinal, cleaning, and automotive products and are also used as fuels. Methanol is found in certain automotive windshield washer fluids. Exposure can occur from consumption of these products. Ethanol exposure also occurs from the consumption of alcoholic beverages and raw bread dough.
- Ethanol has also been used in veterinary medicine to treat ethylene glycol poisoning in dogs and cats.
- Exposure to these alcohols most commonly results in vomiting, CNS depression, and ataxia. Management is predominantly directed at correction of dehydration and acid–base status.

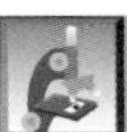

ETIOLOGY/PATHOPHYSIOLOGY

Poisonings arising from exposure to short chain alcohols are occasionally observed in veterinary medicine. Most veterinary cases will involve accidental ingestion of alcoholic beverages (ethanol), raw bread dough, fermented garbage, uncooked pizza dough, rotten apples (ethanol), automotive windshield washer fluids (methanol), or consumer products (ethanol, methanol, isopropanol). Household products that may contain these alcohols can be categorized into medicinal, cosmetic, personal hygiene, or cleaning products.

Consumer products with high ethanol content can include alcoholic beverages, certain mouthwashes (up to 27%), perfumes and colognes (>50%), and hand sanitizers (>60%). Consumer products with high methanol concentrations include model engine fuels (<75%), deicers (>30%), windshield washer fluids (>50%), and varnish and stain removers (>30%). Consumer products with high isopropanol concentrations include engine water removers

Blackwell's Five-Minute Veterinary Consult Clinical Companion: Small Animal Toxicology, Second Edition.
Lynn R. Hovda, Ahna G. Brutlag, Robert H. Poppenga, and Katherine L. Peterson.

Companion website: www.fiveminutevet.com/toxicology

(>50%), deicers (>20%), windshield-coating fluids (>50%), and certain sanitizers (>50%). Products containing >95% of these alcohols are also available.

The US Department of Health and Human Services maintains a searchable household products database that provides information about short chain alcohol concentrations in many household products. This database is available at: http://hpd.nlm.nih.gov/.

Mechanism of Action

The neurotoxic effects of these short chain alcohols are multifactorial. Short-term consumption depresses brain function by altering the balance between inhibitory and excitatory neurotransmission. For example, at some doses ethanol increases the function of the inhibitory neurotransmitter gamma-aminobutyric acid (GABA). These alcohols are also an irritant to mucous membranes and the eyes. The germicidal mechanism of action of alcohols involves denaturation of proteins and disruption of cell membranes.

Methanol is metabolized by hepatic alcohol dehydrogenase to formic acid via formaldehyde. Species with low levels of tetrahydrofolate (e.g., humans and other primates) have slower rates of formate metabolism, resulting in metabolic acidosis and blindness. Dogs and cats have higher rates of formate detoxification and do not develop these signs.

Pharmacokinetics – Absorption, Distribution, Metabolism, Excretion

- Short chain alcohols can be absorbed orally, by inhalation, or by dermal exposure, with oral exposure occurring most commonly.
- Oral absorption occurs rapidly. The highest blood levels are seen after oral dosing, with lower levels after inhalation and lowest levels after dermal application.
- These alcohols rapidly distribute throughout the body and cross the blood–brain barrier and the placenta. Ethanol, methanol, and isopropanol are initially metabolized by hepatic alcohol dehydrogenase to acetaldehyde, formaldehyde, and acetone, respectively. Acetaldehyde is subsequently metabolized to acetic acid, formaldehyde to formic acid, and acetone to acetic acid.
- Excretion of the parent alcohols occurs predominantly through the urine and exhalation. A fraction of the metabolites formed will be excreted in the urine.

Toxicity

Ethanol.

- The LD_{LO} intravenous route for ethanol in dogs is 1.6 mL/kg. The LD_{LO} oral is 5–8 mL/kg.
- The oral LD_{50} of ethanol in rats is 9 mL/kg.

Methanol.

- The oral LD_{50} for methanol in dogs is reported to be 4–8 mL/kg.
- Toxic doses for methanol in canines and felines are approximately the same as for ethanol.

Isopropanol.

- The oral LD_{50} for isopropanol in dogs is reported to be approximately 2 mL/kg of a 70% isopropanol solution (rubbing alcohol).
- In general, isopropanol is considered to be twice as potent a CNS depressant as ethanol.

Systems Affected

- Nervous – CNS depression, ataxia, lethargy, sedation.
- Gastrointestinal – nausea, vomiting.
- Endocrine/metabolic – metabolic acidosis, hypothermia.

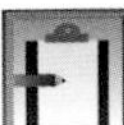

SIGNALMENT/HISTORY

- Canines are more commonly reported to ingest alcoholic products than felines.
- Younger animals tend to chew and drink articles not intended for consumption.

Risk Factors

- A seasonal effect is seen with alcohol toxicosis. Ethanol toxicosis often occurs during holiday seasons (e.g., Christmas, Easter), when pet owners may be baking desserts more frequently. Methanol toxicosis often occurs during the spring and summer, when windshield wiper fluid is more readily available in the garage.

Historical Findings

- Ingestion witnessed by the owner; chewed bottle found by the owner.
- Clinical signs including ataxia, CNS depression, and lethargy are often noted by the pet owner

Location and Circumstances of Poisoning

- Ethanol toxicity often occurs in the kitchen, where baked goods are being made.
- Dogs housed in the garage may be at higher risk for ingestion.
- Chewed bottles may be found in the garage or outdoor environment.

CLINICAL FEATURES

- CNS depression, ataxia, lethargy, and sedation.
- Hypothermia.
- Metabolic acidosis.
- Clinical signs (ataxia and CNS depression) would be expected rapidly (within an hour) if the animal ingested a toxic dose.
- Excessive gas accumulation in the gut, flatulence, bloating, abdominal pain, vomiting, retching, and nausea can occur in animals ingesting fermented bread dough. The smell of ethanol may be obvious on the pet's breath.

- Isopropanol intoxications may be more prolonged compared to ethanol and methanol intoxications because the acetone metabolite is also a CNS depressant.

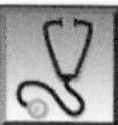

DIFFERENTIAL DIAGNOSIS

- Other toxicants with sedative and/or CNS depressant effects include the following.
    - 2-butoxyethanol
    - Amitraz
    - Barbiturates
    - Benzodiazepines
    - Ethylene glycol
    - Macrolide antiparasitics
    - Marijuana
    - Other volatile alcohols
- Primary neurological disease (e.g., inflammatory, infectious, infiltrative, etc.).
- Primary metabolic disease (e.g., hypoglycemia, hepatic encephalopathy).
- Hypoglycemia (e.g., juvenile hypoglycemia, xylitol toxicosis, hypoadrenocorticism, insulinoma, hepatic tumor, hunting dog hypoglycemia).

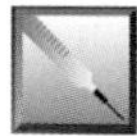

DIAGNOSTICS

Clinical Laboratory

- A PCV/TS, blood glucose, and venous blood gas should be performed to evaluate severity of dehydration and electrolyte and acid–base status.
- In isopropanol toxicosis, an osmole gap may develop.
- Many laboratories are capable of determining ethanol, methanol, or isopropanol levels in blood although ethanol determination is most commonly available as a routine test.
- Blood ethanol concentrations of 87–109 mmol/L (400–500 mg/dL) and above are considered severe and potentially life-threatening in people and are likely similar in companion animals.

Pathological Findings

- There are no specific gross or histological lesions observed in alcohol-poisoned companion animals.

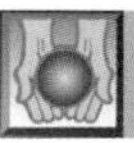

THERAPEUTICS

Detoxification

- Alcohols in general are absorbed very quickly from the gastrointestinal tract so the use of emetics is rarely effective. The administration of medications to cause emesis is generally not recommended because of the rapid onset of CNS depression and risk of aspiration.

- If a large amount of gastric contents is present in a symptomatic patient, gastric lavage may need to be performed under sedation and with an inflated endotracheal tube to prevent aspiration.
- Ethanol and other short chain alcohols are poorly adsorbed by activated charcoal, which is therefore not recommended.
- If dermal exposure to volatile alcohols has occurred, rinse the affected area with a mild detergent shampoo and water.
- Forced diuresis is generally not effective.
- Hemodialysis may be an effective means of enhancing elimination of ethanol from the body and can therefore be beneficial in cases expected to be potentially life threatening or associated with high morbidity.

Appropriate Health Care

- Hospitalization may be required to manage severe CNS depression, metabolic acidosis, and respiratory depression.
- If respiratory function is compromised, a cuffed endotracheal tube should be placed and ventilation supported mechanically as required.
- Maintaining normal body temperature is important.
- Alcohol toxicosis can result in severe CNS depression/coma, and appropriate nursing care is imperative. Patients should be kept in a padded cage and should be turned every 6 hours to prevent atelectasis.

Antidotes

- There are no known antidotes for ethanol or isopropanol. Antidotes used for methanol (e.g., ethanol or fomepizole) toxicosis in humans are not used with dogs and cats since blindness due to formic acid formation has not been reported in these species.

Drugs of Choice

- Therapy should include careful rehydration with dextrose solution to correct hypoglycemia.
- A balanced, isotonic crystalloid IV fluid can be used in symptomatic patients to aid in correction of dehydration.
- In the presence of a severe metabolic acidosis (e.g., pH <7.0, BE ≤ 15 mmHg, HCO_3 <11 mmHg), the judicious use of sodium bicarbonate can be considered.

Precautions/Interactions

- If other substances have been co-ingested, initiate specific treatment for those substances, if available.

Nursing Care

- Provide respiratory support and mechanical ventilation if needed.
- Monitor temperature, heart rate, and respiratory rate.

- Monitor blood pressure and blood glucose frequently and treat appropriately.
- Ophthalmic lubrication may be necessary every 6 hours. Keeping the patient clean and dry is imperative.

Follow-up

- Follow-up is generally unnecessary, as patients are clinically normal once signs resolve.

Activity

- Patients should be restricted from activity until clinical signs resolve, as ataxia and CNS depression will be apparent. Once clinical signs resolve, no exercise restriction is necessary.

Prevention

- Prevent access of pets to obvious or potential sources of alcohol.

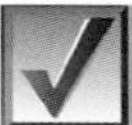

COMMENTS

Client Education

- Prevention is critical. Advise clients that alcohol-containing products are potentially dangerous for their pets. Educate clients about common sources of alcohol available in the home (e.g., kitchen).
- Early treatment is also important. Clients should be taught to contact their veterinarian if an exposure has occurred or an animal is displaying unusual clinical signs.

Patient Monitoring

- Acid–base monitoring is recommended in symptomatic animals.
- Blood glucose concentrations should be monitored frequently.

Expected Course and Prognosis

- Most cases involving mild signs usually resolve with close monitoring and supportive care within a 24-hour period.
- No long-term effects are expected unless brain injury secondary to prolonged respiratory depression and hypoxia has occurred.
- The prognosis is fair to guarded in cases involving metabolic acidosis, severe CNS or respiratory system depression, or aspiration pneumonia.

Abbreviations

See Appendix 1 for a complete list.

Suggested Reading

Keno LA, Langston CE. Treatment of accidental ethanol intoxication with hemodialysis in a dog. J Vet Emerg Crit Care 2011; 21(4):363–368.

Means C. Bread dough toxicosis in dogs. J Vet Emerg Crit Care 2003; 13(1):39–41.

Rayar P, Ratnapalan S. Pediatric ingestions of house hold products containing ethanol: a review. Clin Pediatr (Phila) 2013; 52(3):203–209.

Valentine WM. Short-chain alcohols. Vet Clin North Am Small Anim Pract 1990; 20(2):515–523.

Author: David C. Dorman, DVM, PhD, DABVT, DABT
Consulting Editor: Robert H. Poppenga, DVM, PhD, DABVT

Ethylene Glycol and Diethylene Glycol

DEFINITION/OVERVIEW

- Ethylene glycol (EG) is often used in the manufacture of synthetic fibers and plastic bottles. Most commonly, exposure occurs in animals from ingestion of antifreeze and other automotive chemicals/fluids.
- Diethylene glycol (DEG) can be found in lotions, skin creams, and deodorants as well as in brake fluid, lubricants, wallpaper strippers, and heating/cooking fuel.
- EG intoxication can be successfully treated with early intervention despite a commonly grave prognosis if recognized late in the clinical course of the intoxication.
- Clinical signs of EG intoxication include CNS depression, ataxia, knuckling, nausea, vomiting, polyuria/polydipsia, and hypothermia, depending on the dose and time from ingestion.
- Ethanol or fomepizole treatments should be used as soon as the intoxication is suspected or proven.
- Fomepizole can be used in both dogs and cats with EG intoxication. Cats, however, require a much higher dosage.
- Hemodialysis is highly effective at removing EG and its more toxic metabolites from the patient. Like other treatments, it is best used as early as possible following exposure.
- DEG intoxication, although rare, has similar signs to EG intoxication but without oxalate crystalluria. Both reportedly have a sweet taste which may promote significant ingestion in some animals.

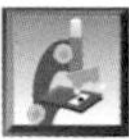

ETIOLOGY/PATHOPHYSIOLOGY

Mechanism of Action

- EG is metabolized by alcohol dehydrogenase into many toxic metabolites. Oxalic acid is of particular note for its high toxicity. Oxalic acid binds calcium to form calcium oxalate crystals which are found in the urine and deposited in the kidneys, causing acute kidney injury (AKI) and failure. Signs of AKI include anorexia, vomiting, lethargy, polyuria with

Blackwell's Five-Minute Veterinary Consult Clinical Companion: Small Animal Toxicology, Second Edition.
Lynn R. Hovda, Ahna G. Brutlag, Robert H. Poppenga, and Katherine L. Peterson.

Companion website: www.fiveminutevet.com/toxicology

potentially rapid progression to oliguria/anuria, and polydipsia. Hypocalcemia is often found in patients with EG intoxication. Toxic metabolites (glycoaldehyde, glyoxylic acid, oxalic acid, and especially glycolic acid) contribute to a severe metabolic acidosis and a large osmolar gap.

- DEG is metabolized through an alternative pathway in the liver to a weak acid that is ultimately filtered by the kidney and does not induce calcium oxalate crystalluria. However, clinical signs can be similar to EG intoxication.

Pharmacokinetics – Absorption, Distribution, Metabolism, Excretion

- EG is rapidly absorbed from the gastrointestinal tract with quick distribution to the blood and tissues. The plasma half-life is 3 hours. Some EG is excreted unchanged in the urine. However, most is metabolized by alcohol dehydrogenase to glycoaldehyde and organic acids.
- DEG has very quick absorption and metabolism, often with complete excretion in 36 hours. Diglycolic acid (DGA) is the presumed nephrotoxic metabolite of DEG.

Toxicity

- A minimum lethal dose for undiluted EG is 6.6 mL/kg in dogs and 1.5 mL/kg for cats. Toxicity of DEG for dogs and cats is not well defined. In adult humans, a mean estimated fatal dose is approximately 1 mL/kg of pure DEG.

Systems Affected

- Gastrointestinal – direct irritation causes vomiting in both dogs and cats.
- Nervous – mental dullness and ataxia can be related to hyperosmolality and cerebral edema.
- Metabolic – metabolic acidosis from the organic acid metabolites is common and severe.
- Renal – with EG, renal failure occurs due to renal epithelial damage from oxalate crystalluria. DGA is believed to be accumulated by renal proximal tubular cells, resulting in cellular dysfunction and cell necrosis.

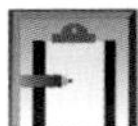

SIGNALMENT/HISTORY

- Clinical signs are dependent upon the species, the amount of food in the stomach (slower absorption if food present), and the amount ingested. Cats are more sensitive to intoxication but are intoxicated less often, likely due to their tendency to be more discriminating than dogs when ingesting products containing EG or DEG.

Risk Factors

- None known.

Historical Findings

- For EG, the most common exposure is from automobile radiator leakage (antifreeze) or windshield deicing agents. However, EG is found in many products in the home or garage (paint solvent, photographic developing solutions, hydraulic brake fluid, motor oil, ink, wood stains).

Location and Circumstances of Poisoning

- Due to the sources of EG and DEG, exposure is often within the home when the animal has access to areas where there are automobiles, workshops, or storage of leaking containers of chemicals.
- Malicious poisoning occurs.

Interactions with Drugs, Nutrients, or Environment

- None known.

CLINICAL FEATURES

- Acute signs (first 30 minutes to 12 hours) are mostly related to gastric irritation (nausea, vomiting) and plasma hyperosmolality (mental dullness, ataxia). After this time, the patient often appears to have recovered until the next phase of clinical signs appears.
- For EG, after 12–24 hours in cats and 36–72 hours in dogs, the signs are consistent with acute oliguric renal failure. These signs are caused by the toxic metabolites binding calcium to form oxalate nephrolithiasis that results in renal tubular epithelial damage and rapidly progressive renal failure.
- Anuric renal failure develops by 72–96 hours post ingestion.
- Painful enlarged kidneys are often found on physical examination.

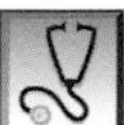

DIFFERENTIAL DIAGNOSIS

- Vomiting – dietary indiscretion, foreign body/obstruction, pancreatitis.
- Ataxia – ethanol, methanol, propylene glycol, xylitol, barbiturate, ivermectin, marijuana.
- High anion gap metabolic acidosis – diabetic ketoacidosis, severe lactic acidosis, other forms of renal failure and uremia.
- Acute renal failure – NSAIDs, leptospirosis, aminoglycoside antibiotics, oxalate-containing plants (lily ingestion in cats), grapes/raisins (dogs), and acute on chronic renal failure.

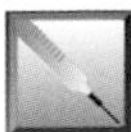

DIAGNOSTICS

- Blood gas – to identify high anion gap metabolic acidosis.

- Serum biochemistry – to quantitate azotemia and electrolyte (particularly calcium) derangements. Occasionally, hyperphosphatemia may be found due to presence of a phosphate rust inhibitor in some commercial antifreeze products.
- Urinalysis – to identify calcium monohydrate or dihydrate oxalate crystalluria as well as measure urine specific gravity (often isosthenuric by 3 hours post ingestion).
- Measured osmolality – to compare to calculated osmolality. High osmolar gaps are commonly found with EG intoxication.
- Serum EG concentration – for confirmation of the presence of the EG or its metabolites. Point-of-care tests for EG are available that provide semi-quantitative glycol concentrations; however, false positives can occur if the patient is treated with drugs with a propylene glycol vehicle (methocarbamol, diazepam, some activated charcoal products). Point-of-care tests can be relatively insensitive (do not detect serum EG concentrations <50 mg/dL). Therefore, false-negative results can occur in some cats or in animals presenting several hours after exposure.
- Wood's lamp examination of vomitus or urine – due to the presence of fluorescent dyes placed in some antifreeze products.
- Abdominal ultrasonography – can aid in identification of hyperechoic kidneys late in the intoxication once calcium oxalate crystals have deposited to a significant level in renal tubules.

Pathological Findings

- Histopathology – the kidneys are the primary target for postmortem diagnosis of EG intoxication and show proximal tubular degeneration and necrosis with intraluminal calcium oxalate crystal deposits. Calcium oxalate crystals may also be found in a wide array of other tissues. DEG causes proximal tubular cell necrosis without crystalluria.

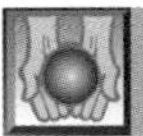

THERAPEUTICS

The goal of therapy is to inhibit absorption, to remove the parent compound and toxic metabolites, and to correct the physiological derangements of AKI. The rapid systemic absorption of EG and DEG following ingestion often precludes effective gastrointestinal decontamination.

Inhibit metabolism

Choose one of the following initial treatments.

Dogs

- Fomepizole: 20 mg/kg IV followed q 12 hours by 15 mg/kg IV for two doses, then 5 mg/kg IV for one dose.
- Ethanol IV CRI: 1.3 mL of 30% ethanol/kg IV bolus followed by 0.42 mL/kg/hour for 48 hours.
- Ethanol IV boluses: 5.5 mL 20% ethanol/kg IV q 4 hours for five treatments, then q 6 hours for four treatments.

Cats

- Fomepizole: 125 mg/kg IV followed q 12 hours by 31.25 mg/kg IV for three doses.
- Ethanol IV CRI: 1.3 mL of 30% ethanol/kg IV bolus followed by 0.42 mL/kg/hour for 48 hours (note: same as dogs above).
- Ethanol IV boluses: 5 mL 20% ethanol/kg IV q 6 hours for five treatments, then q 8 hours for four treatments.

Either drug can be used and they are most effective when used early. The side effects of ethanol require that the patient be hospitalized and monitored closely due to the potential for aspiration pneumonia from recumbency. Fomepizole is often preferred since it does not require such intensive nursing care. However, fomepizole is more expensive than ethanol.

Correct acid–base and electrolyte derangements:

For severe hypocalcemia (*total* less than 7 mOsm/L, *ionized* less than 0.7 mM/L or if symptomatic – muscle twitching/fasciculations, weakness) while monitoring heart rate, EKG, and respiratory rate during treatment.

- Dogs: calcium gluconate 10% 5–15 mg/kg (0.5–1.5 mL/kg) IV over 20 minutes to effect.
- Cats: calcium gluconate 10% 10–15 mg/kg (1.0–1.5 mL/kg) IV over 20 minutes to effect.

For severe metabolic acidosis (pH <7.0, bicarbonate <10 mEq/L) for both dogs and cats.

- Bicarbonate replacement (mEq required = body weight (kg) × base deficit × 0.3).
- Administer 1/3–1/2 of the calculated replacement IV over 30 minutes.
- Recheck blood gas and consider another infusion if pH remains below 7.2 or bicarbonate <12 mEq/L.

Correct fluid imbalances

- Correct dehydration – calculate isotonic fluid replacement and administer this amount IV over 4–6 hours.
- Provide maintenance fluids – calculate hourly isotonic fluid rate and administer at this rate hourly as long as urine output continues.
- Administer estimated abnormal ongoing losses – provide this amount extra each hour as long as polyuria, vomiting, diarrhea, or other fluid losses continue. Reevaluate every 4 hours.

Remove parent compound and metabolites

- In areas near specialty centers skilled at hemodialysis and extracorporeal blood purification, early referral is essential for best patient outcomes only after initial steps directed at the inhibition of EG metabolism are completed by the primary care provider.

Provide supportive care for other symptoms commonly associated with AKI

- Antiemetics, gastrointestinal protectants, and phosphate binders can be used with the above treatments at the clinician's discretion.

Detoxification

- Activated charcoal is not effective for the adsorption of EG. Hemodialysis or peritoneal dialysis are less commonly available but effective options.

Appropriate Health Care

- Treatment with ethanol renders the patient sedate and obtunded whereas fomepizole does not have these side effects. The complete costs for each treatment and hospitalization need to be considered. This is neither a risk-free nor inexpensive intoxication to treat.

Antidotes

- Fomepizole and ethanol act indirectly as antidotes. They do not directly counteract the intoxication but are competitive inhibitors that interrupt metabolism of EG and DEG and thus allow time for urinary excretion of unchanged parent compound.

Precautions/Interactions

- Treatment with ethanol alters the patient's mentation and provides temporary immobilization and sedation. As such, the patient is at higher risk for aspiration pneumonia but is not necessarily sedated sufficiently to allow endotracheal intubation.

Alternative Drugs

- There are no alternative drugs for the treatment of EG and DEG intoxication.

Nursing Care

- Skilled nursing care for the critically ill and recumbent patient must be employed while the patient is treated with ethanol due to the higher risk of aspiration.

Diet

- Food and water should be withheld in the recumbent patient.

COMMENTS

Patient Monitoring

- Recumbent patients need to have detailed and frequent monitoring and treatments with thoughtful and attentive veterinary evaluations over several days.

Prevention/Avoidance

- Removal of the offending substances from the reach of animals is essential to prevent reexposure. Use propylene glycol-based antifreeze products instead of EG-based products.

Possible Complications

- Aspiration pneumonia can be a sequela.
- Hemorrhage is possible due to anticoagulation needed for hemodialysis.
- Prevention of a septic abdomen requires diligent sterile technique and hygiene in patients receiving peritoneal dialysis.

Expected Course and Prognosis

- Prognosis depends mainly on the expediency of appropriate treatment as well as amount ingested and species. Chronic renal impairment can occur even for treated EG-intoxicated patients. A high chance exists that the renal dysfunction will be severe and permanent.
- The sequelae of DEG intoxication are currently unknown.

Abbreviations

See Appendix 1 for a complete list.

DEG = diethylene glycol
DGA = diglycolic acid
AKI = acute kidney injury

See Also

See Appendix 1 for complete list.

Alcohols
Propylene Glycol

Suggested Reading

Bischoff K, Mukai M. Diethylene glycol. In: Peterson M, Talcott P, eds. Small Animal Toxicology, 3rd edn. St Louis, MO: Elsevier, 2013; pp. 543–546.

Connally HE, Thrall MA, Forney SD, et al. Safety and efficacy of 4-methylpyrazole as treatment for suspected or confirmed EG intoxication in dogs: 107 cases (1983-1995). J Am Vet Med Assoc 1996; 209:1880–1883.

Connally HE, Thrall MA, Hamar DW. Safety and efficacy of high-dose fomepazole compared with ethanol as therapy for EG intoxication in cats. J Vet Emerg Crit Care 2010; 20(2):191–206.

Lewis DH, Goggs RA. Possible DEG toxicity in a dog. Vet Rec 2009; 164:127.

Thrall MA, Connally HE, Grauer GF, Hamar DW. Ethylene glycol. In: Peterson M, Talcott P, eds. Small Animal Toxicology, 3rd edn. St Louis, MO: Elsevier, 2013; pp. 551–567.

Authors: Karl E. Jandrey, DVM, MAS, DACVECC; Kate S. Farrell, DVM
Consulting Editor: Robert H. Poppenga, DVM, PhD, DABVT

chapter 8

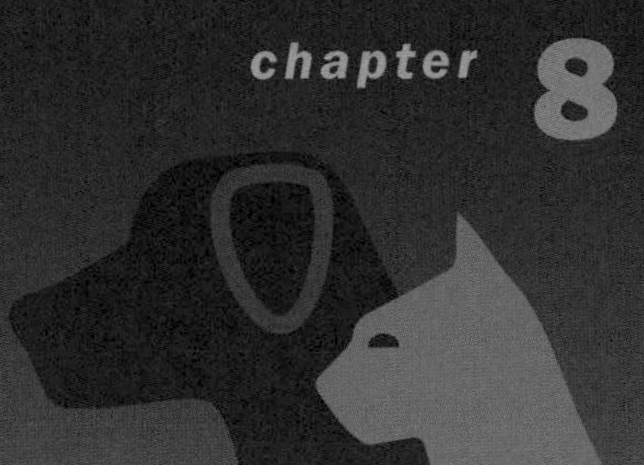

Propylene Glycol

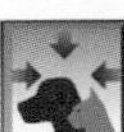

DEFINITION/OVERVIEW

- Propylene glycol (propane-1,2-diol) is an organic compound with the chemical formula $C_3H_8O_2(CH_3CHOHCH_2OH)$.
- It is miscible with water and is used as a carrier for hydrophobic compounds that are relatively insoluble in water.
- It is a colorless, odorless liquid with a wide range of consumer, pharmaceutical, food, and industrial uses.
- Propylene glycol is also used in certain brands of automotive antifreeze. It does not produce the same syndrome as ethylene glycol-based antifreeze products.
- It has been used in veterinary medicine as a source of energy for food-producing animals (cattle, sheep, goats, pigs, poultry).
- Acute clinical effects of oral exposure include ataxia and CNS depression with lactic acidosis.
- For cats, exposure can result in Heinz body anemia.

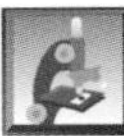

ETIOLOGY/PATHOPHYSIOLOGY

- Propylene glycol has been classified by the US Food and Drug Administration (FDA) as generally regarded as safe (GRAS) and is approved by the agency for use as an anticaking agent, antioxidant, dough strengthener, emulsifier, flavor agent, formulation aid, humectant, processing aid, stabilizer, and thickener, among other uses. Examples of maximum levels, as served, allowed by the US FDA include 5% for alcoholic beverages, 24% for confections and frostings, and 2.5% for frozen dairy products.
- Propylene glycol is used as a vehicle for certain pharmaceutical preparations. Some formulations intended for IV use contain >30% propylene glycol.
- Poisoning arising from exposure to propylene glycol is occasionally observed in veterinary medicine. Most veterinary cases will involve accidental ingestion of concentrated forms of propylene glycol.
- Propylene glycol poisoning in cats has also been associated with its use in moist cat food preparations. The use of propylene glycol in cat food is contraindicated.

Blackwell's Five-Minute Veterinary Consult Clinical Companion: Small Animal Toxicology, Second Edition.
Lynn R. Hovda, Ahna G. Brutlag, Robert H. Poppenga, and Katherine L. Peterson.

Companion website: www.fiveminutevet.com/toxicology

- Household products that may contain propylene glycol can be categorized into medicinal, cosmetic, personal hygiene, or cleaning products.
- Consumer products with high propylene glycol content can include certain soaps (14–20%), leather conditioners (10–30%), stain removers (10–40%), tire sealants (45–50%), and antifreezes (>90%). The US Department of Health and Human Services maintains a searchable household products database that provides information about propylene glycol concentrations in many household products: http://hpd.nlm.nih.gov/.

Mechanism of Action

- The toxicity of propylene glycol is mainly due to the parent compound and not to its metabolites.
- Propylene glycol has an irritant effect on direct contact with eyes, mucous membranes, and possibly after prolonged contact with skin.
- Propylene glycol causes CNS depression similar to that caused by ethanol but it is only one-third as potent. The mode of action of propylene glycol neurotoxicity is poorly understood.
- Propylene glycol is metabolized to l- and d-lactic acid, which results in acidosis.

Pharmacokinetics – Absorption, Distribution, Metabolism, Excretion

- Little is known about the pharmacokinetics of propylene glycol in dogs and cats. It is expected that data derived in people can apply to these species.
- Propylene glycol is rapidly absorbed from the gastrointestinal tract of humans with plasma maximum concentrations observed within 1 hour of ingestion.
- The main metabolic pathway of propylene glycol involves oxidation by alcohol dehydrogenase to form lactaldehyde, and then to lactate by aldehyde dehydrogenase. This step can be saturated following the ingestion of propylene glycol, resulting in delayed metabolism and elimination of the parent compound.
- The lactate formed from metabolism of propylene glycol enters into normal endogenous metabolic biochemical cycles, where it is further metabolized to pyruvate, carbon dioxide, and water. The d-lactate isomer has a greater tendency to accumulate and result in an anion gap.
- In adult humans, approximately 45% of the administered dose of propylene glycol is eliminated through the kidney. The remaining 55% is metabolized through hepatic alcohol dehydrogenase. Approximately 30% is excreted via the kidneys as a glucuronide conjugate.
- The elimination half-life of propylene glycol is estimated to be approximately 2–5 hours in most species.

Toxicity

- The acute oral LD_{50} for propylene glycol in rats is approximately 20 g/kg BW/kg.
- The acute oral LD_{50} for propylene glycol in dogs is approximately 22 g/kg BW/kg. Other authors report the acute LD_{50} for dogs to be as low as 9 mL/kg BW.
- Cats appear to be more sensitive and develop an anion gap with d-lactic acidosis seen at oral doses of 1600 mg/kg BW for 35 days.

- Signs of acute toxicosis have been reported in a dog with a propylene glycol blood concentration of 1100 mg/dL.

Systems Affected

- Nervous – CNS depression, ataxia.
- Gastrointestinal – nausea, vomiting.
- Hematological – Heinz body anemia (cat).
- Endocrine/metabolic – metabolic acidosis, hypothermia.
- Respiratory – increased respiratory rate and effort secondary to metabolic acidosis.

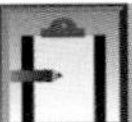

SIGNALMENT/HISTORY

- Canines are more commonly reported to ingest propylene glycol-based products than felines.
- Younger animals tend to chew and drink articles not intended for their consumption.

Risk Factors

- Prolonged elimination half-lives of 10.8–30.5 hours have been reported in preterm human neonates, suggesting that younger animals are likely at greater risk.
- Some metabolites undergo glucuronidation and in cats this is quite limited, thus reducing the effective urinary excretion of these metabolites through the kidney. This results in cats being particularly sensitive to hematological changes, manifesting as Heinz body formation and a reduced lifespan of red blood cells.
- Diabetes mellitus and hyperthyroidism are reported to increase susceptibility to Heinz body anemia, potentially worsening the severity of propylene glycol toxicosis.

Historical Findings

- Ingestion witnessed by the owner; chewed containers found by the pet owner.
- Clinical signs including ataxia, CNS depression, and lethargy are often noted by the pet owner.

Location and Circumstances of Poisoning

- Animals housed in the garage may be at higher risk for ingestion of propylene glycol-based products.
- Iatrogenic poisonings have been suspected following repeated use of drug formulations containing propylene glycol.

CLINICAL FEATURES

- Although propylene glycol is generally regarded as safe, toxicity may involve bradycardia, CNS depression, ataxia, increased anion gap, lactic acidosis, hepatic dysfunction, or kidney injury.

- Cats have been known to also develop Heinz body formation with or without anemia.
- Rarely seen effects include seizures or coma.
- Hypotension and/or cardiovascular collapse can occur.
- Polyuria and polydipsia may also occur.

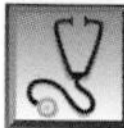

DIFFERENTIAL DIAGNOSIS

- Other toxicants with sedative and/or CNS depressant effects.
- Other agents that produce Heinz body formation with or without anemia in cats (e.g., onion, propofol, acetaminophen, benzocaine products, phenols, methylene blue, d-L methionine, vitamin K_3, naphthalene, zinc, and copper.
- Other toxicants that produce metabolic acidosis, including ethylene glycol.
- Primary neurological or metabolic diseases.

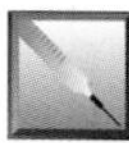

DIAGNOSTICS

Clinical Laboratory

- A PCV/TS, blood glucose, urinalysis, and venous blood gas should be performed to evaluate severity of electrolyte and acid–base status and to rule out other diseases.
- Acute high-dose exposure might increase d-lactic acidemia.
- Heinz body formation in cats can be observed on a peripheral blood smear. Some cats develop anemia with decreased RBC count, increased reticulocyte count, and elevated mean corpuscular hemoglobin concentration.
- Some laboratories are capable of determining propylene glycol levels in gastric contents or blood.

Pathological Findings

- There are no specific acute gross or histological lesions observed in propylene glycol-poisoned companion animals.
- Heinz body formation may be observed in cats.

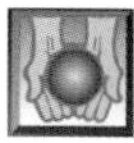

THERAPEUTICS

Detoxification

- Propylene glycol is absorbed relatively quickly from the gastrointestinal tract. Thus the use of emetics may have limited effectiveness.
- If a large amount of gastric contents is present in a symptomatic patient, gastric lavage may need to be performed under sedation and with an inflated endotracheal tube to prevent aspiration.

- Propylene glycol is likely poorly adsorbed by activated charcoal. Therefore activated charcoal and cathartics are rarely recommended.
- If dermal exposure has occurred, rinse the affected area with a mild detergent shampoo and water.
- Forced diuresis is generally not effective.
- Hemodialysis may be an effective means of enhancing elimination of propylene glycol from the body and can therefore be beneficial in cases expected to be potentially life threatening or associated with high morbidity.

Appropriate Health Care

- Hospitalization may be required to manage severe CNS depression, metabolic acidosis, and respiratory depression.
- If respiratory function is compromised, a cuffed endotracheal tube should be placed and ventilation supported mechanically as required.
- Maintaining normal body temperature is important.
- Propylene glycol toxicosis can result in severe CNS depression/coma and appropriate nursing care is imperative. Patients should be kept in a padded cage and should be turned every 6 hours to prevent atelectasis.

Antidotes

- There are no known antidotes for propylene glycol toxicosis. In general, the use of ethanol and other alcohol dehydrogenase inhibitors is not required.

Drugs of Choice

- Therapy should include careful rehydration with dextrose solution to correct hypoglycemia.
- A balanced, isotonic crystalloid IV fluid can be used in symptomatic patients to aid in correction of dehydration.
- In the presence of a severe metabolic acidosis (e.g., pH <7.0, BE ≤15 mmHg, HCO_3 <11 mmHg), the judicious use of sodium bicarbonate can be considered.
- Ascorbic acid can be used in cats as an antioxidant. However, research with cats indicates that common antioxidants (e.g., N-acetylcysteine, d-l alpha-tocopherol, ascorbic acid) are not effective in reducing the hematological effects of propylene glycol.

Precautions/Interactions

- If other substances have been co-ingested (or injected in the case of pharmaceutical agents), initiate specific treatment for those substances, if available.

Nursing Care

- Provide respiratory support and mechanical ventilation if needed.
- Monitor temperature, heart rate, and respiratory rate.

- Monitor blood pressure and blood glucose frequently and treat appropriately.
- Ophthalmic lubrication may be necessary every 6 hours.
- Keep the patient clean and dry.

Follow-up

- Follow-up is generally unnecessary, as patients are clinically normal once signs resolve.

Activity

- Patients should be restricted from activity until clinical signs resolve, as ataxia and CNS depression will be apparent. Once clinical signs resolve, no exercise restriction is necessary.

Prevention

- Prevent access of pets to obvious or potential sources of propylene glycol.
- Do not use propylene glycol as a food additive in cats.

COMMENTS

Client Education

- Prevention is critical. Advise clients that propylene glycol-containing products are potentially dangerous for their pets. Educate clients about common sources of propylene glycol available in the home (e.g., certain automotive antifreezes).
- Early treatment is also important. Clients should be taught to contact their veterinarian if an exposure has occurred or an animal is displaying unusual clinical signs.

Patient Monitoring

- Acid–base monitoring is recommended in symptomatic animals.
- Blood glucose concentrations should be monitored frequently.

Expected Course and Prognosis

- Most exposures are not expected to result in clinical signs.
- Most cases involving mild signs usually resolve with close monitoring and supportive care within a 24-hour period.
- No long-term effects are expected unless brain injury secondary to prolonged respiratory depression and hypoxia has occurred.
- The prognosis can be good even in cases involving metabolic acidosis and moderate CNS depression.
- Monitor RBC morphology, which should return to normal 6–8 weeks post exposure (cats).

Abbreviations

See Appendix 1 for a complete list.

GRAS = generally regarded as safe

Suggested Reading

Bauer MC, Weiss DJ, Perman V. Hematologic alterations in adult cats fed 6% or 12% propylene glycol. Am J Vet Res 1992; 53(1):69–72.

Bischoff K. Propylene glycol. In: Peterson ME, Talcott PA, eds. Small Animal Toxicology. St Louis, MO: Elsevier, 2006; pp. 996–1001.

Claus MA, Jandrey KE, Poppenga RH. Propylene glycol intoxication in a dog. J Vet Emerg Crit Care 2011; 21:679–683.

Fowles JR, Banton MI, Pottenger LH. A toxicological review of the propylene glycols. Crit Rev Toxicol 2013; 43(4):363–390.

Author: David C. Dorman, DVM, PhD, DABVT, DABT
Consulting Editor: Robert H. Poppenga, DVM, PhD, DABVT

Construction and Industrial Materials

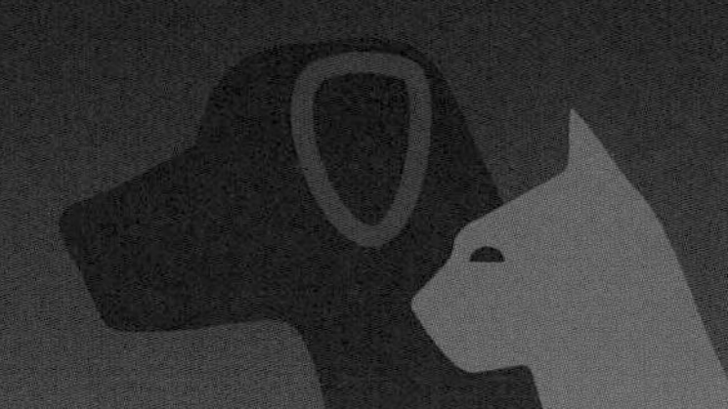

chapter 9

Glues and Adhesives

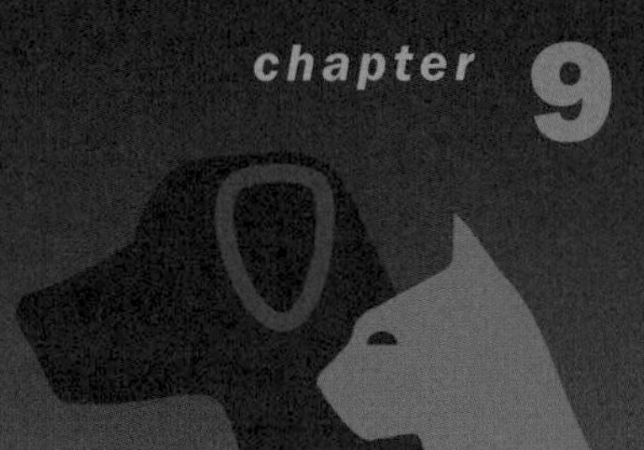

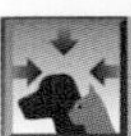

DEFINITION/OVERVIEW

- Cyanoacrylate glues or adhesives, also called instant glues, have uses in the home as well as in the medical field as tissue adhesives. Common brand names include Super Glue and Krazy Glue.
- Cyanoacrylate glue dermal or GI exposure results in local tissue adhesions, skin irritation, and GI irritation. Adhesions and gastroenteritis are usually mild, self-limiting, and easily treated.
- Diisocyanate glues include wood glue, construction glue, and high-strength glues. Gorilla Glue is a common brand name.
- Diisocyanate glue ingestion results in GI irritation and foreign body obstruction due to glue expansion, necessitating surgical intervention. Inhalation may cause airway irritation.
- Polyvinyl acetate (PVA or PVAc) glues or adhesives are typically rubbery, water-soluble glues used on paper, for crafts, and children's activities. Elmer's glue is a common brand name. Ingestions may cause minor gastroenteritis.
- Glue traps, used to trap insects and rodents, do not typically contain insecticides or rodenticides but may contain small amounts of eugenol and do not pose a toxicity concern.

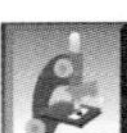

ETIOLOGY/PATHOPHYSIOLOGY

Mechanism of Action

- On contact with the skin or mucous membranes, cyanoacrylate hardens and adheres to surfaces.
- Diisocyanate expands significantly in the moist environment of the GI tract. Inhalation causes irritation to the lungs.

Pharmacokinetics/Absorption

- No significant systemic absorption occurs with the glues described in the Definition/Overview section.

Blackwell's Five-Minute Veterinary Consult Clinical Companion: Small Animal Toxicology, Second Edition.
Lynn R. Hovda, Ahna G. Brutlag, Robert H. Poppenga, and Katherine L. Peterson.

Companion website: www.fiveminutevet.com/toxicology

Toxicity

- Ingestion of glues described in the Definition/Overview section is typically considered a nontoxic ingestion.
- Small amounts of ingested diisocyanate (as little as 0.5 oz) can result in foreign body obstruction.

Systems Affected

- Cyanoacrylate
    - Gastrointestinal: gastroenteritis, oral adhesions.
    - Skin: dermal irritation, adhesions.
    - Respiratory: inhalation irritation, upper airway obstruction (rare).
    - Ophthalmic: corneal irritation, eyelid adhesions.
- Diisocyanate
    - Gastrointestinal: gastroenteritis, foreign body obstruction (common).
    - Skin: dermal irritation, adhesions.
    - Respiratory: tachypnea, coughing, sneezing, airway obstruction.

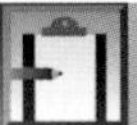

SIGNALMENT/HISTORY

- Dogs are more commonly affected than cats due to chewing behaviors. No breed or sex predilection.
- Younger animals are more commonly affected due to indiscriminate chewing.

Historical Findings

- Owners frequently report a chewed product container or ingestions of material with glue on it. Glue may also be noted on the skin or teeth.
- Anorexia and/or vomiting are commonly reported

Location and Circumstances of Poisoning

- Most exposures occur in the home, garage or work area.

CLINICAL FEATURES

- Cyanoacrylate
    - Clinical signs occur within seconds to minutes of glue exposure.
    - Most common signs include glue adherence to the fur, teeth, tongue or mucous membranes and local tissue adhesions.
    - Vomiting can occur with large ingestions.
    - Oropharyngeal obstruction from glue can cause cyanosis and respiratory distress.

- Diisocyanate
    - Clinical signs occur within 15 minutes up to 20 hours after ingestion.
    - Most common clinical signs are consistent with GI foreign body obstruction and include retching/gagging, vomiting, anorexia, abdominal pain, and abdominal distension. Dehydration can develop with prolonged clinical signs.
    - Tachypnea can be seen with inhalation of fumes or with pain secondary to GI obstruction.

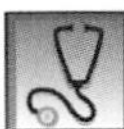

DIFFERENTIAL DIAGNOSIS

- Cyanoacrylate
    - Gastrointestinal signs: foreign body obstruction, gastroenteritis, pancreatitis, inflammatory bowel disease, metabolic disease.
    - Respiratory signs: upper airway obstruction, laryngeal paralysis, lower airway disease.
- Diisocyanate
    - Gastrointestinal signs: foreign body obstruction, food bloat, gastric dilatation and volvulus, gastroenteritis, pancreatitis, inflammatory bowel disease, metabolic disease.

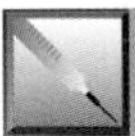

DIAGNOSTICS

- CBC and chemistry: no significant changes expected.
- Abdominal radiographs (4–24 hours after exposure) for diisocyanate ingestion often show a mottled gas and soft tissue opacity within the stomach lumen with gastric distension often resembling food ingestion (Fig. 9.1).

Pathological Findings

- Cyanoacrylate: no specific gross or histopathological findings aside from tissue adhesions.
- Diisocyanate: gross findings include a foreign body present within the stomach. Mucosal congestion, ulceration, and laceration noted on histopathological findings.

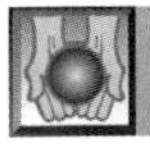

THERAPEUTICS

- Treatment of nonobstructive ingestion involves removal of glue from skin or fur and supportive care for GI symptoms. Surgery for foreign body removal is often needed for diisocyanate ingestion.

Detoxification

- Gastrointestinal
    - Emesis can be performed immediately after exposure with large ingestions but is generally not recommended due to risk for esophageal and GI obstruction.

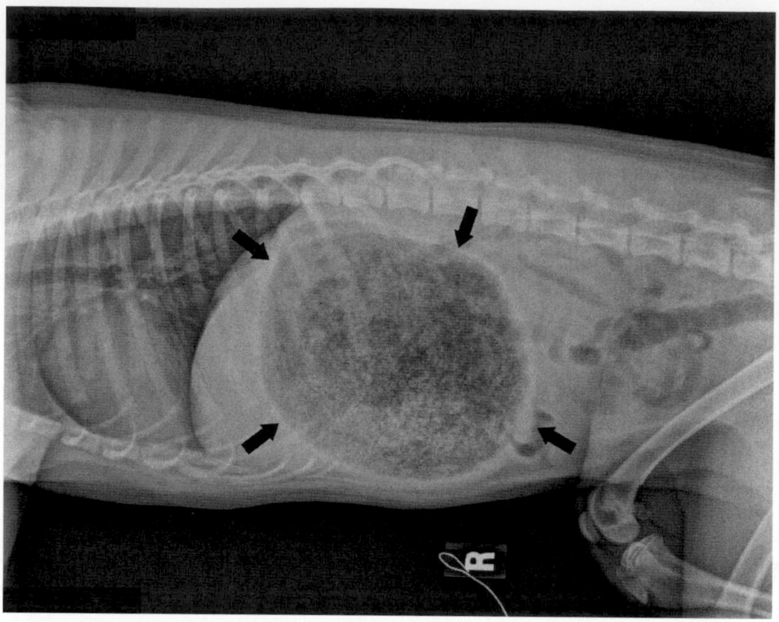

■ **Fig. 9.1.** Abdominal radiograph of a 9-month female Pit Bull Terrier after the ingestion of approximately 1.5 oz of Gorilla Glue 12 hours prior. Surgical extraction yielded a large, firm, glue obstruction, approximately 7–8 inches in diameter. Note the similarity of the glue to food or ingesta. Photo courtesy of Dr Catherine A. Angle.

    - Gastric lavage can be attempted but is generally not successful due to rapid expansion of diisocyanate glue.
    - Activated charcoal is not recommended.
- Respiratory
    - Oxygen therapy as needed.
    - Airway obstruction requires a sedated oral exam for glue removal.
- Ocular
    - Irrigate for 15 minutes with eye wash or room temperature water.
    - Fluorescein stain if indicated.
    - May need sedation or anesthesia for eyelid adhesions.
- Skin
    - Warm, soapy water or vegetable oil rubbed onto fur or teeth to loosen glue adhesions. Remove glue from fur with clippers as needed. Glue not causing morbidity does not need to be removed and will wear off with time.

Drugs and Antidotes of Choice

- Antiemetics can be used once foreign body is ruled out. Maropitant 1 mg/kg SQ q 24 hours.

Precautions/Interactions

- Avoid prokinetics such as metoclopramide until a foreign body obstruction has been ruled out.

Appropriate Health Care

- IV fluids as needed for dehydration and postsurgical care.
- Exploratory laparotomy and gastrotomy needed for dogs with evidence of a gastric obstruction.
- Postsurgical analgesia (i.e., hydromorphone 0.05–0.2 mg/kg IV, IM or SQ q 2–6 hours).

Nursing Care

- Surgical site care.
- Nutritional supplementation as needed postoperatively.

Follow-up

- Recheck postsurgical patients in 10–14 days for suture removal.

COMMENTS

Client Education

- Owners should be educated about the dangers of glue expansion and the high risk of foreign body obstruction.

Patient Monitoring

- Postoperatively, patients should be monitored for hydration, vomiting, diarrhea, appetite, and pain.

Prevention/Avoidance

- Keep pets out of areas where glues and adhesives are being used or stored.

Possible Complications

- Postoperative ileus and incisional dehiscence can occur.
- Gastric rupture can occur with diisocyanate obstruction if left untreated.

Expected Course and Prognosis

- With mild, nonobstructive ingestion, symptoms generally resolve within 24 hours.
- Prognosis is generally good if treated appropriately.
- Up to 75% of patients need surgery after diisocyanate ingestion. Surgery for foreign body removal can prolong and complicate recovery.

Synonyms

- Cyanoacrylate glue: instant glue, Krazy Glue, Super Glue
- Diisocyanate glue: 4,4'-diphenyl methane diisocyanate, diphenylmethyl diisocyanate, diphenylmethane diisocyanate (MDI), methylenedi-p-phenyl diisocyanate, Gorilla Glue

See Also

Foreign Objects

Abbreviations

See Appendix 1 for a complete list.

Suggested Reading

Bailey T. The expanding threat of polyurethane adhesive ingestion. Vet Tech 2004; 426–428.

Fitzgerald KT, Bronstein AC. Polyurethane adhesive ingestion. Topics Compan An Med 2013; 28:28–31.

Horstman CL, Eubig PA, Khan SA, et al. Gastric outflow obstruction after ingestion of wood glue in a dog. JAAHA 2003; 39:47–51.

Lubich C, Mrvos R, Krenzelok EP. Beware of canine *Gorilla glue* ingestions. Vet Human Toxicol 2004; 46:153–154.

Author: Katherine L. Peterson, DVM, DACVECC
Consulting Editor: Ahna G. Brutlag, DVM, MS, DABT, DABVT

chapter 10

Hydrocarbons

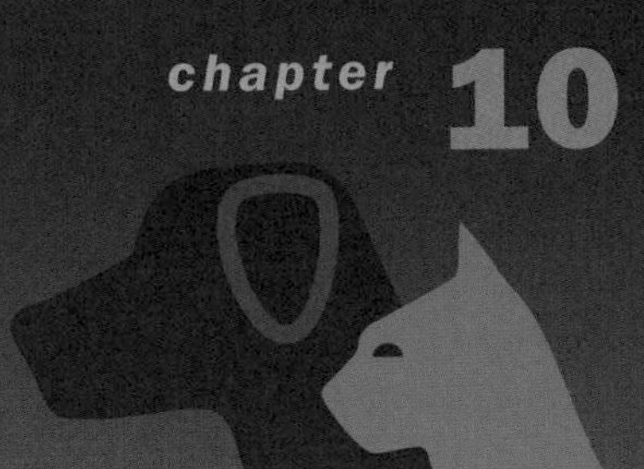

DEFINITION/OVERVIEW

- Hydrocarbons encompass a large group of chemical entities that contain hydrogen and carbon as their main constituents.
- Toxicity of hydrocarbons depends on the volatility and viscosity of the product. Highly volatile compounds lead to CNS signs. Low viscosity compounds pose a significant aspiration risk.
- Hydrocarbons generally belong to one of four categories.
  - Highly volatile – examples include benzene, toluene, and xylene. Toxic effects will result primarily in CNS signs.
  - Intermediate volatility, low to intermediate viscosity – examples include gasoline and kerosene. Toxic effects may result in either CNS or respiratory changes or both. This is the most common hydrocarbon exposure in pets.
  - Low volatility, low viscosity – examples include mineral seal oil in furniture products. These result in severe respiratory changes after aspiration of product or postemesis aspiration.
  - Low volatility, high viscosity – these hydrocarbons pose a lower risk for toxicity unless aspirated. Examples include mineral oil, diesel fuel, and motor oil.
- Toxicity will depend on the specific agent, the route of exposure, the dose, and the duration of exposure.
- Hydrocarbon exposure most often occurs after ingestion and may lead to gastrointestinal irritation, aspiration, and CNS depression. Less commonly reported complications include CNS excitation, dermal irritation or burns, ocular exposure with irritation or burns, cardiovascular effects with arrhythmias and hypotension, and renal or hepatic damage. Rare reports of intravascular hemolysis following ingestion have been noted.

Blackwell's Five-Minute Veterinary Consult Clinical Companion: Small Animal Toxicology, Second Edition.
Lynn R. Hovda, Ahna G. Brutlag, Robert H. Poppenga, and Katherine L. Peterson.

Companion website: www.fiveminutevet.com/toxicology

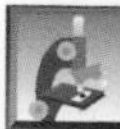

ETIOLOGY/PATHOPHYSIOLOGY

Mechanism of Action

Hydrocarbons predominantly act as irritants to the gastrointestinal tract, skin, eyes, and respiratory tract.

- Intermediate and low viscosity hydrocarbons (kerosene, gasoline, furniture polish containing mineral seal oil) carry the risk for primary aspiration or aspiration post emesis. This can result in respiratory injury and pneumonia.
- Pulmonary edema and/or hemorrhage may develop in severe cases.
- Systemic effects after ingestion of or exposure to hydrocarbons are less common, but may include damage to the liver and kidneys or intravascular hemolysis (rare).
- Inhalation of highly volatile hydrocarbons will not only result in CNS depression, excitation, or cyclical signs of both, but can also lead to cardiac sensitization and arrhythmias.

Toxicity

- Hydrocarbons represent a wide variety of compounds and thus the relative toxicity will vary.
- Oral LD_{50} in rat models shows a wide variability between specific agents.
    - Gasoline: 13,600 mg/kg
    - Kerosene: 15,000 mg/kg
    - Mineral spirits: >5000 mg/kg

Systems Affected

- Gastrointestinal – though poorly absorbed from the GIT, hydrocarbons may have an irritant effect often resulting in vomiting or diarrhea. Signs are typically self-limiting. Vomiting will increase the risk of aspiration.
- Respiratory – direct inhalation of hydrocarbon vapors will lead to respiratory irritation. Signs may include coughing and tachypnea. Direct aspiration or aspiration post emesis may result in aspiration pneumonia and subsequent hypoxemia.
- Nervous – inhalation of vapors or direct aspiration may result in CNS depression and/or agitation. Ataxia, tremors, and rarely convulsions may also occur. Aspiration post emesis may lead to hypoxemia and secondary CNS depression.
- Cardiovascular – inhalation may result in nonspecific arrhythmias (e.g. VPCs) and cardiac sensitization. Compounds that more profoundly affect the CNS will also lead to more significant cardiac abnormalities.
- Skin – in most circumstances hydrocarbons are poorly absorbed through healthy, intact skin. Mild to moderate dermal irritation with erythema and dermatitis may be seen. Caustic injury is rare, but may occur after prolonged exposure.

- Ophthalmic – ocular irritation, rarely ulceration, may occur following ophthalmic exposure. Injury due to self-mutilation may also occur.
- Renal and hepatobiliary – end-organ damage is not typically anticipated with acute ingestion. Chronic exposure may lead to acute renal failure and/or nonspecific liver injury.
- Hematological – rare instances of intravascular hemolysis post hydrocarbon exposure have been reported.

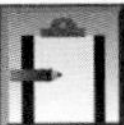

SIGNALMENT/HISTORY

Risk Factors

- Breed sensitivities are not expected.
- Pediatrics, geriatrics, and those animals with concurrent disease are at highest risk for complications.

Historical Findings

- Witnessed exposure.
- Access to storage areas (basement, garages, utility closets), with evidence of chewed containers or spilled product.
- Reports of a strong chemical or fuel odor on the pet's breath, fur coat, or in the vomitus or stool.

Location and Circumstances of Poisoning

- Ingestion – animals are frequently found with spilled material or containers that have been chewed.
- Inhalation –animals may be left in a poorly ventilated area following a spill of a volatile hydrocarbon. Animals with saturated fur coats will continue to inhale the product.

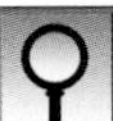

CLINICAL FEATURES

- Signs depend on the route of exposure and may develop minutes to hours following exposure.
- The fur coat and breath may smell strongly of the hydrocarbon.
- Ingestion and oral exposure – mucosal irritation, salivation, vomiting, diarrhea, poor appetite. Vomiting may lead to aspiration. HGE and caustic injury are rare complications.
- Inhalation exposure – CNS depression or agitation, ataxia, coughing, wheezing, gagging, and tachypnea. Monitor for aspiration pneumonia. CNS signs resolve quickly after patient is moved to fresh air and following decontamination of the product from the fur. Cardiac arrhythmias may occur after inhalation of volatile hydrocarbons (gasoline).
- Dermal exposure – erythematous tissue, dermatitis, thermal injury from hot oils and tars.

- Ocular exposure – injected sclera, conjunctival irritation, blepharospasm, lacrimation, pawing at the face. Corneal ulceration is rare.
- Hyperthermia may be noted in cases of aspiration pneumonia.

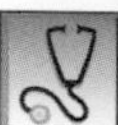

DIFFERENTIAL DIAGNOSIS

- Primary or infectious respiratory disease.
- Primary GI disease including gastroenteritis and ingestion of other GI irritants such as plants, cleaning products, foreign material, essential oils, etc.
- Primary dermal disease, atopic dermatitis, hypersensitivity, external parasites, exposure to other irritants such as household cleaners.
- Toxicities – CNS depressants, hepatotoxins (acetaminophen, xylitol, cycad/sago palm), renal toxins (ibuprofen, grapes/raisins/currants, ethylene glycol).

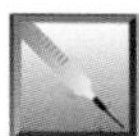

DIAGNOSTICS

- CBC – leukocytosis +/- a left shift may be indicative of pneumonia. Rare instances of hemolytic anemia may be noted.
- Chemistry profile – elevations of BUN, creatinine, ALT, AST, ALP may be noted in more chronic exposures, though are rarely noted in acute exposures. Mild elevations in BUN, creatinine, and total protein may occur secondary to dehydration.
- Urinalysis – a low prefluid urine specific gravity is typically noted in instances of renal failure and would be more common in chronic exposures. Highly concentrated urine samples in lieu of mild azotemia indicate dehydration.
- Radiographs – may indicate evidence of pneumonia either of the right middle lung lobe or multilobular. Evidence of pulmonary edema may develop in severe cases. Radiographic evidence of pulmonary injury may be delayed for up to 8–12 hours.
- ECG – nonspecific tachyarrhythmia, VPCs.
- Pathological postmortem findings – evidence of pulmonary edema, pulmonary hemorrhage, and damage to the pulmonary epithelium and surfactant layers may be noted. Infrequent reports of renal cell degeneration or fatty changes to the liver have been reported.

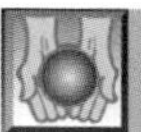

THERAPEUTICS

- Therapy is symptomatic and supportive. Treatment is primarily aimed at preventing aspiration by controlling nausea and managing subsequent respiratory signs with appropriate supportive measures. Aggressive respiratory therapy may be needed in critical cases.

Detoxification

- Bathe the patient with a nonmedicated degreasing shampoo or dish soap to remove the product. Several baths may be necessary.

- Clip the fur to remove thick or dried products such as tar/asphalt. The use of solvents (e.g. mineral spirits) is not recommended.
- In ocular exposure, irrigate eyes, taking care to flush beneath the third eyelid/nictitans. Place an Elizabethan collar to prevent self-trauma.
- Emesis and gastric lavage are typically not recommended due to the increased risk of aspiration.
- Activated charcoal will not bind to hydrocarbons, may increase the risk of nausea, vomiting, and subsequent aspiration, and is not recommended.
- Diuresis with IV fluids is not expected to hasten excretion.

Appropriate Health Care

- Primary care should focus on decontamination and symptomatic and supportive care.
- Critically ill patients may require aggressive respiratory support with a ventilator, stringent monitoring and treatment of cardiac arrhythmias, and management of hypotension. Once stabilized, transfer to a referral center should be considered in critical cases.
- Ocular exposures.
    - Prompt eye irrigation, including beneath the nictitans.
    - Fluorescein stain, slit lamp examination.
- Dermal exposures.
    - Mild irritation: antibiotic ointment or cream, vitamin E oil, and/or skin protectants.
    - Moderate-to-severe dermatitis: topical steroids.
    - Severe dermal compromise (burns and blistering): oral or IV antibiotics.
- Oral exposures.
    - Thorough oral exam for mucosal injury.
    - Irrigation with tepid water.
    - Antiemetics to aid in preventing vomiting and subsequent aspiration.
        - Maropitant 1 mg/kg SQ q 24 hours.
        - Ondansetron 0.1–0.3 mg/kg IV q 8 hours.
    - Gastroprotectants.
        - H2 blockers: famotidine 0.5–1 mg/kg PO, SQ, IM, or IV q 12 hours.
        - Sucralfate: 0.5–1 g PO q 8 hours.
    - Bland, highly digestible diet for 5–7 days.
    - While caustic injury is uncommon, if oral mucosal injury is noted, endoscopy may be needed to evaluate the extent of injury. Consider broad-spectrum antibiotics and pain management in such cases.
    - Animals exhibiting respiratory distress after ingestion or inhalation of hydrocarbons will require hospitalization and aggressive care.
    - Prophylactic use of antibiotics and steroids is controversial.
- Inhalation/respiratory exposure.
    - Thoracic radiographs to determine the extent of pulmonary injury in symptomatic animals. Radiographic changes may be delayed for several hours.
    - Supplemental oxygen or mechanical ventilation as needed.
    - Blood gas analysis to aid in managing acid–base status.

- Beta$_2$-agonists such as albuterol may be needed for bronchodilation.
- Broad–spectrum antibiotics for aspiration pneumonia: ampicillin 5–10 mg/kg IV q 8 hours with enrofloxacin 5–20 mg/kg IV q 12 hours.

- Renal impairment.
  - IV fluid diuresis at 2–3 times a maintenance rate for a minimum of 48 hours or until azotemia resolves.
- Hepatobiliary disease.
  - Hepatoprotectants.
    - S-adenosyl-methione (SAMe): 17–20 mg/kg PO q 24 hours × 28 days.
    - Silymarin/milk thistle: 20–50 mg/kg PO q 24 hours × 28 days.
    - Alternatively, commercial combination products are available and may be dosed and used per patient weight according to manufacturer instructions (e.g. Denamarin).
    - N-acetylcysteine (NAC) may be considered in severe cases. Following dilution to a 5% solution, give a loading dose of 140–280 mg/kg IV through a 0.2 micron filter or PO followed by 70 mg/kg IV or PO q 6 hours for 48–96 hours.

Drugs and Antidote of Choice

- No antidote available.

Precautions/Interactions

- Induction of emesis and gastric lavage are not typically recommended due to increased risk of aspiration.
- Use sympathomimetic agents cautiously if arrhythmias are detected due to sensitization of the myocardium.

Nursing Care

- Frequent assessment of the animal's condition is needed to closely monitor for any respiratory changes.

Follow-up Care

- Owners should be instructed to return to the clinic for reevaluation if current signs worsen or new signs develop. Monitoring for GIT signs and subsequent respiratory signs for 12–24 hours is recommended.

Activity

- No activity restrictions are needed. Convalescing animals may be less active in the immediate recovery phase.

Prevention

- Encourage owners to store hydrocarbons in secure areas that limit patient accessibility.

COMMENTS

Client Education

- Store products in appropriately labeled, original containers with tight, child-proof seals. Store products in secure areas that limit patient accessibility.

Expected Course and Prognosis

- Course and prognosis are dependent upon the type of exposure and the severity of symptoms.
- Animals remaining free of respiratory problems for 12–24 hours following exposure are unlikely to develop such issues.
- Pediatric and geriatric animals or those with concurrent underlying disease may have a more guarded prognosis.
- Hydrocarbon exposure typically results in a moderate-to-high morbidity, low mortality rate.

Abbreviations

See Appendix 1 for a full list.

HGE = hemorrhagic gastroenteritis
NAC = N-acetylcysteine
VPC = ventricular premature complex

See Also

Essential Oils/Liquid Potpourri
Phenols and Pine Oils

Suggested Reading

Dorman DC. Petroleum distillates and turpentine. Vet Clin North Am Small Anim Pract 1990; 20(2):505–513.
Goodwin SR, Berman LS, Tabeling BB, Sundlof SF. Kerosene aspiration: immediate and early pulmonary and cardiovascular effects. Vet Hum Tox 1988; 30(6):521–524.
Lifshitz M, Sofer S, Gorodishcher R. Hydrocarbon poisoning in children: a 5-year retrospective study. Wilderness Environ Med 2003; 14:78–82.
Reese E, Kimbrough RD. Acute toxicity of gasoline and some additives. Environ Health Perspect 1993; 101(suppl. 6):115–131.
Victoria MS, Nangia BS. Hydrocarbon poisoning: a review. Pediatr Emerg Care 1987; 3(3):184–186.

Acknowledgments: The authors and editors acknowledge the prior contributions of Stephen H. LeMaster, PharmD, MPH, who authored this topic in the previous edition.
Author: Holly Hommerding, DVM
Consulting Editor: Ahna G. Brutlag, DVM, MS, DABT, DABVT

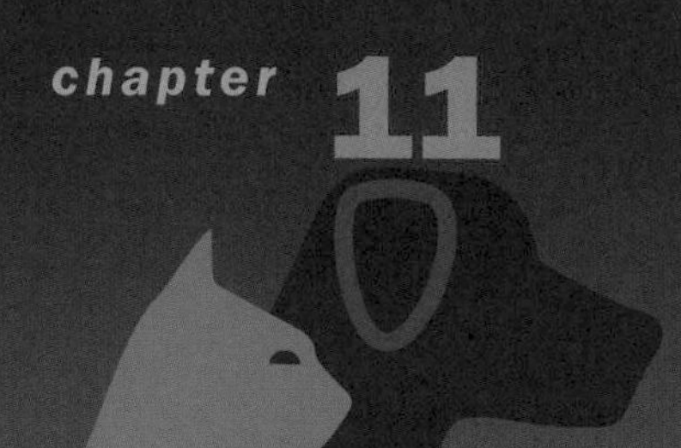

chapter 11

Hydrofluoric Acid

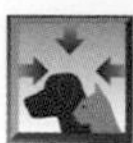

DEFINITION/OVERVIEW

- Highly concentrated hydrofluoric acid (HF) is used in glass etching, polishing of metals, and as an alkylating agent in industrial production. Household products (rust removers and automotive cleaning products) may contain lower concentrations of HF.
- Hydrofluoric acid is a weak acid with most of its toxicity resulting from the fluoride anion.
- HF is corrosive and can cause serious burns to the eyes, skin, and GI tract as well as systemic effects including electrolyte disturbances, respiratory problems, cardiac toxicity, and death.
- Any product containing HF should be considered potentially toxic.

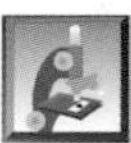

ETIOLOGY/PATHOPHYSIOLOGY

Mechanism of Action

- There are several proposed toxicological mechanisms.
  - HF penetrates deep into tissue and then dissociates.
  - Free fluoride ions chelate with calcium and magnesium to form insoluble complexes that precipitate in tissue leading to pain, necrosis, and bone decalcification.
  - In bone, fluoride replaces the hydroxyl group of hydroxyapatite.
  - Depletion of serum calcium and magnesium disrupts metabolism and may lead to severe hypocalcemia with resulting potassium efflux and hyperkalemia. These disruptions in potassium and magnesium can lead to myocardial irritability and dysrhythmias.
- Fluoride ions bind and inhibit multiple enzyme systems, including acetyl cholinesterase, adenyl cyclase, and Na-K ATPase, which results in excessive cholinergic stimulation and further potassium efflux.

Pharmacokinetics – Absorption, Distribution, Metabolism, Excretion

- HF is readily absorbed via any route of exposure. Systemic absorption occurs readily from the stomach because of its acidic environment.

Blackwell's Five-Minute Veterinary Consult Clinical Companion: Small Animal Toxicology, Second Edition.
Lynn R. Hovda, Ahna G. Brutlag, Robert H. Poppenga, and Katherine L. Peterson.

Companion website: www.fiveminutevet.com/toxicology

- The corrosive effect of HF is almost immediate, but signs may be delayed 12–24 hours.
- Fluoride volume of distribution is 0.5–0.7 L/kg.
- Fluoride is not metabolized by the body.
- It is excreted by the kidney – approximately 90% of fluoride is excreted unchanged in urine.
- A small percentage (5–10%) of absorbed fluoride is excreted in the feces.
- Fluoride elimination half-life is 2–9 hours.

Toxicity

- Corrosive to skin and mucous membranes, especially with concentrations >5%.
  - Systemic toxicosis is possible with low to moderately concentrated products (i.e., even <10% can be harmful).
  - Systemic toxicosis is the most common cause of death following ingestion.
  - Human fatalities have been reported in cases of dermal exposures with highly concentrated HF (70%) affecting 2.5% body surface area.
  - LC_{50} (inhalation) rat: 1278 ppm/1 hour.
  - LC_{50} (inhalation) mouse: 55 ppm/1 hour.
  - LC_{50} (inhalation) guinea pig: 4372 ppm/15 minutes.
  - LC_{50} (inhalation) monkey: 1780 ppm/1 hour.

Systems Affected

- Dermatological – pain (which is often severe, but may be delayed for hours), erythema, burns, edema, erosion/ulceration, and necrosis.
- Gastrointestinal – nausea, vomiting, diarrhea, abdominal pain, gastritis (may be hemorrhagic), dysphagia, corrosive burns to the mouth, throat, esophagus, and stomach.
- Respiratory – cough, dyspnea, bronchospasm, chemical pneumonitis, pulmonary edema (often hemorrhagic), and burns to the upper airways. The onset of lung injury may be delayed for several days.
- Cardiovascular – QTc prolongation, torsade de pointes, ventricular fibrillation, ventricular tachycardia, dysrhythmias, asystole, and cardiac arrest.
- Electrolyte and acid–base – hypocalcemia, hypomagnesemia, metabolic acidosis, and hyperkalemia.
- Bone – decalcification and dissolution.
- Eye – pain, corneal burns, necrosis, and opacification. Conjunctivitis may persist for several months with moderately concentrated solutions.

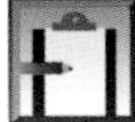

SIGNALMENT/HISTORY

- Any age or breed of animal can be affected.

Risk Factors

- Preexisting renal impairment may lead to further toxicity.
- Preexisting cardiac arrhythmias/disease may increase risk of cardiotoxicity.

Historical Findings

- Exposure (witnessed or suspected) to rust removers, automotive cleaning products, or other products containing HF.
- Clinical signs following topical exposure are often delayed. As a result, HF exposure in animals may not be reported until toxic damage is quite severe.

CLINICAL FEATURES

- Initial signs of vomiting post ingestion; cough, labored breathing, or bronchospasm post inhalation; watery or red eyes following ocular exposure and pain.
- As toxicosis progresses, corrosive GI or respiratory injury may result from ingestion or inhalation, respectively. Electrolyte abnormalities and cardiovascular toxicity may appear due to systemic absorption. Death has occurred within 1–2 hours following ingestion.
- Pain and erythema from dermal exposure may be delayed.
  - Up to 24 hours if HF concentration is <20%.
  - Up to 8 hours if HF concentration is between 20% and 50%.
  - No delay if HF concentration is >50%.
- HF penetrates deeply into tissue, causing widespread necrosis, ulcerations, and scarring.
- In dog studies, fatalities were most often caused by delayed cardiovascular collapse, ventricular fibrillation, and irreversible hyperkalemia.
- Hyperkalemia has been identified as a primary cause of ventricular arrhythmias in dogs. Potassium levels begin to rise slowly at 2 hours post exposure and exponentially at 6 hours.

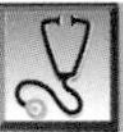

DIFFERENTIAL DIAGNOSIS

- Toxicities.
  - Ammonium bifluoride toxicosis.
  - Aspirin toxicosis.
  - Beta-blocker or calcium channel blocker ingestion.
  - Corrosive injury from other products (acids, alkaline agents, etc.).
  - Tricyclic antidepressant toxicosis.
- Primary cardiac disease.
- Primary respiratory disease.
- Primary metabolic disease.
- Primary mineral deficiencies.

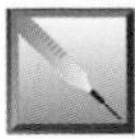

DIAGNOSTICS

- Diagnosis should be made based on history, physical examination, and clinical suspicion.
- Serum electrolyte levels – hypocalcemia, hypomagnesemia, and hyperkalemia.
- ECG – QTc prolongation, torsade de pointes, ventricular fibrillation, and ventricular tachycardia.
- Arterial or venous blood gases may reveal metabolic acidosis.
- Endoscopy should be performed within 12–24 hours after ingestion of large quantities and/or highly concentrated HF products, or if clinical signs (e.g., drooling, stridor, repeated vomiting) persist. Lesion development may be delayed up to 24 hours in burns with HF concentrations <20%.
- Thoracic radiographs should be considered in symptomatic animals post inhalation.
- Urine or serum fluoride levels may be used to confirm HF exposure (serum normal: 0.001–0.047 mg/L) but should not be the only determining factor and may not be useful in assessing need for further treatment. Limited availability in veterinary medicine.

Pathological Findings

- Gross examination at necropsy may reveal GI erosion following ingestion of HF, hemorrhagic pulmonary edema and/or burns to the pulmonary tree following inhalation; severe, deep necrotic damage following dermal exposure; corneal erosion, necrosis, and opacification following ocular exposure.

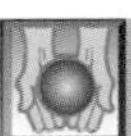

THERAPEUTICS

- Goals of treatment for HF toxicosis include removal from the source of contamination, aggressive decontamination and prevention of additional absorption, assessing the potential for systemic toxicosis by monitoring for cardiac signs, preventing and correcting electrolyte imbalances (especially Ca, Mg, and K) and acidosis, and providing supportive and symptomatic care.
- Treatment and care should be directed at potential toxic clinical signs.

Detoxification

- Dermal – irrigate affected area(s) with copious amounts of lukewarm tap water for at least 30 minutes followed by liberal application of a fluoride-binding calcium gluconate or carbonate 2.5% gel.
- Ingestion – immediately administer a fluoride-binding substance (containing Ca or Mg) such as milk, chewable calcium carbonate tablets, milk of magnesia, or a liquid antacid. If a large volume of fluid was ingested, consider removal via a nasogastric tube if within 1 hour of exposure.

- Ocular – irrigate with water, eye wash, normal saline, or LRS for at least 15 minutes (calcium solutions have not been shown to be more effective than saline for ocular irrigation). Continue irrigation until ocular pH is normal (check with litmus paper). Consult with a veterinary ophthalmologist if initial signs persist.
- Inhalation – administer humidified oxygen and assist with ventilation as needed. Administer 2.5% calcium gluconate by nebulizer to help control respiratory signs.

Drug(s) of Choice

- Initially treat arrhythmias by assessing and correcting for hypocalcemia, hypomagnesemia, and hyperkalemia. Because of its potassium channel-blocking activity, amiodarone is a preferred agent for ventricular arrhythmias. Otherwise, standard cardiac protocols may be used, avoiding agents that may increase the QTc interval (e.g., propranolol and certain calcium channel blockers).
- Hypomagnesemia should be treated with IV magnesium sulfate (0.15–0.3 mEq/kg over 10–20 minutes) followed by a CRI (0.75–1.0 mEq/kg/day).
- Initial doses of calcium can be given while waiting for labs to return.
  - Calcium gluconate 10% (0.50–1.50 mL/kg) can be given as a slow IV bolus over 20–30 minutes. An infusion (0.50–1.50 mL/kg/hour) can be initiated after the bolus to maintain its effect.
  - Calcium chloride 10% (0.15–0.50 mL/kg) may be preferred over calcium gluconate due to a greater concentration of calcium (13.4 mEq vs 4.5 mEq per 10 mL of 10% calcium chloride or gluconate, respectively). Tissue injury secondary to drug extravasation of calcium chloride can be significant. Therefore, calcium gluconate is preferred if a central line cannot be established.
- Administer sodium bicarbonate at 1–3 mEq/kg IV over 30 minutes to shift K^+ intracellularly and/or to treat acidosis.
- For gastrointestinal support, GI protectants (an antacid + sucralfate) may be used.
  - H_2 blockers (injectable therapy may be used while hospitalized if patient is NPO).
    - Famotidine (0.5–1 mg/kg PO q 12 hours × 7–10 days).
    - Omeprazole (0.5–1 mg/kg PO q 24 hours × 7–10 days).
  - Sucralfate.
    - 0.25–1 g PO q 8–12 hours for 7–10 days (ideally premade liquid slurry if esophageal ulceration suspected).
- Provide adequate analgesia.

Precautions/Interactions

- Do not induce vomiting as this may cause further esophageal damage.
- Avoid administering large amounts of liquid or activated charcoal post ingestion as this may induce vomiting.
- Do not perform ocular irrigation more than once since this has been shown to increase corneal damage.

- Intradermal and subcutaneous administration of 10% calcium chloride solution may be damaging to tissues and should be avoided.
- Subcutaneous administration of 10% calcium gluconate in the extremities should be avoided.
- Avoid propranolol and certain calcium channel blockers

Alternative Drugs

- Topical agents such as Epsom salts (magnesium sulfate) and Mylanta (magnesium hydroxide) are additional detoxification options. Calcium acetate soaks and iodine preparations have also shown effectiveness at reducing dermal injuries.
- A 0.5 mL/cm^2 subcutaneous infiltration of 10% calcium gluconate solution is an option if pain continues for >30 minutes after applying calcium gluconate gel, but should be avoided in the extremities.
- Topical corticosteroids can be applied after decontamination in cases of severe dermal inflammation.
- Hexafluorine optical rinse has been shown useful in cases of ocular exposure, with apparent advantages over saline in diminishing HF absorption into the eye. Consult with an ophthalmologist if prolonged signs.
- In canine studies, quinidine sulfate 5–10 mg/kg IV has shown efficacy in stopping K efflux and preventing hyperkalemia and resultant cardiotoxicity.
- Oral or IV corticosteroids and inhaled beta$_2$-agonists may help control bronchospasms.
- Cation exchange resins may be useful for hyperkalemia.
- Hemodialysis may be considered as a last-line option to remove fluoride anions in critical cases of systemic toxicosis or to treat hyperkalemia, although execution in the unstable, compromised patient will be difficult.

Nursing Care

- The animal should be given frequent opportunities to urinate to help excrete fluoride ions if catheterization is not feasible.

Diet

- If oral ingestion or altered level of consciousness, temporarily withhold food and water.

Activity

- Base on clinical signs and severity of exposure.

Surgical Considerations

- In cases of severe dermal necrosis with refractory hypocalcemia, surgical debridement of affected skin region(s) may be necessary.
- Amputation of affected limb(s) may be considered a last resort if the animal fails to respond to other treatment methods.

COMMENTS

Client Education

- Readmit the animal if clinical signs reappear or worsen even after proper treatment.

Patient Monitoring

- Continuous cardiac monitoring is recommended during hospitalization (even if initial ECG is normal) and for up to 48 hours post exposure, depending on the severity of exposure. QTc prolongation commonly precedes dysrhythmias and indicates the presence of hypocalcemia.
- Monitor respiratory function for up to 72 hours after inhalation of HF.
- Serum electrolyte levels (especially serum Ca) should be obtained every 30 minutes in cases of systemic toxicosis or large dermal exposures.
- Animals with well-controlled pain, normal electrolyte levels and ECG readings, and insignificant burns can be sent home after 6 or more hours.

Prevention/Avoidance

- Prevent access to HF-containing products in the home, particularly while cleaning.

Possible Complications

- Pulmonary edema and chronic lung disease.
- Ocular damage, changes in vision, and blindness.
- Scarring.
- Esophageal and GI strictures.
- Hypocalcemia induced by systemic HF toxicosis can lead to coagulation abnormalities, hemorrhage being one of the most common related complications.

Expected Course and Prognosis

- Prognosis depends on HF concentration, route and duration of exposure, and quantity exposed to or ingested.
- Single, small exposures are linked to good prognosis with low risk of long-term effects.
- Larger, multiple, or more severe exposures may require up to 72 hours of monitoring with potential systemic and long-term effects.

Synonyms

Hydrogen fluoride solution, hydrofluoric acid solution, aqueous hydrofluoric acid, fluoric acid solution, HFA, fluorhydric acid

See Also

Acids
Aspirin
Beta Receptor Agonists (Beta-Blockers)
Calcium Channel Blockers

Abbreviations

See Appendix 1 for a complete list.

CRI = continuous rate infusion
HF = hydrofluoric acid
LC_{50} = median lethal concentration

Suggested Reading

Dünser MW, Ohlbauer M, Rieder J, et al. Critical care management of major hydrofluoric acid burns: a case report, review of the literature, and recommendations for therapy. Burns 2004; 30(4):391–398.
Flomenbaum N, Goldfrank L, Hoffman R, et al. Hydrofluoric acid and fluorides. In: Su M, ed. Goldfrank's Toxicologic Emergencies, 8th edn. New York: McGraw-Hill, 2006.
Greenberg MI, Hamilton RJ, Phillips SD, et al. Occupational, Industrial, and Environmental Toxicology, 2nd edn. Philadelphia, PA: Mosby, 2003; pp. 100–101.
Ozcan M, Allahbeickaraghi A, Dündar M. Possible hazardous effects of hydrofluoric acid and recommendations for treatment approach: a review. Clin Oral Invest 2012; 16(1):15–23.
Spoler F, Frentz M, Forst M, et al. Analysis of hydrofluoric acid penetration and decontamination of the eye by means of time-resolved optical coherence tomography. Burns 2008; 34(4):549–555.
Wang X, Zhang Y, Liangfang N, et al. A review of treatment strategies for hydrofluoric acid burns: current status and future prospects. Burns 2014; 40(8):1447–1457.

Acknowledgments: The authors and editors acknowledge the prior contributions of Lauren E. Haak, PharmD, who co-authored this topic in the previous edition.
Authors: Leo J. Sioris, PharmD; Christina Fourré, DVM Candidate
Consulting Editor: Ahna G. Brutlag, DVM, MS, DABT, DABVT

Drugs: Human Prescription

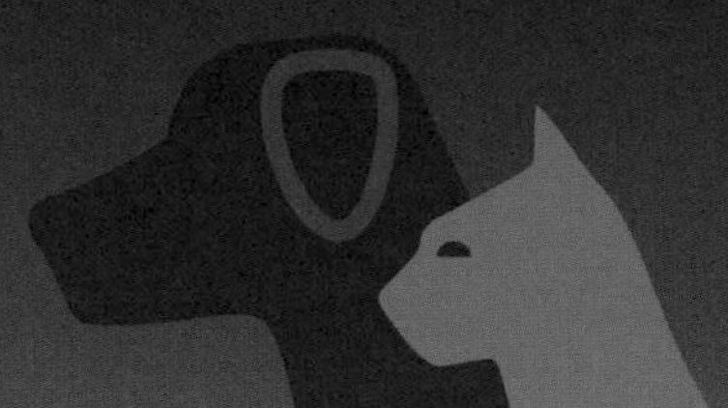

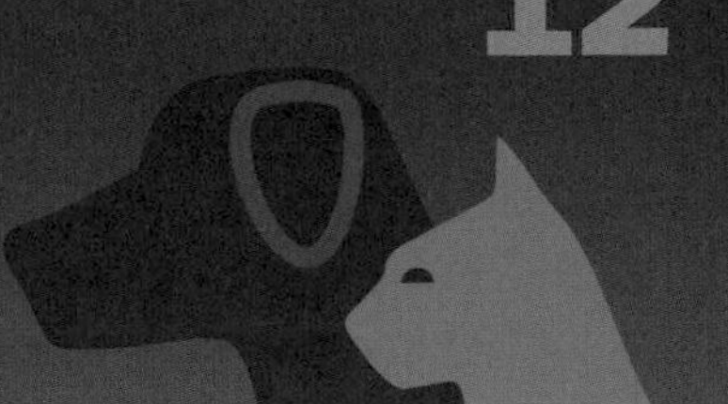

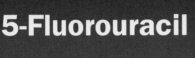

chapter 12

5-Fluorouracil

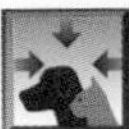

DEFINITION/OVERVIEW

- 5-Fluorouracil (5-FU, Efudex®) is an antineoplastic medication.
- It is most commonly found as a 1% or 5% topical cream, but is also available as a 1%, 2%, and 5% topical solution, and a 50 mg/mL solution for injection.
- 5-FU causes severe GI upset, seizures, and bone marrow suppression.
- Monitor for pulmonary edema and cardiac arrhythmias.
- The onset of seizures can be very rapid or delayed up to 24 hours post exposure. A minimum of 24 hours of hospitalization is required in asymptomatic pets.
- Seizures can be difficult to control and refractory to typical antiepileptics.
- Bone marrow suppression can be seen 5–30 days post exposure.

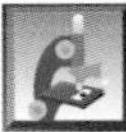

ETIOLOGY/PATHOPHYSIOLOGY

Mechanism of Action

Fluorouracil is an antimetabolite, antineoplastic medication that is metabolized to thymidine. Thymidine blocks the methylation reaction of deoxyuridylic acid to thymidylic acid, creating a thymine deficiency. This interferes with DNA and to a lesser extent RNA synthesis and results in cell death. Rapidly growing cells, such as those in the bone marrow and intestinal crypts, absorb fluorouracil rapidly, resulting in severe GI upset and bone marrow aplasia. 5-FU also has several active metabolites, such as 5-fluorouridine-5'-triphosphate (FUTP). FUTP is slower to cross cell membranes than fluorouracil, resulting in delayed clearance in the bone marrow.

Fluorocitrate inhibits the tricarboxylic acid cycle (TCA cycle), which blocks the gamma-aminobutyric acid (GABA) shunt and causes low levels of GABA in the brain, which can cause seizures. Fluorouracil and its metabolites also result in lamellar splitting of the myelin sheaths in nerve cells, leading to vacuolization of the myelin.

Blackwell's Five-Minute Veterinary Consult Clinical Companion: Small Animal Toxicology, Second Edition.
Lynn R. Hovda, Ahna G. Brutlag, Robert H. Poppenga, and Katherine L. Peterson.

Companion website: www.fiveminutevet.com/toxicology

Pharmacokinetics (all values are for humans, unless otherwise noted)

Absorption

- Reported to be about 6% when used dermally.
- Oral absorption is erratic.

Distribution

- Volume of distribution is 25 L/kg.
- Distributes into intestinal mucosa, bone marrow, liver.
- Crosses the blood–brain barrier and placenta.

Metabolism

- Metabolized in the liver to several active metabolites.

Excretion

- Within 6 hours, 7–20% is excreted unchanged in the urine.
- Expired as carbon dioxide.
- Minor excretion in bile.

Toxicity

- LD_{50} (oral in a rat) 115 mg/kg.
- LD_{50} (oral in dog) 30 mg/kg.
- LD_{50} (oral in rabbit) 18.9 mg/kg.
- Dose of concern is questionable, but considered to be 5.5 mg/kg.
- Margin of safety is very narrow.
- NOEL, LOEL, and MLD are all very close.

Systems Affected

- Gastrointestinal – affects rapidly dividing cells, such as those in the intestinal crypts. Results in vomiting, diarrhea, desquamation and sloughing of the GI tract, and stomatitis.
- Nervous – causes low GABA and splitting and vacuolization of myelin, resulting in seizures, ataxia, tremors, depression, disorientation, head tremors.
- Hepatobiliary – can cause increased liver enzymes.
- Respiratory – pulmonary edema secondary to reversible heart failure.
- Cardiovascular – myocardial ischemia and cardiac arrhythmias, potentially from coronary vasospasm.
- Immune – bone marrow suppression.
- Reproductive – crosses the placenta and is teratogenic and embryotoxic.

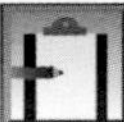

SIGNALMENT/HISTORY

Risk Factors

- Underlying renal or hepatic dysfunction may slow elimination.
- Young animals tend to be more curious and likely to have accidental ingestion.
- Living in areas of high human UV exposure (mountains, large bodies of water), as owners in these areas have increased use of 5-fluorouracil.

Historical Findings

- Owners will typically report an exposure to 5-fluorouracil.
- Often a rapid onset of GI upset will be noted. Cream may be noted in the vomitus, if very early in the course of intoxication.
- Owners sometimes report onset of seizures as early as 30 minutes post exposure.

Location and Circumstances of Poisoning

- Most commonly, pets will chew into a tube of ointment that has been left within reach.
- Occasionally, owners will apply to their pets.
- Rarely, we see an accidental overdose as a part of a chemotherapy regimen.

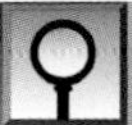

CLINICAL FEATURES

- GI upset is often noted 10 minutes to 5 hours post exposure.
- Seizures can be observed as early as 30 minutes post exposure, but can be delayed up to 24 hours post exposure. The time to onset of seizures does not seem to correlate with their severity.
- Clinical signs often noted are vomiting, diarrhea (often with blood), seizures, ataxia, tremors, depression, disorientation, vocalization, hypothermia, hyperthermia, agitation, hyperesthesia, absent menace response, coma, head tremors, and pulmonary edema.
- Leukopenia, neutropenia, thrombocytopenia, anemia, increased liver enzymes, and metabolic acidosis are also often noted on blood work.

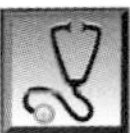

DIFFERENTIAL DIAGNOSIS

- Toxic: sodium fluoroacetate (1080), cycad palms (*Zamia* and *Cycas* spp.), castor bean (*Ricinus communis*), zinc phosphide, metaldehyde, disulfoton, bromethalin, and strychnine toxicoses.
- Metabolic: liver failure, hypoglycemia, hepatic encephalopathy.
- Primary neurological disease: idiopathic epilepsy, neoplasia, meningitis.

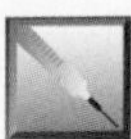

DIAGNOSTICS

- CBC with differential.
  - Baseline, recheck at 12 and 24 hours and then q 24–72 hours for 2 weeks in normal animals or until return to normal in patients with bone marrow suppression (may take up to 30 days).
- Serum chemistry.
  - Baseline, recheck PRN.
  - Increased liver enzymes can be measured, but are typically mild.
- Electrolytes.
  - Baseline, recheck PRN, especially if GI upset is severe.

Pathological Findings

Hemorrhagic colitis, gastric and intestinal ulceration, desquamation of the GI tract, stomatitis, myocardial ischemia, pulmonary edema, congestion of the lungs, liver, thymus, kidney and small intestine.

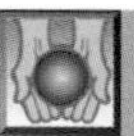

THERAPEUTICS

Objectives of treatment: control seizures, prevent dehydration and sepsis, control pain, treat cardiac arrhythmias and pulmonary edema.

Detoxification

- Emesis is not recommended, due to potential for rapid onset of seizures.
- Activated charcoal with a cathartic, if less than 1 hour post exposure and pet is asymptomatic.
- Hemodialysis, peritoneal dialysis, and fluid diuresis all enhance elimination.

Appropriate Health Care

- IV fluids.
  - Fluid diuresis is recommended to maintain hydration and enhance elimination; reduce or discontinue if pulmonary edema is observed.
- Good nursing care, especially in patients that are recumbent.
- Monitor ECG for arrhythmias.
- Temperature, pulse, and blood pressure should be monitored.
- Respiratory effort and lung sounds should be monitored for indications of pulmonary edema.
- Monitor respirations in heavily sedated or anesthetized animals.

Antidote

- Vistonuridine (uridine triacetate) is used in human medicine as an antidote. However, it is not used in veterinary medicine due to expense and the fact that it has to be administered before CNS signs are seen. Under the orphan drug laws it has to be special ordered, which typically takes 2–3 days. No known cases of its use have been reported in cats and dogs.

Drugs of Choice

- Antiepileptics.
  - Note: seizures can be very difficult to control.
  - Diazepam CRI +/- barbiturates.
    - Pentobarbital 3–15 mg/kg IV slow to effect.
    - Phenobarbital 3–30 mg/kg IV slow to effect.
  - Gas anesthesia.
  - Propofol CRI 0.6 mg/kg/minute.
  - Levetiracetum up to 60 mg/kg IV. Often very helpful for refractory seizures.
- GI protectants.
  - Sucralfate slurry 1g PO q 8 hours for large dogs; 0.5 g PO TID for small dogs and cats.
  - Omeprazole 0.5–1 mg/kg PO q 24 hours.
- Antiemetics.
  - Maropitant 0.1–0.3 mg/kg IV,PO q 8 hours.
- Colony stimulating factors.
  - Filgrastim (Neupogen®) 4–6 µg/kg SQ for neutropenia.
- Opioids for pain control.
  - Buprenorphine 0.005–0.02 mg/kg IM, SQ, IV q 6–12 hours.

Precautions/Interactions

- Hydrochlorothiazide – increases risk of myelosuppression.
- Leucovorin – increases risk of myelosuppression and GI toxicity.
- Levamisole – increases risk of hepatoxicity.
- Metronidazole – reduces clearance and increases serum concentrations of 5-FU and all signs of toxicity.
- Cimetidine – increases peak plasma concentrations of fluorouracil.
- NSAIDS – can increase GI upset and irritation.

Alternative Drugs

- Antiemetics – metoclopramide may be effective in preventing vomiting, but use with caution, as could cause additional CNS signs.

Diet

- Bland, soft diet can be started once seizures have stopped and patient can tolerate it.

Activity

- Activity should be restricted to prevent injury while pets are having seizure activity.

Surgical Considerations

- Patients may have delayed healing time and increased risk of infection due to leukopenia. Excessive bleeding may be a concern due to thrombocytopenia.

COMMENTS

Prevention/Avoidance

Pets should be kept away from 5-fluorouracil. Spills should be cleaned up promptly with pets in another room. Dogs and cats should be prevented from licking skin treated with 5-fluorouracil.

Expected Course and Prognosis

- GI upset typically, but not always, precedes seizures.
- Suppression of one or more cell lines can be noted. Leukopenia and thrombocytopenia are more commonly decreased at day 5–7. Anemia is typically noted around day 9. The nadir for all cell types is typically noted at 9–14 days. Resolution is expected by 30 days post exposure.
- Prognosis is guarded to poor once clinical signs occur.
- 30% of symptomatic dogs died or were euthanized.

Synonyms

Efudex®, Adrucil®, Carac®, Fluoroplex®, 5-FU

Abbreviations

See Appendix 1 for a complete list.

NOEL = no observable effect level
LOEL = lowest observable effect level
MLD = minimum lethal dose
FUTP = 5-fluorouridine-5'-triphosphate

See Also

Sodium Monofluoroacetate (Compound 1080)

Suggested Reading

Frye MM, Forman MA. 5-Fluorouracil toxicity with severe bone marrow suppression in a dog. Vet Hum Toxicol 2004; 46:178–180.

Sayre RS, Barr JW, Bailey EM. Accidental and experimentally induced 5-fluorouracil toxicity in dogs. JVECCS 2012; 22:545–549.

Yashimata K, Yada H, Ariyoshi T. Neurotoxic effects of fluoro-alanine and fluoroacetic acid on dogs. J Toxic Sci 2004; 29:155–166.

Acknowledgment: The authors and editors acknowledge the prior contributions of Lisa L. Powell, DVM, MS, DACVECC, who authored this topic in the previous edition.

Author: Laura Stern, DVM
Consulting Editor: Lynn R. Hovda, RPh, DVM, MS, DACVIM

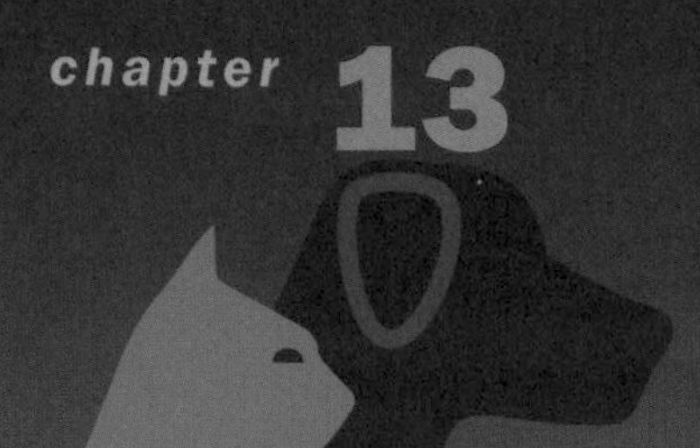

chapter 13 Amphetamines

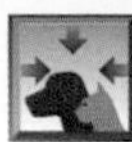

DEFINITION/OVERVIEW

- Amphetamines can be either prescription medications for ADHD or weight loss (Adderall®, Concerta®, Dexedrine®, Focalin®, Ritalin®, Strattera®, Vyvanse®) or illegal drugs (methamphetamine, ecstasy).
- Intoxication stimulates the CNS and cardiovascular systems.

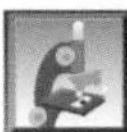

ETIOLOGY/PATHOPHYSIOLOGY

- Amphetamines are sympathomimetic amines. They stimulate the medullary respiratory center and reticular activating system.
- Amphetamines cause stimulation of alpha and beta receptors and release of norepinephrine and serotonin. This increases the amount of catecholamines found in the synapse.
- Clinical signs are stimulatory (agitation, tachycardia, tremors, seizures).
- Amphetamine intoxication in animals is not uncommon, especially in households with ADHD children.

Mechanism of Action

- Amphetamines are stimulants of the CNS and cardiovascular system. They stimulate the medullary respiratory center and reticular activating system.
- Amphetamines increase the concentration of catecholamines at nerve endings by increasing their release and inhibiting their reuptake and metabolism.
- There is also an increase in the presynaptic release of serotonin.

Pharmacokinetics – Absorption, Distribution, Metabolism, Excretion

- Amphetamines are quickly absorbed orally.
- Depending on the formulation, signs can be seen almost immediately, or they can be delayed for several hours (extended-release formulations).
- High lipid solubility leads to high concentrations in the liver, kidneys, and lungs.

Blackwell's Five-Minute Veterinary Consult Clinical Companion: Small Animal Toxicology, Second Edition.
Lynn R. Hovda, Ahna G. Brutlag, Robert H. Poppenga, and Katherine L. Peterson.

Companion website: www.fiveminutevet.com/toxicology

- They cross the blood–brain barrier.
- Metabolism is minimal and most are excreted as the parent compound.
- Amphetamines are eliminated in the urine. Urinary elimination is pH dependent. The half-life varies from 7 to 34 hours (shorter with acidic urine).

Toxicity

- The oral lethal dose in dogs for most amphetamines ranges from 10 to 23 mg/kg. Signs can be seen as low as 1 mg/kg.

Systems Affected

- Nervous – stimulation resulting in agitation and nervousness.
- Neuromuscular – stimulation resulting in tremors and seizures.
- Cardiovascular – stimulation resulting in tachycardia and hypertension.
- Respiratory – stimulation resulting in tachypnea.
- Gastrointestinal – stimulation resulting in vomiting, hypersalivation, and diarrhea.
- Ophthalmic – dilation of the pupils.

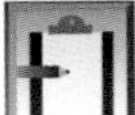

SIGNALMENT/HISTORY

- All species and breeds can be affected.
- The owner may report agitation, tachycardia, panting, tremors, hyperthermia, seizures, and/or death.

Risk Factors

- Animals with preexisting cardiac disease may be more at risk for developing severe signs and fatal arrhythmias.

Historical Findings

- Owners may have evidence of exposure to amphetamines.
- Owners often report agitation (running around), tremors (shaking), and tachycardia (heart racing).

Location and Circumstances of Poisoning

- Most poisonings occur within the home.
- Animals may be given the wrong medication by mistake or may have access to prescription medications.

Interactions with Drugs, Nutrients, or Environment

- Acetazolamide and sodium bicarbonate alkalinize the urine, causing increased renal tubular reabsorption of amphetamines.

- Tricyclic antidepressants (amitriptyline, amoxapine, clomipramine, desipramine, doxepin, imipramine, nortriptyline, protriptyline, trimipramine) enhance release of norepinephrine (hypertension, CNS stimulation).
- Monoamine oxidase inhibitors (clorgyline, isocarboxazide, meclobemide, nialamide, pargyline, phenylzine, procarbazine, rasagiline, selegiline, toloxatone, tranylcypromine) and furazolidone when ingested with amphetamines result in more norepinephrine being made available through inhibition of catecholamine degradation. Greater amounts of norepinephrine increase sympathetic activity.
- Sibutramine when ingested with amphetamines increases blood pressure and heart rate.

CLINICAL FEATURES

- Neurological – acute onset of restlessness and hyperactivity, followed by tremors and seizures.
- Cardiovascular – tachycardia.
- Respiratory – acute onset of tachypnea.
- Ophthalmic – mydriasis.
- Signs can begin within minutes (methamphetamine) or may be delayed for several hours. If signs have been present for a while, hyperthermia and myoglobinuria may be noted.

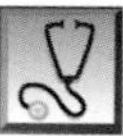

DIFFERENTIAL DIAGNOSIS

- Other stimulants, including the following.
  - Methylxanthines (caffeine, theobromine, theophylline).
  - Nicotine.
  - Serotonergic medications.

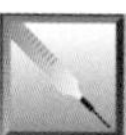

DIAGNOSTICS

- Illicit drug urine test: amphetamines will show up positive on amphetamine and/or methamphetamine tests, although these tests have not been validated in animals.
- Amphetamines can be detected in urine or stomach contents by human hospital laboratories or veterinary diagnostic laboratories.
- ECG – sinus tachycardia, ventricular arrhythmias.
- Blood gas – metabolic acidosis.
- Blood pressure – hypertension.
- Urinalysis – myoglobinuria secondary to rhabdomyolysis.

Pathological Findings

- There are no specific histopathological lesions consistent with this toxicosis.

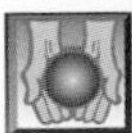

THERAPEUTICS

- Treatment is aimed at controlling life-threatening CNS and cardiovascular signs.

Detoxification

- Emesis if <15 minutes and asymptomatic.
- Gastric lavage if large amounts of pills have been ingested.
- Activated charcoal to reduce absorption if ingestion is over a lethal dose.
- Acidifying urine to 4.5–5.5 pH with either ammonium chloride (100–200 mg/kg/day PO divided QID) or ascorbic acid (20–30 mg/kg PO, SQ, IM or IV) to enhance elimination.

Appropriate Health Care

- Monitor body temperature, respirations, and heart rate.
- Monitor blood pressure.
- Monitor acid–base status.
- ECG for arrhythmias.

Antidotes

- No specific antidote.

Drugs of Choice

- IV fluids to help regulate body temperature and to protect kidneys from myoglobinuria.
- Agitation.
  - Phenothiazine.
    - □ Acepromazine 0.05 mg/kg IV or IM, titrate to effect as needed.
    - □ Chlorpromazine 0.5 mg/kg IV, IM or SQ, titrate up as needed.
  - Cyproheptadine.
    - □ Dogs: 1.1 mg/kg PO or rectally; serotonin antagonist.
    - □ Cats: 2–4 mg total dose per cat.
- Tachycardia.
  - Beta-blockers.
    - □ Propranolol 0.02–0.06 mg/kg IV.
- Tremors.
  - Methocarbamol 50–100 mg/kg IV, titrate up as needed.
- Seizures.
  - Barbiturates to effect.
    - □ Phenobarbital 3–4 mg/kg IV.

Precautions/Interactions

- Diazepam can increase the dysphoria and lead to increased morbidity. It is not recommended for use in amphetamine toxicosis.

Alternative Drugs

- Seizures – inhalant anesthetics (isoflurane, sevoflurane), propofol CRI.

Nursing Care

- Thermoregulation.
- Minimize sensory stimuli.

Follow-up

- No long-term problems are expected in most cases.

Diet

- No diet change is needed, except NPO during severe CNS signs.

Prevention

- Keep all medications out of the reach of pets.

COMMENTS

- Treatment in most cases is very rewarding.
- These animals tend to require large doses of phenothiazines to control their clinical signs.

Client Education

- Monitor appetite and urine color for 24 hours.

Patient Monitoring

- Monitor HR, BP, and urine color, hourly at first and then less often if the animal remains clinically normal.

Prevention/Avoidance

- Keep all medications out of the reach of pets.
- Do not store human and animal drugs in the same area to decrease medication errors.

Possible Complications

- DIC secondary to severe hyperthermia.
- Rhabdomyolysis and secondary renal failure.

Expected Course and Prognosis

- If CNS and cardiac signs can be controlled, prognosis is good.
- Signs may last up to 72 hours with extended-release products.

See Also

Club Drugs (MDMA, GHB, Flunitrazepam, and Bath Salts)
Methamphetamine
SSRI and SNRI Antidepressants

Abbreviations

See Appendix 1 for a complete list.

Suggested Reading

Bloom FE. Neurotransmission and the central nervous system. In: Brunton LL, Lazo JS, Parker KL, eds. Goodman & Gilman's The Pharmacological Basis of Therapeutics, 11th edn. New York: McGraw-Hill Professional, 2006.

Genovese DW, Gwaltney-Brant SM, Slater MR. Methylphenidate toxicosis in dogs: 128 cases (2001–2008). Am Vet Med Assoc 2010; 237(12):1438–1443.

Plumb DC. Plumb's Veterinary Drug Handbook, 8th edn. Ames, IA: Wiley-Blackwell, 2015.

Stern LA, Schell M. Management of attention-deficit disorder and attention-deficit/hyperactivity disorder drug intoxication in dogs and cats. Vet Clin North Am Small Anim Pract 2012; 42(2):279–287.

Author: Tina Wismer, DVM, DABVT, DABT, MS
Consulting Editor: Lynn R. Hovda, RPH, DVM, MS, DACVIM

Angiotensin-Converting Enzyme (ACE) Inhibitors

DEFINITION/OVERVIEW

- Angiotensin-converting enzyme (ACE) inhibitors (ACEIs) are often the initial treatment for hypertension. This group of medications lowers blood pressure by decreasing peripheral vascular resistance. This induces arterial and venous vasodilation.
    - ACEIs commonly used in veterinary medicine include benazepril, captopril, enalapril, imidapril, lisinopril, and ramipril.
- Other indications for use include treatment of mitral insufficiency and congestive heart failure due to dilated cardiomyopathy. ACEIs appear to reduce proteinuria and therefore may be of benefit in the treatment of chronic renal failure or protein-losing enteropathies.
- The primary concern with an overdose is the development of hypotension. The drop in blood pressure will generate weakness and lethargy.
- Other signs of overdose include hypersalivation, tachycardia, GI distress, and renal dysfunction. Hyperkalemia can occur secondary to aldosterone inhibition. A rare adverse effect is the production of a dry cough induced by bradykinin.

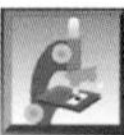

ETIOLOGY/PATHOPHYSIOLOGY

Mechanism of Action

- ACEIs competitively inhibit the conversion of angiotensin I to angiotensin II. Angiotensin II is a powerful endogenous vasoconstrictor; its inhibition leads to systemic vasodilation. There is also a decrease in aldosterone production and a decrease in sympathetic nervous system output.
- ACEIs block the breakdown of bradykinin, which contributes to the decrease in blood pressure but may be responsible for the risk of angioedema.
- Angiotensin II stimulates the kidneys to retain sodium. The decrease in aldosterone leads to a decrease in sodium and water retention and thereby decreased blood volume. This decreases cardiac preload and afterload.

Blackwell's Five-Minute Veterinary Consult Clinical Companion: Small Animal Toxicology, Second Edition.
Lynn R. Hovda, Ahna G. Brutlag, Robert H. Poppenga, and Katherine L. Peterson.

Companion website: www.fiveminutevet.com/toxicology

Pharmacokinetics – Absorption, Distribution, Metabolism, Excretion

- The ACEIs have a rapid oral absorption and are well distributed, except to the CNS. They are metabolized in the liver and excreted by the kidneys.
- Healthy dogs with no underlying cardiovascular or renal impairment are unlikely to experience hypotension if the dose is less than 20 mg/kg.
- Benazepril.
  - In dogs, peak plasma levels occur about 75 minutes after dosing.
  - Liver metabolism is to the active metabolite benazeprilat. Age or hepatic compromise does not seem to alter metabolite levels.
  - The $T_{1/2}$ in healthy dogs is 3.5 hours, but there may be an additional elimination slow phase, which may increase the half-life to 55–60 hours. Benazeprilat is cleared via renal and hepatic routes.
  - $T_{1/2}$ in healthy cats is 16–23 hours.
- Captopril.
  - Rapid absorption in dogs.
  - Food in the stomach will decrease bioavailability by 30–40%.
  - $T_{1/2}$ in dogs is about 2.8 hours but the duration of effect may persist for 4 hours.
  - Renal impairment can greatly extend the $T_{1/2}$ as captopril is renally excreted.
- Enalapril.
  - Is converted in the liver to the active metabolite enalaprilat.
  - Onset of action in dogs is 4–6 hours.
  - Duration of action in dogs is 12–14 hours.
  - 40% is excreted through the kidneys, and 35% is excreted in the feces.
  - $T_{1/2}$ of enalaprilat in dogs is about 11 hours.
  - Severe cardiac disease or renal insufficiency will prolong the $T_{1/2}$.
- Lisinopril.
  - Peak plasma levels in the dog occur about 4 hours after ingestion.
  - $T_{1/2}$ in dogs is 3 hours.
  - The effects last 24 hours, allowing for once-a-day dosing.
- Ramipril.
  - Is converted in the liver to the active metabolite ramiprilat.
  - Effects last 24 hours.
- Imidapril .
  - $T_{1/2}$ is 18–20 hours.

Toxicity

- ACEIs have a fairly wide margin of safety.
- Hypotension is the primary complication of overdose but it is usually mild.
- ACEIs should be used with caution in patients with hyponatremia or sodium depletion.
- ACEIs may have potential for increased hypotensive effects when used with diuretics to treat heart failure. When ACEIs are used with potassium-sparing diuretics, there may be increased hyperkalemic effects.

- Other adverse effects include angioedema, proteinuria, hyperkalemia, bronchospasm, pancreatitis, hepatotoxicity, renal insufficiency, and leukopenia.
  - Benazepril – long $T_{1/2}$ may require prolonged monitoring.
  - Captopril – 6.6 mg/kg every 8 hours may cause renal failure in dogs.
  - Enalapril – 200 mg/kg is a lethal dose in dogs. 100 mg/kg requires prolonged monitoring.
  - Lisinopril, ramipril, imidapril – there are no data available, but the long duration of action necessitates prolonged monitoring in overdose cases.

Systems Affected

- Renal/urological – the renin-angiotensin system is affected, causing a decrease in blood pressure and acute renal failure.
- Cardiovascular – hypotension resulting in tachycardia.
- Gastrointestinal – vomiting and diarrhea.
- Respiratory – bronchospasm.

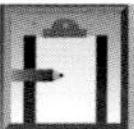

SIGNALMENT/HISTORY

- No specific breed or age predilection.

Risk factors

- Animals with severe CHF or renal insufficiency may be at a higher risk.

Clinical Features

- Most common signs of overdose are hypotension, lethargy, salivation, and tachycardia.
- Secondary signs include vomiting, diarrhea, weakness, cough/bronchospasm, and dysfunction of the renal system.
- Rare potential for skin rashes and neutropenia.
- The onset and duration of signs depend on the particular ACEI ingested.

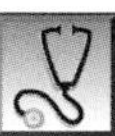

DIFFERENTIAL DIAGNOSIS

- Autonomic insufficiency.
- Acute hypovolemia.
- Benzodiazepine compounds including flunitrazepam.
- Opiate or opioid ingestion.

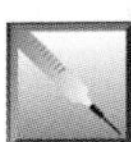

DIAGNOSTICS

- Serum ACEI values are of little use in veterinary medicine.
- Presence of hypotension, systolic BP <90 mmHg or a MAP <60 mmHg.

- Baseline laboratory work should include:
    - CBC, rarely see neutropenia or leukopenia
    - electrolytes, hyperkalemia
    - serum chemistry including liver enzymes, BUN, creatinine, lipase, and amylase
    - urinalysis for early signs for renal disease
    - pathological findings are nonspecific.

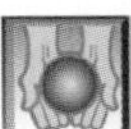

THERAPEUTICS

Detoxification

- Induce emesis only if early after ingestion and the animal is asymptomatic. Potential for hypotension-induced aspiration pneumonia is high.
- Gastric lavage in large ingestions.
- Activated charcoal with a cathartic if no risk of aspiration and GI motility is normal.
- Lisinopril can be removed by hemodialysis.

Appropriate Health Care

- Monitor blood pressure and vital signs every 4 hours. Repeat more often if animal is hypotensive, MAP <60 mmHg.
- Monitor BUN, creatinine, and electrolytes, especially if there is evidence of hypotension or there is preexisting renal insufficiency.
- In human medicine, the recommendations are to observe for a minimum of 6 hours after ingestion if asymptomatic. If symptomatic or hypotensive, observe for 24 hours. If there is significant hypotension, observe for 36 hours as hypotensive episodes may recur up to 36 hours after ingestion.
- In humans, the maximal blood pressure lowering was observed at around 5 hours post ingestion irrespective of the ACEI ingested. If the patient has not had hypotension by 6 hours, they can be considered for discharge.
- Renal impairment due to overdose is due to the systemic hypotension or decreasing glomerular filtration as a consequence of dilation of the efferent arterioles.

Antidotes

- There is no specific antidote available.

Drugs of Choice

- Give IV fluid therapy to maintain renal blood flow. Volume expansion with normal saline is recommended. Maintain urine output and hydration status appropriately.
    - Furosemide CRI at 1–2 mg/kg/hour.
    - Mannitol bolus at 1–2 g/kg slow IV.

- Persistent hypotension.
  - IV crystalloids at 20–30 mL/kg in aliquots. Repeat as needed for volume expansion.
  - Colloids or blood products as needed.
  - Vasopressors.
    - Dopamine at 5–20 µg/kg/min IV CRI.
    - Norephinephrine 0.1–1.0 µg/kg/min IV CRI.
    - Epinephrine 0.1–0.4 µg /kg/min IV CRI.
- Antiemetics.
  - Maropitant 1 mg/kg SQ every 24 hours.
  - Ondansetron 0.1–0.2 mg/kg IV every 8–12 hours.

COMMENTS

Expected Course and Prognosis

- In human medicine, the recommendations are to observe for a minimum of 6 hours after ingestion if asymptomatic. If symptomatic or hypotensive observe for 24 hours. If there is significant hypotension, observe for 36 hours as hypotensive episodes may recur up to 36 hours after ingestion.

Abbreviations

See Appendix 1 for a complete list.

Suggested Reading

Atkins CE, Brown WA, Coats JR, et al. Effects of long-term administration of enalaparil on clinical indicators of renal function in dogs with compensated mitral regurgitation. J Am Vet Med Assoc 2002; 221(5):654–658.

Atkins CE, Keene BW, Brown WA, et al. Results of the veterinary enalapril trial to prove reduction in onset of heart failure in dogs chronically treated with enalapril alone for compensated, naturally occurring mitral valve insufficiency. J Am Vet Med Assoc 2007; 231(7):1061–1069.

Hamlin RL, Nakayama T. Comparison of some pharmacokinetic parameters of 5 angiotensin-converting enzyme inhibitors in normal beagles. J Vet Intern Med 1998; 12:93–95.

Labato MA. Antihypertensives. In: Silverstein DC, Hopper K, eds. Small Animal Critical Care Medicine, 2nd edn. St Louis, MO: Elsevier Saunders, 2015; pp. 840–846.

Lucas C, Christie GA, Waring WS. Rapid onset of hemodynamic effects after angiotensin converting enzyme-inhibitor overdose: implications for initial patient triage. Emerg Med J 2006; 23:854–857.

Acknowledgment: The authors and editors acknowledge the prior contributions of Dr Catherine Adams, who authored this topic in the previous edition.

Authors: Stephanie Kleine, DVM, DACVVA; Jane Quandt, DVM, MS, DACVAA, DACVECC
Consulting Editor: Lynn R. Hovda, RPh, DVM, MS, DACVIM

chapter 15

Atypical Antipsychotics

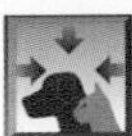

DEFINITION/OVERVIEW

- Atypical antipsychotics are a relatively new class of drugs for use in human medicine. May also be known as second-generation antipsychotics.
- Included are aripiprazole (Abilify®), asenapine (Saphris®), clozapine (Clozaril®), olanzapine (Zyprexa®), paliperidone (Invega®), quetiapine (Seroquel®), risperidone (Risperdal®), and ziprasidone (Geodon®).
- While these medications are commonly used in psychiatric disorders in humans, there is no current labeled use for them in veterinary medicine. Several of them have been used off-label in a limited manner for canine aggression.
- CNS depression or sedation, gastrointestinal disturbances (vomiting) hypotension, and tachycardia are the most common clinical signs noted in a toxicosis.

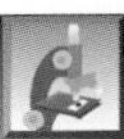

ETIOLOGY/PATHOPHYSIOLOGY

Mechanism of Action

- The exact mechanism of action of the atypical antipsychotics is unknown, but it is postulated that they are primarily antagonists at serotonin (5-HT_2) and dopamine (D_2) receptors.
- Many of the atypical antipsychotics exhibit varying degrees of antagonism at $alpha_1$ and H_1 receptors, which explains why they may cause orthostatic hypotension and somnolence, respectively.
- Risperidone, quetiapine, and paliperidone exhibit antagonism at $alpha_2$ receptors.
- Quetiapine and olanzapine exhibit antagonism at muscarinic receptors and may cause anticholinergic signs.

Pharmacokinetics – Absorption, Distribution, Metabolism, Excretion

- Based primarily on human literature; very little animal information is available.
- All of the atypical antipsychotics have good oral absorption.
- All undergo varying degrees of hepatic metabolism, some through the CYP450 isoenzymes.

Blackwell's Five-Minute Veterinary Consult Clinical Companion: Small Animal Toxicology, Second Edition.
Lynn R. Hovda, Ahna G. Brutlag, Robert H. Poppenga, and Katherine L. Peterson.

Companion website: www.fiveminutevet.com/toxicology

- All of the atypical antipsychotics are excreted in the urine either as unchanged drug or as metabolites. Forced diuresis or hemodialysis is unlikely to be beneficial as these drugs generally are highly protein bound and/or have a large volume of distribution.
- Risperidone (dog).
    - Oral absorption – rapid and extensive.
    - Oral bioavailability 80–100%.
    - Peak plasma parent compound 80 minutes; active metabolite 18 hours.
    - Protein-binding parent compound 92%; active metabolite 80%.

Toxicity

- Aripiprazole.
    - 0.25 and 0.6 mg/kg in a dog – lethargy and hyperactivity, respectively, have been observed.
    - 1.37 mg/kg in a cat – vomiting, lethargy and anorexia have been observed.
- Olanzapine.
    - 0.56 mg/kg in a dog – lethargy and vomiting have been observed.
    - Reported deaths in adult humans at 600 mg, but there have also been patients who have ingested more than 1 g and survived with supportive care.
- Quetiapine.
    - Toxic dose in animals has not been established.
    - Ingestion of 1300 mg in an 11-year-old child resulted in mild toxicosis and no cardiac abnormalities.
    - Adults have survived ingestions of 1200–24,000 mg.
    - One reported fatality in an adult human who ingested 10,800 mg.
- Risperidone.
    - Oral LD_{50} in dogs is 14–24 mg/kg.
    - 0.05 mg/kg in dogs – ataxia, weakness, tachycardia, agitation, hypotension, tremors, seizures have been observed.
    - Studies in the literature have revealed that animals should be able to survive a total dose of at least 5 mg with supportive care.
- Ziprasidone.
    - 0.88 mg/kg in a dog – anxiety, hyperactivity, and tachypnea have been observed.
    - Oral LD_{50} in dogs is 2000 mg/kg.
    - In adult humans, ingestions of up to 4480 mg have not resulted in serious toxicity.
    - Extrapyramidal syndrome (EPS) developed in an adult human after ingesting 12,800 mg.

Systems Affected

- Gastrointestinal – vomiting, diarrhea, hypersalivation.
- Nervous – sedation, depression, ataxia, disorientation, agitation, anxiety, hyperesthesia, tremors, seizures.
- Cardiovascular – hypotension, tachycardia.

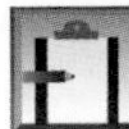

SIGNALMENT/HISTORY

- All breeds or veterinary species can be affected.

Risk Factors

- Animals with the following underlying conditions are at risk.
    - Seizure disorders.
    - Cardiovascular disease.
    - Pregnant or nursing.
    - Patients with significant renal impairment may have reduced drug clearance.

Historical Findings

- Signs typically develop within an hour but may be delayed for up to a few hours, due to the lag in time to peak plasma concentrations or extended release formulations.
- These drugs have long half-lives, so prolonged supportive care may be needed if early decontamination does not occur.

Interaction with Drugs, Nutrients, or Environment

- Drugs that also prolong the QTc interval or widen the QRS interval.
- Metoclopramide may increase the risk for extrapyramidal syndrome.

CLINICAL FEATURES

- The most common signs are vomiting, CNS depression, hypotension, and tachycardia.
- Other signs, occurring less often and which may be drug dependent, include the development of ataxia, agitation, anxiety, hyperactivity, diarrhea, tremors, seizures, and possible arrhythmias.

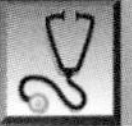

DIFFERENTIAL DIAGNOSIS

- CNS depressants – benzodiazepines, phenothiazines, barbiturates, marijuana, ivermectin, antidepressants, muscle relaxants.
- Cardiovascular drugs – ACE inhibitors, beta-blockers, calcium channel blockers.

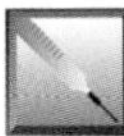

DIAGNOSTICS

- Patient history and clinical signs should be used for diagnosis.
- Serum electrolytes may show hyponatremia, hypokalemia.

Pathological Findings

- No specific findings.

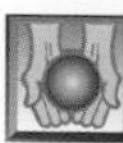

THERAPEUTICS

- The goals of treatment are to prevent absorption, address neurological and cardiovascular status, and provide supportive care.

Detoxification

- Induce emesis if ingestion occurred within the past 30–60 minutes and the dog is asymptomatic.
- If emesis was not induced at home, perform in DVM's office within 60 minutes of ingestion.
    - Note: risperidone may block the emetic effects of apomorphine.
- Activated charcoal with a cathartic may be given for one dose. Generally most beneficial when given within 60 minutes of ingestion.
- Multidose activated charcoal without a cathartic may be considered when signficant ingestion of sustained-release formulations has occurred.

Appropriate Health Care

- If clinical signs are present, hospitalize until asymptomatic, generally about 12–24 hours.
- Maintain hydration and monitor for hypernatremia if using multiple-dose activated charcoal.
- Monitor blood pressure and heart rate.
- Monitor for temperature alterations and treat appropriately.
- ECG for arrhythmias.

Antidotes

- There is no specific antidote available.

Drugs of Choice

- IV fluids to improve renal perfusion and for correction of hypotension.
- Pressor agents only after well hydrated and when hypotension is severe and does not respond to IV fluids. Use of norepinephrine and phenylephrine may be preferred over epinephrine or dopamine due to their beta-adrenergic effects worsening hypotension in the face of drug-induced alpha blockade.
    - Norepinephrine 0.05–0.3 μg/kg/min IV CRI.
    - Phenylephrine 1–3 μg/kg/min IV CRI.
- Agitation and CNS stimulation.
    - Diazepam 0.5–1 mg/kg IV.
    - Phenobarbital 3–5 mg/kg IV PRN.

- Extrapyramidal syndrome.
  - Diphenhydramine 2–4 mg/kg IM or PO.
- Intravenous lipid emulsion (ILE) may be considered in severe cases as at least some of the atypical antipsychotics are lipid soluble.
  - Bolus 1.5 mL/kg of a 20% solution over 3–5 minutes; follow with a 0.25 mL/kg/min CRI for 30–60 minutes.
  - Consider repeating bolus and CRI in 4 hours if serum is clear.
  - If serum is clear or once serum clears, continue repeating the bolus and CRI every 4 hours until animal shows significant improvement or has not responded after three doses.

Precautions/Interactions

- In humans there are many potential drug interactions. While many of them are theoretical and focus on concern for worsening QT interval (not commonly noted in veterinary patients with atypical antipsychotic toxicoses), they include several common medications used in veterinary medicine. These include but are not limited to sodium channel-blocking or potassium-blocking antiarrhythmics, TCAs, dolansetron, ondansetron, phenothiazine tranquilizers, cisapride, ketoconazole, itraconazole, sulfamethoxazole trimethoprim and metronidazole.
- Both atypical antipsychotics and cyproheptadine are antagonists at the serotonin 5-HT_{2A} receptor. Therefore cyproheptadine is unlikely to be helpful in treating atypical antipsychotic toxicoses.
- For those drugs that are metabolized via hepatic CYP450 isoenzymes, there may be interactions with drugs that affect CYP450 (phenobarbital).
- There is some controversy about whether true neuroleptic malignant syndrome, found in human beings and other species, occurs in dogs and cats. Some veterinarians agree, some disagree.

Nursing Care

- Ensure urine output.
- Frequent TPRs.

Prevention

- Pet owners should be advised to keep medications out of the reach of pets, preferably stored in locked cabinets or cabinets located high off the ground.

COMMENTS

Client Education

- Ensure the home environment is safe for the pet's return.
- Readmit if clinical signs recur or worsen even after proper treatment.

Patient Monitoring

- Serum chemistry for renal and hepatic values.
- Electrolytes, especially potassium and sodium.
- ECG as needed.

Prevention/Avoidance

- Store medications in locked or difficult-to-reach cabinets.
- Keep purses and full shopping bags off the floor and away from easy-to-reach places.
- Do not leave medications on countertops that may be accessible to a pet.

Possible Complications

- Rhabdomyolysis if seizures or tremors occur and are left untreated.

Expected Course and Prognosis

- Clinical signs typically develop within 1 hour, but may take up to several hours.
- Signs resolve in 12–24 hours but may be prolonged when sustained-release products have been ingested.
- Prognosis for recovery is excellent, especially with early treatment. Appropriately treated animals rarely die after ingestion of atypical antipsychotics.

Synonyms

Aripiprazole (Abilify®), asenapine (Saphris®), clozapine (Clozaril®), olanzapine (Zyprexa®), paliperidone (Invega®), quetiapine (Seroquel®), risperidone (Risperdal®), and ziprasidone (Geodonv)

Abbreviations

See Appendix 1 for a complete list.

Suggested Reading

Ader M, Kim SP, Catalano KJ, et al. Metabolic dysregulation with atypical antipsychotics occurs in the absence of underlying disease: a placebo-controlled study of olanzapine and risperidone in dogs. Diabetes 2005; 54(3):862–871.

Depoortere R, Barret-Gevoz C, Bardin L, et al. Apomorphine-induced emesis in dogs: differential sensitivity to established and novel dopamine D2/5HT(1A) antipsychotic compounds. Eur J Pharmacol 2008; 597:1–3.

Juurlink D. Antipsychotics. In: Flomenbaum NE, Goldfrank LR, Hoffman RS, et al., eds. Goldfrank's Toxicologic Emergencies, 8th edn. New York: McGraw-Hill, 2006; pp. 1039–1051.

Acknowledgment: The authors and editors acknowledge the prior contributions of Kelly M. Sioris, who authored this topic in the previous edition.

Author: Kirsten E. Waratuke, DVM

Consulting Editor: Lynn R. Hovda, RPh, DVM, MS, DACVIM

chapter 16

Baclofen

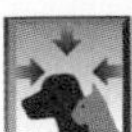

DEFINITION/OVERVIEW

- Baclofen is a centrally acting skeletal muscle relaxant that mimics gamma-aminobutyric acid (GABA) within the spinal cord.
- Baclofen is used to control spasticity and pain in people with multiple sclerosis and spinal disorders.
- It is used extra-label in dogs to treat urinary retention by reducing urethral resistance.
- Clinical signs from overdose can be categorized by affected body systems: CNS, GI, CV, respiratory, and urogenital. Generalized malaise may be noted. The most common body system affected is the CNS.
- The most life-threatening clinical signs are dyspnea, respiratory depression, respiratory arrest, and nonresponsive seizures.

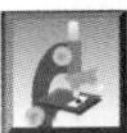

ETIOLOGY/PATHOPHYSIOLOGY

Mechanism of Action

- Baclofen binds to $GABA_b$ receptors and inhibits the influx of calcium, which prevents the release of the excitatory neurotransmitters (glutamate, aspartate, and substance P).
- The $GABA_b$ receptor also opens selective K^+ channels, allowing an outward ion flux. Stimulation of GABA results in hyperpolarization and increased inhibitory tone.
- Baclofen can cause excitatory stimulation that may result in seizure activity.

Pharmacokinetics – Absorption, Distribution, Metabolism, Excretion

- Rapidly and completely absorbed from the GIT.
- Low protein binding and a wide volume of distribution.
- Plasma half-life is 2–6 hours.
- Approximately 80% of the drug is eliminated unchanged in the urine with 20% undergoing deamination in the liver and biliary excretion. There is also some deamination in the renal tubules.

Blackwell's Five-Minute Veterinary Consult Clinical Companion: Small Animal Toxicology, Second Edition.
Lynn R. Hovda, Ahna G. Brutlag, Robert H. Poppenga, and Katherine L. Peterson.

Companion website: www.fiveminutevet.com/toxicology

Toxicity

- In one study, the lowest reported dose with clinical signs was 0.7mg/kg (this animal exhibited CNS depression, dyspnea, and hypothermia).
- In one study, the lowest dose at which death was reported was 2.3 mg/kg.

Systems Affected

- Respiratory – dyspnea, pulmonary edema, respiratory depression, respiratory arrest.
- Nervous – blindness, nystagmus, miosis, ataxia, vocalization, disorientation, coma, seizures.
- Gastrointestinal – hypersalivation, anorexia, vomiting, diarrhea.
- Cardiovascular – bradycardia, hypotension, tachycardia, pallor, arrhythmias.
- Renal/urological – urinary incontinence, urinary retention.
- Endocrine/metabolic – hypothermia.

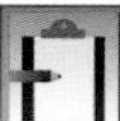

SIGNALMENT/HISTORY

- Any breed or age of dog is susceptible.
- Cats are especially susceptible to toxicity.
- Toxicosis most commonly occurs when the animal ingests the owner's medication.

Risk Factors

- Pet owners with medical conditions (e.g., multiple sclerosis and spinal disorders) are more likely to have baclofen in the house, propagating potential pet ingestion.

Historical Findings

- Evidence of chewed bottle, witnessed ingestion, inadvertent or accidental administration by pet owner.
- Generally, the diagnosis is made based on the history of ingestion coupled with clinical signs.

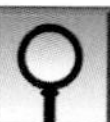

CLINICAL FEATURES

- Clinical signs after acute oral exposure may be rapid, occurring within minutes, or delayed for several hours.
- The duration of clinical signs can vary from several hours to several days due to the slow clearance from the CNS.
- Common clinical signs – vocalization, vomiting, ataxia, disorientation, salivation, depression, coma, weakness, generalized flaccid paralysis, recumbency, seizures, and hypothermia.

- Life-threatening signs – dyspnea, respiratory depression, and respiratory arrest secondary to paralysis of the diaphragm and intercostal muscles.
- Less frequent signs – hypotension, bradycardia, hypertension, cardiac arrhythmias, tachycardia, hyperactivity, agitation, tremors, panting, hyperesthesia, mydriasis, miosis, diarrhea, pulmonary edema, and death.

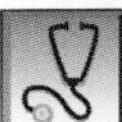

DIFFERENTIAL DIAGNOSIS

- Neuromuscular disease such as lower motor neuron disease (e.g., botulism, polyradiculitis, tick paralysis, *Toxoplasma*, and *Neospora*).
- Primary metabolic disease (renal, hepatic, hepatic encephalopathy, hypoglycemia, hypoadrenocorticism).
- Toxicants.
    - Benzodiazepines
    - Opiates and opioids
    - Barbiturates
    - Sedatives

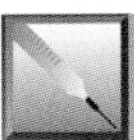

DIAGNOSTICS

- Baseline CBC, chemistry, UA.
- Arterial blood gas analysis to evaluate for hypoxemia, oxygenation, and ventilation.
- Pulse oximetry to evaluate for hypoxemia.
- End-tidal CO_2 to evaluate for hypercapnia or hypoventilation.
- Thoracic radiographs to evaluate for aspiration pneumonia secondary to severe sedation.

Pathological Findings

- No specific lesions associated. May see secondary aspiration pneumonia or atelectasis.

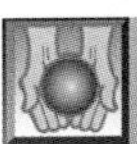

THERAPEUTICS

Detoxification

- Emesis if animal presents within 1 hour of ingestion. Emesis is contraindicated in symptomatic animals.
- Gastric lavage should be considered with large ingestions but should be done with the patient intubated with an inflated endotracheal tube to prevent secondary aspiration pneumonia.
- One dose of activated charcoal with a cathartic may be given.
- Elimination may be enhanced with fluid diuresis.

Appropriate Health Care

- Monitor for cardiac arrhythmias and hypothermia.
- Monitor for hypoventilation and aspiration pneumonia and treat appropriately with mechanical ventilation, oxygen support, IV antibiotic therapy, nebulization and coupage, and appropriate hydration.
- Ventilatory support may be required in those animals with severe respiratory depression and is required with respiratory failure.
- Hemodialysis and hemoperfusion can be used to shorten the serum elimination half-life of baclofen and decrease time to recovery. Hemodialysis is useful for the removal of drugs and toxins with a molecular weight of <1500 Daltons, a low volume of distribution, and minimal (<80%) plasma protein binding. It is the unbound portion of the drug that is removed via dialysis.

Antidote

- No specific antidote is available.

Drugs of Choice

- Atropine 0.02–0.04 mg/kg IM, IV, or SQ as needed for bradycardia.
- Diazepam is used to treat baclofen-induced seizures. The lowest effective dose should be used, due to profound sedation from both drugs.
    - Diazepam 0.25–0.5 mg/kg IV to effect.
    - Diazepam CRI 0.5–1 mg/kg/hour IV to effect.
- Refractory seizures may require treatment with propofol or general anesthesia.
    - Propofol 1–8 mg/kg IV to effect, followed by CRI dose of 0.1–0.6 mg/kg/hour if uncontrolled seizures.
- During drug withdrawal profound agitation may occur, which may necessitate sedation (acepromazine, diazepam, or midazolam).
    - Acepromazine 0.05–0.2 mg/kg, IV, SQ, IM q 4–6 hours PRN.
    - Diazepam 0.1–0.25 mg/kg, IV to effect, PRN.
    - Midazolam 0.1–0.5 mg/kg, IV or IM to effect, PRN.
- Cyproheptadine hydrochloride.
    - Dogs: 1.1 mg/kg PO or rectally q 4–6 hours as needed may help reduce vocalization or disorientation.
    - Cats: 2–4 mg *total* dose q 4–6 hours PRN.
- Intravenous lipid emulsion (ILE).
    - ILE 20% emulsion, administer 1.5 mL/kg IV bolus, followed by 0.25 mL/kg/min for 30–60 minutes (dose is extrapolated from human dosing).
    - The initial bolus can be repeated 1–2 times if no response to the initial bolus is obtained, not to exceed 8 mL/kg/day.

Alternative Drugs

- Flumazenil has been used with limited success in baclofen overdoses but may potentially precipitate seizures. Dose 0.01 mg/kg IV, to effect.

COMMENTS

Nursing Care

- Close patient monitoring with blood gas analysis, pulse oximetry, and $ETCO_2$ may be necessary to evaluate for hypoxemia or hypercapnia; the patient may need to be intubated and ventilated.
- Nursing care, including turning q 6 hours, lubricating eyes, keeping the patient dry and clean, passive range of motion of limbs, and soft bedding may be necessary for intubated or very sedate patients.

Follow-up

- Thoracic radiographs may be warranted to assess for development of aspiration pneumonia.

Client Education

- Clients should be made aware that even though baclofen is used in humans for muscle relaxation, it can be a severe toxin in pets and can lead to serious complications and potential death of the animal.

Possible Complications

- Aspiration pneumonia is a common complication due to clinical signs of vomiting, seizures, and paralysis of the diaphragm and intercostal muscles.

Expected Course and Prognosis

- In one study, ingestion was significantly lower in surviving dogs compared to the nonsurvivors.
- Hospitalized animals may require 5–7 days for a full recovery. Recovery occurs with no residual CNS effects.
- Prognosis is generally good with early and appropriate care but becomes poor with an extended period of time prior to veterinary care. Animals with seizures or aspiration pneumonia have a much more guarded prognosis.

See Also

- Benzodiazepines
- Opiates and Opioids

Abbreviations

See Appendix 1 for a complete list.

Suggested Reading

Khorzad R, Lee JA, Wheelan M, et al. Baclofen toxicosis in dogs and cats: 145 cases (2004–2010). J Am Vet Med Assoc 2012; 241(8):1059–1064.

Scott NE, Francey T, Jandrey K. Baclofen intoxication in a dog successfully treated with hemodialysis and hemoperfusion coupled with intensive supportive care. J Vet Emerg Crit Care 2007; 17:191–196.

Torre DM, Labato MA, Rossi T, et al. Treatment of a dog with severe baclofen intoxication using hemodialysis and mechanical ventilation. J Vet Emerg Crit Care 2008; 18:312–318.

Wismer T. Baclofen overdose in dogs. Vet Med 2004; 99:406–408.

Acknowledgment: The authors and editors acknowledge the prior contributions of Dr Jane Quandt, who authored this topic in the previous edition.

Author: Sarah L. Gray, DVM, DACVECC

Consulting Editor: Lynn R. Hovda, RPh, DVM, MS, DACVIM

chapter 17

Benzodiazepines

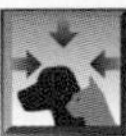

DEFINITION/OVERVIEW

- Several benzodiazepines are commonly used in veterinary medicine – diazepam (Valium®), midazolam (Versed®), alprazolam (Xanax®), and zolazepam found in combination with tiletamine, a dissociative agent (Telazol®).
- Many other benzodiazepines are used in human medicine (see table 17.1).
- Benzodiazepines are used as tranquilizing sedatives. They act as anxiolytics, muscle relaxants, and anticonvulsants.
- Benzodiazepines have a wide margin of safety.
- Common clinical signs of overdose are related to the CNS and include confusion, ataxia, and depression, but paradoxical reactions including agitation and aggression can be seen.

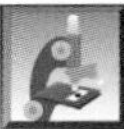

ETIOLOGY/PATHOPHYSIOLOGY

Mechanism of Action

- Benzodiazepines interact with the benzodiazepine receptors that modulate GABA, an inhibitory neurotransmitter.
- Chronic oral use of benzodiazepines in cats can result in fulminant hepatic failure through an unknown mechanism. Toxicity may relate to the cat's inherent deficiency in glucuronide conjugation and glutathione detoxification of reactive intermediates.

Pharmacokinetics – Absorption, Distribution, Metabolism, Excretion

- Well absorbed orally.
- All are highly protein bound and lipid soluble.
- Peak plasma levels generally occur between 30 and 120 minutes.
- Widely distributed to brain, liver, and spleen; poorly to fat and muscle.
- Metabolized in liver to active and inactive metabolites.
- Half-life elimination of diazepam (cat) after IV dosing – 5.46 hours.

Blackwell's Five-Minute Veterinary Consult Clinical Companion: Small Animal Toxicology, Second Edition.
Lynn R. Hovda, Ahna G. Brutlag, Robert H. Poppenga, and Katherine L. Peterson.

Companion website: www.fiveminutevet.com/toxicology

TABLE 17.1. Benzodiazepine drugs currently on the market.

Generic name	Trade name	Peak plasma level in hours (human data)	T ½ in hours (human data)	Speed of onset
Alprazolam	Xanax	1–2	6.3–26.9	Intermediate
Chlordiazepoxide	Librium	0.5–4	5–30	Intermediate
Clonazepam	Klonopin	1–2	18–50	Intermediate
Clorazepate	Tranxene	1–2	40–50	Fast
Diazepam	Valium	0.5–2	20–80	Very fast
Estazolam	Prosom	2	8–28	Fast
Flurazepam	Dalmane	0.5–1	2–3	Fast
Lorazepam	Ativan	2–4	10–20	Intermediate
Midazolam	Versed	0.28–0.83	2.2–6.8	Very fast
Oxazepam	Serax	2–4	5–20	Slow
Quazepam	Doral	1–2	41	Fast
Temazepam	Restoril	1.6–2	3.5–18.4	Fast
Triazolam	Halcion	1–2	1.5–5.5	Fast

- Half-life elimination of nordiazepam (active diazepam metabolite) (cat) after IV dosing – 21.3 hours.
- Conjugated with glucuronide and excreted in urine.
- Duration of action is specific for each benzodiazepine compound.

Toxicity

- Overdose as a single exposure is rarely life threatening in healthy animals.
- Generally, oral diazepam overdoses of >20 mg/kg are considered significant. Other more potent benzodiazepines are proportionately more toxic.
- Chronic exposure of more than one dose may be life threatening in the cat.

Systems Affected

- Nervous – CNS depression, dysphoria, ataxia, excitement, aggression.
- Respiratory – respiratory depression.
- Cardiovascular – bradycardia, hypotension.
- Endocrine/metabolic – hypothermia from sedation.
- Hepatic – fulminant hepatic necrosis (cats only); appears as anorexia, lethargy, vomiting, dehydration, hypothermia, icterus, increased liver enzymes, coagulopathy, hypoglycemia.

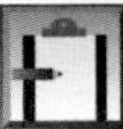

SIGNALMENT/HISTORY

- Any age or breed of dog or cat can be affected.
- Overdose usually occurs due to iatrogenic administration of an improper dose or ingestion of medication.

Risk Factors

- Benzodiazepines present in the household may pose an increased risk of exposure to pets.
- Pediatric, geriatric, or debilitated patients with underlying metabolic disease may have prolonged duration of effects from toxicosis, or even from therapeutic dosing.
- Cats given oral, chronic diazepam for behavior modification treatment may develop acute fulminant hepatic necrosis.

Historical Findings

- Witnessed exposure by pet owner.
- Pet owner may find chewed pill vial or suspect missing pill.
- Clinical symptoms of ataxia, sedation, agitation, and dysphoria may be noted by the pet owner.

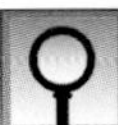

CLINICAL FEATURES

- Common clinical signs include CNS depression, ataxia, confusion, disorientation, agitation, and aggression.
- As ingested dose increases, risks for hypotension, hypothermia, coma, and seizures occur.
- In approximately 40–50% of cases, paradoxical stimulation and excitation occur in both dogs and cats.

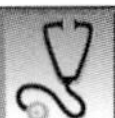

DIFFERENTIAL DIAGNOSIS

- Primary metabolic disease (hepatic encephalopathy, hypoglycemia).
- Primary neurological disease.
- Toxicants.
    - Sedation.
        - Alcohols and glycols (e.g. ethanol, methanol, ethylene glycol)
        - Barbiturates
        - Marijuana
        - Opioids
        - Phenothiazines

- Agitation.
    - Amphetamines
    - Antidepressants (serotonin syndrome)
    - Cocaine
    - Pseudoephedrine

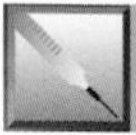

DIAGNOSTICS

- Baseline CBC, chemistry, UA to evaluate underlying metabolic disease.
- The Quick Screen Pro Multi Drug Screening Test is a human testing kit that has been validated by GC/MS for use in animals. It may provide a rapid and accurate diagnosis if the drug is present in high enough concentrations and the time frame is appropriate.
- Urine or serum can be submitted specifically for GC/MS or LC/MS, but the results will take several days to be returned and will only indicate exposure.
- In cats suspected of having acute hepatic necrosis, a coagulation panel should be done to evaluate PT/PTT.

Pathological Findings

- No histological changes are expected in acute overdoses.
- Histology of the feline liver shows severe, acute to subacute, lobular to massive hepatic necrosis.

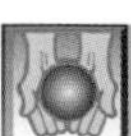

THERAPEUTICS

- For exposures of <20 mg/kg PO diazepam or equivalent for other benzodiazepines, many animals can be monitored at home. Animals should be confined to areas where they cannot injure themselves, e.g., by falling down stairs.
- Treatment consists of general supportive measures, early decontamination, and if necessary, administration of the reversal agent flumazenil.

Detoxification

- Emesis with extreme caution due to rapid onset of signs.
- Activated charcoal with a cathartic × one dose for large ingestions although an increased risk of aspiration should be considered.

Appropriate Health Care

- Monitor body temperature and blood pressure; support appropriately with warming methods and IV fluid therapy. Monitor for severe CNS or respiratory depression; if indicated, consider the use of flumazenil.
- Cats suffering from hepatic failure due to oral diazepam need aggressive treatment.

Antidote

- Flumazenil (Romazicon®) is the specific antidote for benzodiazepine overdose but should be used only in cases where CNS depression or agitation is severe. Flumazenil rapidly reverses the sedative and muscle relaxant effects of the benzodiazepine agonists. Effects are usually seen within 5 minutes. Seizures have been associated with the use of flumazenil.
  - Dose: flumazenil 0.01 mg/kg IV to effect, repeat PRN. If a long-acting benzodiazepine has been ingested, repeated doses of flumazenil may be necessary, due to its short duration of action (1–2 hours).

Drugs of Choice

- IV fluids as needed to treat hypotension, maintain perfusion, and correct dehydration. A balanced crystalloid should be used. If evidence of hepatic failure, LRS should be avoided.
- If the animal is experiencing paradoxical stimulation (e.g., agitation, aggression), treatment with additional benzodiazepines (e.g., diazepam) is contraindicated. An alternative sedative or anxiolytic should be used.
  - Acepromazine 0.05–0.2 mg/kg, IV, SQ, IM PRN.
  - Medetomidine 1–10 µg/kg, IV, SQ, IM PRN.
  - Diphenhydramine 2–4 mg/kg IM or PO.
- Treatment for hepatic failure consists of IV fluid therapy, antibiotic therapy, glucose and potassium supplementation, administration of both water-soluble vitamins (e.g., vitamin B) and vitamin K, nutritional support, hepatoprotectants (SAMe), and potentially, blood plasma transfusions (if coagulopathic or evidence of hemorrhagic shock).

Precautions/Interactions

- CNS stimulants such as caffeine should be avoided.
- Diazepam is not water soluble, and the parenteral formula contains 40% propylene glycol and 10% ethanol. It is very irritating, painful, and poorly absorbed when given IM. Excessive propylene glycol exposure in cats may cause Heinz body formation.

Follow-up

- Cats that survive diazepam-induced acute hepatic necrosis should have liver enzymes checked every 5–7 days until clinically normal.

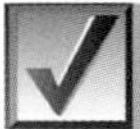

COMMENTS

Client Education

- Owners should be advised not to use their own medicines to treat their pets and to keep them out of the reach of pets.

Patient Monitoring

- While hospitalized, excessively sedate patients should have blood pressure, ECG, TPR, and ventilatory status closely monitored.

Prevention/Avoidance

- Owners should be informed about the risks of benzodiazepines in pets, and keep them out of reach, particularly in the bedroom (sleep aid medication placed on bedroom table).

Expected Course and Prognosis

- Once decontaminated, animals generally only need to be monitored for 4–8 hours. If no clinical signs develop, the patient can be monitored at home. If signs develop, they should be monitored until clinical signs have resolved (typically 8–24 hours depending on the drug involved).
- In those animals experiencing a single overdose exposure, the prognosis is excellent.
- In those cats experiencing idiosyncratic hepatic failure due to repeated doses of oral diazepam, the prognosis is poor to guarded. Based on this, oral chronic use of benzodiazepines should be avoided in cats.

See Also

Ethylene Glycol and Diethylene Glycol
Opiates and Opioids
Nonbenzodiazepine Sleep Aids

Abbreviations

See Appendix 1 for a complete list.

Suggested Reading

Center SA, Elston TH, Rowland PH, et al. Fulminant hepatic failure associated with oral administration of diazepam in 11 cats. J Am Vet Med Assoc 1996; 209:618–625.
Lemke KA. Anticholinergics and sedatives. In: Tranquilli WJ, Thurmon JC, Grimm KA, eds. Lumb & Jones Veterinary Anesthesia and Analgesia, 4th edn. Ames, IA: Blackwell, 2007; pp. 203–239.
Malouin A, Boiler M. Sedatives, muscle relaxants, and opioids toxicity. In: Silverstein DC, Hopper K, eds. Small Animal Critical Care Medicine. St Louis, MO: Elsevier, 2009; pp. 350–356.

Acknowledgment: The authors and editors aknowledge the prior contribution of Jane Quandt, DVM, MS, DACVA, DACVEEC, who authored this chapter in a previous edition.
Author: Eric Dunayer, MS, VMD, DABT, DABVT
Consulting Editor: Lynn R. Hovda, RPh, DVM, MS, DACVIM

chapter 18

Beta$_2$ Receptor Agonists (Albuterol and Others)

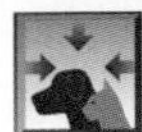

DEFINITION/OVERVIEW

- Albuterol and other beta$_2$ agonist medications are used in human and veterinary medicine to treat bronchoconstriction associated with diseases such as asthma and chronic obstructive pulmonary disease.
- Formulations include immediate- and extended-release tablets, an oral syrup, powders and solutions for inhalation, and pressurized metered-dose inhalers for aerosolization. All are used off-label in veterinary species.
- Overdose often results in tachyarrhythmias, CNS stimulation or lethargy, tachypnea, and hypokalemia.

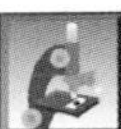

ETIOLOGY/PATHOPHYSIOLOGY

Mechanism of Action

- Activation of beta$_2$ receptors stimulates adenylyl cyclase to produce cyclic adenosine monophosphate (cAMP) which then inhibits phosphorylation of myosin. Inhibition of Na^+/K^+-ATPase also occurs.
- Therapeutically, relaxation of bronchial, vascular, and uterine smooth muscle results.
- Toxicologically, overstimulation of beta$_2$ receptors can cause vasodilation, hypotension, and reflex tachycardia; loss of beta$_2$ selectivity with overdose results in excessive beta$_1$ activity (increased force and rate of contraction); concurrent release of catecholamines further stimulates these receptors.

Pharmacokinetics – Absorption, Distribution, Metabolism, Excretion

- Absorption is generally rapid and complete within minutes with inhalation. Effects are expected within 30 minutes with oral formulations. Peak plasma levels occur within 2 hours in people ingesting immediate-release tablets and within 5–7 hours with extended-release tablets.
- Albuterol is widely distributed. It crosses the blood–brain barrier and also the placenta.

Blackwell's Five-Minute Veterinary Consult Clinical Companion: Small Animal Toxicology, Second Edition.
Lynn R. Hovda, Ahna G. Brutlag, Robert H. Poppenga, and Katherine L. Peterson.

Companion website: www.fiveminutevet.com/toxicology

- Metabolism occurs via hepatic sulfation.
- Excretion is primarily renal with a small amount of fecal elimination. Plasma half-life is ~3–4 hours (range of 1.7–7.1 hours).

Toxicity

- Dogs and cats: signs are expected with exposures >0.1 mg/kg of oral and liquid formulations.
- Dosages associated with metered-dose inhalers are rarely known. Any puncture of a pressurized inhaler warrants immediate veterinary evaluation.
- Rodents: PO LD_{50} >2 g/kg.

Systems Affected

- Cardiovascular.
  - Excessive $beta_2$ stimulation can result in vasodilation, hypotension, and reflex tachycardia.
  - Excessive $beta_1$ stimulation results in severe tachycardia (sinus tachycardia most common) and possibly mild increases in blood pressure.
  - Myocardial hypoxia can lead to more serious arrhythmias – VPCs, ventricular tachycardia, atrioventricular block, etc.
  - Rarely, chordae tendinae may rupture and lead to pulmonary edema.
- Nervous.
  - Excessive beta stimulation of the brain results in anxiety, restlessness, apprehension, agitation, and rarely seizures.
- Respiratory.
  - Beta stimulation can result in bronchodilation, tachypnea/panting.
  - Respiratory alkalosis is possible.
- Neuromuscular/musculoskeletal.
  - Tremors can occur due to excess stimulation of skeletal muscle.
  - Weakness and lethargy can occur due to catecholamine depletion with prolonged/untreated toxicosis, severe hypokalemia, and poor cardiac output.
- Endocrine/metabolic.
  - Intracellular translocation of potassium leading to significant hypokalemia can cause weakness and lethargy, and potentiate arrhythmias.
- Gastrointestinal.
  - Mild vomiting may be seen.
  - Foreign body potential should be evaluated with history of dietary indiscretion.

SIGNALMENT/HISTORY

- No breed or sex predilection.
- No genetic basis for toxicosis.

- Young, indiscriminate, orally fixated, bored and/or inquisitive dogs are typically involved with accidental exposures.
- Cats are uncommonly exposed.

Risk Factors

- Patients with underlying cardiac conditions are at greater risk for significant complications from toxicosis.
- Environmental factors include unattended dogs with access to medications.

Historical Findings

- Owners may report a pounding/racing heart, panting, shaking, weakness, vomiting, bloodshot eyes, and restlessness/hyperactivity.
- History may also include evidence of exposure such as a punctured inhaler or chewed pill vial/drug ampule. See Fig. 18.1.

Location and Circumstances of Poisoning

- Exposures typically occur in unattended household pets with access to medications and a propensity for dietary indiscretion.

Interactions with Drugs, Nutrients, or Environment

The following drugs can exacerbate the toxicosis of beta$_2$ agonist drugs.

- Sympathomimetic drugs such as phenylpropanolamine, pseudoephedrine, phenylephrine, ephedrine, monoamine oxidase inhibitors

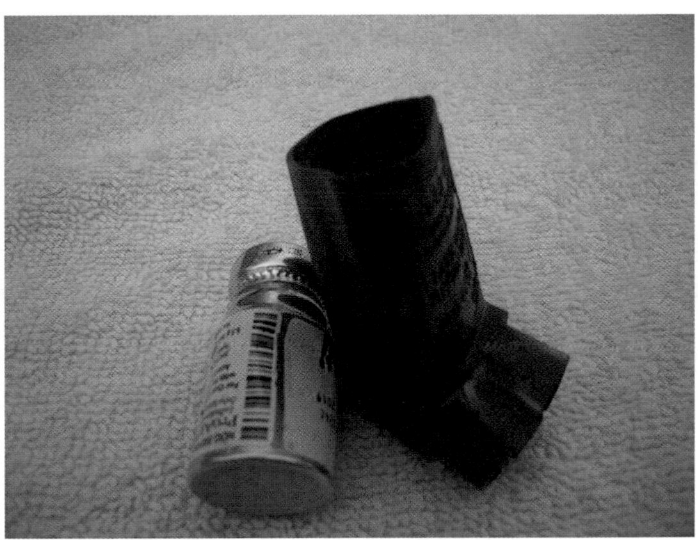

Fig. 18.1. Chewed and discharged inhaler. Photo courtesy Tyne K. Hovda.

- Methylxanthines (caffeine, theobromine)
- Amphetamine-based drugs
- Tricyclic antidepressants
- Thyroid hormones
- Selective serotonin reuptake inhibitors
- Calcium channel blockers
- Cardiac glycosides
- Loop diuretics (hypokalemia)

CLINICAL FEATURES

- Onset of signs within minutes of accidental exposure to inhalers is common. Peak effects may be delayed 2 hours with immediate-release tablets or as long as 5–7 hours with extended-release formulations.
- Physical exam may reveal apprehension, agitation, hyperactivity, weakness, lethargy, sinus tachycardia or other arrhythmias, tachypnea, hyper- or hypotension, changes in pulse quality (weakness, deficits), tremors, hyperthermia, mild vomiting, scleral injection, and/or conjunctivitis.

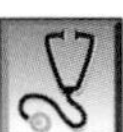

DIFFERENTIAL DIAGNOSIS

- Shock (hypovolemic, septic, cardiogenic).
- Neoplasia.
- Hypokalemia: hyperaldosteronism, diabetic ketoacidosis.
- Intoxications.
    - See Interactions with Drugs, Nutrients, or Environment.
    - Metaldehyde.
    - Hops.

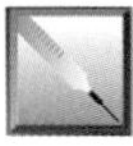

DIAGNOSTICS

- Continuous ECG and intermittent blood pressure monitoring.
- Evaluation of potassium and phosphorus on presentation, with aggressive supplementation, if any significant ECG changes, and as the toxicosis resolves (potential for rebound hyperkalemia).
- Thoracic radiographs if any known underlying cardiac or respiratory disease, if indicated based on auscultation, and/or if patient is dyspneic.
- Acid–base status with lactate determination in severely affected patients.
- CBC/chemistry panel not expected to be significantly abnormal. PCV/TS can guide fluid therapy. Mild hyper- or hypoglycemia may be seen. AST and CK may be elevated from tremors.

Pathological Findings

- Rupture of chordae tendinae and pulmonary edema may be evident grossly.
- Myocardial necrosis and fibrosis are possible histologically.

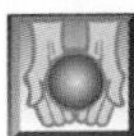

THERAPEUTICS

Detoxification

- Not indicated for exposures to pressurized inhalers or liquid formulations due to rapid onset of signs.
- Induction of emesis is indicated in the asymptomatic patient known or suspected to have ingested a toxic dosage of tablets. Apomorphine (0.03 mg/kg IV or 0.25 mg/kg in conjunctival sac) or 3% hydrogen peroxide PO (1 mL/lb up to maximum of 45 mL) can be used to induce emesis.
- A single dose of activated charcoal may prevent signs if given within 30 minutes of ingestion of immediate-release tablets or within 1–2 hours of ingestion of extended-release tablets.

Appropriate Health Care

- Hospitalization is indicated until HR, rhythm, CNS status, and electrolytes are within normal limits.
- Administer intravenous crystalloids to effect for hypotension. Caution with aggressive fluid therapy if hypertension or significant arrhythmias are present.
- Monitor TPR, heart rhythm, pulse quality, and CNS status.
- Monitor serum potassium and phosphorus, in particular, on presentation, if ECG changes, with aggressive supplementation, and as toxicosis wanes.

Antidote

- No specific antidote exists.

Drugs of Choice

- Beta-blockers (if HR >160 bpm in large dogs or >180–200 bpm in small dogs).
  - Propranolol 0.02 mg/kg IV. Repeat if no response within 20 minutes. This is the preferred beta-blocker due to its nonselectivity (beta$_1$ and beta$_2$ effects).
  - Esmolol 0.25–0.5 mg/kg IV slow bolus then 0.05–1 mg/kg/min CRI to maintain target heart rate.
- Benzodiazepines (PRN for CNS stimulation, tremors).
  - Diazepam, 0.5 mg/kg IV to effect.
  - Midazolam, 0.2–0.4 mg/kg IV or IM to effect.

- Potassium chloride (supplement in IV fluids based on degree of hypokalemia; rate of administration should not exceed 0.5 mEq/kg/hour).
    - 20 mEq/L if K^+ = 3.6–5.5 mEq/L
    - 30 mEq/L if K^+ = 3.1–3.5 mEq/L
    - 40 mEq/L if K^+ = 2.6–3 mEq/L
    - 60 mEq/L if K^+ = 2.1–2.5 mEq/L
    - 80 mEq/L if K^+ <2 mEq/L
- Potassium phosphate, 0.01–0.06 mmol/kg/hour IV in saline or dextrose, if phosphorus <1 mg/dL.
- Lidocaine 2 mg/kg slow IV bolus followed by 30–50 µg/kg/min IV CRI (dog) to effect for ventricular tachycardia.

Precautions/Interactions

- Caution with loop diuretics (worsening hypokalemia).

Alternative Drugs

- Oral beta-blockers may be tried if injectable formulations are not available.
    - Propranolol 0.1–0.2 mg/kg PO q 8 hours (dog); 2.5–10 mg PO (total) q 8 hours (cat).
    - Metoprolol 0.2 mg/kg PO q 12–24 hours (dog); 2–15 mg PO (total) q 8 hours (cat).

Nursing Care

- Catheter maintenance.
- Close monitoring of CV and neuromuscular status.

Diet

- NPO if vomiting.

Activity

- Restrict activity and minimize stimulation.

Surgical Considerations

- Postpone general anesthesia and surgical procedures (for example, non life threatening foreign body removal) until toxicosis wanes.

COMMENTS

Patient Monitoring

- Continuous ECG and intermittent BP monitoring.
- Close monitoring of CNS and neuromuscular status throughout the toxicosis.
- Repeat monitoring of serum potassium and phosphorus as above.

Prevention/Avoidance

- Avoid access to medications for pets (crate or isolate pets when unsupervised; store medications high up or in closed/locked cabinet).
- Follow labeled directions if beta$_2$ agonists are prescribed for a pet.
- Adequately exercise pets prior to being left unattended and/or provide enrichment while alone.

Possible Complications

- Potential for more serious arrhythmias increases with longer duration of significant tachycardia/myocardial hypoxia. Cardiac arrest is possible.
- Potential for a period of catecholamine depletion and prolonged weakness with delayed treatment of stimulatory signs.
- Potential for myocardial necrosis/fibrosis.
- Aggressive supplementation of potassium can result in rebound hyperkalemia as the toxicosis wanes.
- Thermal damage of the oral cavity and subsequent airway compromise has been reported in a Boxer noted to have chewed on a metered-dose inhaler.

Expected Course and Prognosis

- Signs typically resolve within 12–24 hours.
- Prognosis is excellent with prompt treatment in an otherwise healthy patient.

Synonyms

Albuterol = salbutamol

Abbreviations

See Appendix 1 for a complete list.

Suggested Reading

Mackenzie SD, Blois S, Hayes G, Vince AR. Oral thermal injury associated with puncture of a salbutamol metered-dose inhaler in a dog. J Vet Emerg Crit Care 2012; 22(4):494–497.

Mensching D, Volmer PA. Breathe with ease when managing beta-2 agonist inhaler toxicoses in dogs. Vet Med 2007; 369–373.

Sobczak B. Albuterol toxicosis. In: Côté E, ed. Clinical Veterinary Advisor: Dogs and Cats, 3rd edn. St Louis, MO: Elsevier, 2015; pp. 45–46.

Author: Donna Mensching, DVM, MS, DABVT, DABT
Consulting Editor: Lynn R. Hovda, RPh, DVM, MS, DACVIM

chapter 19

Beta Receptor Antagonists (Beta-Blockers)

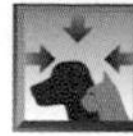

DEFINITION/OVERVIEW

- β-receptor antagonists (generally referred to as "beta-blockers") are class II antidysrhythmics commonly used in animals to treat hypertrophic or hypertrophic-obstructive cardiomyopathy in cats and tachydysrhythmias, systemic hypertension, and glaucoma in cats and dogs.
- This class of drugs has a narrow margin of safety and can cause clinical signs such as bradycardia, hypotension, hypoglycemia, hyperkalemia, and secondary kidney failure.
- Treatment involves supportive care for hypotension and bradycardia and can include IV fluids, atropine, intravenous fat emulsion, high-dose insulin, and dextrose therapy. Vasopressors may be ineffective and may worsen prognosis.

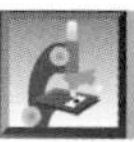

ETIOLOGY/PATHOPHYSIOLOGY

Mechanism of Action

- β-adrenergic antagonists work primarily by blocking the β-adrenergic receptors.
- Negative inotropic and chronotropic actions include decreased sinus heart rate, slowed AV conduction, diminished cardiac output at rest and during exercise, decreased myocardial oxygen demand, reduced blood pressure.
- B_1 receptors are primarily located in the heart, eye, and kidney. Blockade of B_1 receptors results in bradycardia.
- B_2 receptors are found in bronchial smooth muscle, the gastrointestinal tract, pancreas, liver, skeletal muscle, and blood vessels. Blockade of B_2 receptors may result in bronchospasm (especially in cats or dogs with underlying airway disease) and peripheral vasodilation resulting in hypotension.

Pharmacokinetics – Absorption, Distribution, Metabolism, Excretion

- See table 19.1 for human information.

Blackwell's Five-Minute Veterinary Consult Clinical Companion: Small Animal Toxicology, Second Edition.
Lynn R. Hovda, Ahna G. Brutlag, Robert H. Poppenga, and Katherine L. Peterson.

Companion website: www.fiveminutevet.com/toxicology

TABLE 19.1. Human pharmacokinetic information for beta receptor antagonist drugs.

	Adrenergic blocking Activity	Partial agonist activity (ISA)	Membrane stabilizing activity	Vasodilating property	Lipid solubility	Protein binding	Oral bioavailability	Half-life (h)	Metabolism	Volume of distribution (L/kg)
Acebutolol	β_1	Yes	Yes	No	Low	25%	40%	2–4	Hepatic/renal	1.2
Atenolol	β_1	No	No	No	Low	<5%	40–50%	5–9	Renal	1
Betaxolol (ophthalmic and tabs)	β_1	No	Yes	Yes (calcium channel blockade)	Low	50%	80–90%	14–22	Hepatic/renal	NA
Bisoprolol	β_1	No	No	No	Low	30%	80%	9–12	Hepatic/renal	NA
Bucindolol	β_1, β_2	β_2 agonism		Yes (β_2 agonism)	Moderate		30%	8 ± 4.5	Hepatic	NA
Carteolol (ophthalmic)	β_1, β_2	Yes	No	Yes (β_2 agonism and nitric oxide mediated)	Low	30%	85%	5–6	Renal	NA
Carvedilol	α_1, β_1, β_2	No		Yes (α_1 blockade)	Moderate	~98%	25–35%	6–10	Hepatic	115
Celiprolol	α_2, β_1	β_2 agonism		Yes (β_2 agonism)	Low	22–24%	30–70%	5	Hepatic	NA
Esmolol	β_1	No	No	No	Low	50%	NA	~8 min	RBC esterases	2
Labetalol	α_1, β_1, β_2	No	Low	Yes (α_1 antagonism)	Moderate	50%	20–33%	4–8	Hepatic	9

(Continued)

TABLE 19.1. *Continued*

	Adrenergic blocking Activity	Partial agonist activity (ISA)	Membrane stabilizing activity	Vasodilating property	Lipid solubility	Protein binding	Oral bioavailability	Half-life (h)	Metabolism	Volume of distribution (L/kg)
Levobunolol (ophthalmic)	β_1, β_2	No	No	No	NA	NA	NA	6	NA	NA
Metipranolol (ophthalmic)	β_1, β_2	No	No	No	NA	NA	NA	3–4	NA	NA
Metoprolol (long-acting form available)	β_1	No	Low	No	Moderate	10%	40–50%	3–4	Hepatic	4
Nadolol	β_1, β_2	No	No	No	Low	20–30%	30–35%	10–24	Renal	2
Nebivolol	β_1	No		Yes (nitric oxide mediated?)	Moderate	98%	12–96%	8–32	Hepatic	10–40
Oxprenolol	β_1, β_2	Yes	Yes	No	Moderate	80%	20–70%	1–3	Hepatic	1.3
Penbutolol	β_1, β_2	Yes	No	No	High	90%	~100%	5	Hepatic/renal	NA
Pindolol	β_1, β_2	Yes	Low	No	Moderate	50%	75–90%	3–4	Hepatic/renal	2
Propranolol (long-acting form acting)	β_1, β_2	No	Yes	No	High	90%	30–70%	3–5	Hepatic	4
Sotalol	β_1, β_2	No	No	No	Low	0%	90%	9–12	Renal	2
Timolol (ophthalmic)	β_1, β_2	No	No	No	Moderate	60%	75%	3–5	Hepatic/renal	2

- Limited data in dogs and cats.
  - Absorption – oral dosing results in rapid absorption for most drugs.
  - Atenolol – relatively specific B_1 receptor antagonist at higher dosages B_2 blockade can occur.
    - Absorption – reported oral bioavailability in cats up to 90%.
    - Distribution – low protein-binding characteristics (5–15%).
    - Metabolism – minimally biotransformed in the liver.
    - Excretion – 40–50% is excreted unchanged in the urine and the remainder is excreted unchanged in the feces. Reported half-lives: dogs = 3.2 hours; cats = 3.7 hours.
  - Carvedilol – non-selective, β-adrenergic receptor antagonist with selective alpha$_1$-adrenergic blocking activity.
    - Absorption – bioavailability after oral dosing averages about 3–23%.
    - Excretion – elimination half-life was 100 minutes in dogs after oral dosing.
  - Esmolol – primary B_1 antagonist.
    - Absorption – IV injection results in steady-state blood level 5 minutes after bolus; 20 minutes after start of CRI.
    - Distribution – rapidly and widely distributed throughout the body.
    - Metabolism – rapidly metabolized in the blood.
    - Excretion – terminal half-life is about 10 minutes; duration of action after discontinuing CRI is about 20 minutes in the dog.
  - Metoprolol – relatively specific B_1-receptor antagonist; at higher dosages B_2 blockade can occur.
    - Absorption – rapidly and completely absorbed. Large first-pass effect with reduced bioavailability.
    - Distribution – low protein binding of 5–15%.
    - Metabolism – liver.
    - Excretion – primarily excreted in the urine; half-life in dogs is 1.6 hours, cats 1.3 hours.
  - Propranolol – blocks both B_1- and B_2-adrenergic receptors.
    - Absorption – rapid first-pass effect through the liver reduces systemic bioavailability to approximately 2–27% in dogs.
    - Metabolism – primarily liver.
    - Excretion – less than 1% of a dose is excreted unchanged into the urine. Half-life in dogs has been reported to range from 0.77 to 2 hours.
  - Sotalol – nonselective β-receptor antagonist and Class III antiarrhythmic agent. The beta-blocking activity of sotalol is about 30% that of propranolol.
    - Absorption – food may reduce the bioavailability.
    - Distribution – low lipid solubility and virtually no protein binding.
    - Elimination – primarily renal and most of the drug is excreted unchanged. Dogs' half-life is 5 hours.

Toxicity

- Limited published toxicity/overdose information in dogs and cats.
- Anecdotally, doses >2 times the published dose may cause clinical signs.
- Atenolol – therapeutic dose: dogs 0.25–1 mg/kg PO q 12 hours; cats 6.25–12.5 mg total dose PO q 12 hours.
- Carvedilol – therapeutic dose: dogs 0.2 mg/kg PO twice daily initially with slow titration upwards towards a dose of 1.11 mg/kg twice daily.
- Esmolol – therapeutic dose (dogs and cats): initial loading dose of 0.05–0.5 mg/kg (50–500 µg/kg) administered IV as slow bolus over 1–2 minutes, then followed by a constant rate infusion of 10–200 µg/kg/minute. LD_{50} in dogs is approximately 32 mg/kg IV. Dogs receiving doses of 3 mg/kg/minute showed clinical signs.
- Metoprolol – therapeutic dose: dogs 0.2–1 mg/kg, PO q 12–24 hours, titrated up to 6.6 mg/kg q 8 hours; XR formulation 0.4–1 mg/kg PO q 24 hours, cats 2–15 mg total PO q 8 hours.
- Propranolol – therapeutic dose: dogs 0.02 mg/kg IV slowly (up to a maximum of 1 mg/kg). Oral dose: 0.1–0.2 mg/kg initially PO q 8 hours, up to a maximum of 1.5 mg/kg q 8 hours; cats 0.02 mg/kg IV slowly (up to a maximum of 0.1 mg/kg). Oral dose: 2.5 mg (up to 10 mg) total dose per cat q 8–12 hours.
- Sotalol – therapeutic dose: dogs and cats 1–3 mg/kg q 12 hours.

Systems Affected

- Cardiovascular – bradycardia, hypotension.
- CNS – decreased mental status, seizures.
- Endocrine/metabolic – hypoglycemia, hyperkalemia, metabolic acidosis secondary to hypotension, and decreased perfusion.
- Renal/urological – azotemia secondary to hypoperfusion.
- Respiratory – bronchospasm.

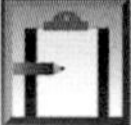

SIGNALMENT/HISTORY

- No breed or sex predilections. Cats may be at increased risk for overdose due to large pill sizes.

Risk Factors

- Animals with preexisting heart conditions or bradyarrhythmias are at increased risk for toxicosis.

Historical Findings

- Clinical signs may include:
    - weakness
    - collapse

- bradycardia
- altered mentation
- seizures.

Location and Circumstances of Poisoning

- Poisoning may occur in the home if the owner or patient is on β-receptor antagonists.
- Iatrogenic toxicity may occur in the clinic, especially with IV administration.

Interactions with Drugs, Nutrients, or Environment

- Animals taking other antiarrhythmics such as calcium channel blockers or digoxin may be at increased risk for bradyarrhythmias to develop.

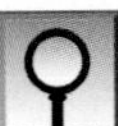

CLINICAL FEATURES

Onset of clinical signs will vary depending on the specific drug and formulation. In general, clinical signs will be noted within 8 hours after exposure with immediate-release formulations.

- Bradycardia
- Decreased pulse quality due to hypotension/cardiogenic shock
- Seizures
- Respiratory compromise/bronchospasm
- Altered mental status/coma

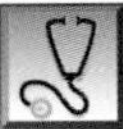

DIFFERENTIAL DIAGNOSIS

- Calcium channel blocker overdose.
- Cardiac disease with secondary arrhythmias.
- Other cardiovascular agent overdose (e.g., clonidine, digoxin toxicosis).
- Sick sinus syndrome of Miniature Schnauzers.
- Baclofen, opiate/opioid, or other sedative toxicosis.

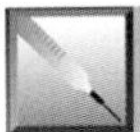

DIAGNOSTICS

- ECG – sinus bradycardia, first-, second-, and third-degree heart block, prolongation of the PR, QRS, and QT complexes.
- Echocardiogram – myocardial depression with negative inotropy.
- Serum biochemistry – may see hypoglycemia, azotemia and elevated liver enzymes can be noted with prolonged hypotension and decreased perfusion.
- Thoracic radiographs should be considered, particularly if any signs of respiratory distress, to assess for intravascular volume status and risk for congestive heart failure.

- Measurement of serum or urine β-receptor antagonist concentrations is not readily available. Serum and urine concentrations do not correlate well with the degree of toxicosis. Therefore, obtaining urine or serum concentrations is not routinely performed.

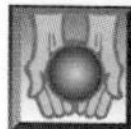

THERAPEUTICS

Detoxification

- Emesis can be performed in asymptomatic animals, typically within 1–2 hours after ingestion.
- Consider gastric lavage with altered mental status or large tablet ingestion.
- Activated charcoal with a cathartic at 1–2 g/kg can be administered within 2 hours after exposure; repeat doses without a cathartic can be considered for sustained- or extended-release formulations.
- Whole-bowel irrigation (GoLytely) can be performed for large ingestion of sustained- or extended-release formulations.
- Hemodialysis may remove water-soluble β-receptor antagonist (atenolol and esmolol).

Appropriate Health Care

- IV fluids (crystalloids and colloids) can be used for initial perfusion and hypotension but this may be ineffective in patients with bradycardia. Care should be taken to prevent fluid overload in animals with cardiogenic shock.
  - Volume resuscitation with IV crystalloid fluid administration for hypotension.
    - □ 20 mL/kg for dogs given over 10–15 minutes.
    - □ 10–15 mL/kg for cats given over 10–15 minutes.
- Close monitoring for fluid overload: frequent assessment of respiratory rate/effort, auscultation of the lungs, pulse oximetry/arterial blood gas analysis.
- Continuous ECG monitoring for assessment of conduction abnormalities.
- Frequent blood pressure monitoring (indirect or direct) for development of hypotension.
- Central line placement – beneficial for frequent blood glucose monitoring (particularly if using HDI therapy) and for guidance of fluid therapy with CVP monitoring.
- Airway protection and ventilatory support (e.g., intubation and positive pressure ventilation) as needed for decreased mental status, respiratory depression, or seizure activity.

Antidote

- Isoproterenol – rarely used synthetic β_1- and β_2-adrenergic agonist. Therapeutic dose (dogs and cats): 0.04–0.08 µg/kg/minute IV infusion.

Drugs of Choice

- Atropine.
  - May be used to treat sinus bradycardia (heart rate ≤50 in dogs, ≤120 in cats).
  - Atropine dose 0.02–0.04 mg/kg IV.
  - Bradycardia is frequently resistant to atropine.
- Calcium gluconate or chloride.
  - Used for hypotension and increased efficacy of HDI therapy.
  - Calcium gluconate 10% (0.05–0.15 mL/kg) can be given as a slow IV bolus over 5–10 minutes. A CRI with doses up to 0.50–1.50 mL/kg/hour can be initiated after the bolus and titrated as needed to maintain its effect. ECG should be monitored for bradycardia or worsening of conduction blockade.
  - Calcium chloride 10% (0.15–0.50 mL/kg) may be preferred over calcium gluconate 10% due to a greater concentration of calcium (13.4 mEq vs 4.5 mEq per 10 mL of 10% calcium chloride or gluconate, respectively). Tissue injury secondary to drug extravasation of calcium chloride can be significant. Therefore, calcium gluconate is preferred if a central line cannot be established.
  - Monitor serum ionized calcium with the goal of maintaining ionized calcium at approximately 1.5–2.0× the normal range (normal range 1.1–1.33 mmol/L).
- Intravenous fat emulsion (IFE).
  - Exact mechanism of how IFE works is not known (see chapter 3, Antidotes and Other Useful Drugs). Adverse effects of IFE may include hyperlipidemia, hepatosplenomegaly, jaundice, seizures, hemolytic anemia, prolonged clotting time, thrombocytopenia, and fat embolism.
  - IFE dose: 1.5 mL/kg IV bolus over 1 minute. Follow immediately with a CRI of 0.25 mL/kg/minute over 30–60 minutes.
  - May repeat IV bolus every 5 minutes until lipemia is detected.
  - If blood pressure continues to drop, may increase infusion up to 0.5 mL/kg/min.
  - Alternative dosing protocol of 1.5 mL/kg every 4–6 hours can also be considered.
  - It is recommended *not to exceed* a total dose of 8 mL/kg based on human literature.
- High-dose insulin (HDI) therapy/dextrose infusion.
  - Also referred to as hyperinsulinemia-euglycemia therapy.
  - Exact mechanism by which HDI works is unknown, but it is thought to improve cardiac inotropy and improves perfusion by increasing cardiac output, rather than affecting vascular tone.
  - Appears to promote the uptake and utilization of carbohydrates as an energy source.
  - May increase intracellular Ca concentrations in myocardial cells, enhancing cardiac contractility and cardiac output.
  - Recommended dose.
    - Check blood glucose (BG) concentration first. Administer glucose if BG is ≤100 mg/dL for dog or ≤200 mg/dL for cat.
    - Administer regular insulin at 1 unit/kg IV bolus. Follow with an intravenous CRI of regular insulin at 2 units/kg/hour. May increase infusion by 1–2 units/kg/hour every 10 minutes up to a maximum dose of 10 units/kg/hour.

    - BG must be carefully monitored every 10 minutes while titrating insulin dosing.
    - Dextrose will need to be administered to maintain normal blood glucose concentration. A concentrated IV infusion of dextrose (often >5% dextrose, possibly upwards of 15–30%) will be needed to maintain BG concentrations. Therefore, the dextrose infusion should be administered through a central line.
    - Once the insulin infusion dose is stabilized, check BG concentrations every 30–60 minutes.
    - Monitor K^+ concentrations every hour. Keep K^+ concentrations in low therapeutic range. Administer potassium chloride if $K^+ \leq 3.0$ mmol/L.
    - When signs of β-receptor antagonist toxicosis have resolved, decrease insulin by 1–2 units/kg/hour. Glucose administration will likely need to be continued for up to 24 hours after the insulin infusion has been stopped.
    - Monitor calcium, glucose, and potassium concentrations hourly while decreasing insulin infusions.
- Glucagon.
  - Traditionally used as a treatment for β-receptor antagonist toxicosis. IFE and HDI are now the preferred treatments when available.
  - Glucagon has a positive inotropic and chronotropic effect on myocardial cells via stimulation of adenyl cyclase.
  - Dose at 0.05–0.2 mg/kg slow IV bolus; an increase in heart rate should be noted within a few minutes of the initial bolus. If a positive response is noted, the bolus should be followed by a continuous infusion of glucagon at 0.05–0.10 mg/kg/hour.
  - Adverse effects of glucagon: nausea, vomiting, transient hyperglycemia.
- Vasopressor therapy: see Precautions/Interactions.

Precautions/Interactions

- Epinephrine/norepinephrine/dopamine/dobutamine – vasopressors are *not* recommended in the treatment of hypotension caused by β-receptor antagonist overdose. Recent literature suggests that vasopressors are less effective than HDI or IFE therapy and may even be potentially harmful.

COMMENTS

Patient Monitoring

- ECG – continuous or intermittent ECG to monitor for heart rate or conduction abnormalities.
- Blood pressure – continuous or intermittent monitoring should be performed.
- Kidney values should be monitored once daily.

Prevention/Avoidance

- Owners should keep pet medications separate from their own to avoid accidental dosing of human β-receptor antagonists.
- Advise clients on the correct dosing to avoid inadvertent overdoses.

Possible Complications

- Renal failure can develop with persistent hypoperfusion.

Expected Course and Prognosis

- Degree and length of clinical signs will be variable depending on class, dose, and formulation (immediate versus extended release).
- Prognosis is typically good with early intervention but guarded to poor if unresponsive to therapy and coma develops.

See Also

Calcium Channel Blockers

Abbreviations

See Appendix 1 for a complete list.

Suggested Reading

DeWitt C, Waksman J. Pharmacology, pathophysiology and management of calcium channel blocker and beta-blocker toxicity. Toxicol Rev 2004; 23:223–238.

Engebretsen KM, Kaczmarek K, Morgan J, et al. High-dose insulin therapy in beta-blocker and calcium channel-blocker poisoning. Clin Toxicol 2011; 49:277–283.

Kerns W. Management of beta-adrenergic blocker and calcium channel antagonist toxicity. Emerg Med Clin North Am 2007; 25:309–331.

Malouin A, King LG. Calcium channel and beta-blocker drug overdoses. In: Silverstein DC, Hopper K, eds. Small Animal Critical Care Medicine. St Louis, MO: Saunders, 2009; pp. 357–362.

Plumb DC. Plumb's Veterinary Drug Handbook, 7th edn. Ames, IA: Wiley-Blackwell, 2011.

Acknowledgment: The authors and editors acknowledge the prior contributions of Kristin M. Engebretsen, PharmD, DABAT and Rebecca S. Syring, DVM, DACVECC, who authored this topic in the previous edition.

Author: Katherine L. Peterson, DVM, DACVECC

Consulting Editor: Lynn R. Hovda, RPh, DVM, MS, DACVIM

chapter 20

Calcipotriene/Calcipotriol

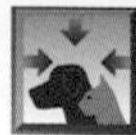

DEFINITION/OVERVIEW

- Calcipotriene/calcipotriol is a synthetic analog of calcitriol, the most active metabolite of cholecalciferol (vitamin D_3).
- It is the active ingredient in aerosol foams, creams, ointments, and scalp solutions used to treat human psoriasis; trade names include Dovonex®, Sorilux®, and Talconex®.
- Calcipotriene in a concentration of 0.005% (50 µg/g) is marketed in 30, 60, and 100 gram tubes and 60 and 120 gram aerosol cans.
  - Talconex also contains 0.05% (0.5 mg/g) of betamethasone propionate.
- Ingestion of even small amounts may result in severe clinical signs in pets.

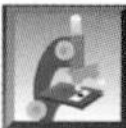

ETIOLOGY/PATHOPHYSIOLOGY

Mechanism of Action

- Calcipotriene has effects similar to cholecalciferol, causing significant elevations in serum calcium and phosphorus levels.
- Untreated, these levels quickly lead to mineralization of soft tissues, including heart, lungs, blood vessels, kidneys, and gastrointestinal tract. Acute renal failure is the most common clinical manifestation.

Pharmacokinetics – Absorption, Distribution, Metabolism, Excretion

- Pharmacokinetic information on calcipotriene in domestic species is lacking.
- In humans, approximately 5–6% of topically applied calcipotriene is systemically absorbed within a few hours, followed by a transient hypercalcemia, and rapid conversion to inactive metabolites.
- Rapidly and well absorbed orally.
- Enterohepatic circulation occurs.
- Significant storage in fat and muscle tissue with slow release is thought to result in a long half-life.

Blackwell's Five-Minute Veterinary Consult Clinical Companion: Small Animal Toxicology, Second Edition.
Lynn R. Hovda, Ahna G. Brutlag, Robert H. Poppenga, and Katherine L. Peterson.

Companion website: www.fiveminutevet.com/toxicology

Toxicity

- Calcipotriene is highly toxic to dogs and cats.
- Pets may be exposed by chewing containers or by licking skin of humans where the product has been applied.
- The minimum acute toxic dose in dogs is 10 μg calcipotriene/kg BW and the acute minimum lethal dose is 65 μg/kg BW. Some references list 1.8–3.6 μg/kg BW as potentially toxic to dogs.
- Dogs treated with 3.6 μg/kg/day for 1 week showed an increase in calcium, phosphorus, BUN, and creatinine; acute renal failure developed.
- Soft tissue mineralization occurs when serum calcium (mg/dL) × serum phosphorus (mg/dL) ≥60 in mature animals or ≥70 in growing, immature animals.

Systems Affected

- Endocrine/metabolic – hypercalcemia, hyperphosphatemia, other electrolyte imbalances secondary to uremia.
- Gastrointestinal – full range of signs including anorexia, vomiting, hypersalivation, constipation, diarrhea, melena, hematemesis, abdominal pain, oropharyngeal erosions.
- Renal/urological – hypercalcemic nephropathy and acute renal failure.
- Cardiovascular – bradycardia, arrhythmias.
- Nervous – decreased neural responsiveness, weakness.
- Musculoskeletal – decreased muscle responsiveness.

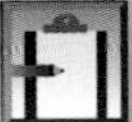

SIGNALMENT/HISTORY

- All breeds and ages of cats and dogs are susceptible to this toxicity.
- Cats and dogs under 6 months of age may be more susceptible.
- Diagnosis is based on history of ingestion, clinical signs, and characteristic laboratory alterations.

CLINICAL FEATURES

- Initial signs include vomiting, depression, anorexia, diarrhea, and polyuria within 24 hours of ingestion.
- Hypercalcemia, hyperphosphatemia, and hypercalcemic nephropathy occur between 18 and 72 hours after ingestion.
- Soft tissue mineralization occurs when serum calcium (mg/dL) × serum phosphorus (mg/dL) ≥60 in mature animals or ≥70 in growing, immature animals.

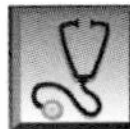

DIFFERENTIAL DIAGNOSIS

- Acute or chronic renal failure.
- Hypercalcemia of malignancy.

- Hypoadrenocorticism.
- Idiopathic hypercalcemia of cats.
- Juvenile hypercalcemia.
- Primary hyperparathyroidism.
- Toxicants.
  - Ethylene glycol.
  - Grapes or raisins.
  - Ingestion of other vitamin D products (rodenticides, high-dose vitamin D supplements).

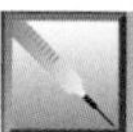

DIAGNOSTICS

- Serum chemistry to include calcium, phosphorus, BUN, and creatinine.
- Urinalysis with specific gravity.
- Toxicosis is serious when the serum calcium is greater than 12.5 mg/dL, serum phosphorus levels are over 7 mg/dL, and hyposthenuria is documented.
- Radiographs or ultrasound may show calcification of renal, gastrointestinal, respiratory, or vascular tissues.
- There is no specific laboratory test for calcipotriol/calcipotriene.
- Neutrophilia may occur, although the cause is unknown.

Pathological Findings

- At necropsy, renal tubular degeneration and necrosis; mineralization of the renal tubules, coronary arteries, gastrointestinal wall, and other soft tissues; hemorrhage of gastric mucosa may all be evident.

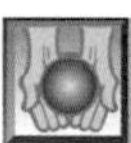

THERAPEUTICS

The goal of treatment is to keep the calcium level at less than 12.5 mg/dL and the phosphorus level at less than 7 mg/dL.

Detoxification

- Early emesis or gastric lavage.
- In cases where the product has been licked, rinse the mouth well for 10–15 minutes.
- Activated charcoal with a cathartic initially, followed by activated charcoal without a cathartic q 8 hours for 1–2 days if GI motility is normal; monitor electrolytes for hypernatremia due to fluid shifts.

Appropriate Health Care

- Obtain baseline serum chemistries, including calcium, phosphorus, BUN, creatinine, and liver enzymes.

- Urinalysis with specific gravity.
- If serum calcium and phosphorus are normal, repeat lab work (at minimum: calcium, phosphorus, BUN, creatinine) in 12 hours. If levels are still within normal limits, repeat the lab work daily for 4 days. If normal at that time, no further treatment necessary.
- In dogs, anorexia is a fairly consistent indication of elevating serum calcium levels; have owners monitor appetite closely and bring in for repeated lab work if any degree of anorexia develops in first 4 days.
- If serum calcium and/or phosphorus are elevated, initiate fluid therapy and continue to monitor blood work as above.
- Phosphorus tends to elevate before calcium.
- If at any time the serum calcium exceeds 12.5 mg/dL, or if the serum calcium × serum phosphorus exceeds 60 (adults) or 70 (growing, immature animals), increase IV fluid rates and begin aggressive medical therapy as indicated later in this chapter.
- Monitor urine output for oliguria or anuria. If urine output is at or less than 0.5 mL/kg/hour, increase fluids or consider other options.
- Monitor blood pressure and treat accordingly.

Antidote

- No specific antidote is available for calcipotriene toxicity.

Drugs of Choice

- Aggressive 0.9% NaCl diuresis at 2–3 times maintenance until calcium levels decrease.
- If urine output decreases in the face of adequate hydration, one or both of the following may be used.
    - Furosemide CRI at 1–2 mg/kg/hour.
    - Mannitol bolus at 1–2 g/kg IV slowly.
- To increase calcium excretion in patients with good urine output.
    - Furosemide 0.5 mg/kg/hr IV or 2.5–4.5 mg/kg PO TID.
    - Dexamethasone 0.2 mg/kg IV q 12 hours or prednisone 2–3 mg/kg PO BID.
- Phosphate binders to keep the calcium × phosphorus product at less than 60 or 70.
- Aluminum hydroxide 2–10 mL PO q 6 hours if phosphorus levels are high.
- Bisphosphonates to inhibit bone reabsorption and minimize hypercalcemia.
    - Pamidronate is the most widely used, although others have been suggested.
    - Pamidronate disodium (Aredia).
        - 1.3–2 mg/kg IV diluted in saline and infused over 2 hours for one dose only.
        - Expect serum calcium and phosphorus levels to decrease in 24–48 hours.
        - Once serum calcium and phosphorus levels have declined to acceptable range, wean off medication and fluids to avoid development of hypocalcemia.
        - If levels decrease and then rebound, a second dose may be needed in 5–7 days. Anecdotally, extremely large ingestions have needed redosing in just 3–4 days. Monitor appetite for anorexia, which may indicate rising calcium levels.

- Antiemetics as needed for persistent vomiting.
    - Dolasetron 0.5–1.0 mg/kg IV q 24 hours.
    - Maropitant 1 mg/kg SQ q 24 hours, not labeled for cats.
    - Ondansetron 0.1–0.2 mg/kg IV q 8–12 hours.
- GI protectants.
    - Famotidine 0.5–1 mg/kg PO, SQ, IM, IV q 12–24 hours (do not use IV in cats).
    - Ranitidine 1–2 mg/kg PO, SQ, IM, IV q 8–12 hours.
    - Cimetidine 5–10 mg/kg PO, SQ, IM, IV q 6 hours.
    - Omeprazole 0.5–1 mg/kg PO daily.
    - Sucralfate 0.25–1 g PO TID × 5–7 days if evidence of active ulcer disease.

Precautions/Interactions

- Thiazide diuretics are contraindicated as they decrease clearance of calcium.
- Bisphosphonates should be used cautiously in combination with calcitonin and then only in refractory cases, as combined use may increase soft tissue mineralization.
- Excessive doses of pamidronate or failure to wean off fluids and medications following normalizing of serum calcium can result in hypocalcemia. Treatment with calcium carbonate, or in severe cases IV calcium gluconate, may be needed.

Alternative Drugs

- Salmon calcitonin (Calcimar®, Micalcin®) at 4–7 IU/kg SQ q 8–12 hours.
    - Currently used less often than pamidronate due to inconsistencies in efficacy and development of resistance after several days of treatment.
    - Used instead of pamidronate. All other treatment recommendations remain the same.

Diet

- Low-calcium diet during times of hypercalcemia.

COMMENTS

Patient Monitoring

- Following normalization of serum levels, recheck calcium and phosphorus levels every third day as needed, then weekly for 3–4 weeks. Calcium and phosphorus levels should be evaluated in all exposed animals regardless of amount ingested.
- Monitor for evidence of GI ulceration secondary to uremia or soft tissue mineralization.

Prevention/Avoidance

- Medications should be kept well out of a pet's reach.
- Do not allow the pet to lick products that have been applied to skin.

Possible Complications

- Cardiac insufficiency and chronic renal failure secondary to calcification.
- Death from cardiac calcification may occur weeks after a presumed recovery.

Expected Course and Prognosis

- The prognosis is good if serum calcium × serum phosphorus is <60 (mature animals) or <70 (growing, immature animals) and aggressive treatment is provided in a timely manner. Soft tissue mineralization is unlikely.
- The prognosis is much more guarded if the serum calcium × serum phosphorus is ≥60 (mature animals) or ≥70 (growing, immature animals) and prolonged for even a few days. The risk of soft tissue mineralization is high.

See Also

Cholecalciferol

Abbreviations

See Appendix 1 for a complete list.

Suggested Reading

Hostutler R, Chew DJ, Jaeger JQ, et al. Uses and effectiveness of pamidronate disodium for treatment of dogs and cats with hypercalcemia. J Vet Intern Med 2005; 19(1):29–33.

Rumbeiha WK. Cholecalciferol. In: Peterson ME, Talcott PA, eds. Small Animal Toxicology, 3rd edn. St Louis, MO: Elsevier, 2013; pp. 489–498.

Saedi N, Horn R, Muffoletto A, et al. Death of a dog caused by calcipotriene toxicity. J Am Acad Derm 2007; 56(4):712–713.

Torley D, Drummond A, Bilsland DJ. Calcipotriol toxicity in dogs. Br J Derm 2002; 147(6):1270.

Acknowledgment: The authors and editors acknowledge the prior contributions of Catherine M. Adams, who authored this topic in the previous edition.
Author: Sharon Gwaltney-Brant, DVM, PhD, DABVT, DABT
Consulting Editor: Lynn R. Hovda, RPh, DVM, MS, DACVIM

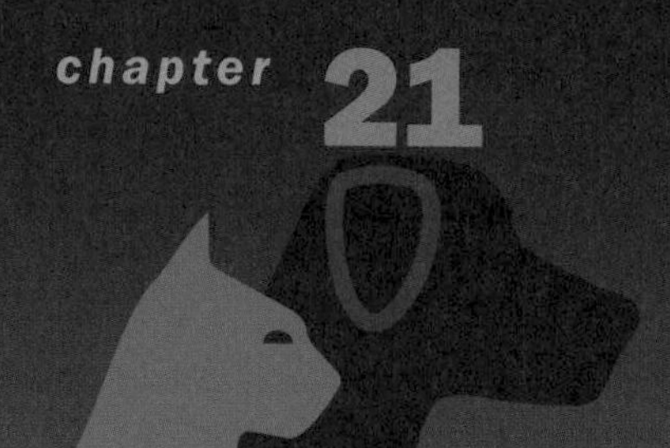

Calcium Channel Blockers

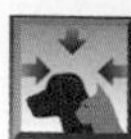

DEFINITION/OVERVIEW

- Calcium channel blockers (CCBs) are medications commonly used in veterinary medicine to treat underlying cardiac disease, tachyarrhythmias, systemic hypertension, and oliguric/anuric renal failure.
- CCB intoxication incidence is increasing in veterinary medicine.
- There are three different classes of CCBs (phenylalkylamines, benzothiazepines, and dihydropyridines) that have varying degrees of effect on the heart and vasculature (table 21.1).
- Common side effects of toxicosis include vomiting, bradyarrhythmias, hypotension, and weakness.

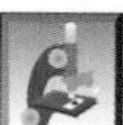

ETIOLOGY/PATHOPHYSIOLOGY

Mechanism of Action

- CCBs inhibit intracellular movement of calcium through L-type voltage-gated slow calcium channels, located predominantly in cardiac (atrial) muscle, vascular smooth muscle, and beta cells of the pancreas.
- Calcium channel blockade results in reduced cardiac automaticity, conduction, contractility, and loss of vascular tone. The degree to which toxicosis affects these functions of the heart and vasculature depends on the class of CCB (phenyalkylamines, benzothiazepines, and dihydropyridines) (see table 21.1).
- Automaticity and conduction: sinoatrial (SA) node depolarization and atrioventricular (AV) node conduction are dependent on activation of L-type calcium channels. Blockade of these channels reduces SA node firing and delays AV conduction.
- Contractility: blockade of L-type calcium channels impairs phase 2 of the action potential in cardiac muscle, ultimately resulting in reduced excitation-contraction coupling of cardiac muscle and reduced force of cardiac contractility.
- Vascular tone: blockade of L-type calcium channels impairs vascular smooth muscle contraction, resulting in vasodilation.

Blackwell's Five-Minute Veterinary Consult Clinical Companion: Small Animal Toxicology, Second Edition.
Lynn R. Hovda, Ahna G. Brutlag, Robert H. Poppenga, and Katherine L. Peterson.

Companion website: www.fiveminutevet.com/toxicology

TABLE 21.1. Relative effects of the three classes of calcium channel blockers (phenylalkylamines, benzothiazepines, and dihydropyridines) on cardiac automaticity, conduction, contractility, and vascular tone.

Class	Drugs	Automaticity	Conduction	Contractility	Vessel tone
Phenylalkylamine	Verapamil	+++	+++	+++	+++
Benzothiazepine	Diltiazem	++++	+++	+	++
Dihydropyridine	Amlodipine Nifedipine Nisoldipine Nimodipine Nicardipine Felodipine Isradipine Clevidipine	+	0	+	++++

Note: Plus signs signify an increasing response, with more plus signs denoting a more inhibitory response. The zero denotes no response.

- Pancreas: hypoinsulinemia and hyperglycemia may occur secondary to CCB administration/overdose because of impaired beta cell function.

Pharmacokinetics – Absorption, Distribution, Metabolism, Excretion

- Verapamil.
  - Absorption – 90% absorption in dogs, low bioavailability (10–23%) due to extensive first-pass metabolism.
  - Distribution – large volume of distribution; extensively protein bound.
  - Metabolism – large first-pass effect. Serum half-lives ranging from 0.8 to 2.5 hours have been reported in dogs.
  - Excretion – primary route in dogs is biliary excretion.
- Diltiazem.
  - Immediate-release formulations.
    - Absorption.
      - Rapid absorption
      - Cats – oral dosing 50–80% bioavailability with peak effect 45 minutes after dosing
      - Dogs – oral dosing may only have 25% bioavailability due to large first-pass effect
      - Peak plasma concentrations occur within 1.5–4.25 hours of ingestion of a therapeutic dose. With toxicosis, clinical signs should be evident within less than 6 hours following ingestion
    - Distribution – approximately 70–75% protein bound.

        - Metabolism.
            - Large first-pass and hepatic metabolism
            - Rapidly metabolized by the liver and undergoes enterohepatic recirculation in dogs
            - Serum half-life for cats is approximately 2 hours, dogs 3 hours; renal impairment may increase half-life
        - Excretion – metabolites are primarily excreted in the feces.
    - Sustained-release (SR), extended-release (XR), controlled-release (CR) formulations.
        - Cats may have improved bioavailability of Dilacor XR, up to 94%.
        - With SR/XR/CR formulations, development of clinical signs of toxicosis may be delayed by as much as 6–12 hours following toxic ingestions.
        - Distribution, metabolism, and excretion are similar to immediate-release formulations.
- Amlodipine.
    - Limited veterinary pharmacokinetic data.
    - Absorption – slow following oral dosing. Peak plasma concentrations and clinical effects are reported 4–9 hours after oral dosing.
    - Distribution – highly protein bound (>90%).
    - Metabolism – slowly metabolized to inactive compounds by the liver. Terminal half-life in dogs is up to 30 hours.
    - Excretion – renal excretion of inactive metabolites.

Toxicity

- Clinical signs can be noted at therapeutic doses.
    - Verapamil.
        - Dog: 0.05 mg/kg IV, 0.5–3 mg/kg PO q 8 hours.
        - Cat: 0.025 mg/kg IV, 0.5–1 mg/kg PO q 8 hours.
    - Diltiazem.
        - Dog: 0.05–0.25 mg/kg IV, 0.5–2 mg/kg PO q 8 hours (IR).
        - Cat: 0.125–0.25 mg/kg IV, 0.5–1.5 mg/kg PO q 8 hours (IR).
        - LD_{50} for diltiazem is 50 mg/kg in dogs.
        - Therapeutic doses for SR/XR/CR formulations in dogs and cats vary depending on the formulation used.
    - Amlodipine.
        - Dog: 0.05–0.4 mg/kg PO q 12 hours.
        - Cat: 0.625–1.25 mg PO q 24 hours.

Systems Affected

- Cardiovascular – bradycardia, AV dissociation, AV conduction blockade (1st-, 2nd-, or 3rd-degree AV block), and hypotension.
- Endocrine – hypoinsulinemia and hyperglycemia.
- Gastrointestinal – vomiting, diarrhea, ileus.

- Hematological – inhibited platelet aggregation.
- Musculoskeletal – diffuse weakness and recumbency secondary to reduced cardiac output and hypotension.
- Nervous – depressed mentation/level of consciousness related to decreased cardiac output, hypotension, and reduced cerebral perfusion. Seizures have been reported.
- Renal/urological – acute renal failure due to decreased perfusion.
- Respiratory – pulmonary edema has been reported, unknown mechanism but may be secondary to fluid therapy, decreased cardiac output, increased vascular permeability.

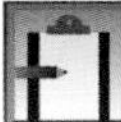

SIGNALMENT/HISTORY

- There are no specific breed or sex predilections for this toxicosis.
- Dogs may be at increased risk for toxicosis, given their propensity to chew into and ingest large quantities of owner's medications.
- Cats may be at increased risk when CR or SR formulations are prescribed to treat underlying hypertrophic cardiomyopathy and dosing errors by pet owners occur.

Risk Factors

- CCB medication in animal's environment.
- Co-administration with β receptor antagonist or other cardiac medications.
- Dosing errors by owner (particularly with cats on SR/XR/CR formulations).
- Liver dysfunction will result in higher serum concentrations and delayed metabolism of the drug.

Historical Findings

- Known dosing error.
- Ingestion of owner's medications by pet (chewed/empty pill vials).
- Acute onset of weakness, lethargy, syncopal episodes.

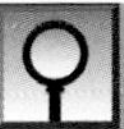

CLINICAL FEATURES

- Bradycardia
- Hypodynamic pulses
- Respiratory distress
- Pulmonary crackles
- Depressed mentation
- Vomiting
- Diarrhea
- Recumbency, weakness
- Syncope, collapse

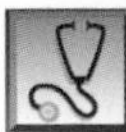

DIFFERENTIAL DIAGNOSIS

- Atrial standstill secondary to hyperkalemia.
- Intrinsic cardiac conduction defects – sick sinus syndrome, AV block, and atrial standstill.
- Toxicants.
    - Baclofen
    - Beta-adrenergic antagonist
    - Opiate and opioid
    - Sedatives

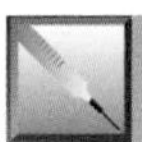

DIAGNOSTICS

- ECG: sinus bradycardia, 1st-, 2nd-, or 3rd-degree AV block, AV dissociation, junctional escape rhythms, idioventricular rhythms, or asystole may be noted following CCB toxicosis.
- Serum ionized/total calcium concentrations: calcium concentrations may remain normal despite CCB intoxication.
- Serum glucose concentrations: hyperglycemia may be noted with toxicosis as a result of suppressed insulin release from beta cells of the pancreas; the extent of hyperglycemia is associated with degree of intoxication.
- Serum lactate concentrations: hyperlactatemia may be noted with toxicosis as a result of impaired cardiac output and glucose entry into cells for aerobic metabolism; the extent of hyperlactatemia is associated with degree of intoxication.
- Thoracic radiographs should be considered, particularly if any signs of respiratory distress, to assess for intravascular volume status and risk of congestive heart failure.
- Serum drug concentrations: concentrations of specific drugs can be measured via high-performance lipid chromatography (HPLC), GCMS, or LC MS/MS.
    - Serum drug concentration results take, on average, about 3 days to obtain and therefore are not clinically useful in the management of toxicities.
    - Therapeutic verapamil concentrations of 300–500 ng/mL are reported for cats and dogs.

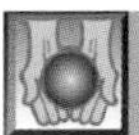

THERAPEUTICS

Detoxification

- Induce emesis if within 2 hours of ingestion and animal is asymptomatic.
- If the animal is deemed too unstable to induce vomiting, and recent ingestion or large number of tablets ingested, gastric lavage should be performed.
- Activated charcoal should be given within 2 hours of ingestion.
    - Because of the abundance of SR and XR CCBs on the market, emesis, gastric lavage, and activated charcoal administration may be useful beyond the first 1–2 hours of ingestion.

- Whole-bowel irrigation with GoLytely can be considered with large ingestion of SR and XR formulations and may be more effective than gastric lavage at removing intact tablets from the intestinal tract.
- CCBs are extensively protein bound, making hemodialysis or hemofiltration ineffective tools for expediting drug elimination following intoxication.

Appropriate Health Care

- A central line IV catheter should be considered in symptomatic patients.
- Intravascular fluid therapy: balanced electrolyte solution should be used as needed to maintain hydration status and support cardiovascular function and perfusion. A fluid bolus of 20–30 mL/kg should be considered in dogs, 10-15 ml/kg in cats with hypotension secondary to toxicosis. Because of the risk for impaired cardiac function, care should be taken to avoid fluid overload.
- Temporary transvenous pacing has been used to increase heart rate and cardiac output. Pacing should be considered when therapies fail to improve heart rate and cardiac output/ peripheral tissue perfusion remains impaired.
- Close monitoring for fluid overload: frequent assessment of respiratory rate/effort, auscultation of the lungs, pulse oximetry/arterial blood gas analysis.
- Continuous ECG monitoring for assessment of conduction abnormalities.
- Frequent blood pressure monitoring (indirect or direct) for development of hypotension.

Antidote

- No specific antidote available.

Drug(s) of Choice

- Calcium infusion: first line of therapy for symptomatic animals. Despite normocalcemia, calcium administration may increase the amount of calcium available for normal cardiac and smooth muscle function.
    - Calcium helps improve myocardial contractility but has little effect on cardiac conduction.
    - Calcium gluconate 10% (0.50–1.50 mL/kg) can be given as a slow IV bolus over 5–10 minutes. A CRI with doses up to 0.05–0.15 mL/kg/hour can be initiated after the bolus and titrated as needed to maintain its effect. ECG should be monitored for bradycardia or worsening of conduction blockade.
    - Calcium chloride 10% (0.15–0.50 mL/kg) may be preferred over calcium gluconate 10% due to a greater concentration of calcium (13.4 mEq vs 4.5 mEq per 10 mL of 10% calcium chloride or gluconate, respectively). Tissue injury secondary to drug extravasation of calcium chloride can be significant. Therefore, calcium gluconate is preferred if a central line cannot be established.
    - Monitor serum ionized calcium with the goal of maintaining ionized calcium at approximately 1.5–2.0 times the normal range (normal range 1.1–1.33 mmol/L).

- Atropine (0.02–0.04 mg/kg IV) can be used to treat bradycardia; heart rate is rarely responsive to atropine.
- Intravenous fat emulsion (IFE).
  - Exact mechanism of how IFE works is not known (see Chapter 3).
  - IFE dose: 1.5 mL/kg IV bolus over 1 minute. Follow immediately with a CRI of 0.25 mL/kg/min over 30–60 minutes.
  - May repeat IV bolus every 5 minutes until lipemia is detected.
  - If blood pressure continues to drop, may increase infusion up to 0.5 mL/kg/min.
  - Alternative dosing protocol of 1.5 mL/kg every 4–6 hours can also be considered.
  - It is recommended *not to exceed* a total dose of 8 mL/kg based on human literature.
- Glucagon.
  - Positive inotropic and chronotropic effect on myocardial cells via stimulation of adenyl cyclase.
  - Dose at 0.05–0.2 mg/kg slow IV bolus; an increase in heart rate should be noted within a few minutes of the initial bolus. If a positive response is noted, the bolus should be followed by a continuous infusion of glucagon at 0.05–0.10 mg/kg/hour.
  - Adverse effects of glucagon: nausea, vomiting, transient hyperglycemia.
- High-dose insulin (HDI) therapy/dextrose infusion.
  - Also referred to as hyperinsulinemia-euglycemia therapy.
  - Exact mechanism by which HDI works is unknown, but it is thought to improve cardiac inotropy and improves perfusion by increasing cardiac output, rather than affecting vascular tone.
  - Appears to promote the uptake and utilization of carbohydrates as an energy source.
  - May increase intracellular Ca concentrations in myocardial cells, enhancing cardiac contractility and cardiac output.
  - Recommended dose.
    - ☐ Check blood glucose (BG) concentration first. Administer glucose if BG is ≤100 mg/dL for dog or ≤200 mg/dL for cat.
    - ☐ Administer regular insulin at 1 unit/kg IV bolus. Follow with an intravenous CRI of regular insulin at 2 units/kg/hour. May increase infusion by 1–2 units/kg/hour every 10 minutes up to a maximum dose of 10 units/kg/hour.
    - ☐ BG must be carefully monitored every 10 minutes while titrating insulin dosing.
    - ☐ Dextrose will need to be administered to maintain normal blood glucose concentration. A concentrated IV infusion of dextrose (often >5% dextrose, possibly upwards of 15–30%) will be needed to maintain BG concentrations. Therefore, the dextrose infusion should be administered through a central line.
    - ☐ Once the insulin infusion dose is stabilized, check BG concentrations every 30–60 minutes.
    - ☐ Monitor K^+ concentrations every hour. Keep K^+ concentrations in low therapeutic range. Administer potassium chloride if K^+ ≤3.0 mmol/L.
    - ☐ When signs of CCB toxicosis have resolved, decrease insulin by 1–2 units/kg/hour. Glucose administration will likely need to be continued for up to 24 hours after the insulin infusion has been stopped.

    - Monitor calcium, glucose, and potassium concentrations hourly while decreasing insulin infusions.
- Vasopressor therapy (dopamine 5–15 µg/kg/min; dobutamine 3–15 µg/kg/min; norepinephrine 0.05–0.3 µg/kg/min) should only be considered when blood pressure has failed to respond to other treatments such as calcium, IFE, or HDI.

Precautions/Interactions

- Beta-blockers: co-administration of beta-blockers and CCB may increase the risk for bradyarrhythmias and conduction blockade. Diltiazem may increase the bioavailability of propranolol.
- Digoxin: CCBs may increase serum concentrations of digoxin, increasing the risk for digoxin toxicosis.
- Cimetidine (and/or ranitidine) may impair hepatic metabolism of CCBs, slowing elimination.
- Co-administration with cyclosporine will result in increased cyclosporine drug levels.

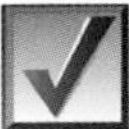

COMMENTS

Patient Monitoring

- ECG: continuous or intermittent ECG to monitor for heart rate or conduction abnormalities.
- Blood pressure: continuous or intermittent monitoring should be performed.
- Kidney values should be monitored once daily.

Prevention/Avoidance

- Owners should keep pet medications separate from their own to avoid accidental dosing of human CCB.
- Advise clients on the correct dosing to avoid inadvertent overdoses.

Possible Complications

- Renal failure can develop with persistent hypoperfusion.

Expected Course and Prognosis

- Degree and length of clinical signs will be variable depending on class, dose, and formulation (immediate versus extended release).
- Prognosis is typically good with early intervention but guarded to poor if unresponsive to therapy and if cardiac pacing is needed.

Abbreviations

See Appendix 1 for a complete list.

See Also

Beta Receptor Antagonists (Beta-Blockers)

Suggested Reading

Costello M, Syring RS. Calcium channel blocker toxicity. J Vet Emerg Crit Care 2008; 18:54–60.

DeWitt C, Waksman J. Pharmacology, pathophysiology and management of calcium channel blocker and beta-blocker toxicity. Toxicol Rev 2004; 23:223–238.

Hayes CL, Knight M. Calcium channel blocker toxicity in dogs and cats. Vet Clin North Am Small Anim Pract 2012; 42:263–277.

Kerns W. Management of beta-adrenergic blocker and calcium channel antagonist toxicity. Emerg Med Clin North Am 2007; 25:309–331.

Lheureux PER, Zahir S, Gris M, et al. Bench-to-bedside review: hyperinsulinaemia/euglycaemia therapy in the management of overdose of calcium-channel blockers. Crit Care 2006; 10:212–218.

Acknowledgment: The authors and editors acknowledge the prior contributions of Kristin M. Engebretsen, PharmD, DABAT and Rebecca S. Syring, DVM, DACVECC, who authored this topic in the previous edition.

Author: Katherine L. Peterson, DVM, DACVECC

Consulting Editor: Lynn R. Hovda, RPh, DVM, MS, DACVIM

Colchicine

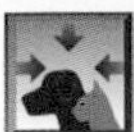

DEFINITION/OVERVIEW

- Alkaloid extracted from *Colchium autumnale* (autumn crocus) or *Gloriosa superba* (glory lily).
- FDA-approved drug for treatment of gout and familial Mediterranean fever in people.
- It has been used in veterinary medicine to treat systemic amyloidosis.
- Colchicine may also be used in treatment of chronic hepatic fibrosis.
- There is a narrow therapeutic index.
- Toxicity causes multiorgan dysfunction, with GI distress often being the first clinical indication of toxicity.
- A high mortality rate is associated with colchicine toxicosis.

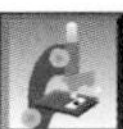

ETIOLOGY/PATHOPHYSIOLOGY

Mechanism of Action

- Colchicine binds to tubulin and interferes with cellular elongation important in cellular mitosis.
- The primary target is rapidly dividing cells.
- It also interferes with intracellular transport and maintenance of cell structure.
- The antifibrotic effects are thought to be due to stimulation of collagenases.

Pharmacokinetics – Absorption, Distribution, Metabolism, Excretion

- There is limited information regarding the pharmacokinetics of colchicine in domestic animals, therefore much of the pharmacokinetic data is derived from people.
- Colchicine is rapidly absorbed from the gastrointestinal tract. It undergoes extensive hepatic first-pass metabolism, resulting in a systemic bioavailability of 25–50%.
- There is extensive distribution of this drug; however, large concentrations of colchicine can be found in leukocytes.
- Metabolism of colchicine occurs in the liver by the cytochrome P450 isoform CYP3A4.
- Colchicine and its metabolites undergo significant enterohepatic recirculation.
- Elimination is primarily through biliary excretion, which is mediated by MDR1. The kidneys also have a role in excretion of colchicine.

Blackwell's Five-Minute Veterinary Consult Clinical Companion: Small Animal Toxicology, Second Edition.
Lynn R. Hovda, Ahna G. Brutlag, Robert H. Poppenga, and Katherine L. Peterson.

Companion website: www.fiveminutevet.com/toxicology

Toxicity

- There is limited information regarding toxic doses in companion animals and some of the information has been extrapolated from people.
- Colchicine has a narrow therapeutic index. There is overlap between the therapeutic and the toxic dose of this drug. Additionally, there is no clear toxic or lethal dose and there may be significant individual variation.
- In people, general dose guidelines have been reported.
  - <0.5 mg/kg has been associated with gastrointestinal toxicity and coagulation disorders.
  - 0.5–0.8 mg/kg has been associated with alopecia, bone marrow aplasia, and a 10% mortality rate.
  - Doses of >0.8 mg/kg have been linked to shock, multiorgan failure, and death.
- Dog.
  - Doses of <0.5 mg/kg have been associated with gastrointestinal distress.
  - The lowest reported lethal dose in a dog is 0.13 mg/kg.

Systems Affected

- Organs with a high cell turnover rate are the most vulnerable.
- Gastrointestinal – gastrointestinal mucosal damage.
- Bone marrow – aplasia.
- Respiratory – acute respiratory distress syndrome.
- Cardiovascular – hypovolemia, dysrhythmias, cardiovascular collapse and death.
- Musculoskeletal – myopathy.
- Renal – acute kidney injury.
- Hepatic – hepatic failure.
- Metabolic – metabolic acidosis, hypokalemia, hyponatremia, hypocalcemia, hypoglycemia.

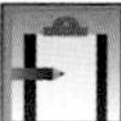

SIGNALMENT/HISTORY

- No age or breed predilection has been identified. However, this drug may be used to reduce the risk of amyloid deposition in Shar Pei fever.

Risk Factors

- An increased risk of toxicity has been identified in people with preexisting hepatic or renal dysfunction.

Interactions with Drugs, Nutrients, or Environment

- Drugs that inhibit CYP3A4 may increase toxicity. These drugs include macrolide antibiotics, cyclosporine, ketoconazole, itraconazole, and natural grapefruit juice.

- Prazosin, vinblastine, quinidine, H_2 blockers, glucocorticoids, and verapamil may alter colchicine clearance.
- Concurrent use of colchicine and statins has resulted in myopathy in people.

Historical Findings

- History of recent colchicine administration.
- Discovery of a chewed pill bottle.
- Discovery of chewed plant material from *C. autumnale* or *G. superba*, which resemble wild garlic or sweet potatoes, respectively.

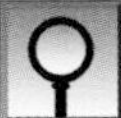

CLINICAL FEATURES

- Limited case reports in dogs have found various clinical signs.
  - Gastrointestinal – inappetence, vomiting, diarrhea, and abdominal pain.
  - Hematological – erythrocyte microcytosis, absence of suspected stress leukogram.
  - Hepatopathy.
    - Increased alanine transaminase, aspartate aminotransferase, alkaline phosphatase, and mild hyperbilirubinemia.
    - Hepatic histology – metaphase arrest and ring mitoses.
  - Myopathy – abnormal posture, lameness, hyperpathia, pain on muscle palpation, increased aspartate aminotransferase and creatine kinase.
- Three-phase clinical course is reported in people.
  - Phase 1.
    - Occurs within 24 hours.
    - Predominantly gastrointestinal signs – nausea, vomiting, diarrhea, abdominal pain, and hypovolemia.
  - Phase 2.
    - Occurs within 7 days of drug exposure.
    - Characterized by multiorgan injury.
    - May initiate DIC, pancytopenia, hemolysis, and metabolic derangements.
  - Phase 3 (recovery phase).
    - Within 7–12 days of drug exposure.
    - Characterized by resolution of organ dysfunction and rebound leukocytosis.
- Myopathy is rare but has also been characterized in people.

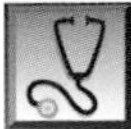

DIFFERENTIAL DIAGNOSIS

- Enterocolitis
- Sepsis

- Heavy metal toxicity (late phase)
- Primary metabolic disease (e.g., hepatic, renal, respiratory)
- Primary neuromuscular disease (e.g., infectious, inflammatory, neoplastic, etc.)

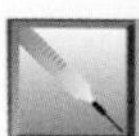

DIAGNOSTICS

- Colchicine plasma concentrations can be measured by liquid chromatography-mass spectrometry but this is not readily available.
- Baseline laboratory work to include:
  - CBC
    - pancytopenia with bone marrow suppression
    - leukocytosis (late phase)
  - serum chemistry including liver enzymes, BUN, and creatinine
  - urinalysis for early signs of renal dysfunction
  - coagulation testing
  - creatine kinase.
- MDR1 loss of function mutation in susceptible breeds.

Pathological Findings

- Hepatic biopsy – inhibition of cell spindle formation is evidenced by metaphase arrest and ring mitoses.
- Muscle biopsy – myocyte vacuolar change in the absence of necrosis or inflammation.

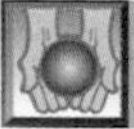

THERAPEUTICS

Detoxification

- Immediate discontinuation of colchicine.
- Induce emesis only if early after ingestion and the animal is asymptomatic.
- Gastric lavage.
- Activated charcoal with a cathartic.

Appropriate Health Care

- Monitor CBC, BUN, creatinine, and liver enzymes.
- Be aware of the potential for multiple organ dysfunction.
- Monitor for development of respiratory and neurological dysfunction.

Antidote

- No specific antidote.

Drugs of Choice

- IV fluid therapy to treat hypovolemia and electrolyte derangements.
- Supportive care addressing specific organ toxicity.

COMMENTS

Expected Course and Prognosis

- Outcome is generally poor as the safety margin is narrow and multiple organs are often affected.

Synonyms

Colchium autumnale (autumn crocus) – meadow saffron, naked lady
Gloriosa superba (glory lily) – climbing lily, flame lily, gloriosa lily, tiger claw

Abbreviations

See Appendix 1 for a complete list.

Suggested Reading

Aghabiklooei A, Zamani N, Hassanian-Moghaddam H, et al. Acute colchicine overdose: report of three cases. Reumatismo 2013; 65:307–311.

Finkelstein Y, AKS SE, Hutso JR, et al. Colchicine poisoning: the dark side of an ancient drug. Clin Toxicol 2010; 48:407–414.

McAlister A, Center SA, Bender H, et al. Adverse interaction between colchicine and ketoconazole in a Chinese shar pei. J Am Anim Hosp Assoc 2014; 50:417–423.

Wagenaar Z. Accidental colchicine poisoning in a dog. Can Vet J 2004; 45:55–57.

Authors: Stephanie Kleine, DVM, DACVAA; Jane Quandt, DVM, MS, DACVAA, DACVECC
Consulting Editor: Lynn R. Hovda, RPh, DVM, MS, DACVIM

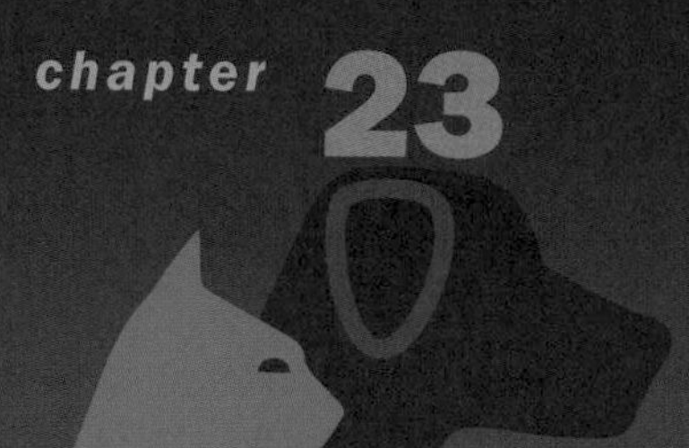

Cyclosporine A

DEFINITION/OVERVIEW

- Cyclosporine is a cyclic lipophilic polypeptide macrolide used as a potent immunosuppressive and immunomodulatory drug.
- It is commonly used to manage canine atopic dermatitis and anal furunculosis, feline allergic dermatoses, and lagomorph (rabbit) sebaceous adenitis.
- There are some uses for neoplasias in conjunction with other chemotherapeutic agents in small animals.
- The margin of safety in both acute and chronic overdosing is wide, with adverse effects usually consisting of mild gastrointestinal distress (diarrhea, vomiting, inappetence).
- Two forms of oral dosing of the medication exist.
    - Vegetable oil-based formulation.
    - Microemulsified formulation.

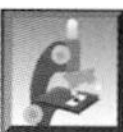

ETIOLOGY/PATHOPHYSIOLOGY

Mechanism of Action

- Both antiinflammatory and antipruritic effects.
    - Calcineurin inhibitor; preferentially suppresses T-lymphocyte activation.
    - Inhibits the antigen-presenting function of the skin immune system.
    - Blocks recruitment and activation of eosinophils, keratinocytic production of cytokines, Langerhans cell function, mast cell degranulation and release of histamine and proinflammatory cytokines.

Pharmacokinetics – Absorption, Distribution, Metabolism, Excretion

- Absorption.
    - Primarily absorbed in the intestine by passive diffusion.
        - Absorption of the vegetable oil-based form in humans and dogs is dependent on biliary secretion.

Blackwell's Five-Minute Veterinary Consult Clinical Companion: Small Animal Toxicology, Second Edition.
Lynn R. Hovda, Ahna G. Brutlag, Robert H. Poppenga, and Katherine L. Peterson.

Companion website: www.fiveminutevet.com/toxicology

    - Absorption of the microemulsified form is not dependent on bile secretion.
    - Oral bioavailablility is 35% in dogs, 25–29% in cats, and <5% in rabbits and guinea pigs.
    - Co-administration of food in dogs decreases bioavailablility.
- Distribution.
  - Lipophilic – large volume of distribution; cyclosporine is distributed widely in skin and adipose tissue, liver, fat and blood cells.
- Metabolism.
  - Metabolized primarily in the liver (cytochrome P450), and to a lesser extent in the intestine and kidney.
    - Dogs metabolize at 2–3 times greater capacity than humans, rabbits and rats.
  - Approximately 30 metabolites of cyclosporine are formed by sulfation, hydroxylation, and demethylation.
- Elimination.
  - Primarily biliary, with minimal renal excretion.
  - Dogs: elimination half-life is 5–12 hours.
  - Cats: elimination half-life varies (6.8–40 hours).

Toxicity

- Wide margin of safety for both acute and chronic overdosing.
- Adverse effects increase with increased dose and duration of ingestion.
- Long-term exposure to cyclosporine is associated with increased incidence of malignant neoplasia.

Systems Affected

- Gastrointestinal – gastroenteritis.
- Rare dermal compromise – pruritus, gingival hyperplasia, other dermatoses.
- Rare hepatic compromise.
- Rare renal compromise.
- Rare lymphoid system compromise.
- Rare hematological compromise.

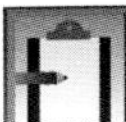

SIGNALMENT/HISTORY

- Any species may be affected.
- Overdose is usually secondary to iatrogenic administration or inappropriate ingestion by pet.

Risk Factors

- Not approved for use in breeding, pregnant or nursing animals – fetotoxic and embryotoxic in rats and rabbits.

- Caution if preexisting renal or hepatic compromise.
- Caution in animals <6 months of age and <1.8 kg BW (safety and efficacy unknown).

Interactions with Drugs, Nutrients, or Environment

- Toxicity may be enhanced in animals concurrently ingesting the following drugs: acetazolamide, allopurinol, amlodipine, azithromycin, azole antifungals, bromocriptine, calcium channel blockers, carvedilol, cimetidine, chloramphenicol, ciprofloxacin/enrofloxacin, cisapride, clarithromycin, clopidogrel, colchicine, corticosteroids, danazol, digoxin, estrogens, fluvoxamine, glipizide/glyburide, grapefruit juice/grapefruit juice powder, imipenem, losartan, valsartan, medroxyprogesterone, metoclopramide, metronidazole, omeprazole, sertraline, tinidazole, vitamin E.

CLINICAL FEATURES

- Common clinical signs include gastrointestinal distress (vomiting, diarrhea, inappetence).
- As ingested dose increases, reported uncommon or rare effects include dermal pruritus, hepatotoxicity, thromboembolism, secondary opportunistic infection, renal dysfunction (in already compromised humans and rats), changes in blood pressure, diabetes mellitus (dog), bone marrow suppression, flaring of latent viral infections (cats).

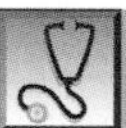

DIFFERENTIAL DIAGNOSIS

- Other gastrointestinal diseases.
- Other toxicants causing mild gastrointestinal signs.

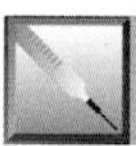

DIAGNOSTICS

- CBC and serum chemistry abnormalities are largely extrapolated from human medicine and may be useful as baseline.

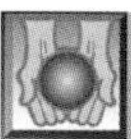

THERAPEUTICS

Detoxification

- Emesis if within 30–45 minutes of witnessed ingestion.
    - Apomorphine for dogs: 0.02–0.04 mg/kg IV or IM, or direct application of the tablet form into the subconjunctival sac.
    - Hydrogen peroxide for dogs: 1–5 mL/kg PO of 3% concentration, not to exceed 45 mL. Xylazine for cats: 0.44mg/kg IM or SQ. Xylazine may be reversed with alpha$_2$-adrenergic antagonists.
        - Yohimbine: 0.1 mg/kg IM, SQ, or IV slowly.
        - Atipamezole (Antisedan): 25–50 μg/kg IM or IV.
- Activated charcoal with a cathartic × one dose.

Appropriate Health Care

- Baseline CBC and chemistry panel, baseline blood pressure.
- Symptomatic and supportive care.

Antidote

- No specific antidote is available.

Drugs of Choice

- Judicious IV fluid use, maintaining hydration and blood pressure as needed.
- Antiemetics if vomiting is severe or persistent.
  - Dolasetron 0.5–1.0 mg/kg IV 24 hours.
  - Maropitant 1 mg/kg SQ q 24 hours.
  - Ondansetron 0.1–0.2 mg/kg IV q 6–12 hours.
- GI protectants as needed.
  - H_2 blockers.
    - □ Famotidine 0.5–1 mg/kg PO, SQ, IM, IV q 12–24 hours (careful IV use in cats).
    - □ Ranitidine 1–2 mg/kg PO, SQ, IM, IV q 8–12 hours.
  - Sucralfate 0.25–1 g PO q 8 hours × 5–7 days if evidence of active ulcer disease.

Nursing Care

- Monitor hydration, as occasionally vomiting and diarrhea may be severe.
- If historically compromised hepatic or renal patient, consider hospitalization to continue to monitor, and do follow-up CBC and chemistry blood work.

COMMENTS

Patient Monitoring

- CBC and chemistry panel as needed.

Expected Course and Prognosis

- Generally excellent prognosis with control of presenting signs (usually only gastrointestinal).

Abbreviations

See Appendix 1 for a complete list.

See Also

Tacrolimus

Suggested Reading

Forsythe P, Paterson S. Cyclosporine 10 years on: indications and efficacy. Vet Rec Focus 2014; March:13–21.

Heinrich N, McKeever P, Eisenschenk M. Adverse events in 50 cats with allergic dermatitis receiving cyclosporine. Vet Derm 2011; 22:511–520.

Kovalik M, Thoday K, van den Broek A. The use of cyclosporine A in veterinary dermatology. Vet J 2012; 193:317–325.

Plumb D. Cyclosporine (systemic). In: Plumb D, ed. Veterinary Drug Handbook, 8th edn. Ames, IA: Wiley, 2015.

Roberts E, VanLare K A, Strehlau G, et al. Safety, tolerability, and pharmacokinetics of 6-month daily dosing of an oral formulation of cyclosporine (ATOPICA for cats©) in cats. J Vet Pharm Ther 2013; 37:161–168.

Vivano K. Update on immunosuppressive therapies for dogs and cats. Vet Clin North Am Small Anim Prac 2013; 43:1152–1153.

Authors: Julie Schildt, DVM, DACVEEC; David R. Brown, PhD
Consulting Editor: Lynn R. Hovda, RPh, DVM, MS, DACVIM

chapter 24

Diuretics

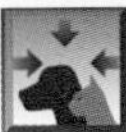

DEFINITION/OVERVIEW

- Diuretic toxicosis is generally confined to plasma volume depletion, with consequent hypoperfusion of critical organs, mainly the kidneys, and electrolyte abnormalities.
- Rehydration is normally sufficient to correct acute diuretic overdosing.

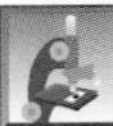

ETIOLOGY/PATHOPHYSIOLOGY

- Diuretics are primarily used in management of congestive heart failure. Aggressive administration can result in prerenal azotemia and if renal perfusion pressure drops sufficiently, intrinsic renal damage may occur (rare).
- Less common complications include electrolyte depletion or excess such as hypokalemia, hypomagnesemia and hyperkalemia (diuretic dependent).

Mechanism of Action

- All diuretics commonly used in veterinary medicine affect electrolyte transfer (and water) across the nephron.
    - Diuretics work in specific sites along the renal tubule, locations vary based on diuretic type.
- See table 24.1 for the mechanism and site of action of most known diuretics.

Pharmacokinetics – Absorption, Distribution, Metabolism, Excretion

- Hydrochlorothiazide.
    - Administered orally.
    - Onset and duration of action – in dogs, onset of action is within 2 hours, with peak plasma concentrations at 2.4 hours. Effects last approximately 12 hours. No data available for cats.
    - Absorption – occurs in the proximal part of the intestine. In humans, approximately 60–80% is absorbed.

Blackwell's Five-Minute Veterinary Consult Clinical Companion: Small Animal Toxicology, Second Edition.
Lynn R. Hovda, Ahna G. Brutlag, Robert H. Poppenga, and Katherine L. Peterson.

Companion website: www.fiveminutevet.com/toxicology

TABLE 24.1. Mechanism of action of various diuretics. Diuretics of veterinary importance are highlighted in bold. Dashes signify that there is no renal location of action.

Classification	Examples	Mechanism	Location
No specific classification	Ethanol Water	Inhibit vasopressin secretion	——
Acidifying salts	$CaCl_2$ NH_4Cl		——
Aquaretics	Goldenrod Juniper	Increase plasma volume	——
Xanthines	Caffeine Theophylline	Inhibit reabsorption of Na^+, increase GFR	Proximal tubule
Osmotic diuretics	Glucose (especially in uncontrolled diabetes), **Mannitol**	Promote osmotic diuresis	Proximal tubule, descending limb
Na-H exchange antagonists	**Dopamine**	Promote Na^+ excretion, increase GFR	Proximal tubule
Carbonic anhydrase inhibitors	Acetazolamide Dorzolamide	Inhibit H^+ secretion, resultant promotion of Na^+ and K^+ excretion	Proximal tubule
Loop diuretics	Bumetanide Ethacrynic acid **Furosemide** Torsemide	Inhibit the Na-K-2Cl symporter	Loop of Henle
Thiazides	Bendroflumethiazide **Hydrochlorothiazide**	Inhibit reabsorption by Na^+/Cl^- symporter	Distal convoluted tubules
Arginine vasopressin receptor 2 antagonists	Amphotericin B Lithium citrate	Inhibit vasopressin	Collecting duct
Potassium-sparing diuretics	Amiloride, **Spironolactone** Triamterene Potassium Canrenoate	Inhibition of Na^+/K^+ exchanger. Spironolactone inhibits aldosterone action. Amiloride inhibits epithelial sodium channels	Cortical collecting ducts

- Distribution – predominantly confined to extracellular space and kidneys, with 40% protein binding.
- Metabolism – no appreciable metabolism.
- Excretion – renally excreted in the urine, unchanged, with 61% being eliminated at 24 hours.
- Elimination half-life – approximately 9 hours in the dog.

■ Furosemide.
- Administered parenterally or orally.
- Onset and duration of action – onset of action is within 30 minutes, and duration of action is approximately 6 hours. Little data exists for cats, but cats generally require lower doses than dogs for comparable degrees of CHF, suggesting an increased sensitivity to furosemide.

  - Absorption – fairly rapid rate of absorption with oral bioavailability of 77% in dogs.
  - Distribution – large volume of distribution, with 90% protein binding.
  - Metabolism – approximately 10% hepatic metabolism.
  - Excretion – 60–90% renal excretion, with the remaining in feces and bile, amount dependent on route of administration.
  - Elimination half-life – 1–1.5 hours.
- Spironolactone.
  - Administered orally.
  - Onset and duration of action – diuretic action takes several days to reach its effect and lasts for several days after cessation.
  - Absorption – rate of absorption is rapid with a variable oral bioavailability of 50% at fasting and up to 90% with a meal.
  - Distribution – large volume of distribution, with 90% protein binding.
  - Metabolism – occurs in liver and kidney, extent is unknown.
  - Excretion – 70% renal excretion, with the remaining in feces and bile.
  - Elimination half-life – 20 hours for the active metabolite canrenone.

Toxicity

- Diuretics have a fairly wide margin of safety.
  - The oral LD_{50} of furosemide in dogs is >1000 mg/kg.
  - Dehydration and electrolyte imbalances are the most common result of toxicity.
  - Most diuretic intoxications do not cause primary nephrotoxicity.

Systems Affected (see table 24.2)

- Cardiovascular – arrhythmias.

TABLE 24.2. Adverse effects and clinical signs associated with diuretics.

Adverse effect	Diuretics	Clinical signs
Hypovolemia	Loop diuretics Thiazides	Thirst, hypotension, azotemia/uremia, oliguric acute renal failure
Hypokalemia	Loop diuretics Thiazides	Muscle weakness, arrhythmias
Hyperkalemia	Spironolactone	Arrhythmias
Hyponatremia	Thiazides Furosemide	Potentially CNS symptoms if severe hyponatremia. Not clinically reported in small animals
Metabolic alkalosis	Loop diuretics Thiazides	Rarely a clinical problem
Hypercalcemia	Thiazides	Only a problem if administered to hypercalcemic patients
Hyperuricemia	Thiazides Loop diuretics	Uric acid retention (dalmatians)
Ototoxicity	Furosemide	Only at supraphysiological doses (20 mg/kg)
Dermatopathy	Spironolactone	Excoriative dermatopathy in cats

- Endocrine/metabolic – electrolyte disturbances.
- Gastrointestinal – vomiting, anorexia secondary to azotemia/uremia.
- Musculoskeletal – weakness due to hypokalemia, hypomagnesemia.
- Skin/exocrine – pruritic excoriative dermatitis with spironolactone in cats.

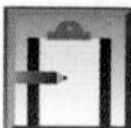

SIGNALMENT/HISTORY

- There are no specific breed or species predispositions to diuretic intoxication.
- Patients with cardiac disease, especially output failure, anorexia and hypodipsia can have an increase in drug effects.

Historical Findings

- Vomiting, anorexia, anuria, depression, and weakness are the most common presenting signs of diuretic toxicosis.

Location and Circumstances of Poisoning

- May be due to continued and/or inappropriate administration in ill CHF patients.
- Many toxicities occur due to misadventure with medication in the house resulting in ingestion of excessive amounts of diuretics.

Interactions with Drugs, Nutrients, or Environment

- Furosemide can increase the potential for aminoglycoside ototoxicity and nephrotoxicity.
- Clinically relevant hyperkalemia is extremely unlikely with potassium-sparing diuretics, even if co-administered with ACE inhibitors.
- Hypokalemia/hypomagnesemia is more likely with co-administration of loop and thiazide diuretics.
- Furosemide can increase the toxicity of digoxin due to hypokalemia and hypomagnesemia.
- Spironolactone can increase digoxin half-life, resulting in increased digoxin concentrations.

CLINICAL FEATURES

- Depression, weakness, lethargy.
- Dehydration.
- Vomiting if severely uremic.
- Arrhythmias on auscultation if severely hypokalemic/hypomagnesemic or severely hyperkalemic.

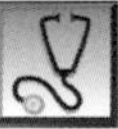

DIFFERENTIAL DIAGNOSIS

- Allergic dermatopathy in cats administered spironolactone.

  - Gastroenteritis (vomiting).
  - Toxicants.
    - □ Digoxin.
    - □ Other toxins that can cause primary renal failure (e.g., NSAIDs, raisins, vitamin D_3/cholecalciferol).
- Primary acute renal failure.

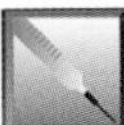

DIAGNOSTICS

- General biochemical analysis should be sufficient to identify dehydration or electrolyte imbalances and any renal concerns.
- Electrocardiography is required to evaluate possible arrhythmias.

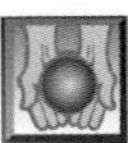

THERAPEUTICS

- Correction of dehydration generally resolves most of the major adverse effects of diuretics.

Detoxification

- Early emesis followed by activated charcoal with cathartic in acute situations.

Appropriate Health Care

- Care should be taken when rehydrating patients that have severe cardiac disease to avoid volume overloading.
- Hourly monitoring of the patient's respiratory rate and effort can help determine if fluid therapy is precipitating CHF recurrence.
- Severe dehydration is best counteracted by judicious fluid administration and cessation of drug administration.

Antidote

- No specific antidote is available.

Drug(s) of Choice

- Intravenous fluid administration will assist with increasing plasma volume and result in increased diuresis and drug excretion.
  - Electrolyte administration may be required in some cases, especially with severe hypokalemia.

- In severely hyperkalemic patients, furosemide and sodium bicarbonate administration can help reduce the hyperkalemia (rarely required with spironolactone toxicity).

Precautions/Interactions

- Aminoglycosides should be used cautiously with furosemide therapy.
- Overly aggressive fluid replacement can precipitate CHF in patients with severe heart disease.

Nursing Care

- Monitor respiratory rate and effort.
- With most electrolyte disturbances, oral supplementation is sufficient for correcting deficits.

Diet

- In cases of chronic hypokalemia, a high-potassium supplement can help minimize recurrence.

Prevention

- Use caution when administering diuretics and the lowest effective dose should be administered.
- Extra vigilance is required when combining diuretics, as the risk of dehydration increases.

COMMENTS

Patient Monitoring

- Monitor urine output.
- Recheck BUN/creatinine 24–48 hours after initial treatment of toxicosis.
- Monitor electrolytes every 4–6 hours until hydration status and electrolyte abnormalities have returned to normal.
- Monitor body weight and PCV to assess correction of hydration deficits.

Prevention/Avoidance

- Clients should be advised to watch for changes in appetite, thirst, or urination while the patient is receiving diuretics. If the patient becomes anorexic or hypodipsic, then the diuretic administration should be suspended and the veterinarian consulted.
- Continued administration of diuretics in anorexic or adipsic patients substantially increases the risk of severe dehydration. Consumption of commercial pet food generally provides sufficient electrolytes to avoid electrolyte depletion.

Expected Course and Prognosis

- Treatment of dehydration due to diuretics is generally straightforward, and if done carefully in heart disease patients, usually results in complete resolution of clinical signs within a few days.

Abbreviations

See Appendix 1 for a complete list.

See Also

Cardiac Glycosides
Veterinary NSAIDs (Carprofen, Deracoxib, Firocoxib, Ketoprofen, Meloxicam, Robenacoxib, Tepoxalin)

Suggested Reading

Aldactazide. Available at: www.rxlist.com/aldactazide-drug.htm

Furosemide. Available at: hwww.rxlist.com/lasix-drug.htm

Khaled KA, Asiri YA, El-Sayed YM. In vivo evaluation of hydrochlorothiazide liquisolid tablets in Beagle dogs. Int J Pharmaceut 2001; 222:1–6.

Kittleson MD. Management of heart failure-drugs used in treating heart failure. Part 2. In: Kittleson MD, ed. Small Animal Cardiovascular Medicine, 2nd edn. Veterinary Information Network. Available at: www.vin.com/Members/proceedings/Proceedings.plx?CID=SACARDIO&PID=12499&O=VIN

MacDonald KA, Kittleson MD, Kass PH, et al. Effect of spironolactone on diastolic function and left ventricular mass in Maine coon cats with familial hypertrophic cardiomyopathy. J Vet Intern Med 2008; 22(2):335–341.

Acknowledgment: The authors and editors acknowledge the prior contributions of Mark Rishniw, MS, PhD, DACVIM, who authored this topic in the previous edition.

Author: Renee D. Schmid, DVM
Consulting Editor: Lynn R. Hovda, RPh, DVM, MS, DACVIM

chapter 25

Minoxidil

DEFINITION/OVERVIEW

- Minoxidil is a potent, directly acting arteriolar dilator. It is used as a prescribed oral medication for the treatment of severe and malignant hypertension in humans.
- Minoxidil also stimulates hair follicles and produces hypertrichosis in humans and animals. Available as an over-the-counter topical formulation, it is applied to the scalp by men and women to slow hair loss and increase hair growth.
- Cats are particularly susceptible to minoxidil toxicosis.
- Cats and dogs can be exposed to minoxidil through topical and oral routes of absorption. The most common poisoning scenario involves minoxidil ingestion during grooming of body areas to which human topical hair loss products have been misapplied. There is also a potential risk for ingestion of minoxidil tablets intended for blood pressure control.

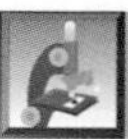

ETIOLOGY/PATHOPHYSIOLOGY

Mechanism of Action

- Minoxidil is a prodrug. It selectively dilates arterioles without affecting venous capacitance after its conversion in the liver to an active, sulfated metabolite. Minoxidil *N-O* sulfate interacts directly and irreversibly with ATP-sensitive potassium channels to lengthen their open time and increase potassium permeability in arteriolar smooth muscle cells. This action limits the availability of calcium required for smooth muscle contraction.
- A small portion of the minoxidil-induced hypotensive effect may involve endogenous vasodilator prostanoids.
- Hypotension caused by systemic vasodilation induces baroreflex activation of the sympathetic nervous system, leading to an increase in heart rate and myocardial oxygen consumption.
- The pathogenesis of cardiac lesions in dogs is unknown, but is thought to result from myocardial hyperperfusion leading to coronary artery and right atrial hemorrhage and necrosis.

Blackwell's Five-Minute Veterinary Consult Clinical Companion: Small Animal Toxicology, Second Edition.
Lynn R. Hovda, Ahna G. Brutlag, Robert H. Poppenga, and Katherine L. Peterson.

Companion website: www.fiveminutevet.com/toxicology

- After topical application, minoxidil affects the hair cycle by stimulating anagen in resting hair follicles and shortening the telogen phase. Sulfotransferases in hair follicles and skin catalyze the formation of minoxidil sulfate, which is more potent in stimulating hair growth than the parent drug. The cellular mechanism of action of minoxidil and its sulfonated conjugate on hair follicles is unknown.

Pharmacokinetics – Absorption, Distribution, Metabolism, Excretion

- Minoxidil is administered as an oral formulation (2.5 or 10 mg tablets) for hypertension. It is also available in topical formulations (2% or 5% in liquid or foam) to stimulate hair growth.
- Minoxidil has high bioavailability (>90%) by the gastrointestinal route. It is rapidly absorbed and eliminated after oral administration, reaching a peak concentration within 2.5 hours, and has a plasma half-life of approximately 2 hours in Beagle dogs. It has lower systemic bioavailability (≈40%) when applied to healthy, intact skin in dogs. There is a dearth of information on the pharmacokinetic profile of minoxidil in cats.
- The peak hypotensive and reflex tachycardic effects of minoxidil occur within 4–8 hours after oral administration to Beagle dogs. The dissociation in time between the peak plasma concentrations and peak cardiovascular effects of minoxidil is attributable to the time-dependent conversion of the parent drug to its active metabolite.
- Minoxidil is rapidly and widely distributed throughout the body and it is not bound to plasma proteins. Studies in rats indicate that it does not cross the blood–brain barrier.
- After oral administration, minoxidil undergoes Phase 1 and Phase 2 metabolism in the liver and other body tissues, including skin and hair follicles. Its Phase 1 metabolite, 4'-hydroxy-minoxidil, is the principal metabolite excreted by dogs, and its Phase 2 glucuronide conjugate is the major metabolite produced in primates, including humans. Biotransformation of minoxidil is limited after its topical administration, and the parent drug is the main compound present at the site of application.
- A relatively minor sulfonated metabolite, minoxidil *N-O* sulfate, represents the biologically active form of the drug. This chemically reactive metabolite is hydrophobic and can accumulate in arteriolar smooth muscle cells, where it produces prolonged (>24 hours) relaxant activity due to its irreversible activation of ATP-sensitive potassium channels.
- It has been hypothesized that cats are more susceptible than dogs to minoxidil toxicity because of their poor ability to conjugate the drug to glucuronic acid, thereby exposing more of it to sulfate conjugation. However, there is no evidence to support this idea.
- Minoxidil and its metabolites are cleared by glomerular filtration and excreted in the urine.

Toxicity

- The toxic signs produced by minoxidil represent extensions of its potent hypotensive action.
- Acute LD_{50} values for dogs and cats have not been published.
- Oral LD_{50} (mice and rats): 1.4–2.5 mg/kg.

- Dogs: in canine studies, short-term administration of oral minoxidil causes a variety of cardiac lesions. However, dermal application of topical minoxidil does not produce these lesions.
- Cats: case literature suggests that topical application of ≤1 mg minoxidil may be lethal to cats. In one published report, two cats died within 90 hours after initial minoxidil exposure. However, ingestion of minoxidil likely occurred during licking of the treated area(s) as 5% minoxidil applied topically for 30 days in a cat did not result in any adverse effects.

Systems Affected

- Cardiovascular – severe and prolonged hypotension with reflex tachycardia, shift in coronary blood flow from endocardium to epicardium, pericardial effusion, and reduced cardiac function.
- Respiratory – dyspnea, cyanosis, pleural effusion and pulmonary edema.
- Renal – salt and water retention.
- Nervous – lethargy, hypothermia.
- Gastrointestinal – potential vomiting with ingestion of large numbers of tablets or hypersalivation with ingestion of topical formulation.

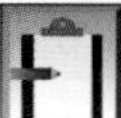

SIGNALMENT/HISTORY

Risk Factors

- Species: cats are more susceptible to minoxidil toxicity than dogs.
- No breed, sex, or age predilection.
- Cats with areas of alopecia where minoxidil may have been applied by the owner.
- Animals with preexisting cardiovascular, respiratory, or renal disease or those receiving antihypertensive or antiadrenergic medications may manifest a more severe toxicosis.

Historical Findings

- Intentional topical application of human hair products containing minoxidil to alopecic areas.
- Ingestion secondary to grooming of fur or hair on other animals or humans to which minoxidil has been applied.
- Spillage of hair loss products resulting in animal contact with minoxidil.
- Ingestion of minoxidil tablets.

Location and Circumstances of Poisoning

- Exposures to minoxidil generally occur in the home after intentional application of hair loss products to pets.

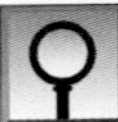

CLINICAL FEATURES

- The onset of minoxidil's cardiovascular action (hypotension with tachycardia) may be delayed for 1–2 hours after initial exposure.
- Animals may not present until severe respiratory signs have developed, which may be days after exposure.
- Once severe signs have developed, death usually occurs within 24 hours.
- For those animals that survive aggressive supportive care, treatment may be prolonged (3–5 days).
- Clinical signs and physical examination findings most commonly noted include the following.
    - Cardiovascular: tachycardia (dogs) or bradycardia (cats), pale mucous membranes, cyanosis, poor pulse quality, muffled heart sounds due to pleural/pericardial effusion.
- Respiratory: dyspnea, tachypnea, crackles and wheezes, decreased lung sounds secondary to pleural effusion.
- Nervous: lethargy, recumbency, hypothermia.
- Gastrointestinal: vomiting or hypersalivation after acute ingestion of tablets or topical formulation.
- Skin: areas of alopecia where topical product may have been applied.
- Death occurs secondary to cardiopulmonary congestion and cardiovascular collapse due to prolonged and severe hypotension.

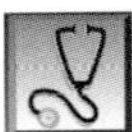

DIFFERENTIAL DIAGNOSIS

- Toxicants.
    - Baclofen, opiates (hypotension with *bradycardia*).
    - Cardiotoxic antineoplastic drugs, such as doxorubicin, cyclophosphamide, 5-fluorouracil.
    - Heavy metals, including copper, cobalt, manganese, nickel, lanthanum.
    - Other antihypertensive drugs, including calcium channel blockers and beta-adrenergic antagonists (hypotension with *bradycardia*).
- Primary respiratory disease.
    - Bronchitis, asthma.
    - Noncardiogenic pulmonary edema (near drowning, acute upper airway obstruction, electrocution, post seizure).
    - Pneumonia, hemorrhage, neoplasia.
    - Pleural effusion (pyothorax, hemothorax, chylothorax, FIP, neoplasia, hypoproteinemia).
- Primary cardiac disease.
- Acute anaphylaxis causing collapse, dyspnea, and hypotension.

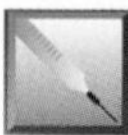

DIAGNOSTICS

- Thoracic auscultation to detect bilateral crackles, wheezes, and rales and assess heart rate (tachycardia or bradycardia).
- Blood pressure monitoring to detect hypotension.
- ECG assessing for tachycardia or bradycardia (especially in cats) and other arrhythmias.
- Monitoring of central venous pressure to assess volume status.
- Echocardiography to help determine if cardiac lesions are present and to help rule out other causes of cardiac disease. Findings with minoxidil toxicosis may include septal thickening, thickening of the left ventricular posterior wall, increased ejection fraction, decreased end-diastolic and systolic volumes and pericardial effusion.
- Thoracic radiography to rule out other causes of respiratory signs. Possible findings include pleural effusion and pulmonary edema.
- Thoracocentesis to characterize fluid and rule out other causes of pleural effusion. Fluid from affected animals is expected to be a transudate.
- Chemistry panel may be normal or liver enzymes (ALT, AST) and BUN may be above normal ranges due to hypotension and decreased perfusion.

Pathological Findings

- Dogs – pathological changes have been reported in the heart and vasculature of dogs treated with multiple oral doses of minoxidil; these include lesions involving the right atrium, left ventricular papillary muscle, and myocardial arteritis. Other reported lesions include subendocardial and papillary muscle necrosis, coronary arterial medial hemorrhage and necrosis, and multifocal to diffusely extensive areas of hemorrhage over the right atrial epicardium.
- Cats – postmortem examination of myocardial tissues from poisoned cats revealed evidence of interstitial edema and acute ischemia, lesions that were different from those seen in dogs.
- Other lesions include pleural effusion, failure of lung collapse due to extensive pulmonary congestion and edema, pericardial effusion, pale streaks interspersed with hemorrhage in the heart chambers extending from epicardial to endocardial surface. Cardiac weights and valvular measurements may be normal. Histologically, marked myocardial interstitial edema in all heart chambers, unevenly distributed areas of myodegeneration, and pleocellular myocarditis.

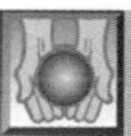

THERAPEUTICS

- The objectives of treatment are decontamination to prevent further toxin exposure in those animals presenting acutely in stable condition.
- In those animals already exhibiting clinical signs, treatment is aimed at stabilization and aggressive supportive care.

- In animals that survive, chronic management may be necessary if significant and permanent cardiac injury has occurred.

Detoxification

- Topical exposure – once patient has been stabilized, bathe areas where minoxidil was applied with liquid dishwashing detergent, even up to 48–72 hours after initial exposure as minoxidil is absorbed slowly by this route.
- Oral exposure – decontamination should only be performed in stable and asymptomatic patients. Induce emesis if ingestion occurred within 1 hour and there are no contraindications. Activated charcoal and cathartic can be considered to reduce further intestinal absorption of minoxidil.

Appropriate Health Care

- Animals should be hospitalized for aggressive cardiovascular and respiratory monitoring.
- Dyspneic animals should receive immediate oxygen supplementation via face mask or oxygen cage. Severely dyspneic animals may require endotracheal intubation and mechanical ventilation.
- Frequent monitoring of respiratory rate/effort, thoracic auscultation, pulse oximetry, blood pressure, and ECG is recommended to allow for adjustments in therapy and response to treatment.
- Thoracocentesis may be beneficial to improve respiratory effort and to allow for diagnostic evaluation in cases of pleural effusion.
- If pulmonary edema is present, diuretics can be given PRN until signs have improved.
- Intravenous crystalloids may be indicated to support blood pressure and facilitate removal of the drug and metabolites in the urine. However, cardiac function must be considered prior to fluid administration.
- Vasopressor agents may be indicated in hypotensive patients.
- Patients may require oxygen supplementation and mechanical ventilation may be necessary in severely affected patients.
- Thermoregulation may be necessary for hypothermic patients.

Antidote

- There is no specific antidote available.

Drugs of Choice

- Furosemide (2 mg/kg IM or IV PRN) or other loop diuretic to reduce fluid and salt retention.
- $Beta_1$-adrenergic receptor antagonists, such as esmolol (loading dose of 0.25–0.5 mg/kg IV over 1–2 minutes, followed by CRI of 10–200 µg/kg/min) or atenolol (0.2–1 mg/kg PO or IV q 12 hours, titrated to effect), to reduce reflex sympathetic activity.

- An $alpha_1$-adrenergic pressor agent such as dopamine (5–20 μg/kg/min IV CRI titrated to effect) or norepinephrine (0.1–0.2 μg/kg/min IV CRI titrated to effect) to maintain blood pressure.

Precautions/Interactions

- Electrolytes, acid–base, and renal values should be monitored in patients receiving diuretic therapy.
- When using diuretics, other potentially nephrotoxic drugs should not be used or used with extreme caution (NSAIDs, ACE inhibitors, aminoglycosides).
- If $beta_1$-adrenergic receptor antagonists are used, blood pressure should be closely monitored and these drugs discontinued if hypotension occurs.

Nursing Care

- Thermoregulatory support may be required for hypothermic patients.

Diet

- A nasoesophageal feeding tube or other means of parenteral nutrition may be necessary in animals with prolonged clinical signs that are unable or unwilling to eat or drink.

COMMENTS

Patient Monitoring

- The extent and type of patient monitoring will depend on the stability of the patient. Certain diagnostics such as thoracic radiographs and echocardiography may not be possible until the patient is stable.
- Patients should be hospitalized for frequent monitoring of respiratory rate/effort, thoracic auscultation, pulse oximetry, blood pressure, and ECG to assess for response to therapy and determine duration of treatment.

Prevention/Avoidance

- Clients should be educated about the toxicity of minoxidil tablets and topical preparations.
- Stress the importance of keeping these medications in secure locations where pets cannot access them.
- Explain that clients should never apply minoxidil or any medication topically unless directed to do so by a veterinarian.
- If topical minoxidil is being used therapeutically, appropriate measures should be taken to prevent oral access to the medication (e-collar, protective covering, etc.). Additionally, if there are other pets in the house, they should be isolated from any pet being treated with minoxidil.

Possible Complications

- In dogs, hypotension and reflex tachycardia lead to significant, irreversible cardiac lesions.
- In cats, death occurs secondary to cardiopulmonary congestion and cardiovascular collapse due to prolonged and severe hypotension.
- For severely affected patients, referral to a 24 hour facility with mechanical ventilation capabilities may be necessary.

Expected Course and Prognosis

- There are limited published data on the prognosis and expected clinical course in affected animals.
- Based on limited published information in cats, once a cat is severely affected prognosis is poor to grave.
- In those animals responsive to therapy, prolonged hospitalization may be necessary.
- For those animals that survive, permanent cardiac damage may be present.

Abbreviations

See Appendix 1 for a complete list.
FIP = feline infectious peritonitis

Suggested Reading

DeClementi C, Bailey KL, Goldstein SC, Orser MS. Suspected toxicosis after topical administration of minoxidil in 2 cats. J Vet Emerg Crit Care 2004; 14:287–292.

Hanton G, Gautier M, Bonnet P. Use of M-mode and Doppler echocardiography to investigate the cardiotoxicity of minoxidil in beagle dogs. Arch Toxicol 2004; 78:40–48.

Herman EH, Balazs T, Ferrans VJ, et al. Divergent effects of propranolol and furosemide pretreatment on acute cardiomyopathy induced by minoxidil in Beagle dogs. Toxicology 1981; 20:155–164.

Mesfin GM, Robinson FG, Higgins MJ, et al. The pharmacologic basis of the cardiovascular toxicity of minoxidil in the dog. Toxicol Pathol 1995; 23:498–506.

Thomas RC, Harpootlian H. Metabolism of minoxidil, a new hypotensive agent II: biotransformation following oral administration to rats, dogs, and monkeys. J Pharm Sci 1975; 64:1366–1371.

Thomas RC, Hsi RS, Harpootlian H, et al. Metabolism of minoxidil, a new hypotensive agent I: absorption, distribution, and excretion following administration to rats, dogs, and monkeys. J Pharm Sci 1975; 64:1360–1366.

Authors: Julie Schildt, DVM, DACVECC; David R. Brown, PhD
Consulting Editor: Lynn R. Hovda, RPh, DVM, MS, DACVIM

Nonbenzodiazepine Sleep Aids

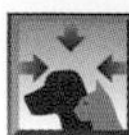

DEFINITION/OVERVIEW

- Three nonbenzodiazepine (NBZD) sleep aids are commonly prescribed in human medicine – eszopiclone (Lunesta®), zaleplon (Sonata®), and zolpidem (Ambien®).
- They have a similar mechanism of action to benzodiazepines (BZD) but are chemically distinct from BZDs.
- NBZD sleep aids are used for induction of sleep in people.
- Common clinical signs of overdose are related to the CNS and include agitation, ataxia, and depression.

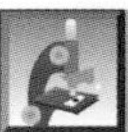

ETIOLOGY/PATHOPHYSIOLOGY

Mechanism of Action

- NBZD sleep aids interact with the type I benzodiazepine receptors that modulate GABA, an inhibitory neurotransmitter. They have strong hypnotic, i.e., sleep-inducing properties, but unlike benzodiazepines, do not have strong antianxiety or anticonvulsive effects.

Pharmacokinetics – Absorption, Distribution, Metabolism, Excretion

- NBZDs are well absorbed orally.
- Depending on the compound, they are moderately (eszopiclone, zaleplon) to highly (zolpidem) protein bound.
- Peak plasma levels generally occur between 60 and 90 minutes.
- Metabolized in liver to mainly inactive or less active metabolites.
- Half-life elimination in humans ranges from 1 to 6 hours depending on drug.
- Mainly excreted in urine.

Toxicity

- Overdose as a single exposure is rarely life-threatening in healthy animals.
- Lower doses generally cause CNS depression while higher doses may cause CNS excitation (paradoxical reaction).

Blackwell's Five-Minute Veterinary Consult Clinical Companion: Small Animal Toxicology, Second Edition.
Lynn R. Hovda, Ahna G. Brutlag, Robert H. Poppenga, and Katherine L. Peterson.

Companion website: www.fiveminutevet.com/toxicology

- Eszopiclone: dosages of >0.37 mg/kg were associated with signs.
- Zaleplon.
  - In dogs, dosages >0.11 mg/kg have been associated with restlessness and hyperactivity.
  - In cats, dosages of >1.25 mg/kg caused paradoxical reactions.
- Zolpidem.
  - In dogs, dosages >0.2 mg/kg cause mild sedation while those >0.6 cause paradoxical reactions.
  - Paradoxical reactions were seen in cats with dosages of >0.34 mg/kg.

Systems Affected

- Nervous – CNS depression, dysphoria, ataxia, excitement, aggression.
- Respiratory – respiratory depression.
- Cardiovascular – bradycardia, hypotension.
- Endocrine/metabolic – hypothermia from sedation.

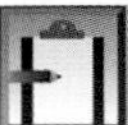

SIGNALMENT/HISTORY

- Any age or breed of dog or cat can be affected.
- Smaller animals are more prone to paradoxical reactions due to higher dosages received.
- Overdose usually occurs due to accidental ingestion of owner's medication.

Risk Factors

- NBZD sleep aids present in the household may pose an increased risk of exposure to pets.
- Pediatric, geriatric, or debilitated patients with underlying metabolic disease may have prolonged duration of effects from toxicosis.

Historical Findings

- Witnessed exposure by pet owner.
- Pet owner may find chewed pill vial or discover that a pill is missing.
- Clinical symptoms of ataxia, sedation, agitation, and dysphoria may be noted by the pet owner.

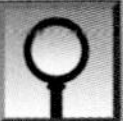

CLINICAL FEATURES

- Common clinical signs include CNS depression, ataxia, confusion, and disorientation.
- As ingested dose increases, risks for paradoxical reactions, hypotension, hypothermia, coma, and seizures occur.
- In approximately 50% of cases, paradoxical stimulation and excitation occur in both dogs and cats.

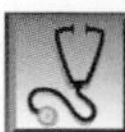

DIFFERENTIAL DIAGNOSIS

- Primary metabolic disease (hepatic encephalopathy, hypoglycemia).
- Primary neurological disease.
- Toxicants.
  - Sedation.
    - Alcohols and glycols (e.g., ethanol, methanol, ethylene glycol).
    - Barbiturates.
    - Marijuana.
    - Opiates and opioids.
    - Phenothiazines.
  - Agitation.
    - Amphetamines.
    - Antidepressants (serotonin syndrome).
    - Cocaine.
    - Pseudoephedrine.

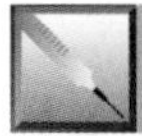

DIAGNOSTICS

- Baseline CBC, chemistry, UA to evaluate underlying metabolic disease.
- While not routinely available, urine or serum can be submitted specifically for GC/MS or LC/MS, but the results will take several days to be returned and will only indicate exposure.

Pathological Findings

- No specific findings are expected.

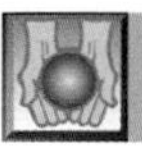

THERAPEUTICS

- Treatment consists of general supportive measures, early decontamination, and if necessary, administration of the reversal agent, flumazenil.

Detoxification

- Emesis with extreme caution due to rapid onset of signs.
- Activated charcoal with a cathartic × one dose for large ingestions although risk of aspiration must be considered.

Appropriate Health Care

- Monitor body temperature and blood pressure; support appropriately with warming methods and IV fluid therapy. Monitor for severe CNS or respiratory depression; if indicated, consider the use of flumazenil.

Antidote

- Flumazenil (Romazicon®) is the specific antidote for benzodiazepine overdose and has been shown to be useful in NBZD sleep aid exposure. It should be used only in cases where CNS depression or agitation is severe. Flumazenil rapidly reverses the sedative effects of the NBZDs. Effects are usually seen within 5 minutes. Seizures have been associated with the use of flumazenil.
- Dose: flumazenil 0.01 mg/kg IV to effect, repeat PRN. Repeated doses of flumazenil may be necessary, due to its short duration of action (1–2 hours).

Drugs of Choice

- IV fluids as needed to treat hypotension, maintain perfusion, and correct dehydration. A balanced crystalloid should be used.
- If the animal is experiencing paradoxical stimulation (e.g., agitation, aggression), treatment with benzodiazepines (e.g., diazepam) is contraindicated. An alternative sedative or anxiolytic should be used.
  - Acepromazine 0.05–0.2 mg/kg, IV, SQ, IM PRN.
  - Medetomidine 1–10 µg/kg, IV, SQ, IM PRN.

Precautions/Interactions

- CNS stimulants such as caffeine should be avoided.
- Co-ingestion of sedative or stimulants may intensify signs.

Follow-up

- No long-term effects expected.

COMMENTS

Client Education

- Owners should be advised not to use their own medicines to treat their pets and to keep them out of the reach of pets.

Patient Monitoring

- While hospitalized, excessively sedate patients should have blood pressure, ECG, TPR, and ventilatory status closely monitored.

Prevention/Avoidance

- Owners should be informed about the risks of NBZD sleep aids in pets, and keep them out of reach, particularly in the bedroom (e.g., tablet placed on bedroom table prior to ingestion).

Expected Course and Prognosis

- Once decontaminated, animals generally only need to be monitored for 2–4 hours.
  - If no clinical signs develop, the patient can be monitored at home.
  - If signs develop, they should be monitored until clinical signs have resolved (typically 12–24 hours depending on the drug involved).
- In those animals experiencing a single overdose exposure, the prognosis is excellent.

Abbreviations

See Appendix 1 for a complete list.

See Also

Benzodiazepines
Ethylene Glycol and Diethylene Glycol
Opiates and Opioids

Suggested Reading

Lancaster AR, Lee JA, Hovda LR, et al. Sleep aid toxicosis in dogs: 317 cases (2004-2010). J Vet Emerg Crit Care 2011; 21(6):658–665.

Richardson JA, Gwaltney-Brant SM, Albertsen JC, et al. Clinical syndrome associated with zolpidem ingestion in dogs: 33 cases (January 1998–July 2000). J Vet Intern Med 2002; 16:208–210.

Author: Eric Dunayer, MS, VMD, DABT, DABVT
Consulting Editor: Lynn R. Hovda, RPh, DVM, MS, DACVIM

chapter 27

Opiates and Opioids

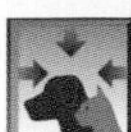

DEFINITION/OVERVIEW

- Opiate and opioid drugs are commonly used to provide analgesia to human and animal patients.
- Technically, opiates are naturally occurring while opioids are semi-synthetic or synthetic. Much blurring occurs and the entire group is often referred to as "opioids."
- Many different opioids with a variety of actions are commercially available (table 27.1).
- Opioids are commonly abused. Abused drugs may include prescribed medications or illicit drugs such as heroin. See chapter 37 on illicit opioids for more information.
- Recuvyra® is a novel, long-acting, highly concentrated (50 mg/mL), transdermal fentanyl solution for dogs.
- Simbadol™ is a long-acting, concentrated (1.8 mg/mL) formulation of buprenorphine meant for subcutaneous injection in cats.

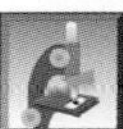

ETIOLOGY/PATHOPHYSIOLOGY

Mechanism of Action

- Opioids exert their effects on different opioid receptors.
- Opioid receptors, designated mu (μ_1 and μ_2), kappa (κ), sigma (σ), delta (δ), and epsilon (ε), are found throughout the body, including the adrenal glands, ANS, CNS (multiple locations), GIT, heart, lymphocytes, kidneys, pancreas, and vas deferens.
- The action of each drug varies depending on the affinity and activity at the opioid receptor, particular receptor, location of the receptor, and other factors such as lipid solubility.
- Affinity and activity.
  - Full agonist (e.g., morphine, codeine, heroin, fentanyl, meperidine, others) – affinity and activity at all important opioid receptors.
  - Full antagonist (e.g., naloxone) – affinity but no activity at opioid receptors; generally used as reversal agents for agonists.

Blackwell's Five-Minute Veterinary Consult Clinical Companion: Small Animal Toxicology, Second Edition.
Lynn R. Hovda, Ahna G. Brutlag, Robert H. Poppenga, and Katherine L. Peterson.

Companion website: www.fiveminutevet.com/toxicology

TABLE 27.1. Human prescription opioids.

Drug name (trade names)	Opioid receptor activity	Routes of administration
Alfentanil (Alfenta)	Mu agonist Short duration	IV
Buprenorphine (Buprenex, Temgesic, Subutex); buprenorphine + naloxone (Suboxone)	Partial mu agonist Dissociates slowly from receptors; long duration of action, difficult to antagonize	IM, IV, sublingual, transdermal patch (Europe)
Butorphanol (Torbugesic)	Mu antagonist Kappa agonist	IM, IV, SQ, nasal spray
Carfentanil (Wildnil)	Mu agonist	IM, PO (if specially prepared)
Codeine (Tylenol with Codeine #3, Robitussin AC)	Mu, delta, and kappa agonist (upon metabolism to morphine)	PO – many combination formulations with acetaminophen for pain and with dextromethorphan or guaifenesin for cough
Diprenorphine (M50–50)	Antagonist – reverses etorphine and carfentanil	IM, IV
Etorphine (M99)	Mu, delta, and kappa agonist (fentanyl analog)	IM
Fentanyl (Duragesic, Actiq, Sublimaze)	Mu agonist Highly lipid soluble Short acting	IM, IV, transdermal patch, PO as lollipop/lozenge or buccal soluble film/tablet
Heroin	Mu, delta, and kappa agonist	Illicit drug
Hydrocodone (Lortab, Lorcet); hydrocodone + acetaminophen (Vicodin); hydrocodone + ibuprofen (Vicoprofen); hydrocodone + aspirin (Lortab-ASA)	Agonist	PO Only available as a combination product in the US
Hydromorphone (Dilaudid)	Mu agonist (morphine derivative)	IM, IV, SQ, PO, rectal suppository
Loperamide (Imodium, Dimor, Lopex)	Acts on receptors in myenteric plexus of large intestines only; no CNS effects	PO
Meperidine (Demerol, Pethidine)	Agonist	IM, IV, SQ, PO
Methadone (Dolophine, Methadose)	Mu agonist	IM, IV, SQ, PO
Morphine (Avinza, Kadian, MS Contin)	Mu, delta, and kappa agonist	IM, IV, SQ, PO (often as extended-release forms), epidural, rectal suppository
Nalbuphine (Nubain)	Mu antagonist Kappa agonist	IM, IV
Nalmefene (Revex, disc. 2008)	Antagonist	IV

(*Continued*)

TABLE 27.1. *Continued*

Drug name (trade names)	Opioid receptor activity	Routes of administration
Naloxone (Narcan); naloxone + buprenorphine (Suboxone); naloxone + pentazocine (Talwin NX)	Antagonist	IV preferred, IM and SQ acceptable. Talwin NX is PO only
Naltrexone (Vivitrol, Revia); naltrexone + morphine sulfate (Embeda)	Antagonist Duration twice as long as naloxone	IM, PO
Oxycodone (OxyContin = controlled-release form); oxycodone + acetaminophen (Percocet and Roxicet); oxycodone + aspirin (Percodan); oxycodone + ibuprofen (Combunox)	Agonist	PO
Oxymorphone (Numorphan, Opana)	Mu agonist	IM, IV, SQ, PO
Pentazocine (Talwin); pentazocine + naloxone (Talwin NX); pentazocine + acetaminphen (Talacen)	Mu antagonist Kappa agonist	IM, IV, SQ Talwin NX and Talacen are PO only
Remifentanil (Ultiva)	Mu agonist Short duration	IV
Sufentanil (Sufenta)	Mu agonist Short duration	IV, epidural
Tapentadol (Nucynta)	Mu agonist	PO
Thiafentanil (A-3080)	Agonist – faster onset and shorter duration than carfentanil	IM
Tramadol (Ultram, Ultram ER, Ryzolt)	Agonist, weak	PO

- Agonist/antagonist (e.g., butorphanol, nalorphine) – affinity at all receptors with activity at only some of them.
- Partial agonist (e.g., tramadol, buprenorphine) – affinity for only some of the opioid receptors.

- Receptor types.
  - Mu receptors, in particular μ_1 receptors, are responsible for the analgesic effects; μ_2 receptors for respiratory depression. Mu agonists may be responsible for euphoria.
  - Kappa receptors produce sedation and dysphoria.
  - Delta receptors are responsible for analgesia at the spinal level.
  - Sigma receptors were originally thought to be responsible for euphoria and psychoactive effects, but that may no longer be the case.
- Location.
  - CNS – location of receptors determines whether excitation or depression occurs.
    - Dog – CNS depression; higher number of opioid receptors in amygdala and frontal cortex.
    - Cat – CNS stimulation and excitation; fewer receptors.

- ◻ CNS receptors located in CTZ – emesis.
- ◻ CNS receptors located in brainstem – cough and respiratory depression.
- ◻ GIT – decreased motility and constipation.

- Dopamine and norepinephrine concentrations play a role as well.

Pharmacokinetics – Absorption, Distribution, Metabolism, Excretion

- Opioids are well absorbed by all routes. They undergo extensive first-pass metabolism which results in a bioavailability of about 25% and a less predictable effect when given orally.
- Recuvyra® is well absorbed via the skin of the dorsal interscapular region. Absorption may vary based on site of application.
- Simbadol® is quickly absorbed after subcutaneous injection but there is a marked delay between plasma concentration and the onset/offset of the analgesic effect.
- Distribution is variable and depends on the particular opioid.
- Opioids undergo hepatic metabolism via hydrolysis, oxidation, and *N*-dealkylation.
    - Morphine's major metabolite is morphine-6-glucuronide, which is a pharmacologically active metabolite. Cats are deficient in glucuronyl-S-transferase, so this may account for their sensitivity.
    - Some of the glucuronides undergo enterohepatic recirculation.
- Elimination is renal.

Toxicity

- Morphine.
    - The minimum lethal SQ dose in the dog is 210 mg/kg, and for the cat 40 mg/kg.
    - The LD_{50} IV dose for the dog is 133 mg/kg.
- Codeine.
    - The intravenous LD_{50} for the dog is 69 mg/kg.
- Meperidine.
    - In the cat, 30 mg/kg has been known to cause seizures.

Systems Affected

- Varies depending on opioid and species involved.
- Respiratory – respiratory depression leading to death.
- CNS – depression (dogs) or excitation (cats).
- Cardiovascular – instability with hypotension; bradycardia.
- Gastrointestinal – decreased GI motility with constipation.
- Ophthalmic – miosis (dogs) or mydriasis (cats generally).
- Renal/urological – urinary retention.
- Endocrine/metabolic – meperidine and tramadol have some serotonergic activity.

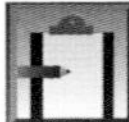

SIGNALMENT/HISTORY

- Any age or breed of dog or cat.
- Cats are particularly sensitive to morphine as at least 50% is metabolized by glucuronidation.
- Opioid overdose is usually through iatrogenic dose miscalculation or accidental ingestion of an oral product or patch.
- Opioid overdose can also occur with accidental ingestion of a human use product.
- Ingestion of spent fentanyl transdermal patches poses a significant risk of toxicosis. Patches worn for 3 days by humans and then discarded still retain 24–84% of the original amount of fentanyl (Fig. 27.1).
- Recent application of Recuvyra® or contact with a dog that has recently received Recuvyra® may pose a significant toxicity risk.
- Recuvyra® is approved for use in dogs only. Cats that have been treated or have come in contact with Recuvyra® should be treated for toxicity for up to 72 hours.
- Simbadol™ has not been evaluated in dogs or moribund cats so exposure to Simbadol may cause toxicity in these patients.

Risk Factors

- Loperamide should be used with caution in those dogs with the ATP-binding cassette (ABCB1-1Δ) polymorphism. Dogs that may exhibit this gene mutation include collies, Shetland sheepdogs, Old English sheepdogs, and other herding type dogs.
- Administration of Recuvyra® to diseased or injured skin may result in more rapid systemic absorption.

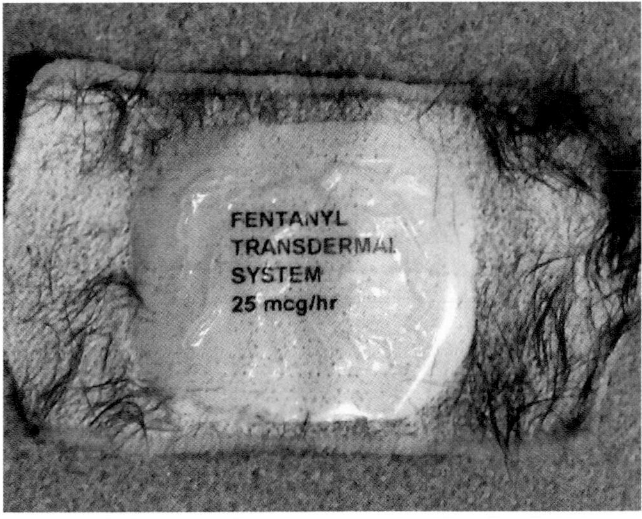

■ **Fig. 27.1.** Fentanyl patch when removed and discarded. Photo courtesy of Christy Klatt.

Interactions with Drugs, Nutrients, or Environment

- Tramadol and meperidine should not be used with tricyclic antidepressants, SSRIs, or monoamine oxidase inhibitors as this may lead to serotonin syndrome.

Historical Findings

- Discovery of a chewed pill bottle, fentanyl patch or lollipops, or the loss of a fentanyl patch that the animal has chewed off.

CLINICAL FEATURES

- CNS – depression and lethargy (dogs), excitation and aggressiveness (cats), ataxia, frank stupor, seizures, coma, death.
- Respiratory – early increasing rate followed by depression; decreased gag response with potential for aspiration pneumonia.
- Gastrointestinal – hypersalivation, vomiting, defecation (dogs), constipation (cats), urination or urinary retention.
- Cardiovascular – bradycardia, possible vasodilation, and hypotension.
- Ophthalmic – miosis (dogs) or mydriasis (more common in cats).
- Thermoregulatory center effects include hypothermia as the most common response; in some clinical cases hyperthermia may occur in cats. Panting may be seen in dogs.

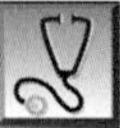

DIFFERENTIAL DIAGNOSIS

- Primary neurological disease (e.g., infectious, inflammatory, neoplastic, etc.).
- Primary metabolic disease (e.g., renal, hepatic, hepatic encephalopathy, hypoglycemia, hypoadrenocorticism).
- Toxicants.
    - Amphetamines/methylphenidate/methamphetamine/MDMA toxicoses.
    - Benzodiazepines.
    - **Cocaine.**
    - Marijuana toxicosis.
- Toxicities resulting in bradycardia include the following.
    - Alpha$_2$ agonist drugs.
    - Barbiturates.
    - Beta agonist blocking drugs.
    - Calcium channel blocking drugs.

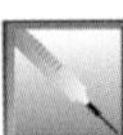

DIAGNOSTICS

- Detection of opioids can be done from urine or serum samples at human hospitals or be submitted to a laboratory for GC/MS or LC/MS.

- The Quick Screen Pro Multi Drug Screening Test is a human testing kit that has been validated by GC/MS for use in animals. It may provide a rapid and accurate diagnosis if the drug is present in high enough concentrations and the time frame is appropriate.
- Baseline CBC, chemistry, and UA, particularly in neonatal and geriatric patients, or those with underlying metabolic disease.
- Blood gas analysis to evaluate adequate oxygenation and ventilation.

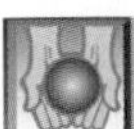

THERAPEUTICS

Detoxification

- If there was recent ingestion and the animal is alert, vomiting should be induced followed by activated charcoal with a cathartic × one dose.
- Gastric lavage if large doses ingested.
- Performing decontamination, even several hours post ingestion, is often effective due to decreased GI motility.
- Removal of fentanyl patches via endoscopy or surgery.

Appropriate Health Care

- Monitor closely for signs of respiratory depression, as this is the most common cause of death with opioid overdoses. If the animal is exhibiting severe respiratory depression leading to hypoxemia and hypercarbia, intubation, oxygen therapy, and positive pressure ventilation via orotracheal intubation may be required. Intubation will also protect the airway from possible aspiration of gastric contents.
- Close patient monitoring of heart rate, blood pressure, body temperature, and ventilation.
    - In cats demonstrating body temperatures >105.5°F, active cooling may be required.
- Be aware of the potential for the development of aspiration pneumonia.
- Monitor for normal urination.

Antidote

- Naloxone is the antidote of choice.
    - The dose is 0.01–0.02 mg/kg IM, IV, SQ. Doses up to 0.04 mg/kg may be required in serious intoxications, but monitor closely for CNS excitement.
    - The effects of naloxone last 30–60 minutes, so repeat doses may be necessary. A continuous IV infusion may be needed to help maintain ventilation.
    - The recommended dose for reversal of Recuvyra® is 0.04–0.16 mg/kg IM every 1 hour.
- If naloxone is not available, butorphanol 0.1–0.2 mg/kg IV, can be used to partially reverse pure μ agonists.

Drugss of Choice

- IV fluid therapy to support blood pressure and treat hypotension.
- Bradycardia is vagally mediated and can be treated with an anticholinergic such as atropine or glycopyrrolate given IM, IV, or SQ.
  - Atropine: 0.02–0.04 mg/kg IV, IM, or SQ.
  - Glycopyrrolate: 0.01–0.02 mg/kg SQ, IM, or IV.

Precautions/Interactions

- Buprenorphine is not reliably reversible with naloxone or butorphanol, due to its high affinity for the μ receptor.
- Simbadol™ may also be difficult to reverse and may require reversal for up to 24–28 hours.
- Recuvyra® has a duration of approximately 72 hours and may require reversal for up to 72 hours.

Nursing Care

- Turn frequently.
- Use eye lubricant as needed.
- Monitor TPR and urine output.

Surgical Considerations

- Ingested fentanyl transdermal patches should be removed by endoscopy or surgery.
- Sticks from fentanyl lollipops may become a foreign object requiring surgical removal.

COMMENTS

Client Education

- Keep all controlled medications out of reach of pets.
- If a pet has had a fentanyl patch placed, the patch should be monitored frequently to ensure that it is still in place. Preventive measures (e.g., e-collar, bandage, tape) should be used to prevent ingestion (Fig. 27.2). If the patch is missing and cannot be found, immediate veterinary attention should be sought.

Patient Monitoring

- Monitor TPR, ventilation, and blood pressure frequently.
- Thoracic radiographs to rule out secondary aspiration pneumonia.
- Pulse oximetry and arterial blood gas analysis to evaluate oxygenation and ventilation.

Possible Complications

- Aspiration pneumonia.

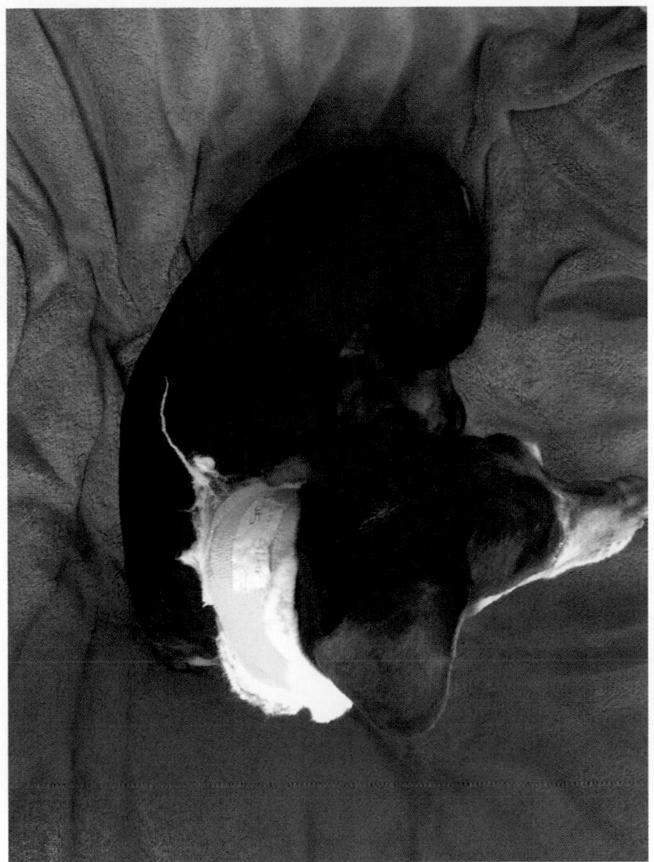

■ **Fig. 27.2.** Appropriately applied and labeled fentanyl patch on miniature dachshund. Photo courtesy of Christy Klatt.

Expected Course and Prognosis

- If the respiratory and cardiovascular function can be maintained, the prognosis is good; if seizures develop, the prognosis is guarded.

See Also

Benzodiazepines
Nonbenzodiazepine Sleep Aids
Opiates and Opioids (Illicit)

Abbreviations

See Appendix 1 for a complete list.

ABCB1-1Δ = ABC binding cassette polymorphism
MDMA = methylenedioxymethamphetamine

Suggested Reading

Freise KJ, Newbound GC, Tudan C, et al. Pharmacokinetics and the effect of application site on a novel, long-acting transdermal fentanyl solution in healthy laboratory Beagles. J Vet Pharmacol Ther 2012; 35:27–33.

Freise KJ, Newbound GC, Tudan C, et al. Naloxone reversal of an overdose of a novel, long-acting transderman fentanyl solution in laboratory Beagles. J Vet Pharmacol Ther 2012; 35:45–51.

Lamont LA, Mathews KA. Opioids, non-steroidal anti-inflammatories, and analgesic adjuvants. In: Tranquilli WJ, Thurmon JC, Grimm KA, eds. Lumb & Jones Veterinary Anesthesia and Analgesia, 4th edn. Ames, IA: Blackwell, 2007; pp. 241–271.

Malouin A, Boiler M. Sedatives, muscle relaxants, and opioids toxicity. In: Silverstein DC, Hopper K, eds. Small Animal Critical Care Medicine. St Louis, MO: Elsevier, 2009; pp. 350–356.

Schmiedt CW, Bjorling DE. Accidental prehension and suspected transmucosal or oral absorption of fentanyl from a transdermal patch in a dog. Vet Anaesth Analg 2007; 34:70–73.

Teitler JB. Evaluation of a human on-site urine multidrug test for emergency use with dogs. J Am Anim Hosp Assoc 2009; 45:59–66.

Acknowledgment: The authors and editors acknowledge Annemarie J. Solon for her assistance with this manuscript.

Authors: Stephanie Kleine, DVM, DAVCAA; Jane Quandt, DVM, DACVA, DACVECC

Consulting Editor: Lynn R. Hovda, RPh, DVM, MS, DACVIM

chapter 28

SSRI and SNRI Antidepressants

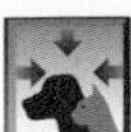

DEFINITION/OVERVIEW

- Toxicosis secondary to the overdose of an SSRI, SNRI, or co-ingestion of two types of serotonergic drugs.
- SSRIs include citalopram (Celexa®), escitalopram (Lexapro®), fluoxetine (Prozac®), fluvoxamine (Luvox®), paroxetine (Paxil®), sertraline (Zoloft®), vilazodone (Viibryd®), vortioxetine (Brintellix®). Most SSRIs are used as antidepressants.
- SNRIs include desvenlafaxine (Pristiq®), duloxetine (Cymbalta®), levomilnacipran (Fetzima®), milnacipran (Ixel®, Savella®), sibutramine (Meridia®, Reductil®) and venlafaxine (Effexor®). SNRIs are used to treat depression, chronic pain, generalized anxiety disorder, fibromyalgia, and obesity.

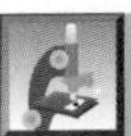

ETIOLOGY/PATHOPHYSIOLOGY

- SSRIs inhibit reuptake of serotonin, a neurotransmitter involved in aggression, anxiety, appetite, depression, migraine, pain, and sleep.
- Excessive stimulation of serotonin receptors leads to serotonin syndrome. Serotonin syndrome is characterized in humans as a combination of symptoms that include at least three of the following: myoclonus, mental aberration, agitation, hyperreflexia, tremors, diarrhea, ataxia, or hyperthermia.
- SNRIs inhibit the reuptake of serotonin but also norepinephrine. Norepinephrine (noradrenaline) acts as both a hormone and neurotransmitter. It is involved in the sympathetic system and can increase blood pressure and heart rate.
- Serotonin syndrome can occur along with cardiovascular signs (tachycardia, hypertension).

Mechanism of Action

- SSRIs: highly selective reuptake inhibitors of serotonin at the presynaptic membrane with little to no effect on other neurotransmitters.
- SNRIs: potent inhibitors of neuronal serotonin and norepinephrine reuptake.

Blackwell's Five-Minute Veterinary Consult Clinical Companion: Small Animal Toxicology, Second Edition.
Lynn R. Hovda, Ahna G. Brutlag, Robert H. Poppenga, and Katherine L. Peterson.

Companion website: www.fiveminutevet.com/toxicology

Pharmacokinetics – Absorption, Distribution, Metabolism, Excretion

- Most forms are well absorbed.
- Peak effects will vary depending on the formulation (immediate vs sustained/extended release).
- Most SSRIs and SNRIs are highly protein bound.
- Most undergo hepatic metabolism.
- Excretion may be renal or fecal.

Toxicity

- Toxic dosage varies widely among commonly available SSRIs and SNRIs and is not well defined in veterinary medicine.

Systems Affected

- Cardiovascular – decreased vascular tone (hypotension), increased heart rate and stroke volume (tachycardia).
- Gastrointestinal – increased smooth muscle contractility (vomiting, diarrhea).
- Nervous – stimulation (agitation, restlessness, seizures) and altered mental status (vocalization, disorientation).
- Neuromuscular – autonomic dysfunction (hyperactivity) and neuromuscular hyperactivity (hyperreflexia, myoclonus, tremors).
- Ophthalmic – increased autonomic function (mydriasis).
- Respiratory – increased bronchial smooth muscle contraction (dyspnea).

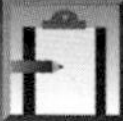

SIGNALMENT/HISTORY

- All species and breeds can be affected.
- There are no age or sex predilections.

Risk Factors

- Household members on SSRIs or SNRIs.

Historical Findings

- Agitation or lethargy
- Dilated pupils
- Vomiting
- Tremors
- Hypersalivation
- Diarrhea
- Seizures
- Nystagmus

Location and Circumstances of Poisoning

- Most poisonings occur within the home.
- Animals may be given the wrong medication by mistake or may have access to prescription medications.

Interactions with Drugs, Nutrients, or Environment

- Any drug that may affect serotonin levels or that is metabolized via CYP enzymes in the liver may lead to drug–drug interactions.
- This list includes lithium, nebivolol, ritonavir, MAO inhibitors (selegiline, isoniazid), TCAs, tryptophan, other SSRIs, other SNRIs, cimetidine, amiodarone, sumatriptan, tramadol, warfarin, tolbutamide (hypoglycemic agent), dextromethorphan, pentazocine, clarithromycin, cyproheptadine, benztropine, terfenadine, class 1C antiarrhythmics (propafenone, flecainide, encainide), desipramine, perphenazine, metoprolol, phenothiazines, theophylline, procyclidine, amitraz, and St John's wort.

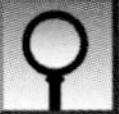

CLINICAL FEATURES

- Onset of signs can be within 1–2 hours for immediate-release products and up to 8 hours for extended/sustained-release products.
- Agitation
- Ataxia
- Mydriasis
- Tremors
- Vomiting
- Disorientation
- Hyperthermia
- Vocalization
- Depression
- Tachycardia
- Hypotension
- Diarrhea
- Blindness
- Seizures
- Hypersalivation
- Death

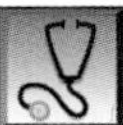

DIFFERENTIAL DIAGNOSIS

- Toxicological: TCAs, MAOIs, 5-HTP, metaldehyde, lead, ethylene glycol, hops, anticholinergics, antihistamines.

- Nontoxicological: meningitis (e.g., rabies, canine distemper), neoplasia, heat stroke, malignant hyperthermia.

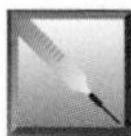

DIAGNOSTICS

- There are no diagnostic tests to confirm serotonin syndrome.
- Testing for individual SSRIs/SNRIs can be performed, but the tests are not clinically useful.
- Note: venlafaxine will give a false positive for PCP on many urine drug screens.
- Blood gas: metabolic acidosis may be seen.

Pathological Findings

- No pathological changes are expected.

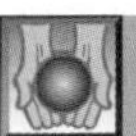

THERAPEUTICS

- Treatment is aimed at controlling life-threatening CNS and cardiovascular signs. Hypotension should be corrected and tremors controlled to decrease the risk of rhabdomyolysis.

Detoxification

- Emesis (if asymptomatic and recent ingestion) or gastric lavage (if large number of pills ingested).
- Activated charcoal with cathartics (if severe signs are expected).

Appropriate Health Care

- Hospitalize.
- Monitor body temperature, respirations, and heart rate.
- Monitor blood pressure.
- Monitor acid–base status.
- ECG for arrhythmias.
- IV fluids to help regulate body temperature and blood pressure and to protect kidneys from myoglobinuria secondary to rhabdomyolysis.

Antidote

- No specific antidote.

Drugs of Choice

- Agitation.

  - Phenothiazine.
    - Acepromazine 0.05 mg/kg IV or IM, titrate to effect as needed.
    - Chlorpromazine 0.5 mg/kg IV, IM or SQ, titrate up as needed.
  - Cyproheptadine.
    - Dogs: 1.1 mg/kg PO or rectally; serotonin antagonist.
    - Cats: 2–4 mg total dose per cat.
- Tachycardia.
  - Beta-blockers.
    - Propranolol 0.02–0.06 mg/kg IV.
- Tremors.
  - Methocarbamol 50–100 mg/kg IV, titrate up as needed.
- Seizures.
  - Benzodiazepines (diazepam 0.5–2 mg/kg IV); see Precautions/Interactions.
  - Barbiturates to effect.
    - Phenobarbital 3–4 mg/kg IV.

Precautions/Interactions

- Avoid tramadol as it can cause additive serotonergic effects.

Alternative Drugs

- Seizures – inhalant anesthetics (isoflurane, sevoflurane), propofol CRI.

Nursing Care

- Thermoregulation.
- Minimize sensory stimuli.

Follow-up

- No long-term problems are expected in most cases.

Diet

- No diet change is needed, except NPO during severe CNS signs.

Prevention

- Keep all medications out of the reach of pets.

COMMENTS

- Treatment in most cases is very rewarding.

Patient Monitoring

- Monitor HR, BP, and urine color, hourly at first and then less often if the animal remains clinically normal.

Prevention/Avoidance

- Keep all medications out of the reach of pets.
- Do not store human and animal drugs in the same area to decrease medication errors.

Possible Complications

- DIC secondary to severe hyperthermia.
- Rhabdomyolysis and secondary renal failure.

Expected Course and Prognosis

- If CNS and cardiac signs can be controlled, prognosis is good.
- Signs may last up to 72 hours with extended-release products.

See Also

Club Drugs (MDMA, GHB, Flunitrazepam, and Bath Salts)
Methamphetamine

Abbreviations

See Appendix 1 for a complete list.

MAOI = monoamine oxidase inhibitor
PCP = phencyclidine (angel dust)

Suggested Reading

Bloom FE. Neurotransmission and the central nervous system. In: Brunton LL, Lazo JS, Parker KL, eds. Goodman & Gilman's The Pharmacological Basis of Therapeutics, 11th edn. New York: McGraw-Hill Professional, 2006.

Fitzgerald KT, Bronstein AC. Selective serotonin reuptake inhibitor exposure. Top Comp Anim Med 2013; 28(1):13–17.

Author: Tina Wismer, DVM, DABVT, DABT, MS
Consulting Editor: Lynn R. Hovda, RPh, DVM, MS, DACVIM

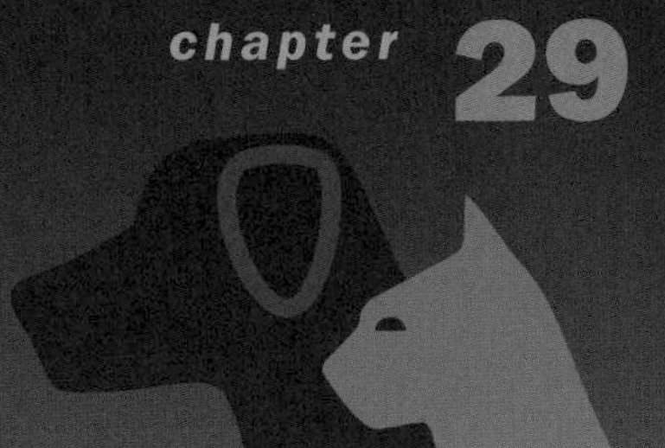

chapter 29

Tacrolimus

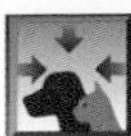

DEFINITION/OVERVIEW

- Tacrolimus is a macrolide antibiotic immunosuppressant produced by *Streptomyces tsukubaensis* that is used to manage immune-mediated disorders and prevent graft versus host disease in transplant patients.
- Tacrolimus is formulated as capsules (0.5 mg, 1 mg, 5 mg), ointments (0.03%, 0.1%), and injectable solutions (5 mg/mL). Aqueous ophthalmic solutions are frequently compounded for veterinary use.

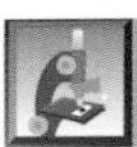

ETIOLOGY/PATHOPHYSIOLOGY

Mechanism of Action

- The immunosuppressive activity of tacrolimus is thought to be due to inhibition of calcineurin which blocks T-lymphocyte activation, thus impeding cell-mediated immunity.
- The mechanisms of the toxic effects of tacrolimus, including intussusception in dogs, are not known.

Pharmacokinetics – Absorption, Distribution, Metabolism, Excretion

- There is minimal systemic absorption following topical (epidermal) application and slight absorption following ocular administration.
- Oral bioavailability of tacrolimus is 9% in dogs. Bioavailability varies considerably among species. Presence of food reduces the rate and extent of absorption.
- Tacrolimus is 99% protein bound, primarily to red blood cells. It is highly lipophilic and distributes widely throughout body.
- Peak plasma levels occur in 0.7 hours in cats and 1.4 hours in dogs.
- Some species (e.g., pig, rat) have significant first-pass metabolism that occurs in the intestine and/or liver

Blackwell's Five-Minute Veterinary Consult Clinical Companion: Small Animal Toxicology, Second Edition.
Lynn R. Hovda, Ahna G. Brutlag, Robert H. Poppenga, and Katherine L. Peterson.

Companion website: www.fiveminutevet.com/toxicology

- Metabolized in liver by demethylation and hydroxylation.
- Excreted primarily in bile; little in urine.
- Undergoes enterohepatic recirculation.
- Half-life of tacrolimus is 10.3 hours in dogs and 20.5 hours in cats.

Toxicity

- In canine transplant studies, doses of tacrolimus of >0.15 mg/kg/day IM have been associated with toxicosis, predominantly the development of intestinal intussusception, in 25–75% of treated dogs.
  - Doses >2 mg/kg/day PO resulted in degenerative changes in pancreas, liver, and kidney.
  - Although necrotizing vasculitis was identified in dogs in one study, when the study was unblinded it was determined that vasculitis had occurred in both control and treated dogs with equal frequency, so necrotizing vasculitis was not considered to be a result of tacrolimus therapy.
- Anecdotal reports from animal poison control centers indicate that clinical signs in dogs may be seen at 0.08 mg/kg PO and deaths have occurred at 3.89 mg/kg PO.
- Toxic effects in cats have not been described. Cats receiving tacrolimus at 0.375 mg/kg q 12 hours for 14 days following renal transplantation did not develop signs that could confidently be attributed to tacrolimus administration.
- While some rabbit breeds appear to tolerate tacrolimus at 1 mg/kg/day, Dutch-Belted rabbits developed toxicosis at dosages >0.08 mg/kg/day IM.

Systems Affected

- Gastrointestinal – vomiting, diarrhea, increased intestinal gas, gastrointestinal hemorrhage, intussusception, pancreatic degeneration, hepatocellular degeneration.
- CNS – lethargy, anorexia, convulsions.
- Renal/urological – renal proximal tubular degeneration, renal failure.
- Cardiovascular – cardiac hypertrophy.
- Respiratory – pulmonary edema, dyspnea.

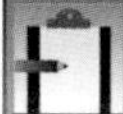

SIGNALMENT/HISTORY

- All ages, sexes, and breeds of dogs are susceptible.
- Cats appear to be more resistant than dogs to toxicosis.
- Dutch-Belted rabbits are much more susceptible than other rabbit breeds.

Risk Factors

- Topical application of tacrolimus to dogs does not appear to pose risk of toxicosis.

Historical Findings

- History of ingestion of tacrolimus capsules, ointments or solutions.

CLINICAL FEATURES

- Dogs.
  - Initial vomiting after ingestion may be severe and may be accompanied by lethargy, anorexia, and diarrhea.
  - Development of further GI signs, including abdominal discomfort, increased intestinal gas, and intussusception, may occur within 3–6 days following exposure.
- Cats: not described.
- Rabbits: anorexia, convulsions, pulmonary edema, heart failure, renal failure, and death occurred within 1 week of initiation of tacrolimus daily therapy; similar signs were reported in acute overdosing of rabbits with tacrolimus.

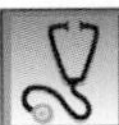

DIFFERENTIAL DIAGNOSIS

- Dogs: infectious/inflammatory gastroenteritis, GI foreign body obstruction, GI neoplasia, gastric dilation/volvulus.
- Rabbits: primary cardiac disease, infectious/inflammatory encephalitis, primary CNS disease, primary renal disease.

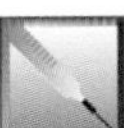

DIAGNOSTICS

- Baseline serum chemistry and CBC.
- Radiography to evaluate gastrointestinal tract for intussusception. Note that evidence of GI abnormality may not be apparent for several days following exposure.
- Tacrolimus blood levels can be measured to confirm exposure, but turnaround time makes usefulness for diagnosis of emergency cases questionable.

Pathological Findings

- Dogs: intussusception, gastrointestinal hemorrhage, renal tubular degeneration, centrilobular hepatocellular degeneration, pancreatic acinar cell degeneration.
- Rabbits: pleural effusion, pulmonary edema, myocarditis, myocardial necrosis, proximal renal tubular necrosis.

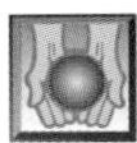

THERAPEUTICS

- The goals of treatment are to minimize absorption, manage clinical signs and monitor for complications (e.g., intussusception, renal injury).

Detoxification

- If ingestion was recent and patient is asymptomatic, emesis may be induced.
  - 3% hydrogen peroxide: 2 mL/kg PO up to maximum of 45 mL; feeding small, moist meal may improve efficacy.
  - Apomorphine (dogs): 0.02–0.04 mg/kg IV, SC, IM.
  - Alpha$_2$-adrenergic agonists (cats).
    - Dexmedetomidine 1–2 μg/kg to 40–50 μg/cat IM.
    - Xylazine 0.44 mg/kg IM.
- If patient has already vomited, manage vomiting and consider a dose of activated charcoal if it can be given without risk of aspiration.

Appropriate Health Care

- If vomiting is protracted, consider antiemetic therapy +/– GI protectants.
- For rabbits, convulsions may be treated with standard anticonvulsants.
- IV fluid therapy as needed to maintain hydration and provide cardiovascular support.

Antidotes and Drugs of Choice

- There is no specific antidote for tacrolimus.
- Antiemetics.
  - Dolasetron 0.5–1.0 mg/kg IV q 24 hours.
  - Maropitant 1 mg/kg SC q 24 hours.
  - Ondansetron 0.1–0.2 mg/kg SC, IV q 8–12 hours.
- GI protectants.
  - Famotidine 0.5–1 mg/kg PO, SC, IM, IV q 12–24 hours (do not use IV in cats).
  - Ranitidine 1–2 mg/kg PO, SC, IM, IV q 8–12 hours.
  - Cimetidine 5–10 mg/kg PO, SC, IM, IV q 6 hours.
  - Omeprazole 0.5–1 mg/kg PO daily.
  - Sucralfate 0.25–1 g PO q 8 hours × 5–7 days if evidence of active ulcer disease.
- Anticonvulsants.
  - Diazepam 0.1–0.25 mg/kg, IV to effect PRN.
  - Phenobarbital 2–4 mg/kg, IV to effect PRN.

Precautions/Interactions

- Avoid drugs that directly alter intestinal motility.

Diet

- Dietary alterations as needed for GI irritation (bland diet, NPO, etc.).

Surgical Considerations

- Surgical reduction of intussusception may be required.

COMMENTS

Patient Monitoring

- Dogs: monitor for abdominal discomfort, abdominal distension, anorexia or other signs that might suggest development of intussusception.
- Rabbits: monitor for evidence of cardiovascular or renal dysfunction.

Prevention/Avoidance

- Secure medications where they cannot be accessed by pets.
- Never apply/administer human medications to pets without consultation with a veterinarian.
- Minimize/discourage licking of site of topical application of tacrolimus.

Possible Complications

- Dogs: intestinal intussusception may occur 2–6 days following oral exposure to tacrolimus.

Expected Course and Prognosis

- Most dogs with tacrolimus toxicosis respond to antiemetics and fully recover within 24 hours.
- Some dogs have occurrence of abdominal pain with increased intestinal gas 2–6 days following initial tacrolimus exposure.
- Less commonly, intestinal intussusception may occur 2–6 days following exposure.

Abbreviations

See Appendix 1 for a complete list.

Suggested Reading

Berdoulay A, English RV, Nadelstein B. Effect of topical 0.02% tacrolimus aqueous suspension on tear production in dogs with keratoconjunctivitis sicca. Vet Ophthalmol 2005; 8(4):225–232.

Chung TH, Ryu M-H, Kim DY, Yoon HY, Hwang CY. Topical tacrolimus (FK506) for the treatment of feline idiopathic facial dermatitis. Austral Vet J 2009; 87(10):417–420.

Giessler GA, Gades NM, Friedrich PF, Bishop AT. Severe tacrolimus toxicity in rabbits. Exp Clin Transplant 2007; 5(1):590–595.

Author: Sharon Gwaltney-Brant, DVM, PhD, DABVT, DABT
Consulting Editor: Lynn R. Hovda, RPh, DVM, MS, DACVIM

Thyroid Hormones (T3 and T4)

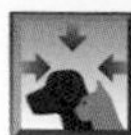

DEFINITION/OVERVIEW

- Hypothyroidism is a common endocrine disease in both humans and dogs. Due to the presence of thyroid supplementation in many homes, the chance of excessive ingestions is fairly high.
- Thyroid supplementation is available in synthetic forms of T3 (liothyronine) and T4 (levothyroxine), as well as natural T3/T4 combinations (desiccated).
- While thyrotoxicosis likely occurs frequently, there is a wide margin of safety with supplementations and the development of significant effects is rare.

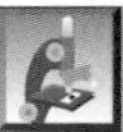

ETIOLOGY/PATHOPHYSIOLOGY

Mechanism of Action

- Thyroid supplementation is used to replace naturally occurring and circulating thyroid hormones.
- The exact mechanism of action is unknown.
- High amounts of thyroid hormones may cause changes to the cardiovascular and neurological systems, with effects generally being mild and short-lived.

Pharmacokinetics – Absorption, Distribution, Metabolism, Excretion

- Absorption – levothyroxine is absorbed in the small intestine. Bioavailability is increased in fasting animals.
- Distribution – levothyroxine is widely distributed throughout the body with highest concentrations in liver and kidney. A small amount of enterohepatic recirculation occurs.
- Metabolism – levothyroxine is deiodinated in peripheral tissues to more active T3 and then further conjugated in the liver.
- Excretion – approximately 30% is excreted in the feces, with the remaining excreted in urine and bile.

Blackwell's Five-Minute Veterinary Consult Clinical Companion: Small Animal Toxicology, Second Edition.
Lynn R. Hovda, Ahna G. Brutlag, Robert H. Poppenga, and Katherine L. Peterson.

Companion website: www.fiveminutevet.com/toxicology

- Peak plasma level.
  - T4: 4–12 hours.
  - T3: 2–5 hours.
- Half-life.
  - T4: 8–16 hours.
  - T3: 5–6 hours.

Toxicity

- Thyroid hormones are minimally toxic to dogs and cats.
- Pets become exposed by ingesting an excessive amount of their own or their owner's oral medication.
- The minimum suggested toxic dose is approximately 1–1.5 mg/kg in healthy dogs.
- Data collected from calls for over 500 thyroid hormone ingestions through the Pet Poison Helpline indicate little concern for ingestions less than 1.4 mg/kg.
- Geriatric animals or those with underlying renal, cardiac or hepatic disease may see effects at lower doses.
- Ingested doses must be converted to a levothyroxine (T4) equivalent.
  - One grain (65 mg) of desiccated thyroid contains approximately 0.1 mg/kg levothyroxine.
  - Liothyronine (T3) is considered to be four times as potent as levothyroxine, so its dose should be multiplied by four.

Systems Affected

- Cardiovascular – tachycardia (HR >160 bpm), hypertension, bradycardia, arrhythmias.
- Gastrointestinal – vomiting, diarrhea, hypersalivation.
- Nervous – agitation, irritability, hyperactivity, tremors, seizures.
- Renal – polyuria/polydipsia.
- Respiratory – panting.

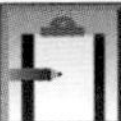

SIGNALMENT/HISTORY

- While there is no breed or age predisposition, animals that are affected with other illnesses are at a greater risk of developing symptomatic toxicity at lower doses.

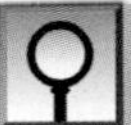

CLINICAL FEATURES

- The majority of thyroid toxicity patients remain asymptomatic due to its wide margin of safety.
- Animals that do become symptomatic will have clinical signs within the first few hours of ingestion.

- The most common clinical signs in symptomatic patients are agitation, irritability, and hyperactivity, with tachycardia seen less frequently.
- Clinical signs may persist for up to 24 hours in symptomatic animals.

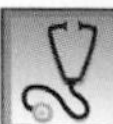

DIFFERENTIAL DIAGNOSIS

- Toxicants.
    - Amphetamine/methamphetamine/methylphenidate.
    - Caffeine/theobromine.
    - SSRI intoxication.

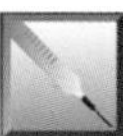

DIAGNOSTICS

- CBC and biochemistry profile to evaluate hydration status and overall health.
- T3 and/or T4 may be evaluated in significant ingestions. Elevations to T3 may occur within 3 hours of ingestion and T4 elevations within 9 hours. However, this is rarely necessary.

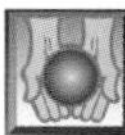

THERAPEUTICS

- The goal of treatment is to perform early decontamination to minimize the occurrence of clinical signs.
- In symptomatic patients, care should be taken to minimize the severity of clinical signs.

Detoxification

- Early emesis, within 1 hour of ingestion ideally, followed by one dose of AC with a cathartic.
    - While there is a small amount of enterohepatic recirculation, the risk of giving multiple doses of AC, such as aspiration pneumonia and hypernatremia, outweighs the benefit of a second dose.

Appropriate Health Care

- For healthy dogs with ingestions <1–1.5 mg/kg, no further therapy should be needed after decontamination.
    - Pet owners can monitor animals at home and if no symptoms greater than mild agitation occur, hospitalization is rarely needed.
- For dogs with >1.5 mg/kg ingestions, or those with underlying disease, hospitalization with close monitoring should be performed.
- Monitor heart rate and blood pressure for tachy- or bradycardia and hypertension.

Antidote

- No specific antidote is available for thyroid hormone toxicity.

Drugs of Choice

- IV fluids to help with hydration and aid in small amount of urinary excretion.
- Antiemetics as needed for vomiting.
  - Maropitant 1 mg/kg SQ q 24 hours.
  - Metoclopramide 0.3 mg/kg SQ q 8 hours.
  - Ondansetron 0.1–0.2 mg/kg IV q 8–12 hours.
- Methocarbamol 55–220 mg/kg IV if tremors develop.
- Sedation with acepromazine 0.05 mg/kg SQ, IM or IV, or butorphanol 0.2–0.4 mg/kg SQ or IM if agitation and/or tachycardia develops.
- Beta-blockers should be used only if persistent tachycardia (>180 bpm) is present and unresponsive to sedation.

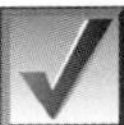

COMMENTS

Patient Monitoring

- Heart rate and blood pressure should be evaluated throughout hospitalization.
- Symptomatic patients should remain hospitalized until clinical signs have resolved and no medical intervention is needed.
- If T3 or T4 levels are monitored, T3 levels should return to normal within 6 days, with T4 remaining elevated for up to 1 month.

Prevention/Avoidance

- Owners should be educated on the importance of keeping medication out of reach of pets, especially with the added appeal of flavored, chewable tablets.

Expected Course and Prognosis

- Thyrotoxicosis has a good to excellent prognosis, even in the symptomatic patient.
- While severe clinical signs such as seizures and cardiovascular abnormalities are possible, their occurrence is rare.

Abbreviations

See Appendix 1 for a complete list.

T3 = triiodothyronine
T4 = thyroxine

Suggested Reading

Ferguson DC. Thyroid hormones and antithyroid drugs. In: Rivere JE, Papich M, eds. Veterinary Pharmacology and Therapeutics, 9th edn. Ames, IA: Wiley-Blackwell, 2009; pp. 735–770.

Reinker LN, Lee JA, Hovda LR, et al. Summary of thyroid hormone ingestion: a review of 593 cases (2004–2010). Pet Poison Helpline internal document.

Rosendale M. Hypothyroid medications. In: Plumlee, KH, ed. Clinical Veterinary Toxicology. St Louis, MO: Mosby, 2004; pp. 320–322.

Author: Renee D. Schmid, DVM

Consulting Editor: Lynn R. Hovda, RPh, DVM, MS, DACVIM

Drugs: Illicit and Recreational

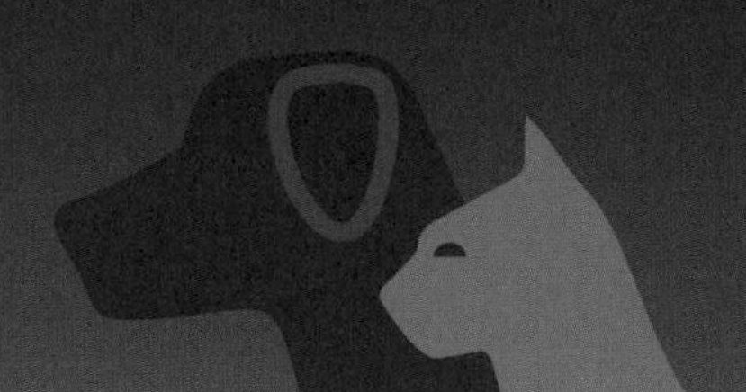

Club Drugs (MDMA, GHB, Flunitrazepam, and Bath Salts)

chapter 31

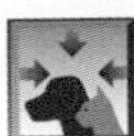 DEFINITION/OVERVIEW

- Toxicosis is caused by ingestion of designer drugs methylenedioxymethamphetamine (MDMA; see Fig. 31.1), gamma-hydroxybutyric acid (GHB), flunitrazepam (Rohypnol or Narcozep), and bath salts or synthetic cathinones (methylone, mephedrone [4-methylmethcathinone], MDPV [methylenedioxypyrovalerone], and many others).
- MDMA, GHB, and bath salts are DEA Schedule I controlled substances; flunitrazepam is a DEA Schedule IV controlled substance.
- MDMA is referred to as "ecstasy"; GHB and flunitrazepam as "date rape drugs"; synthetic cathinones as "bath salts" or "Ivory Snow."
- Animal cases may be the result of malicious poisonings, accidental ingestion of drugs in the environment, or intentional sharing of drugs with a pet.
- Degree of intoxication depends on how much of the drug has been ingested and what other toxic substances may be present as adulterants or contaminants.
- Most common responses to exposure.
    - MDMA – neurological stimulant with possible hallucinations.
    - GHB – signs of CNS depression.
    - Flunitrazepam – sedation, confusion, muscle relaxation, and hallucinations.
    - Bath salts – neurological stimulant and cardiovascular effects.

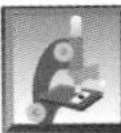 ETIOLOGY/PATHOPHYSIOLOGY

- The incidence of club drug toxicosis is unknown and probably underreported due to the clandestine nature of the chemicals.
- Club or party drugs are used by young adults at all-night dance parties (raves or trances), dance clubs, and bars. MDMA, GHB, flunitrazepam, and bath salts are the most commonly abused drugs, but ketamine, PCP, and methamphetamine are also involved.

Blackwell's Five-Minute Veterinary Consult Clinical Companion: Small Animal Toxicology, Second Edition.
Lynn R. Hovda, Ahna G. Brutlag, Robert H. Poppenga, and Katherine L. Peterson.

Companion website: www.fiveminutevet.com/toxicology

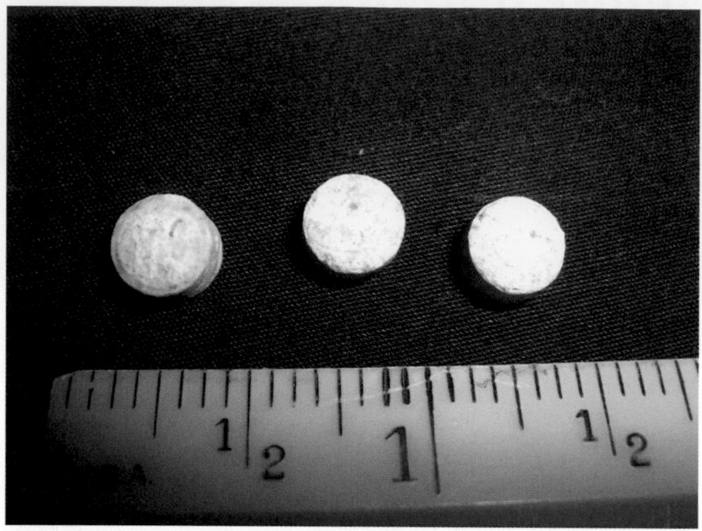

■ **Fig. 31.1.** MDMA (ecstasy) tablets. Photo courtesy of Ahna G. Brutlag.

Mechanism of Action

- MDMA – increases the release of serotonin while also inhibiting the uptake of the neurotransmitter.
- GHB – synthetic GABA derivative; modulates dopamine signaling.
- Flunitrazepam – benzodiazepine drug; acts on chloride channel of GABA (an inhibitory neurotransmitter) receptor in the CNS and increases the frequency of chloride channel opening.
- Bath salts – mechanism of action poorly understood, but appears to be similar to amphetamines and MDMA.

Pharmacokinetics – Absorption, Distribution, Metabolism, Excretion

- MDMA – readily absorbed from GI tract and crosses blood–brain barrier from plasma; metabolized by the liver and excreted by the kidneys.
- GHB – rapidly absorbed from GI tract and distributed across blood–brain barrier; excreted as carbon dioxide through respiratory system.
- Flunitrazepam – absorbed well from the GI tract and metabolized by the liver into two active compounds; excreted by the kidneys.
- Bath salts – rapidly absorbed after snorting or ingestion and excreted in the urine.

Toxicity

- MDMA
    - 3 mg/kg results in hyperactivity and mydriasis.
    - 9 mg/kg results in hypersalivation and circling behavior.
    - 15 mg/kg results in severe clinical signs and death.

- GHB – doses exceeding 50 mg/kg have been associated with death. There is a slim margin between clinical effect and fatal dosing.
- Flunitrazepam – extent of toxicosis is a direct continuation of side effects.
- Bath salts – difficult to measure as most contain multiple and varying substances.

Systems Affected

- Central nervous system – MDMA and bath salts have a stimulatory effect; GHB and flunitrazepam cause CNS depression.
- Hepatobiliary – MDMA may produce liver failure as a result of hyperthermia.
- Renal/urological – renal failure may be seen with MDMA toxicosis secondary to hyperthermia and rhabdomyolysis.
- Cardiovascular – MDMA, GHB, and bath salts intoxication may cause cardiac abnormalities, including arrhythmias.
- Endocrine/metabolic – MDMA and bath salts are associated with hyperthermia; GHB with hypothermia.

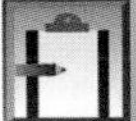

SIGNALMENT/HISTORY

- Dogs are the species most commonly affected by ingestion of a club drug.
- Signs associated with MDMA are similar to those with amphetamines and occur within 45 minutes after ingestion.
    - Hyperactivity and agitation
    - Mydriasis
    - Hyperthermia
    - Tachypnea
    - Hypersalivation
    - Seizures
    - Cardiac arrhythmias
    - Death
- Signs associated with GHB occur within 15–30 minutes after ingestion.
    - Lethargy
    - Hypotonia
    - Tremors
    - Hypothermia
    - Loss of consciousness
    - Respiratory depression
- Signs associated with flunitrazepam occur 20–30 minutes after ingestion.
    - Confusion
    - Sedation
    - Changes in heart rate

- Muscle relaxation
- Memory inhibition that may affect training

■ Signs associated with bath salts occur 15–45 minutes after snorting or ingestion.
- Hyperthermia
- Tachycardia and cardiac arrhythmias
- Vomiting
- Muscle twitching
- Euphoria, confusion, hallucinations

Risk Factors

- Animals in households with young people who attend raves.
- Drug-sniffing police dogs.
- Guard dogs.

Location and Circumstances of Poisoning

- Cases occur anywhere these drugs are available.

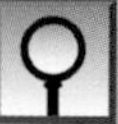

CLINICAL FEATURES

Onset of Clinical Signs

- MDMA signs occur within about 45 minutes after ingestion and may last for 8 hours.
- GHB signs occur within 15–30 minutes of ingestion and resolve within 7 hours.
- Flunitrazepam signs occur within 30–60 minutes and may last up to 8–12 hours.
- Bath salts signs occur within 15–45 minutes and generally last about 2–4 hours but may last days.

Systems Affected

- Nervous system – MDMA and bath salts may cause hyperactivity and seizures; GHB and flunitrazepam may cause lethargy, loss of consciousness, and in severe cases, seizures.
- Cardiovascular – MDMA-associated signs include tachycardia or bradycardia, hypertension, and AV block; bath salts may cause tachycardia, hypertension, and arrhythmias; flunitrazepam may cause changes in heart rate.

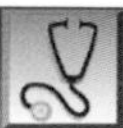

DIFFERENTIAL DIAGNOSIS

MDMA, GHB, Flunitrazepam, and Bath Salts

■ Any disease process that would cause CNS signs.
- Meningitis or meningioencephalitis.
- Severe hepatoencephalopathy.

MDMA and bath salts

- Amphetamines or methamphetamine.
- Cocaine.
- Metaldehyde.

GHB and flunitrazepam

- Benzodiazepines including diazepam and lorazepam.
- Barbiturates.
- Marijuana.
- Opioids.

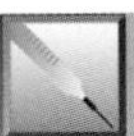

DIAGNOSTICS

- Urine may be sent to a human hospital for toxicological screening to detect MDMA and, in some cases, flunitrazepam and bath salts. GHB is metabolized too quickly to be detected.
- The Quick Screen Pro Multi Drug Screening Test is a human testing kit that has been validated by GC/MS for use in animals. It may provide a rapid and accurate diagnosis for flunitrazepam and perhaps MDMA if the drug is present in high enough concentrations and the time frame is appropriate.

Pathological Findings

- Gross findings include icterus; petechial and ecchymotic hemorrhage; dark, tarry material in the stomach (postmortem); and liver damage (postmortem).
- Histopathological findings include hepatic necrosis and evidence of generalized hemorrhagic disease.

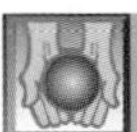

THERAPEUTICS

- Objectives of treatment are to prevent further toxin absorption, provide supportive care, and correct clotting abnormalities.

Detoxification

- Emesis is generally ineffective as the onset of signs is so rapid.
- Activated charcoal with a cathartic × 1 dose

Appropriate Health Care

MDMA and Bath Salts

- Monitor and treat for hyperthermia with cooling vests, blankets, or fluids. Do not overcool. Stop at 103–103.5°F.

- Keep in darkened area and avoid excess stimulation.
- ECG and frequent cardiac monitoring.
- Observe closely for signs of serotonin syndrome.

GHB

- Monitor for hypothermia and use heating methods as needed. Do not overheat.
- Observe for respiratory depression. Be prepared to intubate and ventilate if needed.

GHB and Flunitrazepam

- Monitor closely for signs of excess CNS depression.

Antidotes

- Flunitrazepam: flumazenil, a benzodiazepine antagonist, is the antidote. Dose is 0.01 mg/kg IV (dogs and cats). The half-life of flumazenil is about an hour, so the drug, if effective, may need to be repeated several times.
- MDMA GHB, and bath salts: no specific antidote is available.

Drugs of Choice

- IV fluids at 1.5–2 times maintenance.
- MDMA is a close analog of methamphetamine and specific treatment is the same. Refer to chapter 35 (Methamphetamine) for recommendations.
- Bath salts
    - Seizure control options
        - ☐ Diazepam 0.1–0.5 mg/kg IV.
        - ☐ Propofol 6 mg/kg IV bolus, followed by CRI of 0.1–0.6 mg/kg/min.
        - ☐ Phenobarbital 2–5 mg/kg IV, can be repeated 3× at 4-hour intervals.
    - Tachyarrhythmia propranolol 0.02 mg/kg IV slowly, maximum of 1 mg/kg; repeat in 8 hours if needed.
    - Ventricular dysrhythmia lidocaine 2–4 mg/kg IV over 1–2 minutes; avoid in cats.
- GHB and flunitrazepam: symptomatic and supportive care until signs resolve.

Public Health

- These are all scheduled controlled substances.

COMMENTS

Client Education

- Educate the client on the potential for toxicosis from club drugs.

Prevention/Avoidance

- Remove drugs from the environment or restrict the pet's access to them.

Possible Complications

- Contaminants or deliberate adulterants in the drug mixture.
- Unknown additional drugs ingested in addition to known drug.

Expected Course and Prognosis

- Will depend on quantity and mixture of drugs and time of presentation.
- At lower doses, recovery is probable.
- At higher doses, animal may die within 8 hours of ingestion.

Synonyms

- MDMA: ecstasy, adam, bibs, blue kisses, blue niles, eve, scooby snacks, X, XTC, others
- GHB: liquid ecstasy, G, liquid X, salty water, scoop, soap, others
- Flunitrazepam: circles, forget me pills, R2, roofies, rophies, rope, wolfies, others
- Bath salts: blue silk, cloud 9, ivory wave, legal high, moon dust, white lightening, others

See Also

Cocaine
Amphetamines
Methamphetamine
Opiates and Opioids
PCP (Phencyclidine)

Abbreviations

See Appendix 1 for a complete list.

GHB = gamma-hydroxybutyric acid
MDMA = methylenedioxymethamphetamine
MDPV = methylenedioxypyrovalerone

Suggested Reading

Bischoff K. Toxicity of drugs of abuse. In: GuptaRC, ed. Veterinary Toxicology: Basic and Clinical Principles, 2nd edn. New York: Elsevier, 2012; pp. 469–489.

Kapoor P, Deshmukh R, Kukreja I. GHB acid: a rage or reprieve. J Adv Pharm Tech Research 2013; 4(4):173–178.

Karch SB. A Historical review of MDMA. Open Forensic Sci J 2011; 4:20–24.

Prosser JM, Nelson LS. The toxicology of bath salts: a review of synthetic cathinones. J Med Toxicol 2012; 8:33–42.

Ross EA, Watson M, Goldberger B. "Bath salts" intoxication. N Engl J Med 2011; 365:967–968.

Acknowledgment: The authors and editors acknowledge the prior contributions of Teresa K. Drotar, who authored this topic in the previous edition.

Author: Christy A. Klatt, DVM

Consulting Editor: Lynn R. Hovda, RPh, DVM, MS, DACVIM

chapter 32

Cocaine

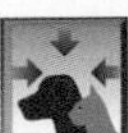 DEFINITION/OVERVIEW

- Solid white powder containing 12–16% cocaine salts and adulterants, which may include lidocaine, caffeine, amphetamines, levamisole, xylazine (Fig. 32.1).
- Free basic alkaloid of cocaine may also be precipitated into "rocks" of crack to be smoked in a process known as "free basing" (Fig 32.2).
- Schedule II drug for topical anesthesia.

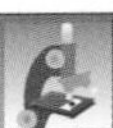 ETIOLOGY/PATHOPHYSIOLOGY

- Cocaine is a natural alkaloid from *Erythroxylon coca* and *E. monogynum*. Grown in Mexico, South America, Indonesia, and the West Indies.
- One of the most commonly abused drugs in the world.

Mechanism of Action

- Sympathomimetic.
  - Blocks NE, serotonin, dopamine reuptake.
  - Increases catecholamine release.
  - Tachycardia, hypertension, and vasoconstriction result.
- Thrombogenic effects.
- NE-mediated hypothalamic effects. Regulates appetite, sleep, and body temperature.

Pharmacokinetics – Absorption, Distribution, Metabolism, Excretion

- Peak plasma concentrations 15–12 minutes after exposure.
- Readily crosses the blood–brain barrier.
- Hydrolyzed by plasma and hepatic esterases to water-soluble metabolites.
- Urinary excretion.
  - 10–20% unchanged.
  - Rest as metabolites.

Blackwell's Five-Minute Veterinary Consult Clinical Companion: Small Animal Toxicology, Second Edition.
Lynn R. Hovda, Ahna G. Brutlag, Robert H. Poppenga, and Katherine L. Peterson.

Companion website: www.fiveminutevet.com/toxicology

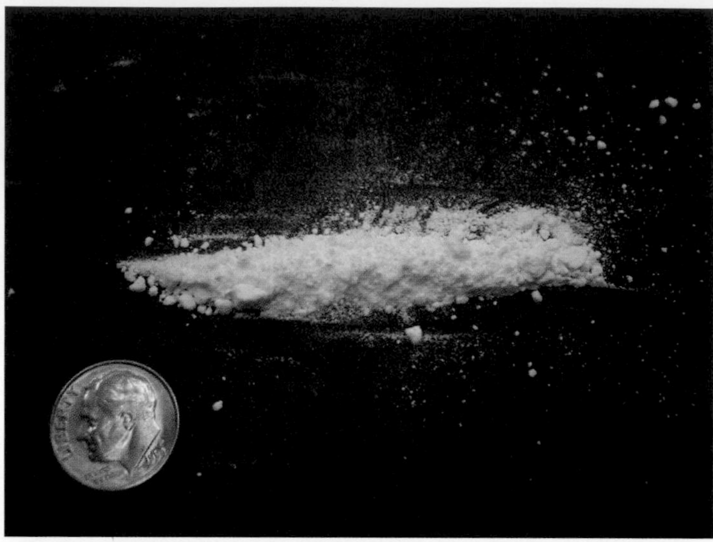

■ **Fig. 32.1.** Cocaine powder. Photo courtesy of Ahna G. Brutlag.

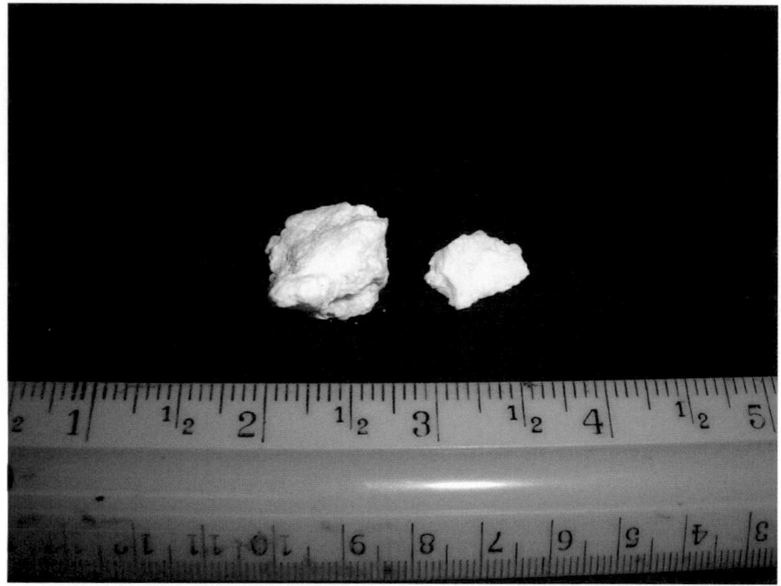

■ **Fig. 32.2.** Crack cocaine. Photo courtesy Ahna G. Brutlag.

Toxicity

Dog

- IV LD_{50}: 3 mg/kg.
- Estimated PO LD_{50}: 6–12 mg/kg.
- Lowest LD: 3.5 mg/kg SQ.

Cat

- Lowest LD: 7.5 mg/kg IV.
- Lowest LD: 16 mg/kg SQ.

Systems Affected

- Nervous
- Cardiovascular

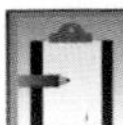

SIGNALMENT/HISTORY

- Dogs most commonly affected.

Risk Factors

- Ingestion of illegal cocaine or crack.
- Police dogs may be predisposed.

Historical Findings

- Access to drugs.
    - Personal use.
    - Guests or party in the home.
- Clients often reluctant to give illegal drug exposure history.

Location and Circumstances of Poisoning

- Neighborhoods with known drug use.

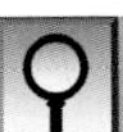

CLINICAL FEATURES

- CNS stimulation
- Hyperactivity, tremors, seizures
- Obtunded mentation
- Bilateral mydriasis
- Hypersalivation
- Ataxia
- Vomiting
- Tachycardia
- Hyperthermia
- Hypertension
- Elevated plasma lactate
- Hypernatremia

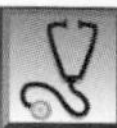

DIFFERENTIAL DIAGNOSIS

- Other stimulant drugs.
  - Amphetamines and methamphetamine.
  - Synthetic cathinones (bath salts).
  - Decongestants (ephedrine, pseudoephedrine, others).
- Other causes of seizures.
  - Strychnine.
  - Metaldehyde.
  - Penitrem A.
  - Caffeine or other methylxanthines.

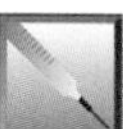

DIAGNOSTICS

- Over-the-counter urine multidrug test kits.
- Urine, plasma, or stomach contents for laboratory confirmation.
  - Thin-layer chromatography.
  - Gas chromatography/mass spectrometry.
- ECG for cardiac effects.

Pathological Findings

- Subendocardial and epicardial hemorrhage.
- Myocardial degeneration.
- Pericardial effusion.
- Pulmonary hemorrhage.

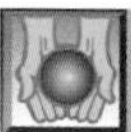

THERAPEUTICS

Detoxification

- Early decontamination if large quantity ingested, vomiting absent.
- Avoid emesis due to seizure potential.
- Sedation and gastric lavage.
- Activated charcoal with cathartic × 1 dose.
- Endoscopic or surgical retrieval if bagged cocaine ingested.

Appropriate Health Care

- Maintain blood volume, pH, and electrolyte balance.
- Prevent and control hyperthermia.
- Maintain adequate airway; monitor respirations.
- Avoid CNS stimulation; dark quiet room.
- ECG monitoring for cardiac effects.

Antidote

- No specific antidote available.

Drugs of Choice

- Seizure control options.
  - Diazepam or midazolam 0.1–0.5 mg/kg IV.
  - Propofol CRI 0.05–0.2 mg/kg/min.
  - Phenobarbital 2–5 mg/kg IV, can be repeated 3× in 4-hour intervals.
- Control life-threatening cardiac arrhythmias.
  - Propranolol 0.02 mg/kg IV slowly, maximum of 1 mg/kg.
  - Esmolol CRI 25–75 µg/kg/minute.
- Antiemetics if needed.
  - Maropitant 1 mg/kg SQ q 24 hours.
  - Ondansetron 0.1–0.2 mg/kg IV q 8–12 hours.
- ILE has been recommended.
  - Initial 1.5 mL/kg IV bolus 20% lipid solution over 5–15 minutes followed by CRI of 0.25 mL/kg/minute over 1–2 hours.
  - Repeat if needed and lipemia absent.

Surgical Considerations

- Cautious surgical or endoscopic removal if whole bags of cocaine are ingested.
- Avoid rupture of the bag.

Prevention

- Proper training and muzzling of police dogs.
- Preventing exposure to illegal drugs.

Public Health

- Illegal drugs are subject to laws concerning drug possession and animal welfare.

COMMENTS

Client Education

- Properly train police dogs.
- Prevent exposure to illegal drugs.
  - Keep animals away from illegal drug stash.
  - Keep them confined during parties where drugs may be used.

Prevention/Avoidance

- Avoid access to illegal drugs.
- Keep animals away from parties and other sources of illegal drugs.
- Muzzle police dogs.

Possible Complications

- Cardiac arrest due to cardiac vasospasm.
- Hyperthermia due to seizures and vasoconstriction.

Expected Course and Prognosis

- Hospitalization 10–30 hours.
- Good prognosis with treatment.
- Ongoing neurological or cardiovascular signs reported.

Synonyms

Cocaine: coke, bernies, snow, dust, blow, nose candy, toot, white lady, star dust, others
Crack cocaine: beamers, rock, crank, flake, ice

See Also

Amphetamines
Methamphetamine

Abbreviations

See Appendix 1 for a complete list.

NE = norepinephrine

Suggested Reading

Bischoff K. Toxicity of drugs of abuse. In: Gupta RC, ed. Veterinary Toxicology: Basic and Clinical Principles, 2nd edn. New York: Elsevier, 2012; pp. 469–489.

Llera RM, Volmer PA. Toxicologic hazards for police dogs involved in drug detection. J Am Vet Med Assoc 2006; 228:1028–1031.

Thomas EK, Drobatz KJ, Mandell CK. Presumptive cocaine toxicosis in 19 dogs: 2004-2012. J Vet Emerg Crit Care 2014; 24:201–207.

Authors: Karyn Bischoff, DVM, MS, DABVT; Hwan Goo Kang, DVM, PhD
Consulting Editor: Lynn R. Hovda, RPh, DVM, MS, DACVIM

chapter 33

LSD (Lysergic Acid Diethylamide)

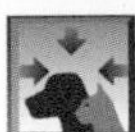

DEFINITION/OVERVIEW

- Lysergic acid diethylamide (LSD) was first synthesized from ergot in 1938.
- Similar compounds are present in other plants.
    - Morning glory seeds (*Ipomea violacia*)
    - Pink morning glory (*Ipomea carnea*)
    - Sleepygrass (*Stipa robusta*)
    - Hawaiian baby wood rose (*Agyreia nervosa*)

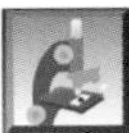

ETIOLOGY/PATHOPHYSIOLOGY

- LSD is used as a recreational drug.
    - Banned by FDA in 1966; currently DEA Schedule I drug.
    - Decline in illegal use over last 20 years.
- LSD is dissolved in water and applied to paper, sugar cubes, gelatin cubes, or other substances for ingestion.
    - Final product in circulation today contains 0.04–0.06 mg per dose.
    - Older products (1960s) contained up to 0.25 mg LSD per sugar cube or dose.
- Difficult to predict effects on individuals.
    - Altered sensory perceptions (visual, auditory) in humans.
    - May cause euphoria or panic.

Mechanism of Action

- Not completely understood.
- Structurally similar to serotonin (5-HT).
- Primarily acts as agonist at 5-HT_{2A} receptors found in cortex.
- Promotes glutamate release.

Blackwell's Five-Minute Veterinary Consult Clinical Companion: Small Animal Toxicology, Second Edition.
Lynn R. Hovda, Ahna G. Brutlag, Robert H. Poppenga, and Katherine L. Peterson.

Companion website: www.fiveminutevet.com/toxicology

Pharmacokinetics – Absorption, Distribution, Metabolism, Excretion

- Data from human subjects are available.
- Rapid gastrointestinal absorption.
- Peak plasma concentrations within 6 hours.
- Highly protein bound.
- Hepatic metabolism.
  - Hydroxylation.
  - Glucuronide conjugation.
- Predominantly fecal elimination.
- Elimination half-life 2–5 hours.
- Clinical signs often last a few hours but may persist for up to 12 hours.

Toxicity

- Effective dose in humans – 0.05–0.20 mg.
- Toxic dose in humans – 0.70–2.80 mg/kg BW.
- Clinical signs seen in cats dosed with IP LSD:
  - 0.0025 mg/kg BW – mild signs
  - 0.0500 mg/kg BW – marked signs.
- Rat IV LD50 – 16 mg/kg BW.

Systems Affected

- Nervous – ranges from excitation to complete disorientation.
- Cardiovascular – tachycardia from stimulation of autonomic nervous system.
- Endocrine/metabolic – malignant hyperthermia reported in humans.
- Ophthalmic – mydriasis.

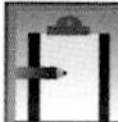

SIGNALMENT/HISTORY

- Young animals, particularly puppies, predisposed to ingesting foreign material.

Risk Factors

- Police dogs used to detect drugs may be more susceptible.

Historical Findings

- Access to drugs.
  - Teenagers in the home.
  - Guests or party in the home.
- Owner may be reluctant to provide a complete history.
- May be combined with other drugs.

Location and Circumstances of Poisoning

- Animals residing in neighborhoods with known drug use.

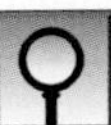

CLINICAL FEATURES

- Disorientation
- Mydriasis
- Vocalization
- Excitation or sedation
- Tachycardia
- Signs reported in cats.
  - Hallucinatory behavior – tracking and pouncing on unseen objects.
  - Compulsive scratching in litter.
  - Bizarre sitting and standing postures.
  - Increased grooming, which may be incomplete.
  - Increased play behavior (chasing tails, pawing, biting, sniffing).
  - Vomiting.
  - Increased defecation.

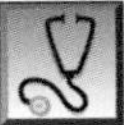

DIFFERENTIAL DIAGNOSIS

- Other hallucinogenic or dissociative drugs.
  - Ketamine
  - MDMA
  - Mescaline
  - PCP
  - Psilocybe spp. mushrooms
  - Salvia (*S. divinorum*)

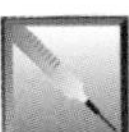

DIAGNOSTICS

- No specific serum chemistry abnormalities.
- Laboratory analysis to confirm exposure. Results will take several days to be returned and cannot be used to guide therapy.
  - Immunoassays
  - HPLC
  - LC/MC
  - TLC

Pathological Findings

- No specific lesion. LSD is not reported as a direct cause of death.

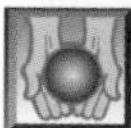

THERAPEUTICS

- Treatment is generally limited to symptomatic and supportive care with close observation until clinical signs have resolved. Up to 12 hours may be required after a large ingestion.

Detoxification

- Gastrointestinal detoxification is not useful due to rapid absorption and onset of clinical signs.

Appropriate Health Care

- Minimize sensory stimulation.
    - Keep in a darkened, quiet area.
    - Avoid excessive restraint.
- Monitor and symptomatic care for tachycardia and hyperthermia.

Antidote

- No specific antidote available.

Drugs of Choice

- IV fluids as needed to stabilize cardiovascular system.
- Diazepam 0.25–0.5 mg/kg IV for anxiety, seizures.
- Haloperidol has been used successfully in humans.

Precautions/Interactions

- Selective serotonin reuptake inhibitors can aggravate CNS effects and should be avoided.

Activity

- Minimize sensory stimulation for 12 hours.

COMMENTS

Client Education

- Most animals will recover within 12 hours if kept in a dark, quiet room.
- Illegal drugs are subject to laws concerning drug possession and animal welfare.

Patient Monitoring

- Monitor heart rate and body temperature regularly over 12 hours post exposure.

Prevention/Avoidance

- Avoid access to illegal drugs.
  - Keep animals away from parties and other possible sources.
  - Police dogs wear a muzzle to prevent ingestion of contraband.
  - Monitor teenagers who might intentionally expose companion animals to drugs.

Possible Complications

- Tachycardia reported in humans.
- Hyperthermia reported in humans. Associated with restraint.
- Injury of animal or caretaker possible because of behavioral changes.

Expected Course and Prognosis

- Deaths have not been directly attributed directly to LSD abuse.
- Fatal accidents are possible due to behavioral changes.

Synonyms

Acid, blotter, dots, purple haze, sugar cubes, window pane

See Also

Club Drugs (MDMA, GHB, Flunitrazepam, and Bath Salts)
Miscellaneous Hallucinogens and Dissociative Agents

Abbreviations

See Appendix 1 for a complete list.

MDMA = 3,4-methylene-dioxymethamphetamine
PCP = phencyclidine

Suggested Reading

Bischoff K. Toxicity of drugs of abuse. In: GuptaRC, ed. Veterinary Toxicology: Basic and Clinical Principles, 2nd edn. New York: Elsevier, 2012; pp. 469–489.

Fantegrossi WE, Murnane KS, Reissig CJ. The behavioral pharmacology of hallucinogens. Biochem Pharmacol 2008; 75:17–33.

Jacobs BL, Trulson ME, Stern WC. Behavioral effects of LSD in the cat: proposal of an animal behavior model for studying the actions of hallucinogenic drugs. Brain Res 1977; 132:301–314.

Volmer PA. Recreational drugs. In: PetersonME, TalcottPA, eds. Small Animal Toxicology, 3rd edn. St Louis, MO: Elsevier, 2013; pp. 309–334.

Authors: Karyn Bischoff, DVM, MS, DABVT; Hwan Goo Kang, DVM, PhD
Consulting Editor: Lynn R. Hovda, RPh, DVM, MS, DACVIM

chapter 34

Marijuana

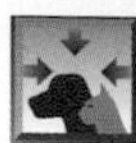

DEFINITION/OVERVIEW

- Marijuana consists of the dried flower buds and subtending leaves and stems of the female *Cannabis sativa* plant. It contains varying concentrations of the psychoactive substance tetrahydrocannabinol or THC.
- It is a popular drug of abuse due to its psychoactive effects.
- It is legal for recreational use in some states, including Washington and Colorado, and also legal for medical use in multiple other states.
- Tetrahydrocannabinol (THC) is the toxin in marijuana. The highest concentration exists in the flower buds and tiny leaves that are produced at the top of the plant (Fig. 34.1).
  - Marijuana refers to any part of the plant but especially to the dried preparations of flower buds and small leaves. The United Nations Office on Drugs and Crime (UNODC) states that the concentration of THC may vary from 5% to 20% in plant materials depending upon species and hydration.
  - Hashish is the resin that is collected from the surfaces of hair-like leaf structures called trichomes. THC concentration in hashish is variable, but generally greater than in the plant itself, usually expected to be about 20% (Fig. 34.2).
  - Sinsemilla is a seedless female *Cannabis* plant that has been carefully manually tended to prevent pollination. Sinsemilla plants produce THC concentrations higher than plants which have been allowed to pollinate and produce seeds.
- Marijuana can be harmful to pets through both ingestion of plant parts and inhalation of smoke when burned. Ingestion may be in the form of fresh or dried plant parts, baked goods which contain plant parts, or food products infused with oil from the plant (for example, green butter).
  - Green butter is made by heating dairy butter with dried plant parts. The resulting product is then used in cooking, baking, or as a spread. The concentration of THC in green butter depends upon which plant parts and quantities were used in the manufacture.
- Dronabinol (Marinol®) and nabilone (Cesamet®) are synthetic cannabinoids commonly prescribed as an antiemetic and/or appetite stimulant in human cancer patients. They may also be prescribed for other medical uses.
- Most common effects from exposure are neurological and gastrointestinal.

Blackwell's Five-Minute Veterinary Consult Clinical Companion: Small Animal Toxicology, Second Edition.
Lynn R. Hovda, Ahna G. Brutlag, Robert H. Poppenga, and Katherine L. Peterson.

Companion website: www.fiveminutevet.com/toxicology

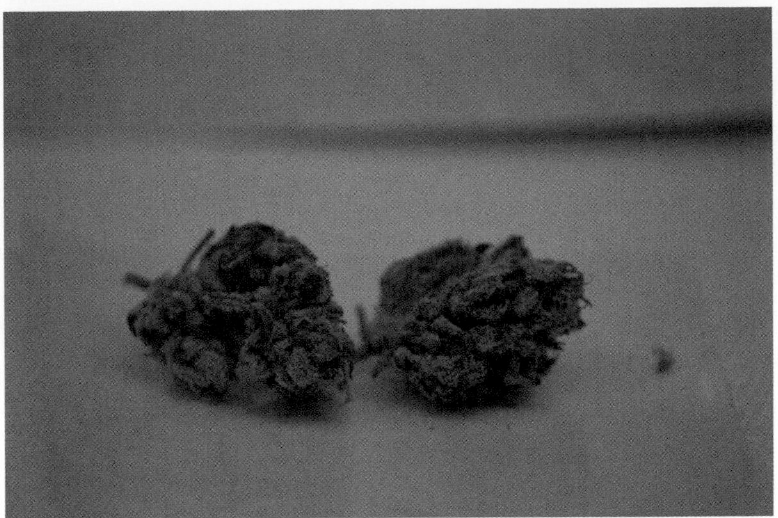

■ **Fig. 34.1.** Marijuana bud (*Cannabis sativa*). Photo courtesy of Seth Wong, TEQ Analytical Labs, Aurora, CO.

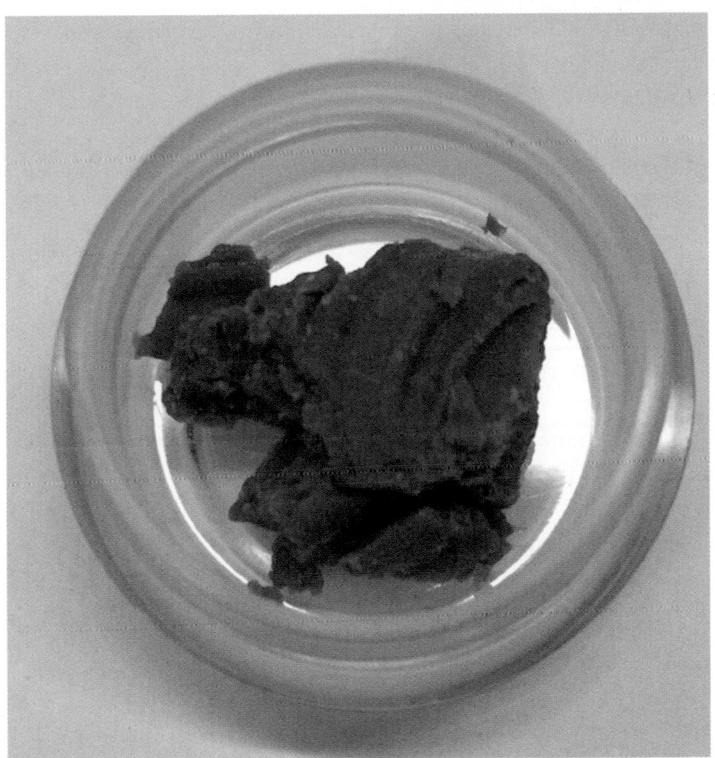

■ **Fig. 34.2.** High-quality hash extract or "wax." Sometimes referred to as "butter" but it is not a butter base. Photo courtesy of Seth Wong, TEQ Analytical Labs, Aurora, CO.

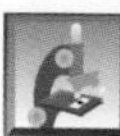

ETIOLOGY/PATHOPHYSIOLOGY

Mechanism of Action

- THC is a CB1 and CB2 receptor agonist.
  - CB1 receptors are located in the CNS.
  - CB2 receptors are located in the periphery, specifically in the immune system.
- Ingestion of marijuana may cause irritation to the mucosa of the gastrointestinal tract, often resulting in vomiting.

Pharmacokinetics – Absorption, Distribution, Metabolism, Excretion

- Marijuana is ingested orally and absorbed through the gastrointestinal tract or inhaled as smoke from burning plant parts and absorbed via the respiratory system.
- Absorption is rapid through both routes The presence of fatty foods increases the rate of absorption with ingestion.
  - Inhalation: 18–50% bioavailability.
  - Ingestion: 5–20% bioavailability.
- Highly distributed to body fat, brain, liver, and kidney.
- Undergoes enterohepatic recirculation.
- Metabolism occurs in the liver; the primary metabolite (11-OH-Δ-9-THC) is more potent than THC and crosses the blood–brain barrier.
- Dogs, unlike humans, have multiple metabolites that are structurally larger and more complex than those present in humans.
- Elimination is through bile via feces (85–90%) and urine (10–15%), although specific amounts vary among species.
- Elimination is typically complete within 5 days.

Toxicity

- Toxicity may occur with ingestion of green butter, cookies or brownies containing green butter or marijuana, hash or hashish, dried marijuana leaves, marijuana plants, or cigarettes containing marijuana.
- Toxicity may also occur through inhalation of second-hand marijuana smoke.
- Toxic dose:
  - Cannot be established in dogs due to variations in purity of the drug and route of exposure.
  - Fatalities have occurred at 3–9 g/kg (toxicological effects can be seen at much lower doses).

Systems Affected

- Nervous – CNS depression, disorientation, ataxia, hyperesthesia, coma; CNS stimulation may occur in some dogs, including vocalization, hyperactivity, and, less commonly, seizures.

- Gastrointestinal – vomiting.
- Cardiovascular – bradycardia or tachycardia.
- Endocrine/metabolic – hypothermia or hyperthermia.
- Respiratory – respiratory depression may occur, but is extremely rare.

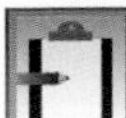

SIGNALMENT/HISTORY

- All animals can be affected, but dogs are more indiscriminate eaters.

Risk Factors

- Exposure to marijuana by ingestion of plant parts or inhalation of smoke.
- Marijuana use by pet owners or family members.
- Police service dogs.

Historical Findings

- Owners are often reluctant to admit pet exposure and may need encouragement to help with diagnosis.
- Some pets may be deliberately poisoned by their owners.

Location and Circumstances of Poisoning

- Cases occur throughout the country as use of marijuana by humans is widespread.
- Despite marijuana's legality for recreational use in Colorado and Washington, the prevalence of exposures resulting in a call to an animal poison center is not significantly more as compared to other states.
- In some animal hospitals in Colorado, there has been a significant increase in total number of marijuana exposures in dogs.

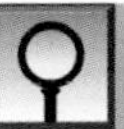

CLINICAL FEATURES

- Onset of clinical signs: 5 minutes–12 hours (most clinical signs occur within 30–60 minutes of exposure).
- Duration of clinical signs: 30 minutes–3 days (average 18–24 hours).
- Systems most commonly affected include the following.
  - Nervous system – ataxia is the most common clinical sign, but may be accompanied by weakness, hyperesthesia, CNS depression, coma, and mydriasis; CNS stimulation occurs more rarely and signs include vocalization, hyperactivity, tremors, and seizures.
  - Gastrointestinal tract – vomiting.

  - Other reported signs include bradycardia or tachycardia, hypothermia or hyperthermia, and urinary incontinence.
- Signs of toxicity often resolve spontaneously without treatment.

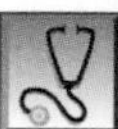

DIFFERENTIAL DIAGNOSIS

- Alcohols
- Hallucinogenic mushrooms
- Human pharmaceuticals with CNS stimulant effects (amphetamines, methylphenidate, and others)
- Human pharmaceuticals with CNS depressant effects (benzodiazepines, opioids, and others)
- LSD
- PCP
- Synthetic cannabinoids
- Xylitol

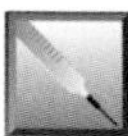

DIAGNOSTICS

- Typically must rely on history from owner. They may not be forthcoming so it is important to use unbiased questioning.
- The use of human on-site urine tests for marijuana has not shown to be effective in dogs as the large number of metabolites may result in a false negative result.
- Gas chromatography/mass spectrometry (GC/MS) is effective in identifying marijuana, but takes several days to perform and is not useful in guiding therapy.

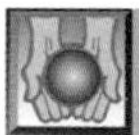

THERAPEUTICS

- The objectives of treatment are to prevent further toxin absorption and provide supportive care. In general, animals will require care for 18–24 hours, but this varies depending on severity of clinical signs.

Detoxification

- Remove from source, especially smoke inhalation.
- Emesis if acute and animal not already vomiting. THC has a strong antiemetic effect but this may occur more often in humans than dogs.
- Activated charcoal with cathartic × 1 for oral exposure. Second dose of activated charcoal with NO cathartic.
- Gastric lavage if the animal has ingested large quantities of baked goods containing marijuana.

Appropriate Health Care

- Warming measures for hypothermia; cooling for hyperthermia.
- Oxygen therapy if respiratory depression occurs.
- Close monitoring of CNS signs.
    - Depression occurs most frequently and is generally not treated.
    - CNS stimulation and behavior hazardous to the animal or handlers may require sedation.

Antidote

- No specific antidote is available.

Drugs of Choice

- IV fluids as needed for dehydration secondary to vomiting.
- Sedation if needed in excited animals.
    - Diazepam 0.25–0.5 mg/kg IV PRN.
    - Chlorpromazine 0.5–1 mg/kg IV PRN.
- Antiemetics if vomiting persists or is severe.
    - Maropitant 1 mg/kg SQ q 24 hours.
    - Ondansetron 0.1–0.2 mg/kg IV q 8–12 hours.
- May consider intralipid therapy for severe cases. See Chapter 3.

Nursing Care

- Turn comatose animals every 4 hours.
- Monitor TPR every 2–4 hours until animal has returned to normal mentation.

Public Health

- Marijuana is an illegal Schedule I substance in most states and presents potential human health risks.

COMMENTS

Client Education

- Educate the client on the toxicity of marijuana in dogs.
- Discuss intentional misuse.
    - Do not intentionally blow smoke in a dog's face.
    - Do not intentionally feed marijuana-laced baked goods.
- Muzzle police dogs if they are indiscriminate eaters.

Prevention/Avoidance

- Eliminate marijuana from the environment.
- Keep dogs out of the area where marijuana use may occur.

Expected Course and Prognosis

- Recovery time will depend on the quantity of toxin ingested or inhaled but is usually complete within 3 days.
- Marijuana toxicity is rarely fatal.
- There have been two documented deaths recently in dogs that ingested baked goods containing green butter. Other causes or contributors of death could not be ruled out.

Synonyms

- Weed, pot, grass, ganja, Mary Jane, reefers, hemp, devil weed, hashish, and a wide variety of others

Abbreviations

- See Appendix 1 for a complete list.

See Also

Club Drugs (MDMA, GHB, Flunitrazepam, and Bath Salts)
Synthetic Cannabinoids

Suggested Reading

Fitzgerald KT, Bronstein AC, Newquist KL. Marijuana poisoning. Top Compan Anim Med 2013; 28(1):8–12.

Garrett ER, Hunt CA. Pharmacokinetics of delta 9-tetrahydrocannabinol in dogs. J Pharm Sci 1977; 66: 395–407.

Janczyk P, Donaldson CW, Gwaltney S. Two hundred and thirteen cases of marijuana toxicoses in dogs. Vet Hum Tox 2004; 46(1):19–21.

Llera RM, Volmer PA. Toxicologic hazards for police dogs involved in drug detection. J Am Vet Med Assoc 2006; 228(7):1028–1031.

Meola SD, Tearney C, Haas S, et al. Evaluation of trends in marijuana toxicosis in dogs living in a state with legalized medical marijuana: 125 dogs (2005-2010). J Vet Emerg Crit Care 2012; 22(6):690–696.

Teitler JB. Evaluation of a human on-site urine multidrug test for emergency use with dogs. J Am Animal Hosp Assoc 2009; 45:59–66.

Acknowledgment: The authors and editors acknowledge the prior contributions of Christy A. Klatt, DVM,, who authored this topic in the previous edition.
Author: Kelly Sioris, PharmD, CSPI
Consulting Editor: Lynn R. Hovda, RPh, DVM, MS, DACVIM

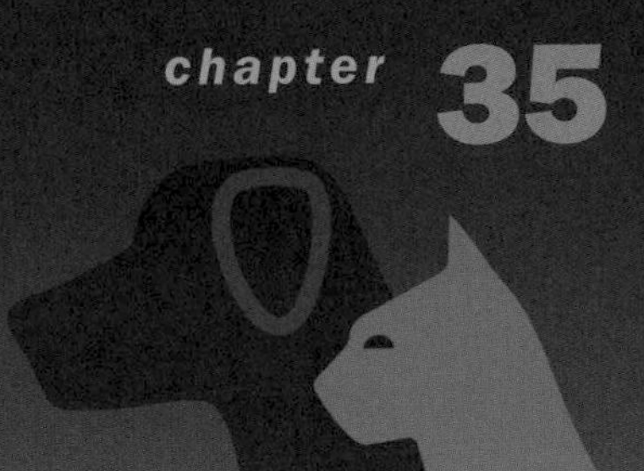

chapter 35

Methamphetamine

DEFINITION/OVERVIEW

- Toxicosis caused by ingestion, and less frequently by inhalation.
- Degree of toxicosis is dependent upon the quantity ingested.
- Most common effects are neurological with cardiac failure and hyperthermia as secondary effects.

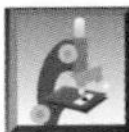

ETIOLOGY/PATHOPHYSIOLOGY

- The manufacture and use of methamphetamine (meth = slang or street name) as a human recreational drug are widespread across the country. Cases of intoxication may be seen nationwide; however, due to the illegal nature of the substance, cases may be underreported.
    - Crystal meth (Fig. 35.1 and Fig 35.2) is smoked.
    - Powdered meth is ingested, snorted, or administered IV.
- The abuse of methamphetamine is growing rapidly, primarily because it can be easily manufactured in basements and other crude laboratories from precursors like ephedrine.
- Pure methamphetamine is rare; it is often cut or adulterated with other potentially harmful substances, including phenylpropanolamine, caffeine, and other compounds.
- Methamphetamine is a DEA Schedule II drug.

Mechanism of Action

- Increased release of catecholamines.
- Inhibition of monoamine oxidase (MAO).
- Probable direct action on dopamine and serotonin receptors.

Pharmacokinetics – Absorption, Distribution, Metabolism, Excretion

- Rapidly absorbed from the gastrointestinal system.
- Peak plasma levels in human beings are reached in 1–3 hours.
- Crosses the blood–brain barrier in high concentrations and is also distributed to the kidneys, liver, and lungs.

Blackwell's Five-Minute Veterinary Consult Clinical Companion: Small Animal Toxicology, Second Edition.
Lynn R. Hovda, Ahna G. Brutlag, Robert H. Poppenga, and Katherine L. Peterson.

Companion website: www.fiveminutevet.com/toxicology

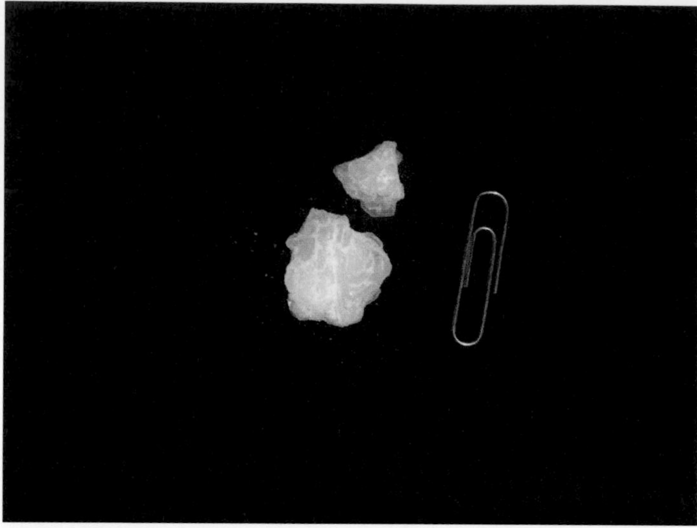

■ **Fig. 35.1.** Crystal meth. Photo courtesy of Ahna G. Brutlag.

- Metabolized in the liver by hydroxylation and deamination and excreted in the urine, with the rate of excretion increasing with acidification of the urine.

Toxicity

- The oral LD_{50} in dogs suggested to be 9 mg/kg.

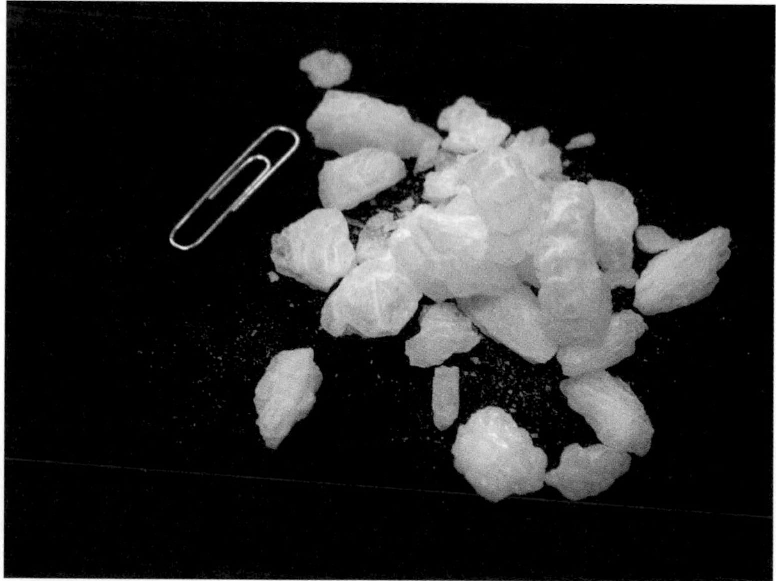

■ **Fig. 35.2.** Contents of plastic bag filled with crystal meth. Photo courtesy of Ahna G. Brutlag.

- Toxicosis in animals may occur by accidental ingestion (oral route) or occasionally by the inhalation of smoke (respiratory route).
- Adulterants may pose a separate toxicosis.

Systems Affected

- Nervous – hyperactivity, tremors, restlessness, seizures, and occasionally ataxia and depression. Hyperthermia is secondary to peripheral vasoconstriction and seizure activity.
- Cardiovascular – tachycardia and premature ventricular contractions.
- Endocrine/metabolic – hyperthermia, liver failure.
- Respiratory – failure and death.
- Renal/urological – renal failure from myoglobinuria secondary to rhabdomyolysis.

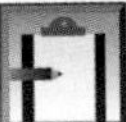

SIGNALMENT/HISTORY

- Dogs are the species most frequently affected, but cats may also be at risk.
- No breed or sex predilection.
- Any age may be affected.
- Signs of exposure include the following:
  - Hyperactivity, restlessness, muscle tremors
  - Seizures
  - Hyperthermia
  - Tachycardia, ventricular premature contractions
  - Disseminated intravascular coagulation (DIC) secondary to hyperthermia
  - Hypersalivation
  - Hypertension
  - Liver or renal failure
  - Respiratory failure

Risk Factors

- Exposure to methamphetamine by drug-sniffing dogs.
- Methamphetamine use or manufacture by family members.

Historical Findings

- History of exposure to or ingestion of methamphetamine.
- Owners are often reluctant to admit the presence of drugs in the home or environment.

Location and Circumstances of Poisoning

- Cases occur throughout the country as use of methamphetamine by humans is widespread.

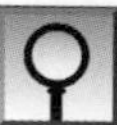

CLINICAL FEATURES

- Onset of clinical signs ranges from 2 minutes to 20 minutes depending on whether intoxication occurred from inhalation or ingestion.
- Duration of acute clinical signs ranges from 3 hours to 8 hours.
- Systems most commonly affected include the following:
  - Nervous system – hyperactivity, long-term neuropsychiatric abnormalities.
  - Cardiovascular system – tachycardia to long-term cardiomyopathy.
- Fatalities are the result of hyperthermia causing cardiomyopathy, respiratory failure, or liver or renal damage.
- In cats, may see signs similar to hallucinations.

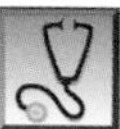

DIFFERENTIAL DIAGNOSIS

- Intoxications such as amphetamines, methylphenidate; herbal products (ephedra, guarana, ma huang); metaldehyde; strychnine.
- Other toxins or disease processes that would cause neurological signs.

DIAGNOSTICS

- Serum chemistry to measure BUN, creatinine, liver enzymes, CK, glucose, and electrolyte abnormalities.
- Urinalysis for evidence of myoglobinuria.
- Venous blood gas analysis for metabolic acidosis.
- If methamphetamine toxicosis is suspected, a urine sample may be submitted for an illicit drug screen at a human hospital.
- The Quick Screen Pro Multi Drug Screening Test is a human testing kit that has been validated by GC/MS for use in animals. It may provide a rapid and accurate diagnosis if the drug is present in high enough concentrations and the time frame is appropriate.

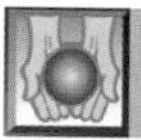

THERAPEUTICS

- Objectives of treatment are to prevent further toxin absorption, control temperature abnormalities by supplying cooling measures, correct hyponatremia, control neurological effects, and provide supportive care.

Detoxification

- Induce emesis if within 2 hours of ingestion and animal is asymptomatic; rapid onset of clinical signs may preclude this.
- Gastric lavage if large dose is ingested.
- Activated charcoal with a cathartic × 1 dose.

Appropriate Health Care

- Monitor closely for signs of hyperthermia and treat with a cooling vest, cool water baths, fans, or ice packs. Do not overcool. Stop at 103–103.5°F.
- ECG for the development of cardiac arrhythmias.
- Monitor blood pressure for hypertension.
- Minimize external stimulation; keep in a darkened area.
- Observe closely for signs of serotonin syndrome and treat as described below.

Antidote

- No specific antidote is available.
- IV fluids at 1.5–2 times maintenance to increase excretion and protect kidneys from myoglobinuria.
- Agitation.
    - Chlorpromazine (0.5–1 mg/kg IV or IM) is preferred due to its benefit in treating serotonin syndrome. Can go as high as 5 mg/kg but need to titrate use against clinical signs.
    - Acepromazine (0.05–1 mg/kg IV, IM, SQ). Begin at low end of dosage range and increase as necessary. The belief that this drug lowers the seizure threshold is not currently supported by recent literature.
    - Diazepam and other benzodiazepines are generally *not* recommended as they may cause dysphoria or paradoxical stimulation.
- Seizures.
    - Chlorpromazine (0.5–1 mg/kg IV or IM) is preferred due to its benefit in treating serotonin syndrome. Can go as high as 5 mg/kg but need to titrate use against clinical signs.
    - Phenobarbital 3–5 mg/kg IV PRN.
    - Propofol: use cautiously in animals with seizures and decrease dose by 25% if animal has already received chlorpromazine or acepromazine.
    - Mask down with sevoflurane if unresponsive to other medications.
    - Avoid diazepam if at all possible and be alert to dysphoria and paradoxical excitation.
- Tremors.
    - Methocarbamol 55–220 mg/kg slow IV titrated to effect. Labeled maximum is 330 mg/kg/day, but in some intoxications this dose may be exceeded. Monitor carefully for severe CNS depression, hypertension, and seizures.
- Tachycardia.
    - Propranolol 0.02 mg/kg slow IV up to a maximum of 1 mg/kg.
- Hypertension: treat with propranolol.
- Arrhythmias.
    - Lidocaine.
        - Dogs: 2–4 mg/kg IV to effect while monitoring ECG. If effective, begin CRI at 25 mcg/kg/min.

        - Cats: 0.25–0.5 mg/kg slow IV while monitoring ECG. If effective, begin CRI at 10–20 mcg/kg/min. Use judiciously in cats.
    - Procainamide.
        - Dogs: 2 mg/kg IV over 3–5 minutes (up to 20 mg/kg IV bolus), followed by 25–50 μg/kg/min CRI.
- Serotonin syndrome (if occurs).
    - Cyproheptadine 1.1 mg/kg (dogs) and 2–4 mg total per cat PO or rectal. Repeat every 4–6 hours as needed.

Public Health

- Methamphetamine and the chemicals used to manufacture it present human health risks.
- Residues from the hair may be a risk to animal caretakers.

Environmental Issues

- Remove the animal from the environment where methamphetamines are cooked or stored.

COMMENTS

Client Education

- Educate the client on methamphetamine toxicosis in pets and stress the need to eliminate it from the animal's environment.

Prevention/Avoidance

- Eliminate methamphetamine from the environment.
- Recovery time will depend on the quantity of toxin ingested or inhaled and the chronicity of exposure. Long-term exposure may result in brain and other neurological damage.

Synonyms

Chalk, crank, glass, ice, meth, pep pill, speed, upper, others

See Also

Amphetamines
Club Drugs (MDMA, GHB, Flunitrazepam, and Bath Salts)
Cocaine

Abbreviations

See Appendix 1 for a complete list.

Suggested Reading

Bischoff K. Toxicity of drugs of abuse. In: GuptaRC, ed. Veterinary Toxicology: Basic and Clinical Principles, 2nd edn. New York: Elsevier, 2012; pp. 469–489.

Dumonceaux GA, Beasley VR. Emergency treatment for police dogs used for illicit drug detection. J Am Vet Med Assoc 1990; 197:185–187.

Pei Z, Zhang X. Methamphetamine intoxication in a dog: case report. BMC Vet Res 2014; 10:139.

Street Drugs: A Drug Identification Guide. Minneapolis: Publishers Group West, 2010.

Volmer PA. Recreational drugs. In: PetersonME, TalcottPA, eds. Small Animal Toxicology, 3rd edn. St Louis, MO: Elsevier, 2013; pp. 309–334.

Acknowledgment: The authors and editors acknowledge the prior contributions of Teresa K. Drotar who authored this topic in the previous edition.

Author: Christy A. Klatt, DVM

Consulting Editor: Lynn R. Hovda, RPh, DVM, MS, DACVIM

chapter 36 Miscellaneous Hallucinogens and Dissociative Agents

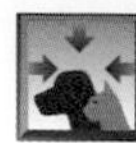

DEFINITION/OVERVIEW

- Several of the remaining hallucinogens and dissociative agents are of concern due to their widespread abuse. They are inexpensive, relatively easy to obtain, and frequently found at parties and in homes where pets live.
  - Hallucinogens.
    - Lysergic acid amide substances (LSAs) are closely related to LSD and provide a similar experience.
      - Seeds from morning glory plant – *Ipomoea* spp. (Fig. 36.1)
      - Seeds from Hawaiian baby woodrose plant – *Argyreia nervosa*
      - Endophyte infected sleepy grass – *Stipa robusta*
    - Salvia – *Salvia divinorum*.
  - Dissociative agents.
    - Ketamine (DEA Schedule III) is a prescription injectable medication often obtained by theft from veterinary clinics. It is gaining popularity as a club drug, and many consider it the ideal substance of abuse as it provides the effects of LSD, opiates, and cocaine in one drug.
- Others worthy of mention but not addressed further in this chapter.
  - Hallucinogens.
    - Jimson weed (thornapple).
      - Seeds from the *Datura stramonium* plant are chewed or powdered and smoked for hallucinogenic properties. The plant is found in ditches and unimproved land throughout the United States. The powerful anticholinergic alkaloids found in the seeds are responsible for the effects. Clinical signs include diaphoresis, decreased salivation, hyperthermia, and psychoactive effects
    - Nutmeg.
      - Seeds from the fruit of an evergreen tree (*Myristica fragrans*) are chewed or powdered and smoked for hallucinogenic properties. The tree is native to the South Pacific, Trinidad, and Grenada. In human beings, the toxic

Blackwell's Five-Minute Veterinary Consult Clinical Companion: Small Animal Toxicology, Second Edition.
Lynn R. Hovda, Ahna G. Brutlag, Robert H. Poppenga, and Katherine L. Peterson.

Companion website: www.fiveminutevet.com/toxicology

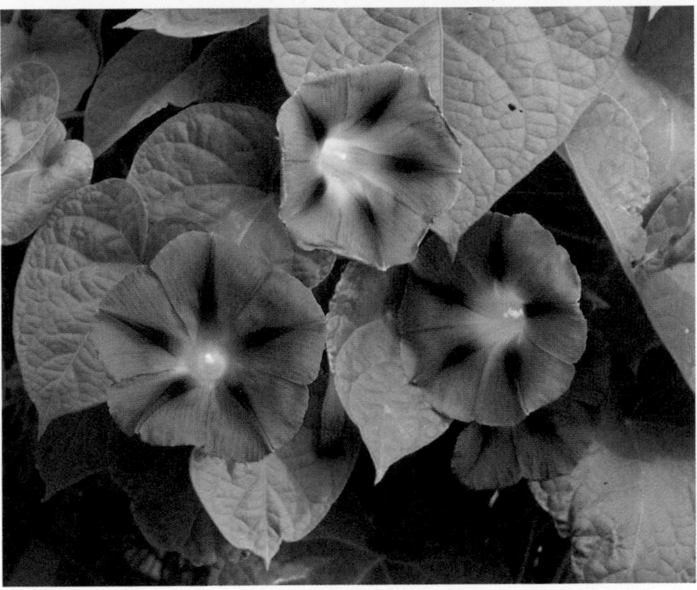

■ **Fig. 36.1.** Morning glory (*Ipomoea spp.*). Photo courtesy of Tyne K. Hovda.

dose is estimated to be three whole nutmegs or 10–15 g (about one tablespoonful) of the dried spice. Clinical signs include decreased salivation, hypothermia, and vomiting

- □ Peyote (mescaline).
  - ◦ The peyote cactus (*Lophophora williamsii*) contains the hallucinogen mescaline. The cactus is found in northern Mexico and the southwestern United States. Crowns or tops of the cactus are harvested and dried; ingestion is generally by chewing on the dried pieces or brewing them and drinking the liquid. In some countries, peyote oil and cream compounded for topical use are heated and concentrated into dry peyote. Clinical signs include early vomiting, diaphoresis, and mydriasis followed by a 12-hour period of psychoactivity resembling that of LSD (Fig. 36.2).
- □ Psilocybin (magic mushrooms or shrooms).
  - ◦ Psilocybin and psilocin are psychoactive agents found in many species of hallucinogenic mushrooms. The mechanism of action is unknown but may be serotonergic in nature. Mushrooms can be ingested directly, brewed into tea, or dried and chewed. Clinical signs are similar to LSD.

- Dissociative agents.
  - □ Dextromethorphan (DMX, triple C, skittles [gelatin capsules]).
    - ◦ Readily available in nonprescription cough syrups and cold remedies. The mechanism of action is very similar to ketamine and phencyclidine. In human beings, approximately 360 mg causes a mild stimulant effect and >1500 mg a completely dissociative state.

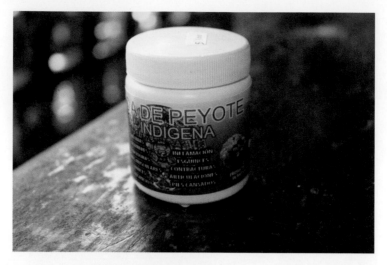

■ **Fig. 36.2.** Peyote oil sold in Mexico. Photo courtesy of Lynn R. Hovda.

ETIOLOGY/PATHOPHYSIOLOGY

- LSAs.
    - Plants are grown throughout the USA and seed packages can be purchased online and in most nurseries.
    - Seeds are germinated, soaked in water, and crushed before ingestion or they are not effective.
- Ketamine.
    - DEA Schedule III drug.
    - Liquid form is odorless, flavorless, and colorless and often added to party punches or individual drinks.
    - It can also be dried and powdered for smoking and inhalation.
- Salvia.
    - Not the same common salvia plant that can be purchased at nurseries and grown in gardens throughout the United States.
    - Leafy green plant native to the Sierra Mazateca region of Mexico.
    - Seeds generally purchased on the internet from specific Salvia divinorum sites.
    - Grown outside in United States in warm, subtropical climates (California and Hawaii); can be grown inside anywhere.
    - Most common forms are the dried leaves, which are chewed or smoked, and the fluid extract, which can be ingested or added to drinks.

Mechanism of Action

- LSAs.
    - Incompletely understood.

- Many act as antagonists at serotonin receptors.
- Action at 5-HT_{2A} receptor may be responsible for hallucinogenic effects.

■ Ketamine.
- Incompletely understood.
- Antagonizes the action of glutamate at the NMDA receptor by binding at site independent of glutamate.
- Inhibits the biogenic amine reuptake complex (NE, dopamine, serotonin).

■ Salvia.
- Salvorin-A is the active toxin.
- Kappa (κ) receptor agonist; no effect on 5-HT_{2A} receptors.

Pharmacokinetics – Absorption, Distribution, Metabolism, Excretion

■ LSAs.
- Little is reported; presumed to follow LSD.
- Clinical signs in 60–90 minutes with a duration of action of several hours.

■ Ketamine.
- Well absorbed IM and IV.
- Poorly absorbed orally, high first-pass effect.
- Distributed to brain, liver, lung, and other tissues.
- Undergoes hepatic metabolism by demethylation or hydroxylation.
- Renal excretion.
- T½ cat = 67 minutes after IM dose.

■ Salvia.
- Smoking.
  - □ Onset time of 20 seconds to 2 minutes (human beings).
  - □ Duration of action is 30–60 minutes.
- Oral or chewed.
  - □ Well absorbed through oral mucosa.
  - □ Chew is kept in mouth much like a tobacco chew, and both onset and duration of action depend on potency of leaves.
- Metabolism unknown.
- T½ in nonhuman primates is 56 minutes.

Toxicity

■ LSAs.
- 1/10 as potent as LSD.
- 150–300 seeds associated with clinical effects in human beings.

■ Ketamine.
- Species dependent.
- Cats – 20 mg/kg IM is sedative dose.
- Dogs – 5–10 mg/kg IM has resulted in seizures.

- Salvia.
    - Not studied in animals.

Systems Affected

- LSAs.
    - CNS – primarily hallucinations with bizarre behaviors.
    - Ophthalmic – mydriasis.
    - Musculoskeletal – rhabdomyolysis.
- Ketamine.
    - CNS – wide variety of signs from ataxia to hallucinations to bizarre or violent behaviors.
    - Musculoskeletal – increased muscle tone, spasms, and rigidity.
    - Ophthalmic – vertical, horizontal, or rotary nystagmus, fixed stares.
- Salvia.
    - CNS – purely a "psychedelic" experience.

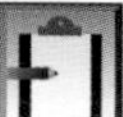

SIGNALMENT/HISTORY

- All species are affected with no particular breed predilection.
- Cats and dogs respond differently to ketamine.

Historical Findings

- The owners are often very reluctant to provide any information regarding these substances, although some may discuss salvia freely.

Location and Circumstances of Poisoning

- Homes and parties where illicit drugs are used.
- Dogs and cats may be exposed by inhaling smoke, drinking leftover "party" punch, chewing on seed packages, digging up and mouthing plants, or finding a stash of "chews."

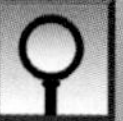

CLINICAL FEATURES

- LSAs.
    - Similar to LSD.
    - Primarily CNS signs including disorientation, vocalization, depression, or excitation. Cats have exhibited very bizarre postures and behaviors. Onset of signs in 1–2 hours with recovery in 6–8 hours.
- Ketamine.
    - Cats – forelimb extensor rigidity, opisthotonus, glazed and dazed staring expression. Hypersalivation with ingestion. Recovery in 10–12 hours.

    - Dogs – CNS excitation with seizures. May develop rhabdomyolysis secondary to seizures.
- Salvia.
    - Clinical signs generally include abnormal mentation and vocalization.
    - Very rapid onset of signs with recovery expected in 1–2 hours.

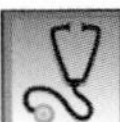

DIFFERENTIAL DIAGNOSIS

- Club drugs such as GHB, PCP, and MDMA.
- CNS diseases with dissociative effects.
- Hepatic encephalopathy.
- Intoxications.
    - Club drugs such as GHB, PCP, MDMA, and synthetic cathinones (bath salts).
    - LSD.
    - Opiates or opioids.

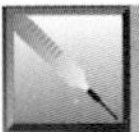

DIAGNOSTICS

- Very limited, difficult to find in serum or urine in routine hospital-based tests.
- LC/MS and GC/MS are useful tools but have a long turnaround time.
- Seeds or plant pieces found in emesis may help with diagnosis.

Pathological Findings

- No specific lesions.

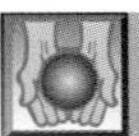

THERAPEUTICS

Detoxification

- Onset of signs is rapid and emesis is not advised.
- Gastric lavage in large doses, especially when plants or seeds have been ingested.
- Activated charcoal plus a cathartic × one dose may be useful.

Appropriate Health Care

- Keep in a dark, quiet area and minimize excess stimulation. Monitor closely for early signs of self-mutilation or psychosis and treat accordingly.
- Monitor body temperature for hyperthermia and treat with cooling vest, cool baths, etc. Do not overcool. Stop when temperature reaches 103–103.5°F. Rarely, hypothermia may develop.
- Baseline labs should include BUN, creatinine, and CK.

Antidote

- No specific antidote is available.

Drugs of Choice

- IV fluids as needed to replace losses and protect kidneys if rhabdomyolysis occurs.
- Seizures, excitation, muscle rigidity.
  - Diazepam 0.25–0.5 mg/kg IV.
  - Phenobarbital 3–5 mg/kg IV PRN.
  - Mask down with sevoflurane if seizures are severe.

Precautions/Interactions

- SSRIs and clomipramine should not be used as they can aggravate the mental changes that occur with intoxication.

Activity

- Minimize activity and limit restraint until clinically normal.

COMMENTS

Client Education

- Keep these and other illicit substances out of animal's reach and environment.
- Muzzle drug-sniffing dogs if need be.
- Educate users about harmful potential to animals.

Patient Monitoring

- Watch closely for the development of self-mutilation or other bizarre physical behaviors and sedate appropriately.

Possible Complications

- None expected with a single exposure.
- Repeated exposures in human beings have resulted in "flashbacks" and permanent psychosis.

Expected Course and Prognosis

- Prognosis is excellent with supportive care. The onset of seizures or rhabdomyolysis complicates treatment and lowers the prognosis for a complete recovery.

Synonyms

LSAs: heavenly blues, flying saucers, pearly gates
Ketamine: special K, cat valium, green K
Salvia: diviner's sage, shepherdess' herb, Mexican mint, Sally D

See Also

Antitussives and Expectorants (Dextromethorphan)
Club Drugs (MDMA, GHB, Flunitrazepam, and Bath Salts)
LSD (Lysergic Acid Diethylamide)
PCP (Phencyclidine)

Abbreviations

See Appendix 1 for a complete list.

MDMA = methylenedioxymethamphetamine
NMDA = *N*-methyl-D-aspartic acid

Suggested Reading

Street Drugs. Long Lake, MN: Publishers Group, 2010; pp. 3–80.

Bischoff K. Toxicity of drugs of abuse. In: GuptaRC, ed. Veterinary Toxicology: Basic and Clinical Principles, 2nd edn. New York: Elsevier, 2012; pp. 469–489.

Halpern JH. Hallucinogens and dissociative agents naturally growing in the USA. Pharmacol Ther 2004; 102:131–138.

Johnson MW, MacLean KA, Reissig CJ, et al. Human psychopharmacology and dose-effects of salvinorin A, a kappa opioid agonist hallucinogen present in the plant *Salvia divinorum*. Drug Alcohol Depend 2011; 115(1):150–155.

Rosenbaum CD, Carreiro SP, Babu KM. Here today, gone tomorrow… and back again? A review of herbal marijuana alternatives (K2, Spice), synthetic cathinones (bath salts), kratom, *Salvia divinorum*, methoxetamine, and piperazines. J Med Toxicol 2012; 8(1):15–32.

Volmer PA. Recreational drugs. In: PetersonME, TalcottPA, eds. Small Animal Toxicology, 3rd edn. St Louis, MO: Elsevier, 2013; pp. 309–334.

Author: Lynn R. Hovda, RPh, DVM, MS, DACVIM
Consulting Editor: Ahna G. Brutlag, DVM, MS, DABP, DABVT

chapter 37

Opiates and Opioids (Illicit)

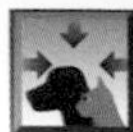

DEFINITION/OVERVIEW

- The opiate and opioid group includes more than 25 different drugs; most are legal prescription drugs.
- Several of these drugs are abused for their psychoactive effects. Among the most frequently abused are opium, morphine, codeine, heroin, oxycodone, hydromorphone, meperidine, and fentanyl.
- Heroin, a morphine derivative, is perhaps the most widely abused because it is inexpensive and more available than other opiates or opioids.
  - Often sold as "black tar heroin," a sticky black substance or "Mexican brown powder," a white to dark brown powder (Fig. 37.1).
  - Generally contains fillers or additives such as sugar, starch, talcum powder, quinine, strychnine, levamisole, or others.
- Animals can be exposed in a variety of different manners.
  - Drug-detecting dogs in active service are at the highest risk for accidental intoxication either by inhalation or ingestion.
  - Puppies have been used as "pack dogs" to transport heroin and cocaine; bags were surgically placed in their abdomens prior to shipping the dogs into the United States.
  - Sporadic cases of malicious heroin injections exist. Staffordshire terriers received at Scottish rescue centers were deliberately injected with heroin by drug dealers to make them more aggressive and attack police officers.
  - Rarely, animal owners want to "share" their experiences with pets.
- Clinical signs vary depending on the species, but death, when it occurs, is generally from respiratory depression and arrest.

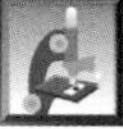

ETIOLOGY/PATHOPHYSIOLOGY

- Opiates – natural opium, morphine, codeine, and other alkaloids are derived from the seeds and sap of the poppy plant (*Papaver somniferum*). See Fig. 37.2.

Blackwell's Five-Minute Veterinary Consult Clinical Companion: Small Animal Toxicology, Second Edition.
Lynn R. Hovda, Ahna G. Brutlag, Robert H. Poppenga, and Katherine L. Peterson.

Companion website: www.fiveminutevet.com/toxicology

■ **Fig. 37.1.** Black tar heroin. Photo courtesy of Lynn R. Hovda.

- Opioids – broad term covering all compounds with morphine-like activity.
  - Heroin, oxycodone, and hydromorphone are semi-synthetic derivatives.
  - Meperidine and fentanyl are strictly synthetic drugs.
- Exposure in animals generally occurs from ingestion, inhalation, or rupture of implanted abdominal packets.

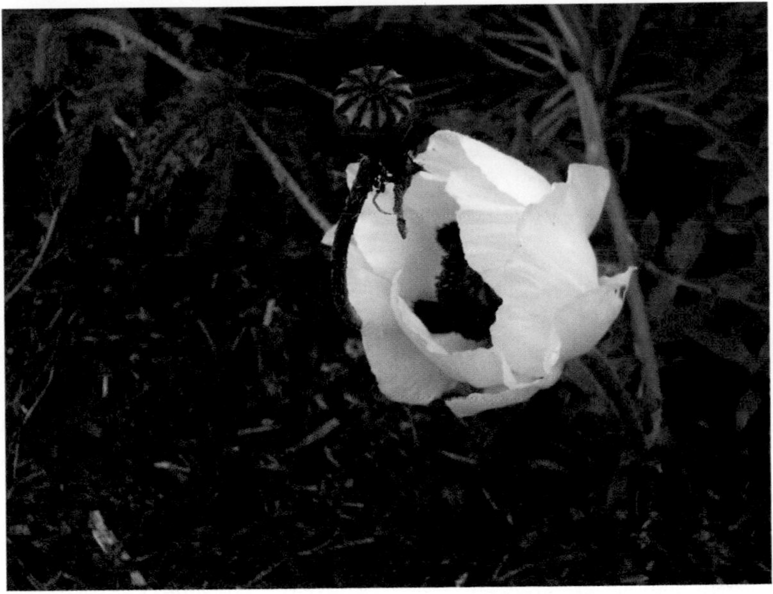

■ **Fig. 37.2.** White opium flower (*Papaver somniferum*). Photo courtesy of Lynn R. Hovda.

Mechanism of Action

- Varies depending on the particular drug.
  - Full agonist – morphine, codeine, heroin, fentanyl, meperidine
  - Full antagonist – naloxone
  - Agonist/antagonist – butorphanol, nalorphine
  - Partial agonist – tramadol, buprenorphine
- Both opiates and opioids bind to opioid receptors.
- Major opioid receptors, designated mu (μ_1 and μ_2), kappa (κ), sigma (σ), delta (δ), and epsilon (ε) are found throughout the body, including the adrenal glands, PNS (peripheral nervous system), CNS (multiple locations), GIT, heart, lymphocytes, kidney, pancreas, and vas deferens.
  - CNS – location of receptors determines whether excitation or depression occurs.
  - Dog – CNS depression; higher number of opioid receptors in amygdala and frontal cortex.
  - Cat – CNS stimulation and excitation.
  - CNS receptors located in CTZ – emesis.
  - CNS receptors located in brainstem – cough and respiratory depression.
  - GIT – decreased motility and constipation.
- Mu receptors, in particular μ_1 receptors, are responsible for the analgesic effects; μ_2 receptors for respiratory depression.
- Kappa receptors produce sedation and dysphoria.
- Sigma receptors were originally thought to be responsible for euphoria and psychoactive effects, but are likely involved in spinal anesthesia.
- Gamma receptors do not appear to mediate analgesia.
- Dopamine and norepinephrine concentrations are likely to play a role as well.

Pharmacokinetics – Absorption, Distribution, Metabolism, Excretion

- Absorption.
  - Oral absorption is generally rapid and occurs in the small intestine.
  - Subcutaneous absorption is rapid.
- Distribution.
  - Well distributed to most organ systems (CNS, intestine, kidney, liver, lungs, placenta, spleen, and skeletal muscle).
  - Liphophilic drugs, including heroin, cross the blood–brain barrier (BBB) more efficiently.
- Metabolism.
  - Readily metabolized in liver by hydrolysis, oxidation, and *N*-dealkylation.
  - Morphine undergoes glucuronidation to morphine-6-glucuronide, an active metabolite.
  - Enterohepatic recirculation of morphine and its metabolite occurs.
- Excretion.
  - Renal, primarily as metabolites.
  - Some biliary excretion via feces.

Toxicity

- Very limited animal data available.
- Codeine: IV LD50 in dogs – 69 mg/kg.
- Heroin – minimum lethal dose:
  - Dog – 25 mg/kg SQ.
  - Cat – 20 mg/kg PO.
- Morphine – minimum lethal dose parenterally:
  - Dog – 110–210 mg/kg SQ.
  - Dog – 133 mg/kg IV LD_{50}.
  - Cat – 40 mg/kg BW given SQ.
- Meperidine:
  - >20 mg/kg BW causes excitation in cats.
  - 30 mg/kg BW causes seizures in cats.

Systems Affected

- Varies depending on drug and species involved.
  - Respiratory – respiratory depression leading to death.
  - CNS – depression or excitation.
  - Cardiovascular – instability with hypotension; heart block and other arrhythmias with propoxyphene overdose.
  - Gastrointestinal – decreased GI motility with constipation.
  - Ophthalmic – miosis or mydriasis (species variation).
  - Endocrine/metabolic – meperidine and tramadol have some serotonergic activity.

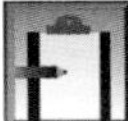

SIGNALMENT/HISTORY

- All breeds and ages are susceptible.
- Cats and dogs present with different clinical signs when exposed to the same opiate or opioid, primarily due to the location of opioid receptors in the CNS.

Risk Factors

- Age.
  - Pediatric animals may have an incomplete BBB and show more severe signs, especially with highly lipophilic substances such as fentanyl and heroin.
  - Neonatal animals may have underdeveloped liver systems and be unable to adequately metabolize opiates or opioids.
  - Geriatric animals may have impaired liver and renal systems, causing inadequate metabolism and excretion of drugs.
- Cats, due to their lack of glucuronyl transferase, may inefficiently metabolize morphine.
- Police dogs, airport dogs, and other narcotic dogs in active service are at a greater risk of exposure.

Historical Findings

- These drugs are illicit and the owners may not provide an accurate history.

Location and Circumstances of Poisoning

- Intoxication can occur anywhere these drugs are found.
- Some dogs have been used as "drug mules" to illegally smuggle heroin or codeine across national borders.

Interactions with Drugs, Nutrients, or Environment

- Many of the drugs, especially heroin, are "cut" with or contain additives such as sugar, starch, dry or powdered milk, chalk, talcum powder, quinine, strychnine, or levamisole.
- Co-ingestion/administration with tramadol, tricyclic antidepressants, selective serotonin reuptake inhibitors, or monoamine oxidase inhibitors may lead to serotonin syndrome.

CLINICAL FEATURES

- Dogs:
  - CNS – early excitation followed by lethargy, ataxia, frank stupor, seizures, coma, death.
  - Respiratory – tachypnea followed by bradypnea.
  - Gastrointestinal – hypersalivation, vomiting, defecation, urination.
  - Cardiovascular – hypotension, arrhythmias related to propoxyphene metabolite.
  - Ophthalmic – miosis.
  - Endocrine/metabolic – hypothermia, decreased pain response, possible serotonin syndrome.
- Cats:
  - CNS – aggression, excitation, seizures, or depression.
  - Respiratory – variable early on, but eventually bradypnea.
  - Gastrointestinal – stasis with lack of emesis, constipation.
  - Cardiovascular – hypotension and arrhythmias.
  - Ophthalmic – mydriasis (more common), miosis.
  - Endocrine/metabolic – hypothermia, decreased pain response, possible serotonin syndrome.

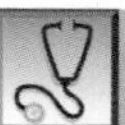

DIFFERENTIAL DIAGNOSIS

- Various encephalopathies.
- CNS depressants:
  - Alcohols
  - Amitraz

    - Barbiturates
    - Benzodiazepines
    - Ethylene glycol
    - Marijuana
    - Synthetic cannabinoids
- CNS stimulants:
    - Amphetamines/methylphenidate/methamphetamine/MDMA
    - Cocaine
    - Metaldehyde
    - Strychnine

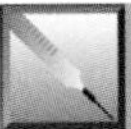

DIAGNOSTICS

- Urine and serum can be submitted to human hospitals for analysis or to a laboratory for GC/MS or LC/MS/MS. Both take several days for results to be returned and will not provide information rapidly enough to guide therapy.
- The Quick Screen Pro Multi Drug Screening Test is a human testing kit that has been successfully used in animals. It may provide a rapid and accurate diagnosis if the drug is present in high enough concentrations and the time frame is appropriate.

Pathological Findings

- No specific findings.

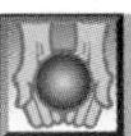

THERAPEUTICS

- The goal of therapy is to provide early decontamination, careful use of an opioid antagonist, and supportive care.

Detoxification

- Induce emesis either at home or in veterinarian's clinic if no clinical signs have developed. Emesis may be successful for 1–2 hours after ingestion due to decreased GI motility.
- Drug-detecting dogs may have ingested bags full of narcotics; be careful that these are not ruptured. Surgical removal may be necessary.
- Gastric lavage if large doses ingested or clinical signs preclude emesis.
- Activated charcoal with cathartic × 1 dose. Repeat doses of activated charcoal may be necessary for drugs such as morphine that undergo enterohepatic recirculation.

Appropriate Health Care

- Hospitalize and monitor closely for CNS and respiratory depression. Be prepared to intubate and ventilate if needed.

- Heart monitor with ECG as needed.
- Monitor body temperature and treat accordingly. Warm but do not overheat.
- Monitor urine output and fluid status.

Antidotes and Drugs of Choice

- Naloxone, a pure opioid antagonist, may be used to reverse CNS and respiratory depression. It has no effects on the GI signs seen in dogs.
    - 0.01–0.04 mg/kg BW IV or IM.
    - The high end of the dosage range may be needed in massive overdoses.
    - Duration of action is generally 45–90 minutes.
    - If effective, dose may need to be repeated.
- IV fluids as needed to replace losses and correct hypotension.
- Diazepam 0. 25–0.5 mg/kg IV as needed for seizures.
- Arrhythmias.
    - Lidocaine.
        - Dogs: 2–4 mg/kg IV to effect while monitoring ECG.
        - Cats: 0.25–0.5 mg/kg slow IV while monitoring ECG. Use judiciously in cats.
    - Procainamide.
        - Dogs: 2 mg/kg IV over 3–5 minutes (up to 20 mg/kg IV bolus), followed by 25–50 µg/kg/min CRI.
        - Cats: 1–2 mg/kg IV once, followed by 10–20 µg/kg/min IV CRI.

Precautions/Interactions

- Naloxone is ineffective for seizures caused by normeperidine, tramadol, or propoxyphene toxicity and may exacerbate signs.
- Naloxone will not reverse propoxyphene-induced cardiotoxicity.

Alternative Drugs

- If naloxone is not available, butorphanol 0.05–0.1 mg/kg IV may be used to partially reverse pure mu agonists.

Surgical Considerations

- Cautious surgical removal of packets in GIT or abdomen of drug-packing dogs.

COMMENTS

Client Education

- Animals should be kept away from parties where these drugs are used. Personal stashes should be locked up and kept out of reach.

- Party drinks and other goodies should be cleared away before animals have access to the area.
- Police and active drug-detecting dogs that are voracious eaters should wear a muzzle.
- Naloxone should be available for police and drug-detecting dogs in active service.

Patient Monitoring

- Baseline labs with attention to BUN, creatinine, and CK, especially if seizures occur.
- Blood gases as needed.
- ECG in the event of arrhythmias.

Expected Course and Prognosis

- The onset of signs is rapid, occurring within 30–120 minutes. The duration of signs depends on the particular opiate or opioid ingested or inhaled.
- The prognosis is generally excellent, especially when naloxone has been used to reverse the signs.
- Death rarely occurs.

Synonyms

Heroin – dope, heaven, Lady Jane, skag, smack, speedball
Fentanyl – China white, tango and cash

See Also

Opiates and Opioids

Abbreviations

See Appendix 1 for a complete list.

GC/MS = gas chromatography/mass spectrometry
LC/MS/MS = liquid chromatography/mass spectrometry/mass spectrometry
MDMA = methylenedioxymethamphetamine

Suggested Reading

Bischoff K. Toxicity of drugs of abuse. In: Gupta RC, ed. Veterinary Toxicology: Basic and Clinical Principles, 2nd edn. New York: Elsevier, 2012; pp. 469–489.

Daily Record. Revealed: Drug dealers injecting dogs with heroin to make them more aggressive. www.daily-record.co.uk/news/scottish-news/revealed-drug-dealers-injecting-pet-1366869

French, D. The challenges of LC-MS/MS analysis of opiates and opioids in urine. Bioanalysis 2013; 5(22):2803–2820.New York Daily News. Colombian vet arrested for implanting heroin inside puppies to smuggle to U.S. www.nydailynews.com/news/world/vet-arrested-implanting-heroin-puppies-article-1.1552806

Volmer PA. Recreational drugs. In: Peterson ME, Talcott, eds. Small Animal Toxicology, 3rd edn. St Louis, MO: Elsevier, 2013; pp. 309–333.

Author: Lynn R. Hovda, RPh, DVM, MS, DACVIM
Consulting Editor: Ahna G. Brutlag, DVM, MS, DABT, DABVT

chapter 38

PCP (Phencyclidine)

DEFINITION/OVERVIEW

- PCP (1-[phenylcyclohexyl] piperidine), or phencyclidine, was introduced in the 1950s as a human surgical anesthetic but was discontinued a few years later because of disagreeable and often violent side effects such as hallucination, mania, delirium, and disorientation.
- It was marketed in 1967 as a veterinary anesthetic (Sernylan) but withdrawn in 1978 because of similar side effects, long half-life, and potential as a drug of abuse.
- Currently a DEA Schedule II synthetic drug.
- Easily synthesized in clandestine laboratories in both the powder and liquid form.
- More than 80 known analogs. Ketamine, one of the analogs, is widely used in veterinary medicine, but it has a shorter half-life and 1/10 to 1/20 potency of PCP.

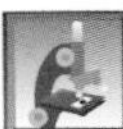

ETIOLOGY/PATHOPHYSIOLOGY

Mechanism of Action

- Dissociative agent, but the precise mechanism is not fully understood.
- Inhibits glutamate at NMDA receptors in the cerebral cortex, thalamus, and limbic system.

Pharmacokinetics – Absorption, Distribution, Metabolism, Excretion

- PCP is a weak base with poor gastric absorption and significant intestinal absorption.
- Inhaled PCP is absorbed via the respiratory system.
- Highly lipophilic.
    - Crosses the blood–brain barrier.
    - Partitions to the CNS, which may increase half-life.
- Metabolism varies with species.
    - In dogs, 68% of a single dose is metabolized in the liver and 32% is excreted unchanged by the kidney.
    - In cats, 88% is excreted unchanged by the kidney.

Blackwell's Five-Minute Veterinary Consult Clinical Companion: Small Animal Toxicology, Second Edition.
Lynn R. Hovda, Ahna G. Brutlag, Robert H. Poppenga, and Katherine L. Peterson.

Companion website: www.fiveminutevet.com/toxicology

Toxicity

- Oral administration.
  - Severe signs of toxicosis.
    - Dogs 2.5–10.0 mg/kg BW PO.
    - Cats 1.1–12.0 mg/kg BW PO.
  - Lethal PO dose in dogs is 25 mg/kg BW.
- IV administration – clinical signs can occur in dogs at 1 mg/kg BW IV.
- IM administration in dogs.
  - 2 mg/kg BW – muscle incoordination.
  - 5 mg/kg BW – immobilization and seizures.

Systems Affected

- Nervous – variable, from depression to stimulation; may last several days.
- Neuromuscular – tremors, loss of motor function.
- Cardiovascular – tachycardia, hypo- or hypertension, arrhythmias.
- Endocrine/metabolic – hyperthermia.
- Musculoskeletal – rhabdomyolysis.
- Renal/urological – acute renal failure secondary to myoglobinuria.

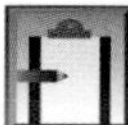

SIGNALMENT/HISTORY

Risk Factors

- Ingestion of illegal PCP.
- Police dogs may be predisposed.

Historical Findings

- Access to drugs.
  - Teenagers in the home.
  - Guests or party in the home.
- Owners may be reluctant to give a complete history.

Location and Circumstances of Poisoning

- Animals residing in neighborhoods with known drug use.
- May be combined with other drugs.

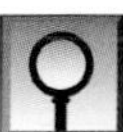

CLINICAL FEATURES

Acute

- Behavioral effects vary depending on dosage.
  - Depression at low dose.
  - Stimulation at high dose with the potential for seizures.

- General signs include hypertension, tachycardia, nausea, vomiting, hypersalivation, fever, sweating, and convulsion.
- Dogs dosed with PCP showed muscular rigidity, facial grimacing, increased motor activity, head weaving, stereotyped sniffing behaviors, jaw snapping, salivation, blank staring, incoordination, nystagmus, coma, tonic-clonic convulsions, and hyperthermia.
- Cardiovascular effects include tachycardia, hypertension, and cardiac arrhythmias.

Chronic

- Not reported.

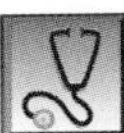

DIFFERENTIAL DIAGNOSIS

- Hallucinogenic mushrooms.
- Ketamine.
- LSD.
- Marijuana and synthetic cannabinoids.

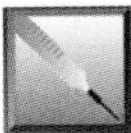

DIAGNOSTICS

- Serum chemistry may show acidosis, hypoglycemia, electrolyte imbalances, and increases in CPK and AST.
- Urine, blood, plasma, or gastric contents for laboratory analysis.
    - Urine is the most commonly analyzed sample. PCP may be detected for more than 2 weeks after exposure.
    - Blood concentrations do not correlate with clinical findings.
- PCP and ketamine may cross-react in immunoassays.

Pathological Findings

- Nonspecific.
- Subendocardial and epicardial hemorrhage.

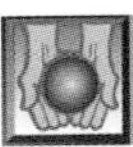

THERAPEUTICS

- Treatment of poisoning is generally symptomatic and supportive.

Detoxification

- Emesis only if very recent ingestion of large doses. Use with caution, as animals may develop seizures at any time.
- Activated charcoal with a cathartic × 1 dose.

Appropriate Health Care

- Monitor for urine output and adjust IV fluids as needed.
- Monitor for hyperthermia and treat accordingly.

- Monitor blood pressure and treat accordingly.
- Obtain baseline BUN, creatinine, and blood glucose. Repeat as needed.
- Keep animal in a darkened, nonstressful environment and do not overstimulate.

Antidote

- No specific antidote is available.

Drugs of Choice

- IV fluids to correct hypoglycemia and electrolyte abnormalities. IV rate, at a minimum, should be 2 times maintenance to ensure adequate urine output and stabilize the cardiovascular system.
- After rehydration, forced diuresis with mannitol or furosemide can be used to increase the rate of clearance.
    - Furosemide CRI at 1–2 mg/kg/hour.
    - Mannitol bolus at 1–2 g/kg slow IV.
- Seizures.
    - Diazepam 0.25–2.0 mg/kg IV.
    - Phenobarbital 2–5 mg/kg IV, can be repeated up to twice at 20-minute intervals.

Precautions/Interactions

- Phenothiazine tranquilizers exacerbate anticholinergic effects, and produce hypotension.

Activity

- Minimize sensory stimulation.
- Dark, quiet room.

COMMENTS

Client Education

- Police dogs can wear a muzzle to prevent ingestion of illegal drugs.
- Prevent exposure to illegal drugs.
    - Keep animals away from illegal drug stash.
    - Keep animals confined during parties where drugs may be used.

Patient Monitoring

- Monitor body temperature regularly over 12 hours post exposure.
- Monitor BUN, creatinine, CK, and blood glucose.

Possible Complications

- Self-induced trauma or rhabdomyolysis may complicate treatment.

Expected Course and Prognosis

- Depends on the clinical condition of the animal at the time of presentation.
- Prognosis is generally good with early decontamination, monitoring, and supportive care.
- Dogs injected IM with low dose of PCP.
    - 1 mg/kg – recovered in a little over 1 hour.
    - 5 mg/kg – recovered within 2 hours.
- Poor prognosis if self-induced trauma or rhabdomyolysis is evident.

Synonyms

Angel dust, angel hair, boat, dummy dust, jet fuel

See Also

Marijuana
Miscellaneous Hallucinogens and Dissociative Agents

Abbreviations

See Appendix 1 for a complete list.

Suggested Reading

Bischoff K. Toxicity of drugs of abuse. In: Gupta RC, ed. Veterinary Toxicology: Basic and Clinical Principles, 2nd edn. New York: Elsevier, 2012; pp. 469–489.
Ortega J. Phencyclidine for capture of stray dogs. J Am Vet Med Assoc 1967; 150:772–776.
Volmer PA. Recreational drugs. In: Peterson ME, Talcott PA, eds. Small Animal Toxicology, 3rd edn. St Louis, MO: Elsevier, 2013; pp 309–334.

Authors: Karyn Bischoff, DVM, MS, DABVT; IIwan Goo Kang, DVM, PhD
Consulting Editor: Lynn R. Hovda, RPh, DVM, MS, DACVIM

chapter 39 Synthetic Cannabinoids

 DEFINITION/OVERVIEW

- Synthetic cannabinoids have become increasingly prevalent in the United States in the past 10 years.
- Typically manufactured in clandestine labs.
- Known by many different brand or street names including, but not limited to, K2, Spice, Buddha, Black Magic, Cloud, Crazy Monkey and Happy Shaman.
- Structures are not related to THC.
- Most common synthetic cannabinoids contain JWH-018, JWH-081, JWH-250, JWH-073, CP-47, HU-210, or PB-22.
- New compounds frequently become available, making these substances difficult to regulate; known synthetic cannabinoids are Schedule I substances.
- Limited information is known regarding the clinical effects in companion animals.

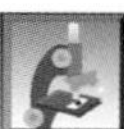 ETIOLOGY/PATHOPHYSIOLOGY

Mechanism of Action

- The exact mechanism of action of most synthetic cannabinoids is unknown and may vary among compounds.
- Strong CB1 and CB2 agonists. May be up to 28 times more potent than marijuana, resulting in more severe clinical effects.
    - CB1 receptors are concentrated in the CNS, specifically the brain and spinal cord.
    - CB2 receptors are located in the periphery.

Toxicity

- A specific toxic dose has not been established, but due to the potency of synthetic cannabinoids, clinical signs will likely occur with smaller amounts as compared to marijuana.
- The current pharmacokinetic properties of these agents are not known, but are being studied.

Blackwell's Five-Minute Veterinary Consult Clinical Companion: Small Animal Toxicology, Second Edition.
Lynn R. Hovda, Ahna G. Brutlag, Robert H. Poppenga, and Katherine L. Peterson.

Companion website: www.fiveminutevet.com/toxicology

- Absorption is rapid following ingestion of most known substances.
- The metabolism of these chemicals is not known; there may be up to 13 metabolites of JWH-018 that are excreted in urine.

Systems Affected

- Cardiovascular – bradycardia.
- Gastrointestinal – vomiting.
- Nervous – ataxia, drowsiness, agitation, hyperesthesia.
- Neuromuscular – twitching, tremors, seizures.
- Ophthalmic – mydriasis.

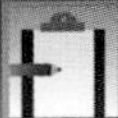

SIGNALMENT/HISTORY

- All animals can be affected, but dogs are more indiscriminate eaters and more likely to ingest them.

Risk Factors

- Exposure to synthetic cannabinoids by ingestion or possibly through inhalation.
- Synthetic cannabinoid use by owners or family members.

Historical Findings

- Owners may be reluctant to admit pet exposure and may need encouragement to help with diagnosis.

Location and Circumstances of Poisoning

- Cases occur throughout the country.
- DEA Schedule I but easily obtainable on the internet.

CLINICAL FEATURES

- Signs are similar to marijuana ingestions, but may be more severe.
- Signs may vary due to multiple different compounds.
- Most common signs are ataxia, drowsiness, vomiting, twitching, mydriasis, agitation, and hyperesthesia.
- Signs may develop within 30 minutes of ingestion or inhalation.

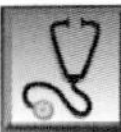

DIFFERENTIAL DIAGNOSIS

- Alcohols
- Hallucinogenic mushrooms

- Human pharmaceuticals with CNS depressant effects (benzodiazepines, opioids, and others)
- Marijuana
- Recreational plants and drugs
- Other CNS stimulants (amphetamines, methylphenidate, and others)

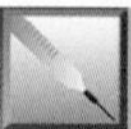

DIAGNOSTICS

- Typically must rely on history from owner. This may not be forthcoming so it is important to use unbiased questioning.
- There is currently no urine test that may be used in a clinical setting.

Pathological Findings

- No specific findings.

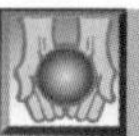

THERAPEUTICS

- The objectives of treatment are to prevent further toxin absorption and provide supportive care.

Detoxification

- Remove from source.
- Emesis if acute, animal is alert, and has not vomited.
    - Many animals may have already vomited.
    - Drowsiness is a common sign and may put animal at risk for aspiration.
- Activated charcoal with cathartic × 1 for oral exposure. Consider a second dose of activated charcoal with NO cathartic if animal is alert and airway not compromised.

Appropriate Health Care

- Hospitalization for all symptomatic animals.
- Monitor CNS and neurological status.

Antidote

- No specific antidote is available.

Drugs of Choice

- IV fluids as needed.

- Twitching.
  - Methocarbamol 55–220 mg/kg IV, labeled maximum of 330 mg/kg/day. The maximum amount may need to be exceeded in some poisonings; the animal should be monitored for severe CNS depression, seizures, and hypotension.
- Seizures or agitation.
  - Diazepam 0.25–0.5 mg/kg IV PRN.
  - Chlorpromazine 0.5–1 mg/kg IV PRN.

COMMENTS

- Synthetic cannabinoids also pose a significant human health risk so pet owners may be at risk of toxicosis if they also were exposed prior to veterinary clinic visit.

Prevention/Avoidance

- Educate pet owner on toxicity of synthetic cannabinoids.
- Eliminate synthetic cannabinoids from the environment.
- Keep pets out of the area where synthetic cannabinoid use may occur.

Expected Course and Prognosis

- Toxicity is rarely fatal, but may be more prevalent than marijuana due to potency.
- Pharmacokinetic profiles of these chemicals are not known, so hospitalization time may vary considerably.
- Recovery time has typically been less than 24 hours.

Synonyms

K2, Spice, Buddha, Black Magic, Cloud, Crazy Monkey, Happy Shaman, Skunk, Stinger, Mr Nice Guy, others

See Also

Marijuana
Club Drugs (MDMA, GHB, Flunitrazepam, and Bath Salts)

Abbreviations

See Appendix 1 for a complete list.

THC = tetrahydrocannabinol

Suggested Reading

Castaneto MS, Gorelick D, Desrosiers N, et al. Synthetic cannabinoids: epidemiology, pharmacodynamics, and clinical implications. Drug Alcohol Depend 2014; 144:12–41.

Gugelmann H, Gerona R, Li C, et al. 'Crazy Monkey' poisons man and dog: human and canine seizures due to PB-22, a novel synthetic cannabinoid. Clin Toxicol 2014; 52(6):635–638.
Sioris KM, Keyler D. K2 and K9s. Clin Toxicol 2014; 52:710.

Author: Kelly Sioris, PharmD, CSPI
Consulting Editor: Lynn R. Hovda, RPh, DVM, MS, DACVIM

Drugs: Over the Counter

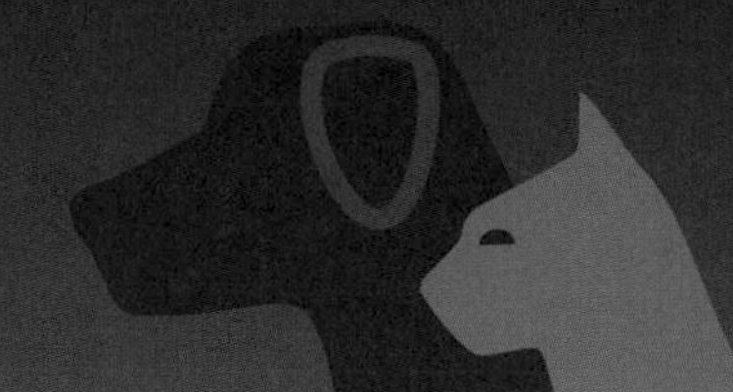

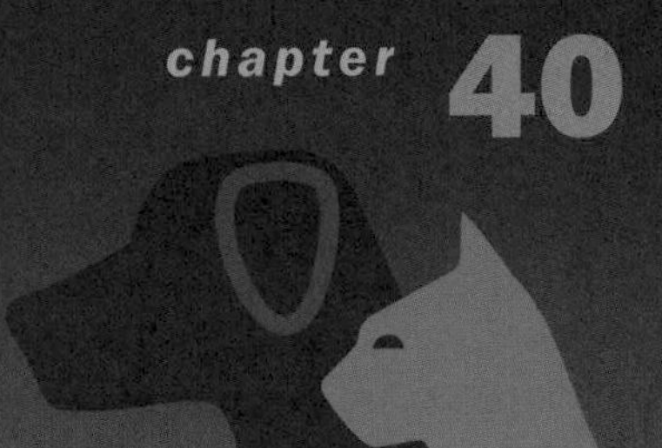

chapter 40

Acetaminophen

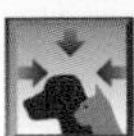 DEFINITION/OVERVIEW

- Acetaminophen (N-acetyl-p-aminophenol), also known as Tylenol, paracetamol, and APAP, is an OTC analgesic and antipyretic medication.
- It has only weak antiinflammatory effects, and is not used to treat inflammation.
- Accidental exposure or deliberate administration in dogs and cats can result in toxicosis due to a narrow margin of safety, particularly in cats. It has some limited uses as an analgesic in dogs, but requires careful veterinary supervision.
- Accumulation of toxic metabolites and oxidative injury results when metabolic pathways for glucuronidation and sulfation are absent or depleted, and glutathione is depleted.
- Clinical signs are related to methemoglobinemia (MetHb) and hepatoxicity and can result from both acute and chronic exposures.
- Common clinical signs include lethargy, respiratory distress, brown mucous membranes from MetHb, and vomiting, icterus, and coagulopathies from hepatotoxicosis.

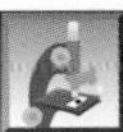 ETIOLOGY/PATHOPHYSIOLOGY

Mechanism of Action

- Acetaminophen interferes with the endoperoxide intermediates of arachidonic acid conversion, and possibly COX-3 inhibition.
- Although the exact mechanism is unknown, acetaminophen increases the pain threshold by inhibition of chemical mediators that sensitize pain receptors.
- Antipyretic effects are centrally mediated at the level of the hypothalamus due to inhibition of prostaglandin synthesis.

Pharmacokinetics – Absorption, Distribution, Metabolism, Excretion

- Rapid absorption occurs in the stomach and small intestine after oral administration; peak blood levels are reached within 30–60 minutes.
- Poor plasma protein binding leads to wide systemic distribution.

Blackwell's Five-Minute Veterinary Consult Clinical Companion: Small Animal Toxicology, Second Edition.
Lynn R. Hovda, Ahna G. Brutlag, Robert H. Poppenga, and Katherine L. Peterson.

Companion website: www.fiveminutevet.com/toxicology

- Metabolism in the liver is completed by three pathways: glucuronidation, sulfation, and cytochrome P450-mediated oxidation.
- Part of the drug is metabolized into nontoxic conjugates by the glucuronidation and sulfation pathways, while some is excreted unchanged in the urine or metabolized to a toxic metabolite, N-acetyl-para-benzoquinoneimine (NAPQI) via the cytochrome P450 enzyme pathway.
- NAPQI is normally detoxified by conjugation with glutathione (GSH) in the liver.

Toxicity

- The toxic dose to induce MetHb in dogs is approximately 100–200 mg/kg, with hepatotoxic doses higher. Some report hepatotoxicity at doses between 100 and 600 mg/kg. For cats, the toxic dose has been reported as low as 10 mg/kg.
- Glucuronidation and sulfation elimination pathways become saturated as the drug dose increases and more of the drug is converted into NAPQI. NAPQI accumulates as cellular stores of GSH are depleted, leading to oxidative injury.
- Cats are more sensitive to the toxic effects due to a deficiency in glucuronyl transferase, an enzyme required to metabolize acetaminophen via the glucuronidation pathway.
- Due to this deficiency, the sulfation pathway is quickly saturated, leaving more drug to be metabolized to NAPQI by the cytochrome P450 enzyme pathway and quickly depleting glutathione.

Systems Affected

- Hemic/lymphatic/immune.
  - Heinz body and MetHb formation, with subsequent hemolytic anemia, result from binding of NAPQI and associated oxidative injury to the RBCs and Hb molecules.
  - MetHb is most commonly seen in cats but has been reported in dogs.
  - MetHb is a nonfunctional complex formed from Hb by the oxidation of Hb iron from the ferrous to the ferric state.
  - Coagulopathy can occur as a consequence of end-stage hepatic failure.
- Hepatobiliary – binding of NAPQI to hepatocyte membranes leads to hepatocellular death and central lobular necrosis.
- Cardiovascular – collapse, shock, death, brown mucous membranes.
- Gastrointestinal – vomiting, anorexia, and diarrhea secondary to hepatoxicity.
- Nervous – hepatic encephalopathy secondary to hepatotoxicity.
- Renal/urological – renal tubular necrosis.
- Respiratory – tachypnea, dyspnea, tissue hypoxia due to MetHb impairing RBC oxygen-carrying capacity.
- Skin/exocrine – facial or paw edema, icterus.

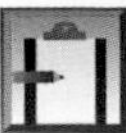

SIGNALMENT/HISTORY

Risk Factors

- No known risk factors exist in animals but smoking is considered a risk factor in humans. Therefore, pets in households with smokers may have increased risk of toxicity due to inhalation of second-hand smoke, which increases risk of oxidative cellular injuries.

Historical Findings

- History of exposure to or ingestion of drug.
- Lethargy, brown mucous membranes, respiratory distress, edema of the face and paws in cats.
- Lethargy, anorexia, vomiting, diarrhea in dogs.
- History may include a nonspecific ailment.
- Acetaminophen may be present with other medications in prescription analgesics and OTC multisymptom cold and allergy products, and a thorough history must be obtained from the owner about the exact contents/ingredients.

Location and Circumstances of Poisoning

- Intoxication may result from deliberate and accidental administration to pets.
- Access to medications may lead to intoxication.

CLINICAL FEATURES

- Pets may present with either syndrome; however, cats commonly present with MetHb while dogs present with hepatotoxicity and associated GI and CNS signs.
    - Hepatotoxicity – hepatic failure, anorexia, nausea, vomiting, lethargy, abdominal pain, icterus, hepatic encephalopathy, coma.
    - Methemoglobinemia – shock (tachycardia, tachypnea, hypothermia, weakness, collapse), brown mucous membranes, respiratory distress, cyanosis, lethargy, depression, coma, edema of face and paws.

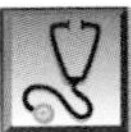

DIFFERENTIAL DIAGNOSIS

- Anemia
    - Oxidative damage (Heinz bodies) to RBCs may result from other oxidants, such as onion, garlic, and zinc. Zinc toxicosis may also reveal a metallic foreign body on radiographs.
    - IMHA is diagnosed with the presence of spherocytes and/or autoagglutination; blood is not discolored brown with IMHA.

  - *Mycoplasma felis* may be present on blood smear.
  - Respiratory distress or cyanosis may be due to primary cardiac or respiratory disease.
  - Facial and paw edema may result from hypersensitivity reactions or trauma.
- Hepatic failure (e.g., drug-induced, neoplasia, copper storage disease, etc.).
- Hepatitis, cholangiohepatitis, hepatotoxicity (e.g., *Amanita* mushrooms, NSAIDs, aflatoxins, xylitol, etc.).

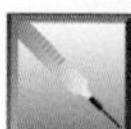

DIAGNOSTICS

- CBC, chemistry profile, and UA are indicated. Abdominal imaging may be indicated if other differentials are considered (to rule out primary liver disease).
- CBC may reveal MetHb recognized as dark brown blood and Heinz body anemia.
- Serum chemistry profile may reveal elevated ALT, AST, and total bilirubin.
- Hypoglycemia and a prolonged PT/PTT time may be present in cases of severe hepatic dysfunction.

Pathological Findings

- Centrilobular hepatic necrosis.
- Proximal renal tubular necrosis.

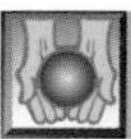

THERAPEUTICS

Detoxification

- Induce vomiting within 2 hours of ingestion if the patient is asymptomatic.
- Administer activated charcoal (1–3 g/kg) without a cathartic once, if ingestion occurred <2 hours earlier. Acetaminophen does not undergo significant enterohepatic recirculation, so multiple doses of activated charcoal are not routinely recommended and may interfere with oral administration of N-acetylcysteine (NAC).

Appropriate Health Care

- Minimize stress.
- Provide supplemental oxygen as indicated.
- Institute IV fluid therapy to provide hemodynamic support and treat for shock.
- Administer packed red blood cells as indicated.

Drugs and Antidotes of Choice

- Limit formation of the toxic metabolite, NAPQI, by providing glutathione substrates.
  - N-acetylcysteine (NAC) 140 mg/kg IV initial dose, followed by 70 mg/kg IV q 4–6 hours for 7–17 doses. NAC may be more effective given PO but may require a feeding

tube because the odor and taste are offensive. NAC provides a substrate for sulfation, replenishes glutathione stores, and binds directly to NAPQI, the toxic metabolite.

- Antioxidant therapy.
  - S-adenosyl-methionine (SAMe) 18 mg/kg/day PO may reduce oxidative damage.
  - Ascorbic acid (vitamin C) 30 mg/kg PO, SQ, IV q 6 hours acts as an antioxidant to reduce MetHb to Hb.
- Increase oxygen-carrying capacity.
  - Administer pRBC IV, 10–15 mL/kg as needed, or whole blood IV, 20 mL/kg as needed to effect.

Precautions/Interactions

- Activated charcoal may adsorb orally administered NAC, reducing its effect. If treating with oral NAC, separate administration of NAC and activated charcoal by at least 2 hours.

Alternative Drugs

- FFP 10–15 mL/kg IV is indicated if a coagulopathy is present (based on PT/PTT) due to severe hepatic dysfunction.
- Vitamin K 2.5–5 mg/kg/day, SQ or PO, q 12–24 hours can be administered to support production of factors II, VII, IX, and X.
- Methylene blue, 1.5 mg/kg, IV × 1–2 doses, has been used to treat MetHb, but it can cause Heinz bodies and MetHb, particularly in cats. It should be reserved for patients with severe MetHb.

COMMENTS

Client Education

- Acetaminophen should never be administered to cats, and only to dogs with direct veterinary supervision.

Prevention/Avoidance

- Acetaminophen is commonly available in homes, and appropriate pet proofing and client education are important to prevent inadvertent or iatrogenic intoxication.

Expected Course and Prognosis

- Evidence of improvement includes resolving respiratory distress, normalization of mucous membrane color, improvement of laboratory values, resolving facial and paw edema, and improved mentation.
- Generally, a good prognosis is associated with ingestion of a low dose and prompt medical attention.
- Severe hepatic damage and coma represent a poor prognosis.

Synonyms

Tylenol toxicosis, paracetamol toxicosis

Abbreviations

See Appendix 1 for a complete list.

APAP = N-acetyl-p-aminophenol
COX = cyclooxygenase
FFP = fresh frozen plasma
GSH = glutathione
Hb = hemoglobin
IMHA = immune-mediated hemolytic anemia
MetHb = methemoglobinemia
NAC = N-acetylcysteine
NAPQI = N-acetyl-para-benzoquinoneimine
NSAID = nonsteroidal antiinflammatory
pRBC = packed red blood cells
PT = prothrombin time
PTT = partial thromboplastin time

Suggested Reading

Alwood AJ. Acetaminophen. In: SilversteinDC, HopperK, eds. Small Animal Critical Care Medicine. St Louis, MO: Saunders, 2009.

Aronson LR, Drobatz K. Acetaminophen toxicosis in 17 cats. J Vet Emerg Crit Care 1996; 6:65–69.

McConkey SE, Grant DM, Cribb AE. The role of para-aminophenol in acetaminophen-induced methemoglobinemia in dogs and cats. J Vet Pharmacol Ther 2009; 32:585–595.

Richardson JA. Management of acetaminophen and ibuprofen toxicoses in dogs and cats. J Vet Emerg Crit Care 2000; 10:285–291.

Taylor NS, Dhupa N. Acetaminophen toxicity in cats and dogs. Compend Contin Educ Pract Vet 2000; 22:160–169.

Wallace KP, Center SA, Hickford FH. S-adenosyl-L-methionine (SAMe) for the treatment of acetaminophen toxicity in a dog. J Am Anim Hosp Assoc 2002; 38:246–254.

Acknowledgment: The authors and editors acknowledge the prior contributions of Danielle Babski, DVM, and Amie Koenig, DVM, DACVIM, DACVECC, who authored this topic in the previous edition.

Author: John H. Tegzes, MA, VMD, DABVT
Consulting Editor: Ahna G. Brutlag, DVM, MS, DABT, DABVT

Antitussives and Expectorants (Dextromethorphan)

chapter 41

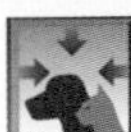

DEFINITION/OVERVIEW

- Antitussives include a variety of OTC and prescription medications designed to help reduce coughing in those with upper respiratory infections or other similar illnesses.
- Dextromethorphan (DXM) is the most popular and widely available OTC antitussive.
- Available as a single-agent product or in combination with other OTC cough and cold medications, including analgesics (e.g., acetaminophen, ibuprofen, aspirin), decongestants (e.g., phenylephrine, pseudoephedrine), and antihistamines (e.g., diphenhydramine, chlorpheniramine).
- Available in tablet, capsule, or liquid forms in various dosage strengths between 5 and 60 mg of DXM per dose.
- DXM has been used in veterinary medicine as an antitussive and to treat repetitive behavior in dogs. The recommended dose is 1–2 mg/kg PO q 6–12 hours.

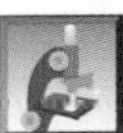

ETIOLOGY/PATHOPHYSIOLOGY

Mechanism of Action

- Dextromethorphan is the d-isomer of 3-methoxy-N-methylmorphinan, a synthetic analog to codeine and structural analog to ketamine.
- At therapeutic doses, it exerts antitussive effects by binding to the delta-opiate receptor.
- DXM exhibits no effects on kappa or mu opiate receptors that normally impart analgesic effects.
- In overdose, it antagonizes N-methyl-D-aspartate (NMDA) glutamate receptors and prevents reuptake of serotonin (SE).

Pharmacokinetics

- Rapidly absorbed orally; oral bioavailability in dogs is 11%.
- Serum levels peak approximately 2–4 hours post ingestion. Absorption and development of clinical signs may occur more rapidly with liquid products.

Blackwell's Five-Minute Veterinary Consult Clinical Companion: Small Animal Toxicology, Second Edition.
Lynn R. Hovda, Ahna G. Brutlag, Robert H. Poppenga, and Katherine L. Peterson.

Companion website: www.fiveminutevet.com/toxicology

- Extensively (>90%) metabolized. Undergoes significant first-pass metabolism to the active metabolite dextrorphan and 3-methoxymorphinan in the liver via CYP-450 system.
- Half-life: 2–4 hours, but may be longer with overdose.
- Metabolites are conjugated with sulfate and glucuronide moieties and excreted in urine; little of the parent compound (<1%) recovered in urine.

Toxicity

- Canine therapeutic dose: 1–2 mg/kg PO q 6–12 hours.
- LD_{50}, SQ dog: 157 mg/kg, LD_{50}, IV cat: 19.8 mg/kg.
- Toxicity is largely dose dependent.
- Primarily affects the CNS.
- Resultant behavioral effects can have secondary effects on cardiovascular and other systems.

Systems Affected

- Nervous – highly variable effects including depression or agitation, unprovoked aggressive behavior, apparent hallucinations, tremors, and seizure activity.
- Cardiovascular – tachycardia (if agitated) or bradycardia (if sedated).
- Respiratory – tachypnea (if agitated) or hypoventilation (if sedated). Respiratory arrest is uncommon.
- Musculoskeletal – staggering gait, "robot" rigidity to the gait (humans).
- Endocrine/metabolic – hyperthermia secondary to neuromuscular effects.
- Renal – renal impairment secondary to prolonged tremors, seizures, and/or hyperthermia.
- Gastrointestinal – nausea, vomiting, diarrhea.

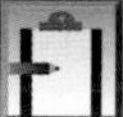

SIGNALMENT/HISTORY

Risk Factors

- No breed sensitivities identified.
- Brachycephalic breeds may be at greater risk of developing respiratory difficulty due to their anatomy.
- Neonatal or geriatric pets or those with underlying health conditions may have an increased risk for severe toxicity.

Historical Findings

- Witnessed exposure.
- Discovery of chewed tablets or spilled bottles of cough and cold products (e.g., cough syrup, decongestants, antihistamines).
- Owners may report behavioral changes such as excessive sedation or agitation (or both). Changes may be abrupt and difficult to predict.
- Unexpected aggressive behavior due to the presumed presence of hallucinations.

Locations and Circumstances of Poisoning

- Exposures most likely to occur in the home.
- Evidence of exposure often readily identifiable (e.g., spilled bottles, owner administered, etc.).

Interactions with Drugs, Nutrients, or Environment

- Animals receiving other agents with sedative properties (e.g., antihistamines, tricyclic antidepressants, some analgesics, etc.) may experience more profound sedation due to additive effects.
- If ingested with sedatives, antihistamines, narcotics, illicit substances, etc., toxicity may be enhanced.

CLINICAL FEATURES

- Clinical features vary widely based on the amount of DXM consumed.
- Effects from intoxication can be gradual, over a period of a few hours.
- Overall neurological status may vary from sedated to highly agitated.
- Ataxia is common.
- Tremors or seizure activity may occur.
- Tachycardia or bradycardia (depending on level of agitation/sedation).
- Body temperature may be elevated secondary to agitation, tremors, or seizure activity.
- Anticholinergic co-ingestions (e.g., antihistamines) may result in generalized erythema, dry mucous membranes, and dilated pupils.
- Stimulant co-ingestions (e.g., decongestants) may result in tachycardia, agitation, or tremors.
- Some animals may develop serotonin syndrome due to DXM's ability to inhibit reuptake of SE. Serotonin syndrome is the overstimulation of SE receptors in the CNS, GIT, cardiovascular, and respiratory systems. Clinical signs associated with serotonin syndrome include tremors, seizures, hyperesthesia, hyperthermia, hypersalivation, and death.
- Respiratory arrest is uncommon with DXM alone.

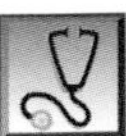

DIFFERENTIAL DIAGNOSIS

- Other toxicities.
  - Recreational/street drugs (e.g., stimulants, sedatives, hallucinogens).
  - Other prescription and nonprescription drugs (e.g., antihistamines, amphetamines, benzodiazepines, sedatives), chocolate/caffeine/methylxanthines.
- Primary metabolic disorders (e.g., hypoglycemia, hepatic disease resulting in hepatic encephalopathy, renal disease, etc.).
- Primary neurological disease resulting in ataxia, sedation, behavioral changes, etc.

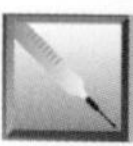

DIAGNOSTICS

- Commercially available urine drug screens may show false-positive results for phencyclidine (PCP).
- DXM serum levels are not widely available or helpful in establishing diagnosis.
- Renal indices, BG, and electrolytes should be assessed in any symptomatic animal. Assess upon presentation and monitor as needed if tremors, seizures, DIC, or severe hyperthermia develop.

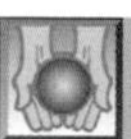

THERAPEUTICS

- No well-established or accepted antidote exists.
- Overall approach to treatment involves early GI decontamination (if presenting shortly after ingestion) and supportive care for subsequent signs that arise.
- Determine if other common cold and flu products were also ingested (e.g., acetaminophen, antihistamines, etc.).

Detoxification

- Induce emesis if recent ingestion (<30 minutes) and patient is asymptomatic. Emesis initiated later (>1 hour) may trigger seizure activity, so judicious decontamination should be performed.
- In asymptomatic patients, a single dose of activated charcoal with a cathartic within the first hour post ingestion may be beneficial.
- Decontamination in the symptomatic animal is often not necessary, as the drug is already absorbed. Additionally, it may also put the patient at risk for aspiration pneumonia.
- No evidence that fluid diuresis is specifically beneficial to enhance elimination.

Appropriate Health Care

- Treatment is largely symptomatic and supportive following decontamination.
- Symptomatic animals require inpatient hospitalization for 24 hours, or until clinical signs resolve.
- Assess vital signs (including TPR, blood pressure, and mental/behavioral status).
- Establish IV access in any symptomatic animal.
- Agitation, hyperactivity, and tachycardia can be treated with phenothiazines.
- Benzodiazepines can also be used in animals not responding to these agents (see Precautions/Interactions).
- Seizure activity can be treated with standard doses of anticonvulsants.
- Closely monitor body temperature in any agitated/hyperactive animal. Hyperthermia should be treated as needed with cooling measures (e.g., water misting and fans, cooling blankets, etc.) if the temperature exceeds 105.5°F. Reassess body temperature frequently. Cooling measures should be discontinued at 103.5°F.

- Metabolic derangement such as acid–base imbalance or glucose metabolism is secondary to overall toxicity and should be managed supportively.
- IV fluids should be used to maintain hydration and perfusion, and ensure adequate urine output.

Drugs and Antidote of Choice

- Naloxone (0.02–0.04 mg/kg IV, IM or SQ) may be beneficial to reverse sedative effects, though effects are not uniform. Duration of effect is 30–60 minutes, necessitating frequent reassessment and possible redosing.
- Acepromazine (0.05–0.1 mg/kg IV, IM, or SQ) to control restlessness and agitation. Start at low end of range and increase as needed to effect. Chlorpromazine may also be used as an alternative.
- Cyproheptadine (1.1 mg/kg, PO or rectally, q 6–12 hours for dogs; 2–4 mg total per cat, PO or rectally q 6–12 hours) for serotonin syndrome. Cyproheptadine is a specific serotonin antagonist. Generally given orally, but can be administered rectally (same dose) in animals with severe signs or those recently administered activated charcoal.

Precautions/Interactions

- Benzodiazepines should generally be avoided if serotonin syndrome is present.

Nursing Care

- Monitor vital signs routinely, including body temperature, HR, RR, and blood pressure.
- Prevent unnecessary agitation by sequestering animal in quiet, dark area to decrease sensory stimulation.
- Monitor hydration status and urine output.
- Mental status of animal may wax and wane. Ensure measures are taken to provide for safety of animal and staff.

Follow-up

- Typically not needed unless end-organ damage has occurred, requiring monitoring until resolution.

Prevention

- Encourage owner to store DXM and all other prescription and nonprescription medications out of reach of animals.

COMMENTS

- Many cough and cold products contain multiple active ingredients; instruct owner to provide packaging of product to ensure accurate and complete identification.

- Cases can typically be managed with supportive care; ensure animal remains well hydrated and sedated (if signs of agitation are present) as needed until effects pass.
- Observe closely for evidence of serotonin syndrome and treat with sedatives and cyproheptadine as needed if present.

Expected Course and Prognosis

Symptomatic animals require 24-hour hospitalization until symptoms resolve.

- Animals that present asymptomatic and remain so for 8 hours can be sent home for close observation over the following 24 hours.
- Young and otherwise healthy animals typically do well with symptomatic and supportive care.

Complications

- Renal impairment can occur if agitation, hyperthermia, or any seizure activity is not addressed quickly and aggressively with IV fluids.

See Also

Acetaminophen
Aspirin
Decongestants (Pseudoephedrine, Phenylephrine)
Decongestants (Imidazolines)
Human NSAIDs (Ibuprofen, Naproxen)

Abbreviations

See Appendix 1 for a complete list.

BP = blood pressure
DIC = disseminated intravascular coagulation
DXM = dextromethorphan
NMDA = N-methyl-D-aspartate
PCP = phencyclidine
SE = serotonin

Suggested Reading

Barnhart JW. Urinary excretion of dextromethorphan and three metabolites in dogs and humans. Toxic App Pharm 1980; 55:43–48.

Dodman NA, Shuster L, Nesbitt G, et al. The use of dextromethorphan to treat repetitive self-directed scratching, biting, or chewing in dogs with allergic dermatitis. J Vet Pharmacol Ther 2004; 27(2):99–104.

Kukanich B, Papich MG. Plasma profile and pharmacokinetics of dextromethorphan after intravenous and oral administration in healthy dogs. J Vet Pharmacol Ther 2004; 27(5):337–341.
Liang IE, Boyer EW. Dissociative agents: phencyclidine, ketamine and dextromethorphan. In: Shannon MW, Borron SW, Burns M, eds. Haddad and Winchester's Clinical Management of Poisoning and Drug Overdose, 4th edn. New York: Saunders, 2007.

Acknowledgment: The authors and editors acknowledge the prior contributions of Stephen H. LeMaster, PharmD, MPH, who authored this topic in the previous edition.
Author: Jacinda Christie, DVM
Consulting Editors: Ahna G. Brutlag, DVM, MS, DABT, DABVT

chapter 42

Aspirin

DEFINITION/OVERVIEW

- Aspirin, also known as acetylsalicylic acid (ASA), is a common OTC NSAID and antipyretic medication.
- Therapeutic indications in veterinary medicine include pain management for osteoarthritis in dogs and antithrombotic therapy in dogs and cats.
- Toxic effects are dose dependent, ranging from GI side effects to multiple organ failure and death.

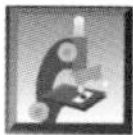

ETIOLOGY/PATHOPHYSIOLOGY

Mechanism of Action

- Nonselective prostaglandin inhibitor.
- ASA causes irreversible inhibition of COX that is needed to produce thromboxane, prostacyclin, and other prostaglandins.
- Inhibition of thromboxane and prostacyclin disrupts platelet aggregation and therefore can alter hemostasis.
- Inhibition of PGE_2 production disrupts normal GI and renal blood flow.
- Salicylates alter the Krebs cycle, which leads to organ dysfunction from uncoupling of oxidative phosphorylation.

Pharmacokinetics – Absorption, Distribution, Metabolism, Excretion

- ASA is easily and rapidly absorbed in the stomach and proximal small intestine.
- ASA is metabolized by the liver, intestines, and RBCs to salicylic acid.
- Salicyclic acid is highly protein bound (70–90%) and conjugated with glucuronate and glycine.
- Conjugated forms of salicyclic acid are excreted in urine.
- Half-life of aspirin at 25 mg/kg dose: dog 7–8 hours, cat 38–45 hours.
- Cats have a prolonged half-life due to decreased amounts of glucuronate.

Blackwell's Five-Minute Veterinary Consult Clinical Companion: Small Animal Toxicology, Second Edition.
Lynn R. Hovda, Ahna G. Brutlag, Robert H. Poppenga, and Katherine L. Peterson.

Companion website: www.fiveminutevet.com/toxicology

- When large quantities of ASA are ingested, glucuronate conjugation is saturated, thereby decreasing the excretion rate.
- Excreted metabolites of ASA lower the urinary pH, enabling renal tubular reabsorption and therefore prolonging the half-life.

Toxicity

- Intoxication is dose dependent.
- Mild toxicity (≤50 mg/kg) is usually limited to GI side effects such as vomiting, inappetance, and/or diarrhea.
- Significant toxicity has been reported with doses of 100–500 mg/kg in dogs and multiple doses of 80 mg/kg in cats.
- Exposures to ≥100 mg/kg may have the potential for death.
- Chronic administration of 23 mg/kg PO q 8 hours for ≥6 days produced gastric lesions in an experimental dog model.
- Enteric-coated aspirin tablets are less likely to lead to GI ulceration/intoxication.

Systems Affected

- Gastrointestinal – vomiting, hematemesis, diarrhea, melena, GI ulceration/erosions.
- Hematological – anemia from GI hemorrhage, primary bone marrow suppression, or Heinz body formation (cats).
- Renal/urological – azotemia, ARF, anuria, sodium retention, fluid overload.
- Hepatobiliary – hepatopathy induced by aspirin has been documented with high doses in cats.
- Respiratory – respiratory depression secondary to muscle weakness from hypokalemia and CNS depression, pulmonary edema.
- Nervous – CNS depression, seizures, cerebral edema (rare), coma and death.

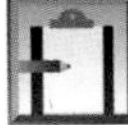

SIGNALMENT/HISTORY

- Intoxication in small animals occurs by accidental ingestion of patient's or owner's medication, complications from prescribed chronic administration, or well-meaning attempts of the pet owner that exceed therapeutic dosages.

Risk Factors

- Cats and other pets with coagulation disorders, underlying renal disease, concurrent steroid or NSAID administration, and hypoalbuminemia may be more susceptible to toxicity.

Historical Findings

- Owners may report that their pet is currently receiving prescription aspirin or concurrent NSAID therapy.

- Owners may report that they medicated their pet with OTC medications containing ASA/ aspirin-related products (such as Pepto-Bismol).
- Chewed bottle or other container found by owner at home.

Interactions with Drugs, Nutrients, or Environment

- Animals on steroid therapy or prescription NSAIDs at the time of ingestion will have an increased risk of GI side effects, including vomiting, diarrhea, and ulcer formation.
- Old and/or expired ASA degrades into salicylic and acetic acid, which does not need to be further conjugated by the liver to have a toxic effect.

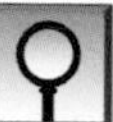

CLINICAL FEATURES

- Usually apparent within several hours after ingestion if acute intoxication; however, some clinical signs may not be apparent for days (e.g., septic peritonitis from GI perforation).
- Dehydration from excessive GI loss (e.g., vomiting, diarrhea, melena) may be noted on exam.
- Abdominal pain may be noted secondary to GI cramping, GI ulceration, or septic peritonitis from GI perforation.
- Pale mucous membranes, prolonged CRT, and poor femoral pulse quality may be present secondary to anemia or hypovolemia.
- Altered mentation from obtundation to severe coma.
- Anemia from gastrointestinal blood loss.
- Elevated anion gap.
- Heinz body anemia in cats.
- Tachypnea, increased respiratory effort, or dyspnea.
- Pulmonary crackles on auscultation if pulmonary edema is present.

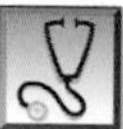

DIFFERENTIAL DIAGNOSIS

- Other substances containing salicylates, such as Pepto-Bismol, headache remedies, Ben-gay, oxycodone with aspirin combinations, and oil of wintergreen may cause salicylate intoxication with similar findings.
- NSAID toxicosis.
- Primary or secondary coagulopathy (e.g., thrombocytopenia, etc.).
- Primary gastrointestinal disease.
- Metabolic disease (e.g., renal, hepatic, hypoadrenocorticism).

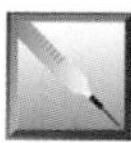

DIAGNOSTICS

- Baseline blood work (PCV/TS) is recommended to evaluate for anemia secondary to hemorrhage from the GIT.

- If anemia is present with no evidence of blood loss, a blood smear to screen for the presence of Heinz bodies should be performed, particularly in cats.
- An electrolyte panel should be performed to check for hypokalemia and hypernatremia.
- A blood chemistry should be performed to assess both kidney and liver function parameters.
- Increased liver enzymes (e.g., ALP, AST, ALT, and GGT) can be seen with hepatotoxicity.
- Baseline renal values and urinalysis should be considered, with repeat values performed 24–48 hours after presentation to help monitor for development of ARF.
- Blood gas analysis will usually show a respiratory alkalosis early on with progressive metabolic acidosis as poisoning progresses.
- An increased anion gap is also commonly seen due to increased lactate and ketone production along with the presence of salicylates themselves.
- Thoracic radiographs are indicated to evaluate for pulmonary edema if dyspnea, tachypnea, or hypoxemia is observed and/or pulmonary crackles are auscultated.
- Blood glucose should be initially evaluated and monitored. Care should be taken when evaluating a patient's glycemic status as neuroglycopenia can be present with a normal glucose reading on blood and/or serum.
- Patients exhibiting bleeding tendencies and/or liver insufficiency warrant evaluation of the hemostatic system, which may include platelet count, PT, PTT, ACT, BMBT, or rarely TEG.

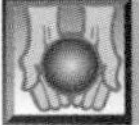

THERAPEUTICS

Detoxification

- Emesis is indicated if ingestion occurred up to several hours before presentation, provided the patient is asymptomatic and able to protect their airway.
- If emesis is unsuccessful and there was high-dose exposure, then gastric lavage should be considered (only if ingestion was within 1–2 hours before and/or an abdominal radiograph confirms the presence of gastric contents). If performed, should be done with airway protected via intubation.
- Activated charcoal with a cathartic is recommended whether or not emesis or gastric lavage is successful in cases where there has been a massive overdose or ingestion of sustained-release or enteric-coated tablets.
- Repeated doses of activated charcoal without a cathartic should be given orally every 6–8 hours for 24 hours to prevent enterohepatic circulation.

Appropriate Health Care

- Aggressive IV fluids should be used to prevent dehydration, promote renal and GI perfusion, and vasodilate renal vessels.
- Peritoneal and/or hemodialysis should only be considered for patients who develop ARF, fluid overload, or persistent acidosis, or have deterioration of their neurological status.

- Urine alkalinization therapy, with target urine pH within 7.5–8.0 and systemic pH within 7.35–7.5. This is usually attained by adding 1–2 mEq/kg of sodium bicarbonate, diluted with sterile water in a 1:1 ratio and administered as a bolus slowly IV. Once target range is reached, repeat urine and blood pH q 2–4 hours.

Antidotes

- No antidote.

Drugsof Choice

- Treatment consists of decontamination, supportive care, and gastric protectants.
- Misoprostol (2–5 µg/kg, PO q 8 hours) has been the most effective drug shown to help prevent GI ulcer formation due to NSAID administration and should be part of therapy to treat aspirin toxicosis from the first day and used up to 5–6 days.
- GI protectant (e.g., sucralfate 250–1000 mg, PO q 6–8 hours).
- Proton pump inhibitors (e.g., pantoprazole 1 mg/kg, IV q 24 hours or omeprazole 0.5–1 mg/kg, PO q 24 hours).
- H_2 blockers (e.g., famotidine 0.5 mg/kg, IV or PO q 12 hours).
- Consider antiemetics such as maropitant (1 mg/kg, SQ q 24 hours) for persistent vomiting if contraindications such as a GI perforation/septic abdomen have been ruled out.

Nursing/Supportive Care

- If hypovolemic, the patient should be volume resuscitated with balanced crystalloid solutions. In severely hypoproteinemic patients, the addition of a synthetic colloid (e.g., Hetastarch) may be necessary and/or enteral nutrition using liquid feedings via a nasoesophageal tube.
- If the patient has severe blood loss (typically from the GIT), hemoglobin-containing solutions may be necessary, including whole blood or packed red blood cell transfusions.
- If presumptive hepatopathy with concurrent coagulopathy is present, consider vitamin K_1 supplementation and/or S-adenosyl-methionine (SAMe) supplementation.
- Oxygen supplementation via oxygen cage, nasal cannula, or oxygen mask if hypoxemia present due to pulmonary edema.

Precautions/Interactions

- Concurrent NSAIDs or steroid should be avoided.
- Other protein-bound drugs may alter metabolism of aspirin.

Diet

- A highly digestible, bland diet is generally recommended for those patients showing GI signs such as vomiting and/or diarrhea. Once signs have resolved, they can be slowly weaned on to their regular diet.

Surgical Considerations

- If a GI ulcer causing excessive hemorrhage and/or possible associated perforation is suspected, abdominal exploration may be recommended to provide definitive diagnosis and treatment.

COMMENTS

Monitoring

- Electrolytes to monitor for hypokalemia.
- Blood glucose may be normal with neuroglycopenia.
- Acid–base status to help guide alkanization therapy and help offset progressive metabolic acidosis.
- Monitor respiratory effort/rate in case pulmonary edema develops from toxicity. Pulse oximetry or arterial blood gas monitoring may be useful in determining if hypoxemia is present.
- Urine output (UOP) quantification can facilitate decisions for ongoing fluid therapy needs and possibly provide information that may raise a concern for the development of oliguric (<0.5 mL/kg/hour) or anuric ARF. For those with significant toxicity exposure and concern for ARF, urinary catheter placement should be done to monitor UOP.
- Urinalysis may provide evidence of renal damage (e.g., casts prior to the development of azotemia).
- Monitor neurological status; if cerebral edema suspected, mannitol should be administered (0.5–1.0 g/kg, IV over 20 minutes).

Prevention/Avoidance

- Prevention includes refraining from using ASA for treatment as analgesic/antiinflammatory in pets, and having any aspirin in the house secured in out-of-reach locations in cabinets or drawers. This medication should never be left out on nightstands, in purses, or on countertops within reach of pets.

Possible Complications

- Chronic renal damage may be a problem for those dogs and/or cats that develop azotemia after toxic exposure.

Expected Course and Prognosis

- Prognosis varies depending on amount ingested. With lower doses (≤50 mg/kg), prognosis likely good with supportive care for GI side effects. With higher exposures (≥50 mg/kg), prognosis can be poor to guarded if multiple organ dysfunction develops, to fair if patient is treated aggressively and early.

Synonyms

- Salicylate toxicity, acetylsalicylic acid toxicity, ASA toxicity, NSAID toxicity, nonsteroidal antiinflammatories

Abbreviations

See Appendix 1 for a complete list.

Suggested Reading

Alwood AJ. Salicylates. In: Silverstein DC, Hopper K, eds. Small Animal Critical Care Medicine. St Louis, MO: WB Saunders, 2009.

Curry SL, Cogar SM, Cook JL, Nonsteroidal anti-inflammatory drugs: a review. J Am Anim Hosp Assoc 2005; 41:298–309.

Khan SA, McLean M. Toxicology of frequently encountered nonsteroidal anti-inflammatory drugs in dogs and cats. Vet Clin North Am Small Anim Pract 2012; 42(2):289–306.

Papich MG. An update on nonsteroidal anti-inflammatory drugs (NSAIDS) in small animals. Vet Clin North Am Small Anim Pract 2008; 38(6):1243–1266.

Author: Megan Kaplan, DVM, DACVECC
Consulting Editor: Ahna G. Brutlag, DVM, MS, DABT, DABVT

Decongestants (Pseudoephedrine, Phenylephrine)

chapter 43

DEFINITION/OVERVIEW

- Pseudoephedrine (PSE) and phenylephrine (PE) are decongestants commonly used by humans for their vasoconstrictive effects. PSE and PE are most commonly found in cough/cold preparations, allergy and asthma medications (PSE), diet pills (PSE), nasal sprays (PE), and hemorrhoid preparations (PE).
- When present in cough/cold or allergy medications, the presence of PE or PSE is often indicated by a "-D" suffix in the name (e.g. Claritin-D).
- In veterinary medicine, PE has been used IV to treat hypotension and shock, intranasally to treat sinusitis, and intraocularly for treatment of ocular disorders and as a diagnostic aid (e.g. Horner's syndrome). Oral PSE has been used as an aid in increasing urethral sphincter tone and as a decongestant.
- PSE and PE are sympathomimetic drugs with alpha- and beta-adrenergic properties.
- Clinical signs of toxicosis include CNS stimulation, tachycardia, hypertension, decreased appetite, vomiting, mydriasis, and seizures.

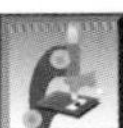

ETIOLOGY/PATHOPHYSIOLOGY

Mechanism of Action

- PE and PSE stimulate both alpha- and beta-adrenergic receptors by increasing norepinephrine levels.
  - PE stimulates beta-adrenergic receptors only at high doses.
  - Pharmacological effects include increased vasoconstriction, heart rate, blood pressure, and coronary blood flow; mild CNS stimulation; increased urethral tone (PSE); and decreased nasal congestion and appetite.
- PSE is a stereoisomer of ephedrine (from *Ephedra* spp.; see chapter 78, Ephedra/Ma Huang).

Blackwell's Five-Minute Veterinary Consult Clinical Companion: Small Animal Toxicology, Second Edition.
Lynn R. Hovda, Ahna G. Brutlag, Robert H. Poppenga, and Katherine L. Peterson.

Companion website: www.fiveminutevet.com/toxicology

Pharmacokinetics – Absorption, Distribution, Metabolism, Excretion

- In humans, PE is extensively metabolized in the GI tract and liver, resulting in a relatively low oral bioavailability. Peak plasma levels are achieved within 30 minutes and the half-life is 2–3 hours. PE crosses the BBB and placenta, and passes into the milk. PE is excreted primarily unchanged via the urine, with higher excretion rates in acidic urine.
- PSE is well absorbed orally in dogs with bioavailability of 58% and peak plasma levels achieved within 24 minutes. Onset of action is generally less than 30–60 minutes and the half-life is approximately 1.5 hours. PSE is poorly bound to plasma proteins (~20%) and crosses the BBB and placenta, and passes into the milk. It is partially metabolized to norpseudoephedrine, an active metabolite. PSE is excreted via the urine, primarily as parent drug, in a pH-dependent fashion.

Toxicity

- The low bioavailability of PE makes it less toxic orally than other sympathomimetics.
    - Hemorrhoid medications may have higher toxicity as their ointment bases may enhance oral transmucosal absorption, bypassing GI first-pass metabolism.
    - Hypertension was noted in dogs that ingested 7 mg/kg and 11.9 mg/kg of PE from hemorrhoidal preparations. Hypertension was not reported in dogs ingesting unknown amounts of PE in nasal spray or ocular drops nor in dogs ingesting tablet or capsule forms in dosages ranging from 0.23 to 30 mg/kg.
- PSE has a very narrow window of safety in veterinary medicine, with therapeutic dosages in dogs of 1–2 mg/kg (some dogs show mild signs at therapeutic doses), and moderate-to-severe clinical signs possible at 5–6 mg/kg. Dosages of 10–12 mg/kg have caused fatalities in dogs.

Systems Affected

- Cardiovascular – peripheral vasoconstriction leads to increased systemic vascular resistance and hypertension with tachycardia or reflex bradycardia. Beta-adrenergic stimulation results in tachycardia, increased contractility/output, and tachyarrhythmias.
- Nervous – stimulation results from endogenous catecholamine release and adrenergic stimulation.
- Metabolic/endocrine – hyperthermia secondary to adrenergic effects (severe).
- Ophthalmic – alpha-adrenergic stimulation causes mydriasis.
- Hemic – DIC (sequela to prolonged seizure activity and hyperthermia).
- Renal – myoglobinuria (sequela to prolonged seizure activity and hyperthermia).

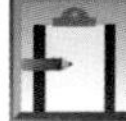

SIGNALMENT/HISTORY

- All species or breeds susceptible. Dogs may be at increased risk of accidental exposure due to their inquisitive nature and indiscriminate eating habits.

Risk Factors

- Animals with underlying conditions such as cardiovascular disease, seizure disorders, renal insufficiency, narrow-angle glaucoma, or concurrent disease predisposing to hypertension (e.g., immune-mediated hemolytic anemia, hyperthyroidism).

Historical Findings

- Intentional exposures due to owners medicating patients with OTC products containing decongestants (e.g., Claritin-D versus regular Claritin).
- Accidental ingestion of owner medication by pets.
- Acute onset of restlessness, pacing, agitation.

Interactions with Drugs, Nutrients, or Environment

- PE and PSE can enhance the CNS and/or cardiovascular toxicity of other sympathomimetics (e.g., phenylpropanolamine), methylxanthines (e.g., caffeine, theobromine), and MAO inhibitors (e.g., selegiline).

CLINICAL FEATURES

- Signs generally occur within 30–60 minutes of exposure but can be delayed if extended-release products are ingested.
- Clinical signs of PE toxicosis in dogs have included vomiting, lethargy, diarrhea, bradycardia, tachycardia, trembling, and hypertension.
  - Signs reported to an animal poison control center in dogs exposed to PE include vomiting (83%), lethargy (8%), hyperactivity (5%), trembling (5%), panting (3%), diarrhea (3%), bradycardia (2%), tachycardia (2%), and hypertension (1%).
- Clinical signs of PSE toxicosis can include hyperactivity, agitation, mydriasis, vomiting, tachycardia, hypertension (+/-reflex bradycardia), ventricular arrhythmias, hyperthermia, cyanosis, hypersalivation, tremors, and possible seizures. Rarely, cerebral hemorrhage may be seen.
- Animals that exhibit severe or sustained CNS signs and hyperthermia typically have a poorer prognosis.

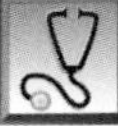

DIFFERENTIAL DIAGNOSIS

- Intoxications: amphetamines, baclofen, methylxanthines, nicotine, and phenylpropanolamine.

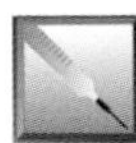

DIAGNOSTICS

- Minimum baseline blood work, including blood glucose, potassium, and venous blood gas, should be performed.

- Geriatric patients or those with underlying metabolic disease should have more extensive blood work done, including CBC, serum chemistry panel, and creatine kinase.
- Patient history and clinical signs may assist in diagnosis.
- PSE will frequently cause a positive reaction for amphetamines in many OTC urine drug test kits for humans.

Pathological Findings

- No specific pathological lesions are expected.

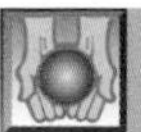

THERAPEUTICS

- The goals of treatment are to prevent absorption, support the cardiovascular and neurological systems, and provide supportive care.

Detoxification

- Induce emesis if ingestion occurred within the previous 30 minutes and the pet is asymptomatic.
- If emesis was not induced at home, and the patient is asymptomatic, prompt emesis should be performed by the veterinarian.
- Activated charcoal with a cathartic may be given for one dose in asymptomatic patients.
- Multidose activated charcoal may be given to animals ingesting sustained-release formulations.
- Acidifying the urine may enhance excretion of PSE and phenylephrine. *Note: severely symptomatic animals may already be acidotic, so evaluation of acid–base status is recommended.*

Appropriate Health Care

- IV fluid therapy should be administered to aid in perfusion and excretion of the drug, maintain hydration, and help cool the patient (if hyperthermic).
- Cooling measures for hyperthermia; cooling measures should be discontinued at 103.5°F.

Drugs of Choice

- In patients demonstrating agitation or anxiety, sedation should be used (see Precautions/Interactions).
- Acepromazine 0.02–1.0 mg/kg, IV, IM, or SC PRN to effect; select dose based on severity of signs and titrate to effect.
- Chlorpromazine 0.5–1 mg/kg, IV or IM PRN to effect; select dose based on severity of signs and titrate to effect. Cumulative dosages up to 10–15 mg/kg have been necessary.
- In patients with tachycardia (dog >180 bpm; cat >220 bpm), a fast-acting beta-blocker should be used.
    - Propranolol 0.02 mg/kg IV slowly, up to a maximum of 1 mg/kg.
    - Esmolol 0.25–0.5 mg/kg, IV slow load, then 10–200 µg/kg/min CRI.

    - Carvedilol 0.5 mg/kg PO q 12 hours was used to successfully manage tachycardia and hypertension in a dog that ingested 50 mg/kg PSE and whose CNS signs persisted for 2 days.
- With severe toxicity, seizures may be seen and should be treated with anticonvulsant therapy (see Precautions/Interactions).
    - Phenobarbital 4 mg/kg, IV × 4–5 doses to effect PRN.

Precautions/Interactions

- Benzodiazepines are not recommended as they may exacerbate signs.

Alternative Drugs

- Urinary acidification in dogs can be used to aid in excretion but must be done with caution.
- Ammonium chloride 50 mg/kg, PO q 6 hours.
- Ascorbic acid 20–30 mg/kg, SC, IM or IV q 8 hours.

Nursing Care

- Regulate body temperature, heart rate, and respiratory rate frequently.
- Ensure appropriate urine output (1–2 mL/kg/hour) and treat accordingly.
- Minimize stimulation or excitement.
- Monitor blood pressure and heart rhythm (with continuous ECG monitoring).

COMMENTS

Patient Monitoring

- Animals should be monitored in the clinic for 18–24 hours, or until clinical signs resolve.
- If the product was sustained release, the patient should be monitored for 24–72 hours, or until clinical signs resolve.

Prevention/Avoidance

- Pet owners should be advised to keep medications out of the reach of pets, preferably stored in locked cabinets or cabinets located high off the ground.
- Keep purses, gym bags, full shopping bags, etc. out of reach of pets.
- When recommending OTC allergy medications for use in pets, instruct owners to avoid products with a "-D" suffix in the name (e.g., Benadryl-D).

Possible Complications

- DIC, rhabdomyolysis, and myoglobinuria (with subsequent ARF) may occur with prolonged, untreated tremors/seizures or hyperthermia.

Expected Course and Prognosis

- The earlier the animal is treated, the better the prognosis.
- Signs generally resolve within 1–24 hours for regular formulations, and within 24–72 hours for sustained-release formulations.
- Animals that exhibit severe or sustained CNS signs and hyperthermia typically have a poorer prognosis.
- Animals with DIC or myoglobinuria have a poorer prognosis and will need aggressive therapy, including 24-hour care, aggressive IV fluid therapy, FFP transfusions, and aggressive monitoring.

Synonyms

Ephedrine, ephedra; methamphetamine; weight loss supplements, Sudafed

See Also

Amphetamines
Methamphetamine
Phenylpropanolamine
Ephedra/Ma Huang

Abbreviations

See Appendix 1 for a complete list.

PE = phenylephrine
PSE = pseudoephedrine

Suggested Reading

Bischoff K, Mukai M. Toxicity of over-the-counter drugs. In: Gupta RC, ed. Veterinary Toxicology: Basic and Clinical Principles, 2nd edn. New York: Elsevier, 2012; pp. 443–468.

Kang MH, Park HM. Application of carvedilol in a dog with pseudoephedrine toxicosis-induced tachycardia. Can Vet J 2012; 53:783–786.

Wegenast C. Toxicology Brief: Phenylephrine ingestion in dogs: What's the harm? http://veterinarymedicine.dvm360.com/toxicology-brief-phenylephrine-ingestion-dogs-whats-harm

Acknowledgment: The authors and editors acknowledge the prior contributions of Kelly M. Sioris, PharmD, and Dean Filandrinos, PharmD, who authored this topic in the previous edition.

Author: Sharon Gwaltney-Brant, DVM, PhD, DABVT, DABT
Consulting Editor: Ahna Brutlag, DVM, MS, DABT, DABVT

chapter 44

Decongestants (Imidazolines)

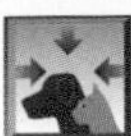

DEFINITION/OVERVIEW

- Imidazolines are a class of drugs commonly found in OTC nasal decongestants and ophthalmic preparations for the relief of redness and inflammation due to their topical vasoconstrictive activity.
- They are from a broader class of drugs known as sympathomimetics.
- Examples include oxymetazoline, tetrahydrozoline, naphazoline, and tolazoline.
- While generally safe and well tolerated in adult humans, oral overdoses in children have resulted in significant toxicosis. This is because overdosed amounts of the drug tend to have a central effect.
- The central action of the drug leads to significant CNS depression.

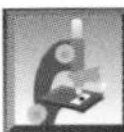

ETIOLOGY/PATHOPHYSIOLOGY

Mechanism of Action

- Imidazolines are sympathomimetic compounds specific to alpha$_2$-adrenergic receptors.
- Oxymetazoline and naphazoline have no effect on histamine H_1 and H_2 receptors.
- Tetrahydrozoline and tolazoline may influence H_2 receptors but not H_1.
- Imidazolines do not influence beta-adrenergic receptors.
- While imidazolines may bind to both central and peripheral receptors, central binding tends to predominate in overdose situations.
  - Central receptor binding will result in the inhibition of norepinephrine, resulting in decreased sympathetic response. Common side effects of this binding are hypotension, bradycardia, and lethargy.
  - Peripheral receptor binding will result in vasoconstriction (topical application) and hypertension.

Pharmacokinetics – Absorption, Distribution, Metabolism, Excretion

- Information on companion animal pharmacokinetics is limited.
- Systemic absorption may follow topical administration.

Blackwell's Five-Minute Veterinary Consult Clinical Companion: Small Animal Toxicology, Second Edition.
Lynn R. Hovda, Ahna G. Brutlag, Robert H. Poppenga, and Katherine L. Peterson.

Companion website: www.fiveminutevet.com/toxicology

- Imidazolines are readily absorbed from the GIT.
- The half-life of most imidazolines is 2–4 hours (humans).
- Widely distributed throughout the body. Though imidazoline receptors have been found in the brain, human studies have shown that their concentrations there were relatively low.
- Metabolism is not well understood but is thought to be (partly) hepatic.
- Imidazolines are eliminated, mostly unchanged, in the urine.

Toxicity

- Imidazolines have a narrow safety margin.
- Oxymetazoline oral LD_{50} (mice): 10 mg/kg
- No therapeutic dose known in veterinary literature

Systems Affected

- Gastrointestinal – vomiting/GI irritation.
- Nervous – may present as lethargic (most common) or agitated. Lethargy can progress to the point of coma.
- Cardiovascular – initial hypertension progressing to severe hypotension, bradycardia, weakness/lethargy, prolonged CRT, and hypoperfusion.
- Neuromuscular – animals may develop tremors or seizures.
- Respiratory – depression.
- Ophthalmic – miotic pupils.

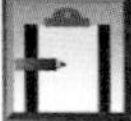

SIGNALMENT/HISTORY

Risk Factors

- Animals with renal insufficiency may have reduced drug clearance, resulting in more severe or prolonged clinical signs.
- Neonates and geriatric animals may be more severely affected.
- Drugs of this class have a narrow safety margin and unknown therapeutic range.

Historical Findings

- Witnessed ingestion or administration.
- Discovery of chewed nasal decongestant or “eye-drop” containers.
- The owner may find the animal vomiting, lethargic or in a state of collapse.

Location and Circumstances of Poisoning

- Exposures generally occur in the home due to unsecured medications.

Interactions with Drugs, Nutrients, or Environment

- Potentially fatal in combination with other drugs in this class or those exhibiting adrenoreceptor activity (e.g., clonidine, medetomidine, xylazine, tizanidine, detomidine, etc.). Clinicians should not attempt to induce vomiting in a cat exposed to imidazoline with any of these agents.
- Drugs with the capability of causing CNS depression, such as opioids, barbiturates, or other sedatives/anticonvulsants, may exacerbate toxicosis.
- Drugs with the capability of causing bradycardia, such as beta-blockers, may exacerbate toxicosis.

CLINICAL FEATURES

- Onset of symptoms is generally rapid (within 15 minutes).
- Animals may present with initial hypertension and agitation but will likely progress to depression and bradycardia.
- Cardiovascular collapse may be noted.

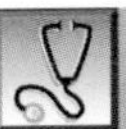

DIFFERENTIAL DIAGNOSIS

- Dependent on the stage of toxicosis.
- Toxicities – amphetamines, cocaine, other CNS stimulants (early stages).
- Toxicities – sedatives, opioids, tranquilizers (later stages).
- Primary cardiac disease resulting in bradycardia, hypotension, syncope, etc.
- Trauma or blood loss leading to collapse.

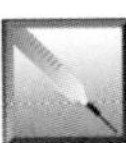

DIAGNOSTICS

- ECG – may show tachycardia or bradycardia depending on stage of presentation.
- Blood pressure monitoring – may vary between hypertension and hypotension, trending toward hypotension.
- Chemistry panel – in severe cases, blood glucose and electrolytes (especially potassium) should be monitored.
- As these cases may be critically ill, 24/7 intensive care (along with the ability to perform blood pressure monitoring) is essential.

Pathological Findings

- No specific gross or histopathological findings.

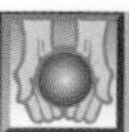

THERAPEUTICS

Detoxification

- It is NOT recommended to induce vomiting due to the rapid absorption and onset of clinical signs.
- Often, patients present already symptomatic due to rapid onset of signs rendering a risk instead of a benefit. If a patient presents asymptomatic and in the early stages of ingestion, activated charcoal with a cathartic may be administered once.

Appropriate Health Care

- Hypotension – aggressive IV fluids (e.g., a balanced electrolyte crystalloid at 20–30 mL/kg IV over 20–30 minutes, repeat 2–3x as needed) should be used to correct hypotension, as needed to effect. Diuresis does not enhance drug elimination.
- If patient does not respond to crystalloids, consider colloids such as Hetastarch (5 mL/kg IV aliquots; repeat 1–2x as needed).
- If patient is persistently hypotensive, vasopressors may be necessary (e.g., dopamine, 5–20 µg/kg/min IV CRI).
- Frequent monitoring of TPR, HR, blood pressure, mentation, and UOP.

Drugs and Antidotes of Choice

- No specific antidotes are available; however, $alpha_2$-adrenergic antagonists may be helpful. They may need to be administered multiple times during the course of treatment as their half-life may not be as long as the imidazoline agent.
    - Yohimbine, 0.1 mg/kg IV, to reverse severe sedation and bradycardia.
    - Atipamezole, 50 µg/kg, to reverse severe sedation and bradycardia. Give one quarter of the dose IV and the remaining three-quarters of the dose IM to avoid worsening hypotension. Another one quarter to one half dose may be considered IV if patient has not responded in 30–60 minutes.
- Atropine, 0.01–0.02 mg/kg IV, IM, SQ, as needed for bradycardia.While atropine may be considered, there is potential for it to cause a significant increase in mean arterial pressure. Fluids and alpha antagonists are typically the mainstay of treatment.
- Diazepam, 0.5–1 mg/kg IV, as needed for tremors and seizures.
- Antiemetics if vomiting is protracted (e.g., maropitant, 1 mg/kg SQ q 24 hours).

Precautions/Interactions

- Do not induce vomiting in symptomatic animals.
- Do not attempt to induce vomiting in a cat exposed to imidazolines with xylazine or medetomidine. This may exacerbate toxicosis.
- Any drug that may decrease blood pressure (e.g., beta-blockers, acepromazine, ACE inhibitors) should be used cautiously.

Alternative Drugs

- Naloxone, 0.011–0.022 mg/kg IV or IM q 1 hour or PRN, may also be used. The mechanism is currently unknown so success is unpredictable.

Follow-up

- Generally minimal in uncomplicated cases or cases in which clinical signs are easily controlled.

Diet

- Animal may return to normal diet at discharge or may be given several days of bland diet if GI irritation is persistent.

Activity

- Patient should be kept quiet and secure while symptomatic but may return to normal activity with successful resolution of the case.

Surgical Considerations

- No surgical considerations unless the animal has ingested large amounts of the container, and radiographic evidence or clinical signs of foreign body obstruction are present.

Prevention

- Imidazolines are not intended for use in companion animals.
- Imidazolines are readily available in multiple OTC preparations and their toxicity is widely underestimated for this reason. Owners and clinicians may not make the connection between exposure and symptoms.

COMMENTS

Client Education

- Secure all medications, even OTCs, so they cannot be accessed by pets or children.
- Imidazolines are readily available in multiple OTC preparations and their toxicity is widely underestimated for this reason. This allows for dogs (most commonly) or cats to chew on bottles out of exploration/curiosity. Owners and clinicians are often unaware of the severity of toxicity, or may not make the connection between exposure and symptoms.
- Do not advise clients to use medicated OTC nasal sprays or eyedrops in their pets without educating them about the dangers of imidazolines.

Patient Monitoring

- Observation may be required for as long as 24–36 hours if the product is a sustained-release formulation.

Expected Course and Prognosis

- Generally good if treated early.

Synonyms

Oxymetazoline, naphazoline, tetrahydrozoline, tetrizolina, tetryzoline, xylometazoline

Abbreviations

See Appendix 1 for a complete list.

ACE = angiotensin-converting enzyme
UOP = urine output

Suggested Reading

Daggy A, Kaplan R, Roberge R, Akhtar J. Pediatric Visine (tetrahydrozoline) ingestion: case report and review of imidazoline toxicity. Vet Hum Toxic 2003; 45(4):210–212.

Eddy O, Howell JM. Are one or two dangerous? Clonidine and topical imidazolines exposure in toddlers. J Emerg Med 2003; 25(3):297–302.

Fitzgerald KT, Bronstein AC, Flood AA. Over-the-counter drug toxicities in companion animals. Clin Tech Small Anim Pract 2006; 21(4):215–226.

Giovannoni, MP, Ghelardini C, Vergelli C, Piaz VD. Alpha-2 agonists as analgesic agents. Med Res Rev 2009; 29(2):339–368.

Acknowledgment: The authors and editors acknowledge the prior contributions of Nancy M. Gruber, DVM, who authored this topic in the previous edition.

Author: Kirsten E. Waratuke, DVM
Consulting Editor: Ahna G. Brutlag, DVM, MS, DABT, DABVT

Human NSAIDs (Ibuprofen, Naproxen)

chapter 45

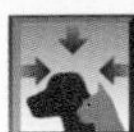

DEFINITION/OVERVIEW

- NSAIDs have antiinflammatory, analgesic, and antipyretic properties.
- OTC NSAIDs, such as ibuprofen and naproxen sodium, are a common source of poisoning for dogs, cats, and ferrets.
- Because pet owners are familiar with how NSAIDs affect themselves and these products are readily available, pet owners may administer NSAIDs to their pet when it is exhibiting signs of illness.
- Animals may intentionally ingest these medications in large quantities.
- Effects of NSAID toxicosis in veterinary patients include GI irritation/ulceration/perforation, ARF, and acute CNS impairment.

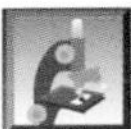

ETIOLOGY/PATHOPHYSIOLOGY

- Ibuprofen (trade names: Advil®, Midol® [older formulations], Nuprin®) is available in both OTC and Rx formulations. It comes in 50, 100, 200, 300, 400, 600, and 800 mg tablets and as 40 mg/mL and 100 mg/5 mL oral suspensions. It is also frequently included in OTC combination flu/cold remedies.
- Naproxen sodium (trade names: Aleve®, Anaprox®, Menstridol®, Napralen®, Naprosyn®) is available in both OTC and Rx formulations. It comes in 200, 220, 250, 275, 375, 500, and 550 mg tablets, 375 and 500 mg controlled/delayed-release tablets, and as a 25 mg/mL, 40 mg/mL, 125 mg/5 mL, and 375 mg/15 mL oral suspension.

Mechanism of Action

- Ibuprofen (2-[p-isobutylphenyl] propionic acid) and naproxen sodium have antiinflammatory, analgesic, and antipyretic properties.
- NSAIDs inhibit the conversion of arachidonic acid to prostaglandins by inhibition of COX enzymes. Specific prostaglandin inhibition is useful to reduce inflammation, but inhibition of prostaglandins that serve beneficial effects may also be inhibited unless the NSAID is selective.

Blackwell's Five-Minute Veterinary Consult Clinical Companion: Small Animal Toxicology, Second Edition.
Lynn R. Hovda, Ahna G. Brutlag, Robert H. Poppenga, and Katherine L. Peterson.

Companion website: www.fiveminutevet.com/toxicology

- Prostaglandins have many other beneficial functions in the body, such as maintaining blood flow to the kidneys and mucosa of the GIT, stimulating intestinal epithelial cell repair and turnover, and stimulating bicarbonate buffer secretion in the stomach. These functions are also interrupted by nonselective COX inhibitors.

Pharmacokinetics – Absorption, Distribution, Metabolism, Excretion

- NSAIDs are well absorbed from the GIT (close to 100% bioavailability) and highly protein bound with a low volume of distribution. Because of the high degree of protein binding, very little of the parent drug is excreted intact through the kidneys.
- NSAIDs are predominantly metabolized in the liver to inactive compounds; however, there is extensive enterohepatic recirculation.
- There are marked differences in clearance and half-life of these drugs between species.
    - Ibuprofen: rapidly absorbed after oral dosing (within 30 minutes to 1.5 hours); the plasma half-life in the dog is 2–2.5 hours.
    - Naproxen sodium: rapidly absorbed after oral dosing, with 68–100% bioavailability. It has a very long half-life in dogs (74 hours).

Toxicity

Ibuprofen

- GI signs >50–125 mg/kg (dogs); >50 mg/kg (cats). Note: GI irritation or ulceration has been reported in dogs at doses as low as 5–6 mg/kg/day with chronic administration.
- Renal signs: >175 mg/kg (dogs).
- CNS signs: >400 mg/kg (dogs).
- Cats are more sensitive to the toxic effects of ibuprofen and exhibit signs of toxicity at approximately half the doses noted above due to limited hepatic glucuronidation. Renal signs are most commonly reported in cats, with or without GI signs.
- The toxic dose of ibuprofen in ferrets is not known – acute CNS signs are most commonly reported in ferrets with or without GI or renal signs.

Naproxen sodium

- There is little information on the dosages at which clinical signs of toxicity occur; however, it is noted that as little as 5 mg/kg can produce GI signs in dogs. Doses >25 mg/kg can cause ARF.
- Naproxen has a very long half-life and appears to have a very narrow therapeutic window in animals.

Systems Affected

- Gastrointestinal – anorexia, vomiting (± hematemesis), diarrhea (± melena, hematochezia), GI irritation, GI ulceration, gastric or duodenal perforation, abdominal pain, septic peritonitis.

- Renal/urological – ARF (oliguric or anuric).
- Nervous – acute ataxia, altered mentation, and seizures (with extremely high doses of ibuprofen).
- Cardiovascular – hemorrhagic shock secondary to severe GIT ulceration, septic shock secondary to septic peritonitis from a ruptured GIT ulcer.
- Hemic/lymphatic/immune – anemia (with concurrent panhypoproteinemia) secondary to severe GIT ulceration; thrombocytopathia may occur as a result of altered platelet aggregation.

SIGNALMENT/HISTORY

- Cats, dogs, and ferrets have been documented to develop signs of toxicosis associated with overdose of these medications. Cats are more sensitive to ibuprofen than dogs.
- There are no breed or sex predilections for this toxicosis.

Risk Factors

- Underlying intestinal or renal pathology.
- Dehydration.
- Concurrent use of other NSAIDs or corticosteroids.
- Animals with liver disease (delays metabolism).
- Geriatric and neonatal animals at higher risk for toxicity.
- Hypoalbuminemia increases the risk for toxicity due to degree of protein binding.
- Inappropriate dosing by pet owner.

Historical Findings

- Witnessed NSAID ingestion, owner administration of NSAID to pet, chewed container found in household.
- Clinical signs secondary to NSAID administration may be detected by the pet owner, including anorexia, vomiting (± hematemesis), diarrhea (± melena), weakness, abdominal pain, and sudden onset of CNS signs (e.g., altered mentation, seizures).

Interactions with Drugs, Nutrients, or Environment

- Co-administration of more than one NSAID, such as an OTC medication, in addition to prescribed NSAID by a veterinarian may result in more severe clinical signs.
- Co-administration of an NSAID with corticosteroids may result in more severe clinical signs.

CLINICAL FEATURES

Gastrointestinal

- GI signs will usually develop within 2–6 hours of ingestion.

- Signs of GI hemorrhage, ulceration, or perforation may be delayed 12 hours to 4–5 days following ingestion.
- With ibuprofen, lower doses (50–100 mg/kg in dogs) are usually associated with milder signs (e.g., inappetance, abdominal pain, vomiting, diarrhea), while higher doses (>100 mg/kg) are more likely to cause bleeding, ulceration, and/or perforation.
- Clinical signs may include anorexia, abdominal pain, hypersalivation/nausea, melena on rectal examination, vomiting, and diarrhea.

Renal

- ARF may develop as early as 12 hours following ingestion but may be delayed 3–5 days following exposure.
- Clinical signs may include depressed mentation, oliguria/anuria, pain on renal palpation (normal to enlarged kidney size), vomiting, uremic breath, and anorexia.

Neurological

- Neurological signs are often noted within 1–2 hours of exposure when extremely high doses are ingested.
- Clinical signs might include decreased mentation (e.g., obtundation, stupor, coma), respiratory depression, seizures, and delayed or absent PLRs.

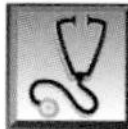

DIFFERENTIAL DIAGNOSIS

- Primary GI disease – IBD, neoplasia, gastroenteritis, nonspecific gastritis.
- Secondary GI disease.
  - Veterinary prescription NSAID toxicosis.
  - Aspirin toxicosis.
  - Ethylene glycol toxicosis.
  - Gastric ulceration/bleeding secondary to ulcerated gastric masses, thrombocytopenia/thrombocytopathia, gastric foreign bodies.
- Primary metabolic disease – renal.
  - Toxins: lily ingestion (cats), ethylene glycol ingestion; grapes/raisins ingestions (dogs).
  - Chronic renal failure or acute-on-chronic renal failure.
  - ARF secondary to hypoxia, ischemia.
  - Ureteral obstruction.
  - Urethral obstruction.
  - Uroabdomen.
  - Pyelonephritis.
- Primary metabolic disease – hepatic: hepatic encephalopathy, hypoadrenocorticism, hypoglycemia.

- Primary neurological disease – intracranial disease (e.g., infectious, inflammatory, neoplastic, vascular).
- Secondary neurological disease – ethylene glycol ingestion, hepatic encephalopathy.

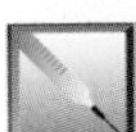

DIAGNOSTICS

- Baseline lab work.
    - CBC, chemistry profile, UA, and USG (prefluid therapy) if >50 mg/kg ibuprofen was ingested.
    - Baseline renal values should be obtained on admission. Repeated renal values should be checked at 24 and 48 hours following ingestion of nephrotoxic doses of ibuprofen. With naproxen, renal values should be monitored q 24 hours for 72 hours (minimum).
    - Baseline and serial PCV/TS should be followed daily in hospitalized animals with clinical GI signs, evidence of GI hemorrhage, or cardiovascular instability.
- Radiographs and/or abdominal ultrasound should be considered when abdominal pain or significant GI signs are present to rule out GIT perforation/septic peritonitis.

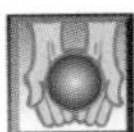

THERAPEUTICS

Detoxification

- Typically, for emesis to be effective, it should be induced within 30 minutes of ingestion (due to rapid GI absorption).
- If large amounts of tablets were ingested, emesis within 3–6 hours of ingestion may be effective as ibuprofen has been shown to form gastric concretions that may result in delayed breakdown and/or gastric emptying.
- If the animal has CNS signs, emesis should be avoided to prevent aspiration. Instead, secure the airway and perform gastric lavage.
- Administer activated charcoal (2–4 g/kg) without a cathartic.
- Activated charcoal (1 g/kg) without a cathartic should be repeated q 4–6 hours for 24–48 hours (due to extensive enterohepatic recirculation).
- IV fluids at maintenance to 1.5 times maintenance enhance renal elimination.

Appropriate Health Care

- Supportive care.
    - Intubation ± mechanical ventilation if acute CNS signs or respiratory depression.
    - Urine output should be monitored in animals exposed to a nephrotoxic dose of NSAIDs.
        - □ An indwelling urinary catheter and closed collection system should be used if oliguric (<1 mL/kg/hour).
        - □ CVP monitoring is useful to determine extent of volume expansion.

- □ If volume depleted and oliguric, IV fluid boluses (10 mL/kg over 30 minutes) can be used to expand the intravascular volume.
- □ If volume expanded and oliguric, furosemide (1–2 mg/kg IV) and/or mannitol (1 g/kg, IV, over 15 minutes) can be administered to encourage urine production.

Drugs and Antidotes of Choice

- Gastroprotection (5–7 days ibuprofen, 2 weeks for naproxen).
  - Misoprostol (2–5 μg/kg, PO q 8 hours).
  - H_2 blockers (e.g., famotidine 0.5 mg/kg, PO, IV, SQ q 12 hours).
  - Proton pump inhibitors (e.g., omeprazole 0.7–1.4 mg/kg, PO q 12–24 hours or esomeprazole 0.7 mg/kg, IV q 12–24 hours).
  - Sucralfate (0.25–1 g, PO q 6–8 hours).
- Antiemetics for protracted vomiting (e.g., maropitant 1 mg/kg SQ once daily for up to 5 days).
- IV fluid therapy should be used to maintain euvolemia, hydration, and renal perfusion.
  - Fluid diuresis (at least 6 mL/kg/hour of an isotonic crystalloid) should be performed for 48 hours with ibuprofen ingestions approaching nephrotoxic doses (exceeding 175 mg/kg [dogs] or 50 mg/kg [cats]).
  - Following toxic doses of naproxen, fluid diuresis should ensue for 72 hours.
- If hypoproteinemia results, artificial colloid therapy (e.g., Hetastarch at 1–2 mL/kg/hour) should be considered to maintain colloid osmotic pressure.
- Blood transfusion with pRBC as needed to maintain PCV ≥15–20% if gastric hemorrhage noted.
- Seizures should be treated with anticonvulsants. Diazepam should be used to stop ongoing seizures (0.25–0.5 mg/kg, IV, to effect PRN). Intravenous phenobarbital loading (4 mg/kg, IV q 2–12 hours × 4–5 doses) should be used when cluster seizures occur.

Precautions/Interactions

- Sucralfate should be dosed at least 2 hours prior to other oral medications.
- Other NSAIDs, aspirin, or corticosteroids should be withheld from any animal with signs of toxicosis for 7–14 days, depending on the severity of toxicity.

Follow-up

- Renal values (e.g., BUN, creatinine, phosphorus) should be determined at time of admission. Recheck blood work should be performed at 24 and 48 hours in dogs ingesting a nephrotoxic dose of ibuprofen and for at least 72 hours following naproxen ingestion.

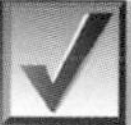

COMMENTS

Client Education

- Ibuprofen and naproxen sodium are not recommended for use in veterinary patients because of the risk for GI adverse events and toxicity.

- Prescription and OTC NSAIDs should be kept out of reach of pets. Care should be taken to find and pick up any dropped medications, since as little as 1 tablet of 200 mg ibuprofen can be toxic to cats, ferrets, and small to moderate-sized dogs.

Patient Monitoring

- Appetite, vomiting, diarrhea, melena.
- Renal parameters (e.g., BUN, creatinine, phosphorus).
- Monitor PCV/TS daily to evaluate for severity of blood loss, hemodilution, and hydration status.
- Urine output.

Prevention/Avoidance

- Pet owners should be instructed never to administer OTC NSAIDs to their pets unless under direct instruction of their veterinarian.
- There are several NSAIDs that have been specifically formulated and undergone extensive FDA testing and approval for veterinary patients. Veterinary-approved COX-selective NSAIDs may reduce the toxic side effects from NSAIDs. Whenever possible, veterinarians should recommend these medications instead of human OTC NSAIDs.

Possible Complications

- Severe gastrointestinal hemorrhage.
- Acute renal failure.

Expected Course and Prognosis

- Prognosis is variable depending on the dose ingested and the duration of time elapsed from ingestion to admission to a veterinary clinic.

See Also

Aspirin
Veterinary NSAIDs (Carprofen, Deracoxib, Firocoxib, Ketoprofen, Meloxicam, Robenacoxib, Tepoxalin)

Abbreviations

See Appendix 1 for a complete list.

COX = cyclooxygenase
CVP = central venous pressure
IBD = inflammatory bowel disease
NSAID(s) = nonsteroidal antiinflammatory drug(s)
pRBC = packed red blood cells
Rx = prescription

Suggested Reading

Khan SA, McLean MK. Toxicology of frequently encountered nonsteroidal anti-inflammatory drugs in dogs and cats. Vet Clin Small Anim 2012; 42:289–306.

Lees P, Landoni MF, Giraudel J, Toutain PL. Pharmacodynamics and pharmacokinetics of nonsteroidal anti-inflammatory drugs in species of veterinary interest. J Vet Pharmacol Ther 2004; 27:479–490.

Papich M. An update on nonsteroidal anti-inflammatory drugs (NSAIDs) in small animals. Vet Clin Small Anim 2008; 38:1243–1266.

Acknowledgment: The authors and editors acknowledge the prior contributions of Rebecca S. Syring, DVM, DACVECC, who authored this topic in the previous edition.
Author: John H. Tegzes, MA, VMD, DABVT
Consulting Editor: Ahna G. Brutlag, DVM, MS, DABT, DABVT

chapter 46

Nicotine and Tobacco

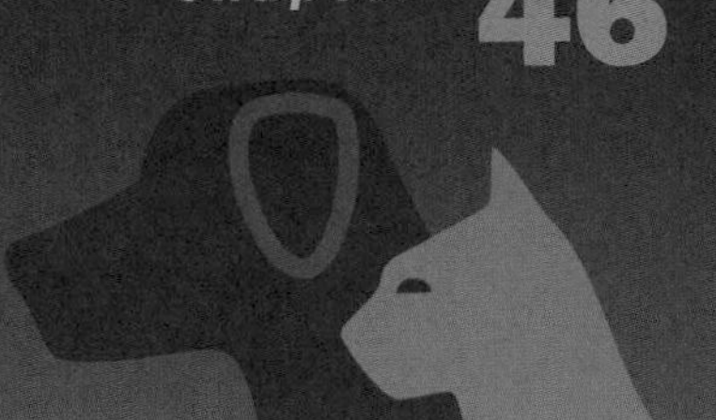

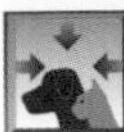

DEFINITION/OVERVIEW

- Nicotine is a rapid-onset, dose-dependent nicotinic ganglion depolarizer.
- Clinical signs develop rapidly, often within 1 hour of ingestion, and can last 1–2 hours for mild exposures and 18–24 hours for severe cases.
- CNS stimulation followed by depression is common.
- Nicotine is available in many products, including chewing tobacco, cigarettes, cigars, bidis, and nicotine replacement products including patches, gum, electronic cigarettes, "E-juice" or "E-liquid" (liquid nicotine refills for e-cigarettes), nasal sprays, and inhalers. For nicotine content of common products, see table 46.1.
- Paper wrapping of cigars and bidis may also contain tobacco with nicotine.
- Ingested cigarette butts may also cause intoxication.
- Some types of nicotine gums contain xylitol, which is also toxic to dogs.
- Although no longer legally used or sold in the United States, 0.05% to 4% nicotine sulfate spray or dust and 40% concentrated nicotine solution (e.g., Black Leaf 40) could be a rare source of nicotine toxicity.

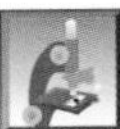

ETIOLOGY/PATHOPHYSIOLOGY

Mechanism of Action

- Low-dose and early high-dose intoxications result in widespread nervous system excitation due to depolarization and stimulation of nicotinic receptors in autonomic ganglia and neuromuscular junctions, as well as in the CNS, spinal cord, and adrenal medulla.
- Persistent ganglionic and neuromuscular junction depolarization and blockade from high-dose intoxication lead to progressive and pervasive nervous system depression.

Blackwell's Five-Minute Veterinary Consult Clinical Companion: Small Animal Toxicology, Second Edition.
Lynn R. Hovda, Ahna G. Brutlag, Robert H. Poppenga, and Katherine L. Peterson.

Companion website: www.fiveminutevet.com/toxicology

TABLE 46.1. Average nicotine content of selected products.

Nicotine-containing product	Average nicotine content (mg/g)	Average nicotine content per typical unit	Notes
Bidi cigar/cigarettes	15–25	4.7 mg per cigarette	Content varies widely, even within the same brand Usually flavored (e.g., cherry, mint, chocolate) Unfiltered rolled tobacco rolled in tobacco-containing paper Usually imported from India
Cigarettes	11–30	13–30 mg per cigarette; 5–7 mg per cigarette butt	Content varies widely, even within the same brand Average commercial brand product (United States)
E-liquid, ready to use	6–36 mg/mL		
E-liquid, do-it-yourself concentrate	Up to 200 mg/mL		
Cigars	NA	100–444 mg per cigar	Wrapped in tobacco-containing paper Cigar size is extremely variable
Wet chewing tobacco	7–16	NA	Some products flavored
Nicotine patches	NA	7–114 mg per patch	Dose absorbed is dependent on whether patch is intact or has been broken or chewed
Nicotine gum	NA	2–4 mg per piece	May contain xylitol

NA, not available.

Pharmacokinetics – Absorption, Distribution, Metabolism, Excretion

- Slowly absorbed in the acidic gastric environment. Much more quickly absorbed in the small intestine
- Eliminated via the kidneys.
- E-liquid is readily absorbed through the skin and mucous membranes as well as via ingestion.

Toxicity

- Canine (oral) LD_{50}: 9–12 mg/kg. However, reports of dogs tolerating significantly higher doses have been made.
- Clinical signs have been reported at doses as low as 1 mg/kg.
- Severe clinical toxicosis is rarely seen, likely due to multiple factors.
    - Spontaneous vomiting often occurs soon after ingestion due to central vomition center stimulation.

- Nicotine absorption is slow in the acidic gastric environment.
- Nicotine-containing products have limited palatability (with the possible exception of flavored chewing tobacco and other products with taste improvement additives such as e-liquid and gum).

Systems Affected

- Gastrointestinal – hypersalivation, vomiting (common shortly after ingestion), diarrhea.
- Nervous – stimulation followed by depression, hyperexcitability, agitation, depression, ataxia, tremors, seizures (rare).
- Cardiovascular – tachycardia, hypertension, reflex bradycardia, cardiac arrest.
- Respiratory – tachypnea, cyanosis.
- Ophthalmic – mydriasis.

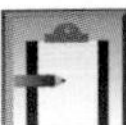

SIGNALMENT/HISTORY

- Indiscriminate chewers/eaters, especially puppies.
- No breed or sex predilection.

Risk Factors

- Preexisting cardiovascular or renal disease.
- Neonatal and geriatric animals may be more severely affected.
- Presence of nicotine products in the environment.
- Access to ashtrays, purses, or backpacks.

Historical Findings

- Witnessed ingestion.
- Discovery of chewed nicotine-containing products (e.g., cigarettes, cigars, smoking cessation patches or gums, etc.).
- Discovery of nicotine-containing products in the vomitus or stool.
- The owners may report vomiting, hyperexcitement, or depression.

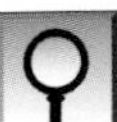

CLINICAL FEATURES

- Signs may begin within minutes of ingestion.
- Duration of signs in mild cases is 1–2 hours; in severe cases, 18–24 hours.
- Signs are initially consistent with CNS excitement, including tremors, ataxia, weakness, sensory disturbances, and possibly seizures.
- Stimulatory signs progress to CNS depression, descending weakness, and paralysis in high-dose intoxications.

- Simultaneous activation of parasympathetic and sympathetic ganglia at low doses can result in the following clinical signs.
    - Bradycardia, paroxysmal atrial fibrillation, and possible cardiac arrest from profound parasympathetic vagal stimulation.
    - Tachycardia, hypertension, and ventricular arrhythmias from adrenal and ganglionic sympathetic stimulation.
    - Tachypnea and panting from stimulation of the brainstem respiratory center.
    - Mydriasis.
- Gastrointestinal signs include hypersalivation, vomiting, and diarrhea.
- Death can result from paralysis of skeletal respiratory muscles, central respiratory depression and subsequent arrest, or cardiovascular collapse.

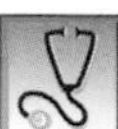

DIFFERENTIAL DIAGNOSIS

- Primary cardiac disease resulting in tachycardia, bradycardia, syncope, etc.
- Primary neurological disease.
- Severe hypoglycemia (e.g., insulin overdose, insulinoma, iatrogenic, hunting dog, sepsis, hepatic disease, etc.).
- Neuromuscular disease (e.g., tick paralysis).
- Toxicities – chocolate/caffeine/methylxanthines, amphetamines, cocaine, carbamates, phenylpropanolamine, pyrethrins/pyrethroids, organophosphates, strychnine, tremorgenic mycotoxins, xylitol.

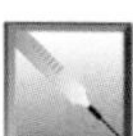

DIAGNOSTICS

- Nicotine analysis of serum, gastric contents, or urine is available but rarely clinically useful due to the need for rapid diagnosis and treatment.
- ECG – monitor symptomatic animals for tachyarrhythmias, ventricular arrhythmias, atrial fibrillation, etc.
- Baseline CBC, chemistry, UA to rule out underlying health concerns (e.g., renal disease) which may prolong recovery.

Pathological Findings

- Gross and histopathological findings are nonspecific.

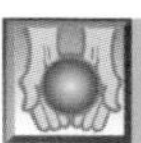

THERAPEUTICS

Detoxification

- Gastrointestinal decontamination is the mainstay of therapy.
    - Induce vomiting (nicotine is an emetic so vomiting may already have occurred) with recent ingestions.

- Administer activated charcoal with a cathartic once if patient is asymptomatic and at low risk for aspiration; for sustained-release products (e.g., transdermal patches), consider two additional doses of activated charcoal (without cathartic) every 4–6 hours.

Appropriate Health Care

Treatment is symptomatic and supportive.

- Sedation for agitation, tachycardia, hypertension.
- IV fluids for hypotension – a balanced electrolyte crystalloid can be administered in small aliquots (i.e., 20–30 mL/kg IV over 20–30 minutes, repeat 2–3× to effect) until blood pressure improves. IV fluids may also speed elimination of nicotine from the kidneys.
- Supplemental oxygen and artificial respiration for respiratory distress.
- Antiemetic therapy/gastrointestinal support.
    - Maropitant, 1 mg/kg, SQ q 24 hours.
    - Ondansetron, 0.1–0.2 mg/kg, IV, IM, SQ q 6–12 hours.
- Acidification of the urine may facilitate excretion.

Antidotes

- No antidote available.

Drugs of Choice

Sedation/anxiolytics

- Acepromazine, 0.05–0.1 mg/kg IM, SQ, IV, or butorphanol, 0.1–0.5 mg/kg IM, SQ, IV, for agitation, tachycardia, hypertension.

Cardiovascular support

- Atropine, 0.02–0.04 mg/kg IV or IM, as needed for bradycardia (dog <50 bpm, cat <120 bpm).
- Beta-blockers (e.g., propranolol, 0.02–0.06 mg/kg, IV slowly to effect) for hypertension or tachycardia unresponsive to sedation (dog >180–190 bpm, cat >220–230 bpm).

Neurological support/anticonvulsant therapy

- Diazepam, 0.25–1 mg/kg IV to effect.
- Phenobarbital, 2–16 mg/kg IV as needed.

Precautions/Interactions

- Avoid antacids (e.g., H_2 blockers) as alkalization of stomach contents hastens absorption.

Nursing Care

- Regular monitoring of heart rate, blood pressure, ECG, and CNS status.

Surgical Considerations

- Removal of extended-release nicotine patches from the GIT prevents continuous release and absorption.
- Endoscopy to remove intact transdermal patches in the stomach or proximal intestine.
- Surgery to remove intact patches from the distal intestine.

Environmental Issues

- Outdoor areas with large numbers of littered cigarette butts may pose a threat for nicotine ingestion as well as a potential foreign body risk.

COMMENTS

Client Education

- Inform staff and clients that some tobacco products are wrapped in tobacco-containing papers so ingestion of the paper alone may be toxic.
- Remind owners that nicotine products can be flavored, making them more appealing to pets. This warning applies to nicotine gums as well, which may also contain xylitol (see chapter 71, Xylitol).
- Advise owners not to leave ashtrays/cigarette butts, packs of cigarettes, smoking cessation drugs (e.g., gums, patches), e-liquid, or other nicotine-containing products in reach of pets.
- Many pets are exposed to nicotine with "purse digging."

Patient Monitoring

- Regular monitoring of heart rate, blood pressure, ECG, and CNS status while hospitalized.
- Once the animal is asymptomatic and stable without intervention, the pet may be discharged.

Expected Course and Prognosis

- Prognosis for low-dose ingestions is excellent.
- Prognosis for high-dose exposures is poor unless treatment is initiated early and the animal can be stabilized within the first 4 hours after ingestion.

See Also

Amphetamines
Chocolate and Caffeine

Cocaine
Decongestants (Imidazolines)
Ephedra/Ma Huang
Foreign Objects
Metaldehyde
Methamphetamine
Mycotoxins – Tremorgenic
Organophosphorus and Carbamate Insecticides
Phenylpropanolamine
Pyrethrins and Pyrethroids
Strychnine

Abbreviations

See Appendix 1 for a complete list.

Suggested Reading

Brutlag AG. Topical toxins. In: Ettinger SJ, Feldman EC, eds. Textbook of Veterinary Internal Medicine, 7th edn. St Louis, MO: Elsevier, 2010; pp. 565–568.

Davis B, Dang M, Kim J, Talbot P. Nicotine concentrations in electronic cigarette refill and do-it-yourself fluids. Nicotine Tob Res 2014; doi:10.1093/ntr/ntu080.

Malson JL, Sims K, Murty R, Pickworth WB. Comparison of the nicotine content used in bidis and conventional cigarettes. Tob Control 2001; 10(2):181–183.

Plumlee KH. Nicotine. In: Peterson ME, Talcott PA, eds. Small Animal Toxicology, 3rd edn. St Louis, MO: Saunders, 2013; p. 683.

Acknowledgment: The authors and editors acknowledge the prior contributions of Carey L. Renken, MD, who authored this topic in the previous edition.
Author: Jean Ihnen, DVM
Consulting Editor: Ahna G. Brutlag, DVM, MS, DABT, DABVT

Vitamins and Minerals

DEFINITION/OVERVIEW

- Vitamins, in the form of single nutrient formulations, multivitamins, and prenatal vitamins, are readily available in many homes. However, there is a paucity of veterinary literature describing toxicosis resulting from vitamin and mineral ingestion in small animals.
- In the United States, a multivitamin/mineral supplement is defined as a supplement containing three or more vitamins and minerals but does not include herbs, hormones, or drugs. Each nutrient is at a dose below the tolerable upper level determined for humans by the Food and Drug Board and the maximum daily intake to not cause a risk for adverse health effects.
- Among the common vitamins and minerals found within readily available multivitamin, prenatal, and single nutrient formulations, the most dangerous ingredients resulting in toxicosis following acute ingestion are vitamin A, vitamin D_3, and iron.
- Management of patients who have ingested any vitamin or mineral containing medication entails calculation of amount consumed, emesis, specific antidote therapy if indicated, monitoring, and supportive care.
- Prognosis following vitamin and/or mineral toxicosis depends on ingested ingredient(s), health status of the pet, prompt and appropriate care, and response to treatment.

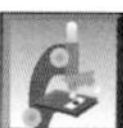

ETIOLOGY/PATHOPHYSIOLOGY

Mechanism of Action

- Common ingredients found within commercially available multivitamins in the United States may include the following items, though in variable amounts depending on the manufacturer and formulation.
    - Vitamin A
    - Vitamin B_1 (thiamine)
    - Vitamin B_2 (riboflavin)
    - Vitamin B_3 (niacin)
    - Vitamin B_6 (pyridoxine)

Blackwell's Five-Minute Veterinary Consult Clinical Companion: Small Animal Toxicology, Second Edition.
Lynn R. Hovda, Ahna G. Brutlag, Robert H. Poppenga, and Katherine L. Peterson.

Companion website: www.fiveminutevet.com/toxicology

- Vitamin B_{12} (cobalamin)
- Vitamin C (ascorbic acid)
- Vitamin D_3 (cholecalciferol)
- Vitamin E
- Biotin
- Calcium
- Copper
- Folic acid
- Iodine
- Iron
- Magnesium
- Pantothenic acid
- Phosphorus
- Zinc

- Many formulations are available in order to appeal to the vast array of consumer demands (e.g., adult, children, men, women), health needs, desired dosing regimen, and preferred formulation type (e.g., tablets, capsules, powders, liquids, gummies, and chewables; Fig. 47.1). Vitamin and mineral supplements labeled "high potency" are required to have 100% of the recommended daily value for at least two-thirds of the ingredients contained within the supplement, as dictated by the Food and Drug Administration.
- Prenatal vitamins, which are recommended for women of childbearing age who are attempting to become pregnant or are known to be pregnant, may contain many of the same ingredients found in multivitamins but tend to have higher compositions of folic acid, calcium, and iron However, as with multivitamins, the composition and nutrient amount vary greatly by manufacturer.
- All commercial pet foods contain added vitamins and minerals, in amounts to provide necessary nutrients and withstand manufacturing and storage impacts. Pet foods that have been certified by the Association of American Feed Control Officials (AAFCO) are guaranteed to meet minimal nutrient requirements for given stages of life. Therefore, additional supplementation of vitamins and minerals for pets being fed a high-quality balanced diet is not necessary.
- Although by definition, vitamins should not contain additional herbs or drugs, many do. Labels should be read carefully. For example, words like "active metabolism" may indicate that the product contains significant amounts of caffeine. The following is a list of common added ingredients that could potentially cause clinical signs.
  - Caffeine (guarana, green tea)
  - Citrus aurantium (synephrine)
  - Fluoride
  - Methionine
  - Thioctic acid (alpha-lipoic acid)
  - Tryptophan
  - Xylitol (as a sweetener)
  - 5-HTP

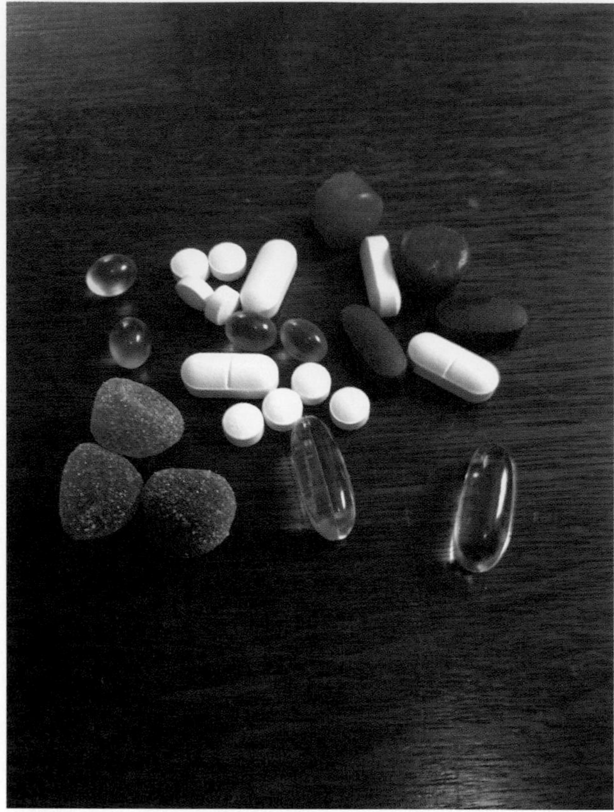

■ **Fig. 47.1.** An assortment of vitamin and mineral supplements in different shapes, sizes, and formulations. Photo courtesy of Ahna G. Brutlag.

Pharmacokinetics – Absorption, Distribution, Metabolism, Excretion

- Vitamin absorption depends mostly on the solubility of the vitamin: fat-soluble vitamins require bile salts and fat in order to be passively absorbed in the duodenum and ileum, whereas water-soluble vitamins require active transport for uptake from the GIT.
- Mineral absorption depends on solubility, density, and mineral–mineral interactions in both the GIT and tissue storage level.
- Please see box 47.1 for further information on distribution, metabolism, and excretion of vitamins and minerals.

Toxicity

- Of the common vitamins and minerals contained within single nutrient supplements, multivitamin/multimineral supplements, and prenatal supplements, **vitamins A, D_3**, and **iron** are the most likely to cause significant clinical signs.
- The remaining vitamins and minerals are likely to cause mild GIT signs, such as vomiting, diarrhea, and anorexia, when ingested in large quantities. Specific vitamin or mineral toxicity is otherwise uncommon.

BOX 47.1. Information on distribution, metabolism, and excretion of vitamins and minerals. For further detail, the reader is referred to a veterinary nutrition textbook.

- **Vitamin A** is stored in the liver and can undergo enterohepatic circulation. Cats require preformed vitamin A, since they lack an enzyme necessary for β-carotene cleavage.
- **Vitamin B_1 (thiamine)** is absorbed primarily in the jejunum after intestinal phosphatases hydrolyze thiamine to free thiamine. Active, carrier-mediated transport is the primary mechanism of absorption; however, passive diffusion is also utilized during periods of increased thiamine intake. It is transported in red blood cells and plasma to the tissues.
- **Vitamin B_2 (riboflavin)** requires hydrolysis prior to absorption in the GIT. Absorbed riboflavin is bound in approximately equal percentages to albumin and globulin. Excess riboflavin is renally excreted.
- **Vitamin B_3 (niacin)** is readily absorbed by the mucosa of the stomach and small intestine and is taken up by tissues, where it is often required for cofactor synthesis. Excessive amounts are excreted by the kidneys following methylation.
- **Vitamin B_6 (pyridoxine)** is absorbed via passive diffusion in the small intestine, but only small quantities are stored. Products of vitamin B_6 metabolism are renally excreted.
- **Vitamin B_{12} (cobalamin)** absorption depends on both intake and GIT function, as it undergoes several transformations (hydrolysis, intrinsic factor binding, ileal absorption, protein-bound transport, and cell surface receptor-mediated uptake) in order to be utilized.
- **Vitamin C (ascorbic acid)**, though not technically a vitamin, can be synthesized from glucose by cats and dogs. Additional vitamin C is absorbed by passive diffusion. It is transported by albumin, distributed throughout the body, and excreted via urine, feces, and sweat.
- **Vitamin D (D_3, cholecalciferol)** can be synthesized by the skin after exposure to UV light. It is also absorbed in the small intestine, using bile salts, and subsequently transported with vitamin D binding protein to tissues where it is contained within lipid deposits.
- **Vitamin E** is absorbed in the small intestine by passive diffusion; however, it is absorbed with poor efficacy. Absorption can be increased by consuming fats at the same time. Transport to circulation is facilitated by the lymphatics. There is minimal metabolism of vitamin E, and the majority of it is fecally excreted.
- **Biotin** is released via protein hydrolysis in order to permit intestinal absorption and subsequent transfer from the blood to the tissues. In addition, intestinal microbes synthesize approximately half of the biotin requirements. Excessive biotin is excreted by the kidneys.
- **Calcium** absorption is variable in the GIT and can be achieved using three possible mechanisms. In the duodenum and jejunum, there is an active, transcellular method using a vitamin D-dependent, calcium-binding protein. The other two methods are passive and facilitated absorption, which are primarily localized to the distal GIT. Most calcium in dietary supplements is in the form of calcium salts, which are poorly absorbed by the GIT.
- **Copper** can be absorbed along the entire length of the GIT, though most is absorbed within the small intestine, by both active and passive mechanisms. The liver is the main site of copper metabolism, and excretion is via feces and bile.
- **Folic acid (folate)** is hydrolyzed in the intestine before enterocyte absorption. There are no folate reserves in the body; therefore, it must be ingested daily in the diet.
- **Iodine** within the plasma is trapped by the thyroid glands to ensure adequate supplies of thyroid hormone.
- **Iron** must be ionized in order to be absorbed. It is absorbed into mucosal cells lining the intestinal lumen, particularly in the duodenum and jejunum. The absorbed iron is then transferred to ferritin or transferrin. No distinct mechanism for iron excretion exists, which contributes to toxicosis with iron ingestion.
- **Magnesium** is absorbed is either actively or passively from the intestines, depending on the intraluminal concentration. The kidney is essential for magnesium homeostasis and is responsible for filtration, excretion, and reabsorption of this mineral.
- **Pantothenic acid** is released via protein hydrolysis within the intestinal lumen. Most of the vitamin is contained within erythrocytes.
- **Phosphorus** is well absorbed in the intestines, particularly when found in animal-based ingredients. Calcium and phosphorus absorption, metabolism, and hemostasis are under the delicate and intricate control of hormonal and renal influences.
- **Zinc** absorption is not completely understood, though the majority of absorption occurs in the duodenum, jejunum, and ileum. The liver is responsible for zinc metabolism, and excretion of excess zinc occurs via the feces.

- **Vitamins** E, K, B_2, B_3, and B_6 are considered to be minimally toxic. No toxicosis has been associated with supplements containing **pantothenic acid**, **folic acid**, **biotin**, and **zinc**.
- **Calcium**, **phosphorus**, **iodine**, and **magnesium** may be associated with specific clinical signs or end-organ damage (see Systems Affected).
- Massive ingestion of capsules or tablets can result in bezoar formation and may require gastric lavage for removal.
- **Vitamin A** – for acute vitamin A toxicosis, clinical signs are usually associated with ingested amounts that exceed 10–1000× the daily requirement.
- Vitamin C (ascorbic acid) – large doses greater than 1 g/kg can cause urine calcium oxalate crystals.
- **Vitamin D_3** – ingested doses < 0.1 mg/kg can cause mild GIT signs, whereas doses > 0.1 mg/kg can lead to hypercalcemia and ARF. To calculate the amount of vitamin D_3 ingested, it is important to note that 1 IU of vitamin D_3 equals 0.025 μg or 0.000025 mg of vitamin D_3. See chapter 113 on vitamin D_3/cholecalciferol.
- **Iron** – in dogs ingesting less than 20 mg/kg of elemental iron, no clinical signs have been reported. When amounts between 20 and 60 mg/kg of elemental iron are consumed, mild clinical signs may be seen. Doses above 60 mg/kg may cause severe clinical signs, and death may result from doses between 100–200 mg/kg. See chapter 95 on iron toxicosis.

Systems Affected

- Gastrointestinal
    - Vomiting –may be seen with ingestion of any vitamin or mineral.
    - Diarrhea – may be seen with ingestion of any vitamin or mineral.
    - Anorexia – may be seen with ingestion of any vitamin or mineral.
    - Gastrointestinal bleeding – seen with iron toxicosis.
    - Gastrointestinal strictures – late complication seen with iron toxicosis.
    - Hematochezia – associated with vitamin B_3 (niacin) toxicosis.
- Nervous
    - Flaccid paralysis – associated with magnesium toxicosis.
    - Tremors/convulsions – associated with vitamin A and B_3 toxicosis.
    - Paralysis – seen with vitamin A toxicosis.
    - Ataxia – seen with vitamin B_6 (pyridoxine) toxicosis.
    - Abnormal reflexes – associated with vitamin B_{12} (cobalamin) toxicosis.
- Musculoskeletal
    - Lameness – associated with calcium and vitamin D_3 toxicosis.
    - Soft tissue calcifications – associated with phosphorus and vitamin D_3 toxicosis.
    - Cervical spondylosis – seen with vitamin A toxicosis.
    - Long bone fractures – seen with vitamin A toxicosis.
- Renal/urological
    - ARF – seen with vitamin D_3 toxicosis.
    - Uroliths – seen with vitamin C, calcium, phosphorus, and magnesium toxicosis.

- Endocrine/metabolic
  - Hypercalcemia – seen with calcium and vitamin D_3 toxicosis.
  - Secondary hyperparathyroidism – seen with phosphorus toxicosis.
- Hemic/lymphatic/immune
  - Coagulopathy – associated with vitamin A and E toxicosis.
  - Anemia – seen with vitamin A toxicosis.
- Hepatobiliary
  - Hepatitis/increased liver enzymes/decreased hepatic function – seen with vitamin A and copper toxicosis.
- Cardiovascular
  - Hypotension and bradycardia – associated with vitamin B_1 (thiamine) toxicosis.
- Skin/exocrine
  - Rough haircoat – associated with chronic iodine toxicosis.

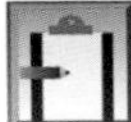

SIGNALMENT/HISTORY

- There are no breed, sex, or age predilections for nutritional supplement toxicosis.
- While no mean age has been reported, it is likely that younger animals are more frequently affected given their increased incidence of ingesting foreign objects.
- Some pet owners may give high doses of vitamins based on internet searches, or the theory that "more is better."

Risk Factors

- Animals living in homes or areas where vitamin or mineral supplements are stored.
- Animals with renal disease could be at increased risk of more severe consequences after vitamin D_3 or calcium ingestion.

Historical Findings

- Ingestion of vitamin or mineral supplements may be witnessed by the owner, or suspected based on damaged packaging or spilled supplements.
- Owners may witness vomiting (which may or may not contain supplements), diarrhea, and neurological changes.

Location and Circumstances of Poisoning

- Ingestion often occurs when plastic baggies are used to store medications temporarily.
- Ingestion often occurs when dogs chew on weekly plastic pill holders, which are not pet-proof.

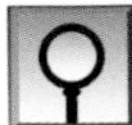

CLINICAL FEATURES

- Gastrointestinal – vomiting, diarrhea, anorexia, GIT bleeding, hematochezia.
- Nervous – abnormal reflexes, ataxia, tremors, convulsions, flaccid paralysis, paralysis.

- Musculoskeletal – lameness, soft tissue calcification, cervical spondylosis, long bone fractures.
- Renal/urological – pain on abdominal (specifically, kidney or bladder) palpation.
- Cardiovascular – bradycardia, poor pulse quality.
- Skin/exocrine – rough haircoat.

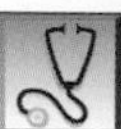

DIFFERENTIAL DIAGNOSIS

- Vomiting, diarrhea, anorexia, and GIT bleeding due to other primary or secondary GIT disease.
- ARF.
- Liver dysfunction or failure.
- Ataxia, tremors, and paralysis due to other primary or secondary neurological disease.

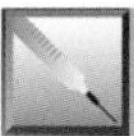

DIAGNOSTICS

- A baseline CBC and serum chemistry should be considered in most animals where **multivitamin/multimineral/prenatal supplement** ingestion is suspected, especially when the ingested amount is unknown.
- In animals known to have ingested near-toxic or toxic amounts of **vitamin D_3** and calcium, total calcium, ionized calcium, BUN, creatinine, and urinalysis (including urine specific gravity) should be measured.
- For patients ingesting near-toxic or toxic amounts of **vitamin A** and **copper**, special attention should be directed toward liver enzymes and measures of liver function (e.g., BUN, glucose, albumin, and cholesterol).
- For animals ingesting toxic or near-toxic doses of **vitamin A**, a complete coagulation panel (e.g., PT, PTT, platelets, and d-dimers) should be measured.
- For patients with severe tremors from **multivitamin** ingestion, serum AST and CK, as well as blood lactate, should be monitored.
- For patients ingesting 1 g/kg of **vitamin C**, baseline chemistry and urinalysis should be obtained.
- For any patient ingesting elemental **iron** at toxic or near-toxic doses, serum iron concentration and total iron-binding capacity should be measured. See chapter 95 for more information about iron toxicity.

Pathological Findings

- Gross or histopathological lesions seen in animals that have ingested multivitamins/multiminerals/prenatal supplements will depend on the ingested dose of a particular vitamin or mineral.
- Gross necropsy findings in pets that have ingested toxic amounts of vitamin or mineral supplements may include whole or partial tablets or capsules within the GIT, GIT

bleeding (iron), GIT stricture formation (iron), soft tissue mineralization (calcium, phosphorus), long bone fracture (vitamin A), cervical spondylosis (vitamin A), nephroliths/uroliths (calcium, phosphorus, vitamin C), renomegaly due to ARF (vitamin D_3), and hepatomegaly associated with hepatitis (copper).

- Histopathological lesions seen in pets ingesting toxic amounts of vitamin or mineral supplements include GIT ulceration (iron), fibrous tissue deposition within the GIT (iron), acute tubular necrosis (vitamin D_3), hepatitis (copper), and soft tissue calcification (phosphorus, calcium).
- For more detailed information on the gross and histopathological lesions associated with iron toxicity, see chapter 95.

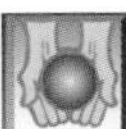

THERAPEUTICS

- If an animal is healthy and did not ingest a toxic or near-toxic amount of any vitamin or mineral, no further action is needed aside from monitoring by the owner.
- If an animal is found to have ingested a toxic or near-toxic dose of any vitamin or mineral, or if there is preexisting hepatic or renal dysfunction, emesis should be induced, and activated charcoal with a cathartic should be administered. For the most dangerous vitamin and mineral toxicoses (vitamins A and D_3), repeat doses of activated charcoal (without a cathartic) may be considered. Activated charcoal does not bind to iron well. See chapter 95 for more information on iron toxicosis.
- Intravenous fluids should be used to manage hydration and prevent hypovolemia in any patient showing clinical signs associated with vitamin or mineral toxicosis.
- Electrolytes, renal values, clotting times, and liver enzymes/measures of liver function should be monitored as indicated by the toxicosis and any underlying disease process.

Detoxification

- In patients presenting with recent, suspected, or confirmed multivitamin or multimineral toxicosis, emesis should be induced as quickly and safely as possible.
- For neurologically inappropriate patients who have ingested multivitamins, initial treatment should be aimed at managing neurological signs, such as paralysis, tremors, or convulsions. Appropriate sedation, intubation (to protect the airway), and gastric lavage should be considered to facilitate decontamination if the supplements are still suspected to be within the stomach.
- As massive ingestion may result in a gastric bezoar, gastric lavage may be indicated for decontamination.

Appropriate Health Care

- In general, fluid therapy (either IV or SQ, depending on the severity of the toxicosis and clinical symptoms) should be used to manage hydration and prevent hypovolemia. Twenty-four hours of fluid diuresis should be considered in large **vitamin C** overdoses.

- Aggressive IV fluids and medications to increase calciuresis may be necessary for patients with **vitamin D_3** toxicosis; see chapter 113.
- With **vitamin D_3** toxicosis, aggressive monitoring of renal values, electrolytes, and assessment for hydration (e.g., skin turgor, chemosis, peripheral edema, PCV/TS, weight, urine output) should be performed in all patients where there is concern for hypercalcemia-induced ARF, especially if furosemide has been given.
- Gastroprotectants and antiemetics may be necessary with multivitamin toxicity, including the following.
  - Famotidine 0.5–1.0 mg/kg IV q 12–24 hours.
  - Pantoprazole 0.7–1 mg/kg IV over 15 minutes q 24 hours.
  - Sucralfate suspension 0.5–1 g PO q 8 hours, administered 30–60 minutes after any medication aimed at decreasing gastric acid production.
  - Ondansetron 0.1–0.2 mg/kg IV q 8–12 hours.
  - Maropitant 1 mg/kg SQ q 24 hours.
- For patients with tremors or convulsions, body temperature, patient comfort, hydration, and blood lactate should be closely monitored.
- For patients with severe tremors or convulsions secondary to vitamin or mineral supplement toxicosis, they should be controlled with diazepam (0.5–1 mg/kg IV) or midazolam (0.2–0.5 mg/kg IV). For patients with ongoing tremors or convulsions, a diazepam (0.25–1 mg/kg/hour) or midazolam (0.1–0.5 mg/kg/hour) CRI may be needed.

Drugs and Antidotes of Choice

- In patients at risk of **iron** toxicosis or those that are showing clinical signs, chelation therapy and gastroprotectants are indicated. See chapter 95 for more information.
- In cases of **vitamin D_3** toxicosis, pamidronate (a bisphosphonate), may be given for hypercalcemia. See chapter 113 for more information.

Follow-up

- The need for follow-up care will depend on extent of end-organ damage or dysfunction and response to therapy.
- If there are derangements in liver or kidney values, patients will likely require follow-up blood work 5–10 days after discharge and may require more long-term monitoring if abnormalities persist.

Diet

- For patients with any neurological compromise, vomiting, or regurgitation, oral food and water should be withheld until the patient is neurologically appropriate and GIT signs have resolved.

Prevention

- Proper storage of vitamin and mineral supplements in an area inaccessible to pets will help prevent toxicosis.

- Clients should be advised that pets being fed an AAFCO-approved, balanced commercial diets do not require additional vitamin or mineral supplementation; therefore, they should not administer any nutritional supplements unless specifically instructed by a veterinarian.

COMMENTS

Client Education

- Clients should be educated on the mechanism of action of the specific vitamin or mineral toxicosis, as well as being given recommendations for safe storage.
- Clients should be informed that children are also at risk of vitamin or mineral toxicosis if large doses are ingested.
- Information about the gradual reintroduction of a bland diet, monitoring for ongoing GIT and neurological signs, and general observation instructions should be provided.
- For patients with persistent renal, hematological, or hepatic derangements, clients should be given clear instructions about frequency of follow-up monitoring, possibility of permanent end-organ injury, and dietary or medication adjustments that are required based on organ dysfunction.

Patient Monitoring

- For patients with hypercalcemia, serum total and ionized calcium should be monitored every 12–24 hours, and more frequently if therapy to treat hypercalcemia is being used. Electrolytes (e.g., sodium, potassium, and chloride) should be monitored every 12–24 hours if furosemide therapy is used.
- For patients at risk for or those with ARF, renal values and PCV/TS should also be measured at least every 12–24 hours. Urine output should be measured every 2–4 hours. Patients should be weighed every 6–8 hours to help assess fluid balance.
- For coagulopathic patients, clotting times should be measured at least every 24 hours and more frequently if being treated with FFP to assess success of therapy.
- In patients with hepatic failure, blood glucose should be monitored every 2–4 hours and supplemented as needed.
- In patients with elevations in liver enzymes, after baseline values are obtained, reassessment should be performed every 3–7 days depending on clinical course.
- Neurological status should be monitored every 2–4 hours, as well as body temperature, gag reflex, and blood lactate in any patient with tremors, paralysis, or other neurological impairment.
- For patients with iron toxicosis, serum iron concentration and total iron-binding capacity should be measured at presentation and during chelation therapy. See chapter 95 for monitoring the patient with iron toxicosis.

Prevention/Avoidance

- Education about proper storage and handling of vitamin and mineral supplements will help prevent reexposure.

Possible Complications

- ARF
- Chronic renal failure after resolution of ARF
- Liver failure/hepatitis
- GIT hemorrhage
- GIT stricture
- Paralysis, tremors

Expected Course and Prognosis

- For patients that did not consume a toxic amount of any vitamin or mineral, owners can expect self-limiting GIT signs that should resolve on their own within 12–48 hours.
- There are four stages associated with **iron** toxicosis: the first stage starts within 6 hours of iron ingestion, and the fourth stage may not be seen for 2–6 weeks after ingestion. Without aggressive supportive care, monitoring, and chelation therapy, acute iron poisoning is potentially lethal in animals. For more specific information about the prognosis and clinical course expected with iron toxicosis, please see chapter 95.
- For patients with hypercalcemia secondary to vitamin D_3 toxicity, prognosis and clinical course will depend on how soon treatment for hypercalcemia is initiated and response to therapy. For patients that develop ARF secondary to hypercalcemia, even though aggressive care is absolutely warranted, a guarded prognosis must be given.
- The prognosis for vitamin A toxicosis is likely favorable with appropriate treatment and supportive care.

Synonyms

Multivitamin toxicosis, multimineral toxicosis, prenatal vitamin/mineral toxicosis, vitamin or mineral supplement toxicosis

See Also

Calcium Supplements
Cholecalciferol
Iron

Abbreviations

See Appendix 1 for a complete list.

AAFCO = Association of American Feed Control Officials
FFP = fresh frozen plasma

Suggested Reading

Albretsen A. The toxicity of iron, an essential element. Vet Med 2006; 82–90.

Gross KL, Wedekind KJ, Cowell CS, et al. Nutrients. In: Hand MS, Thatcher CD, Remillard RL, et al., eds. Small Animal Clinical Nutrition, 4th edn. Marceline, MO: Walsworth, 2000.

Khan SA. Vitamin A toxicosis. In: Cote E, ed. Clinical Veterinary Advisor, 3rd edn. St Louis, MO: Mosby, 2015; pp. 1071–1072.

McKnight KL. Ingestion of over-the-counter calcium supplements. Vet Tech 2006; 446–447, 451.

Murphy LA. Toxicities from over the counter drugs. In: Kahn CM, ed. Merck Veterinary Manual, 9th edn. Whitehouse Station, NJ: Merck, 2005.

Acknowledgment: The authors and editors acknowledge the prior contributions of Dana L. Clarke, VMD, and Justine A. Lee, DVM, DACVECC, who authored this topic in the previous edition.

Author: Charlotte Means, DVM, MLIS, DABVT, DABT

Consulting Editor: Ahna G. Brutlag, DVM, MS, DABT, DABVT

Drugs: Veterinary Prescription

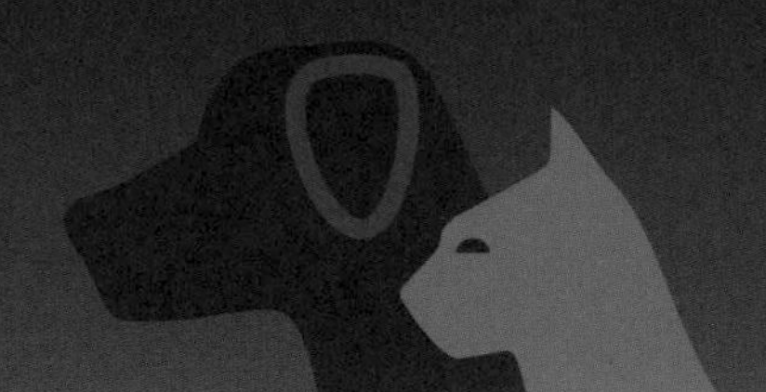

chapter 48

$Alpha_2$-Adrenergic Agonists

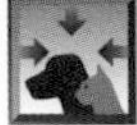

DEFINITION/OVERVIEW

- $Alpha_2$-adrenergic agonists are a widely used class of sedatives in veterinary medicine. They produce dose-dependent sedation, analgesia, and muscle relaxation.
  - The most commonly used $alpha_2$-adrenergic agonists in the veterinary setting are the injectable products xylazine, detomidine, romifidine, and dexmedetomidine.
- $Alpha_2$-adrenergic agonists are also used in human medicine as antihypertensive agents, to treat glaucoma, in the treatment of the abuse of alcohol, narcotics, and cocaine, and as an aid in smoking cessation.
  - Human $alpha_2$-adrenergic agonists include medications and formulations: clonidine (tablet and patch), brimonidine (ophthalmic solution and topical gel), guanfacine (tablet), and tizanidine (tablet).
- All drugs in this class can be rapidly and completely reversed with $alpha_2$ antagonists.

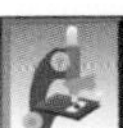

ETIOLOGY/PATHOPHYSIOLOGY

Mechanism of Action

- These agents have agonist actions on the alpha-adrenergic receptors.
  - $Alpha_1$ receptors produce arousal, excitement, and increased locomotor activity.
  - $Alpha_{2A}$ receptors mediate sedation, supraspinal analgesia, centrally mediated bradycardia, and hypotension.
  - $Alpha_{2B}$ receptors mediate the initial increase in vascular resistance and reflex bradycardia.
  - $Alpha_{2C}$ receptors mediate hypothermia.
- Receptor selectivity ratios, $alpha_2/alpha_1$, are as follows.
  - Xylazine 160:1
  - Detomidine 260:1
  - Romifidine 340:1
  - Brimonidine 1000:1
  - Dexmedetomidine 1620:1
- There is inhibition of norepinephrine and dopamine storage and release.

Blackwell's Five-Minute Veterinary Consult Clinical Companion: Small Animal Toxicology, Second Edition.
Lynn R. Hovda, Ahna G. Brutlag, Robert H. Poppenga, and Katherine L. Peterson.

Companion website: www.fiveminutevet.com/toxicology

Pharmacokinetics – Absorption, Distribution, Metabolism, Excretion

- Alpha agonists are well absorbed across the oral mucosa or sublingually.
- There is rapid absorption following IM administration and rapid onset with IV administration.
- The agents are highly water soluble.
- The volume of distribution of dexmedetomidine is 0.9 L/kg.
- Elimination is via biotransformation in the liver to inactive metabolites excreted primarily in the urine.
- The half-life of dexmedetomidine is 40–50 minutes in dogs and 1 hour in cats.

Toxicity

- Dogs exposed to very small amounts of brimonidine ophthalmic solution from puncturing the bottle have showed clinical effects including hypotension and bradycardia.
- Clonidine doses as low as 0.01 mg/kg have caused lethargy, ataxia, and bradycardia in dog cases reported to the ASPCA Animal Poison Control Center (APCC).
- Toxicosis from the injectable veterinary alpha$_2$-adrenergic agonists has been seen with 2–5 times the normal IV dose and 10 times the normal IM dose.
- Intensity and duration of effect are dose dependent.

Systems Affected

- Cardiovascular – **hypotension** common. Initial brief period of hypertension caused by activation of peripheral postsynaptic alpha$_2$ receptors. This leads to vascular smooth muscle contraction and vasoconstriction, with reflex **bradycardia**. Cardiac output can decrease by 30–50%.
- Sinus bradycardia and atrioventricular (AV) block can be seen following administration of alpha$_2$ agonists.
- Nervous – **CNS depression** as evidenced by sedation and anxiolysis. Analgesia (somatic and visceral) and muscle relaxation. **Hypothermia** may occur as a result of depression to the thermoregulatory center, muscle relaxation, and decreased shivering.
- Gastrointestinal – **vomiting** is common immediately following administration. There may be decreased GI secretions in addition to varying effects on intestinal muscle tone.
- Urinary – increased urine output due to action of antidiuretic hormone on the renal tubules and collecting ducts producing dilute urine.
- Endocrine – transient hypoinsulinemia and hyperglycemia due to receptor-mediated inhibition of insulin release from the pancreatic beta cells.
- Respiratory – depression, decreased respiratory rate, and possible apnea can occur.

SIGNALMENT/HISTORY

- Any age or breed of dog or cat.
- Xylazine comes in two concentrations, 20 mg/mL and 100 mg/mL, and overdose can occur when the 100 mg/mL is mistakenly used in place of 20 mg/mL.

Location and Circumstances of Poisoning

- Toxicosis from the injectable veterinary alpha$_2$-adrenergic agonists most often occurs in a veterinary setting due to iatrogenic administration of an improper dose.
- Toxicosis from the human alpha$_2$-adrenergic agonists most often occurs in the owner's home and is due to a pet chewing on the owner's pills, patch, or bottle of ophthalmic solution.

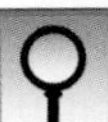

CLINICAL FEATURES

- The onset of clinical signs is rapid (seconds to minutes).
- The duration of signs depends on the drug. However, as all are easily reversible, signs typically only last until the reversal agent is administered.
- CNS depression, ataxia, sedation, and hypothermia. May see muscle twitching.
- Bradycardia, AV block, decreased myocardial contractility and cardiac output, initial hypertension followed by hypotension. Pale (or cyanotic) oral mucous membranes may also be seen.
- Decreased respiratory rate with possible apnea.
- Vomiting.
- Death may occur from circulatory failure and severe pulmonary congestion.

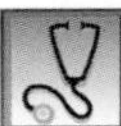

DIFFERENTIAL DIAGNOSIS

- Intoxication with beta-blockers, calcium channel blockers, ivermectin, marijuana, and opioids.

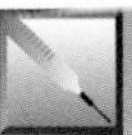

DIAGNOSTICS

- ECG – sinus bradycardia and second-degree AV block.
- Blood glucose – hyperglycemia due to decreased insulin.
- Blood pressure – hypertension followed by hypotension.

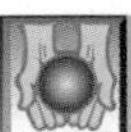

THERAPEUTICS

- All drugs can be rapidly reversed with alpha$_2$ antagonists.
- Overall, treatment consists of general supportive care, protection of the airway, and potentially, mechanical ventilation.
- Monitor heart rate and rhythm, blood pressure, body temperature, urine output, and glucose levels.

Detoxification

- If the alpha$_2$-adrenergic agonist was a pill or patch and was ingested, induction of emesis is recommended within 30 minutes, if the patient is asymptomatic.

- Activated charcoal, given early for a pill or patch ingestion, may reduce the amount of systemically absorbed drug. Absorption is rapid.
- Clinical signs following exposure to brimonidine ophthalmic solution are usually due to absorption across the oral mucosa so emetics and activated charcoal are not warranted.

Appropriate Health Care

- Reversal with IM atipamezole.
- IV crystalloid fluids to treat hypotension and increased urination.
- IV anticholinergic therapy such as atropine or glycopyrrolate to treat severe bradycardia and hypotension. Atropine may increase myocardial oxygen demand, as well as potentiate GI stasis, so use with caution.

Antidotes and Drugs of Choice

- The $alpha_2$ agonists can be rapidly and completely antagonized by $alpha_2$ antagonists.
- There are three available antagonists: atipamezole (Antisedan®), yohimbine, and tolazoline.
- Atipamezole is highly selective for the $alpha_2$ receptors and does not create significant hypotension.
  - Atipamezole is marketed as the reversal agent for dexmedetomidine but will also reverse all other $alpha_2$ agonist drugs.
  - It is recommended to give atipamezole IM due to the potential to create excitement and tachycardia. It can be given IV in emergency situations.
  - Reversal should take into consideration the amount of agonist given and the time duration since the agonist was administered.
  - Dose for detomidine or dexmedetomidine – give the same amount of atipamazole as was given of detomidine or dexmedetomidine.
  - Dose for other $alpha_2$ agonist drugs – 50 μg/kg, give one-quarter to one-third of the dose IV and the rest IM to avoid furthering hypotension; if not improved in 30–60 minutes, can try a little more IV.
- Yohimbine (0.025–0.1 mg/kg IV slowly to effect for dogs) and tolazoline (4 mg/kg IV slow for dogs) produce variable effects and also antagonize $alpha_1$ receptors. This may lead to hypotension.
- Antagonism results in enhanced sympathetic outflow.
- It is better to underdose the antagonist, as side effects from an overdose include excitement, muscle tremors, hypotension, tachycardia, salivation, and diarrhea. Large doses of antagonists will also reverse analgesia.
- An additional dose of the antagonist may be needed if the clinical signs reoccur. The half-life of atipamezole is longer than yohimbine so may need less frequent dosing.

Nursing Care

- Monitor the patient for bradycardia and hypotension.
- Monitor for respiratory depression and hypoventilation.
- Watch fluid balance due to increased urination.

COMMENTS

Patient Monitoring

- ECG and heart rate
- Blood pressure
- Blood glucose
- Urination

Prevention/Avoidance

- Be aware of proper dosing and drug concentration.
- Inform owners of the risk their alpha$_2$ agonist drugs present to their pets if ingested, especially brimonidine ophthalmic solution.

Expected Course and Prognosis

- The prognosis for alpha$_2$ agonist overdose is excellent with proper supportive care and prompt use of a reversal agent.

Synonyms

Alpha$_2$-adrenergic agonist intoxication, alpha$_2$-adrenergic agonist poisoning

See Also

Amitraz
Decongestants (Imidazolines)

Abbreviations

See Appendix 1 for a complete list.

Suggested Reading

Lemke KA. Anticholinergics and sedatives. In: Tranquilli WJ, Thurmon JC, Grimm KA, eds. Lumb & Jones Veterinary Anesthesia and Analgesia, 4th edn. Ames, IA: Blackwell, 2007; pp. 203–239.

Mensching D. Nervous system toxicity. In: Gupta RC, ed. Veterinary Toxicology: Basic and Clinical Principles, 2nd edn. Amsterdam: Elsevier, 2012; pp. 212–213.

Welch SL, Richardson JA. Clinical effects of brimonidine ophthalmic drops ingestion in 52 dogs. Vet Hum Toxicol 2002; 44:34–35.

Acknowledgment: The authors and editors acknowledge the prior contributions of Jane Quandt, DVM, MS, DACVA, DACVECC, who authored this topic in the previous edition.
Author: Camille DeClementi, VMD, DABT, DABVT
Consulting Editor: Ahna G. Brutlag, DVM, MS, DABT, DABVT

chapter 49

Ivermectin/Milbemycin/Moxidectin

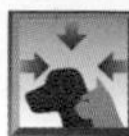

DEFINITION/OVERVIEW

- Ivermectin, milbemycin, selamectin, doramectin, eprinomectin, moxidectin, and abamectin are macrocyclic lactone derivatives used either as anthelmintics and heartworm preventatives in veterinary medicine (see Fig. 49.1) or as environmental pesticides (e.g., abamectin, an insecticide).

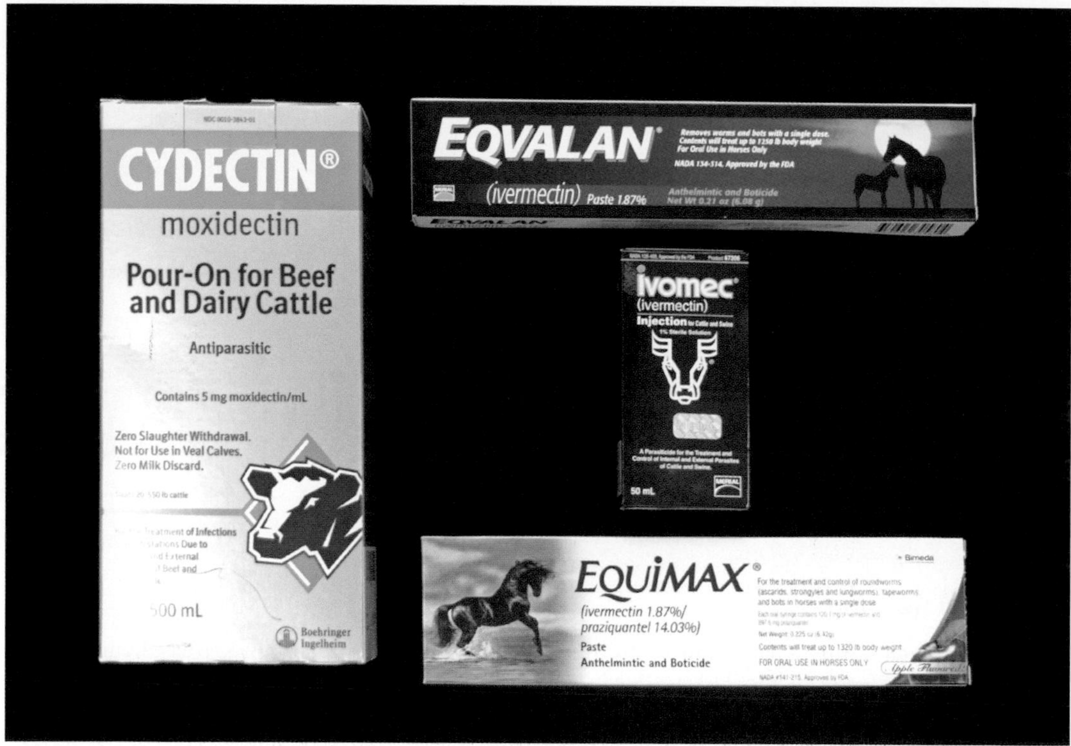

■ **Fig. 49.1.** Selected large animal products containing macrocyclic lactones. Because of the high concentration of macrocyclic lactones in large animal formulations, very small volumes can be toxic to dogs and cats, especially those with defective P-glycoprotein function.

Blackwell's Five-Minute Veterinary Consult Clinical Companion: Small Animal Toxicology, Second Edition.
Lynn R. Hovda, Ahna G. Brutlag, Robert H. Poppenga, and Katherine L. Peterson.

Companion website: www.fiveminutevet.com/toxicology

- Toxicosis can occur when small animals ingest formulations intended for use as pesticides, for use in large animals or when excessive amounts of products for small animals are consumed. In addition, when animals that are sensitive to these drugs due to MDR1 (multidrug resistance) gene mutations (in dogs, this is known as the MDR1 or ABCB1-1Δ mutation; in cats, it is known as ABCB11930_1931del TC), even therapeutic amounts of these drugs can result in toxicosis.
- Clinical signs of toxicosis include lethargy, ataxia, hypersalivation, mydriasis, blindness, and seizures. Toxicosis can be fatal, especially in sensitive breeds.
- Treatment entails decontamination, activated charcoal administration, intensive monitoring, and supportive care. The use of intravenous lipid emulsion (ILE) therapy has also been explored.
- With appropriate supportive care, prognosis for recovery is often good. However, intensive respiratory, cardiovascular, and neurological monitoring, mechanical ventilation, and prolonged hospitalization may be necessary.

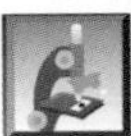

ETIOLOGY/PATHOPHYSIOLOGY

Mechanism of Action

- Ivermectin, selamectin, doramectin, and eprinomectin are antiparasitic drugs that belong to a class of compounds known as avermectins.
- Milbemycin and moxidectin, which is a derivative of milbemycin, belong to the milbemycin group of antiparasitics.
- Abamectin is an insecticide or pesticide licensed under several different trade names for indoor and outdoor use to control insects such as roaches or ants.
- The avermectins and milbemycins are similar in structure, mechanism of action, and effectiveness, and are collectively known as macrocyclic lactones.
- Macrocyclic lactones are fermentation products from *Streptomyces* species. They are highly lipophilic and have excellent activity against nematodes and arthropods.
- Selective toxicity toward arthropod and helminth parasites and sparing mammalian hosts depend on an intact BBB. In particular, P-glycoprotein must be present and functional. Toxicosis in veterinary species results when the drug binds to postsynaptic GABA-gated chloride channels in the CNS, which results in inhibition of neuronal impulse transmission. In most veterinary patients, P-glycoprotein's drug efflux function prevents toxicosis when macrocyclic lactones are used at therapeutic doses.

Pharmacokinetics – Absorption, Distribution, Metabolism, Excretion

- Absorption after oral administration is rapid. Peak plasma concentrations occur at 2 hours after moxidectin administration and 4 hours after ivermectin administration.
- Absorption after SQ drug administration is slower than orally. However, there is better bioavailability after SQ administration.
- They are highly lipophilic and extensively distributed to various tissues, especially fat. Moxidectin has a higher volume of distribution compared to ivermectin.

- The lipophilic nature of these drugs, combined with low plasma clearance, contributes to their long persistence in the body. Moxidectin has an approximately eight-fold longer elimination half-life than ivermectin.
- Canine ivermectin half-life: 3.3 days; moxidectin: 25.9 days.
- Ivermectin and moxidectin are primarily eliminated unchanged in the feces via P-glycoprotein-mediated biliary and enterocyte excretion.
- Although specific pharmacokinetic information about milbemycin, doramectin, eprinomectin, and abamectin in dogs and cats is not available, their similar structure and mechanism of action likely indicate similar pharmacokinetics to other macrocyclic lactones.

Toxicity

- While there are dosage levels at which animals have been described to show clinical signs after ingestion, it is important to remember that each animal's reaction can be variable, especially if P-glycoprotein dysfunction is present due to either genetic mutations or drug–drug interactions (ketoconazole, spinosad, and potentially other drugs are potent P-glycoprotein inhibitors) (see Signalment/History). It is important to note that all FDA-approved heartworm prevention products have been tested for safety in dogs with the MDR1 mutation and are considered safe in these dogs if used at the manufacturer's recommended dose. Review of the drug's package insert will often provide additional safety/toxicology information.

Ivermectin

- For dogs with normal P-glycoprotein function, dosages up to 2.5 mg/kg can be tolerated without clinical signs. Doses ≥2.5 mg/kg may cause mydriasis.
- Tremors can be seen at ≥5 mg/kg; severe tremors and ataxia at ≥10 mg/kg.
- Reported fatalities at 40 mg/kg.
- The reported LD_{50} in experimental Beagle models is 80 mg/kg.
- Dogs affected by the P-glycoprotein deletion can tolerate doses up to 0.1 mg/kg.
- The LD_{50} in ivermectin-sensitive Collies is 0.15–0.2 mg/kg.
- Cats can tolerate oral doses of 0.75 mg/kg, though some reports indicate they are tolerant of higher doses.
- Clinical signs of ivermectin toxicosis in cats and kittens has been reported at doses of 0.3–0.4 mg/kg.

Moxidectin

- No clinical signs at 0.9 mg/kg, which is 300 times higher than the oral pharmacological dose.
- Clinical signs were observed in a Collie after 0.09 mg/kg.

Milbemycin

- Beagles ingesting 100 mg/kg of milbemycin were reported to show no adverse clinical signs, which is 200 time the monthly oral pharmacological dose.

- Hypersalivation, ataxia, mydriasis, and depression were observed in some Collies at dosages of 5 mg/kg and all Collies at the 10 mg/kg dose in one study.
- Information about toxicosis of milbemycin in cats is not available.

Systems Affected

Nervous

- Toxicosis primarily affects the CNS by binding to GABA-gated channels, which causes cell membrane hyperpolarization and subsequent inhibition of neuronal depolarization.
- Severity of CNS signs increases with dose.

Ophthalmic

- Ophthalmic changes include mydriasis, central blindness, multifocal retinal edema, retinal folds, and changes in the ERG.

Gastrointestinal

- Hypersalivation, vomiting, anorexia, diarrhea.

Respiratory

- Severe progression of neurological impairment secondary to macrocyclic lactone ingestion can cause hypoventilation and respiratory failure.
- In vomiting patients, or those with neurological compromise that are unable to protect their airway, aspiration pneumonia is a possible complication of this toxicosis.

Cardiovascular

- In patients with a significant microfilaria burden, anaphylactic shock after sudden microfilaria death can cause severe hypotension and shock.

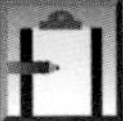

SIGNALMENT/HISTORY

- Dogs and cats of any age, breed, or sex can be affected by this toxicosis.
- Toxicosis is more commonly reported in dogs.
- Pediatric animals are thought to be at higher risk for developing toxicosis due to incomplete development of the BBB.
- Many breeds of dogs, in particular Collies, Australian Shepherds, Longhaired Whippets, Silken Windhounds, Shetland Sheepdogs, German Shepherds and similar breeds, harbor a 4-base pair deletion of the MDR1 gene (current nomenclature ATP-binding cassette 1 or ABCB1) known as the MDR1 mutation or ABCB1-1Δ mutation. Dogs with this mutation have either no (MDR1 mutant/mutant) or decreased (MDR1 mutant/normal) P-glycoprotein in the BBB, resulting in increased CNS penetration and neurotoxic effects of macrocyclic lactones.
- Approximately 5% of cats have a 2-base pair deletion mutation of the MDR1 (ABCB1) gene. Affected cats display the same sensitivity to macrocyclic lactones as dogs affected by the MDR1 mutation.

Risk Factors

- Use of macrocyclic lactone antiparasitic therapies.
- Access to large animal macrocyclic lactone formulation.
- Ingestion of feces from large animals recently treated with macrocyclic lactones.
- Mutations in the MDR1 (ABCB1) gene (dogs or cats).
- Concurrent administration of drugs that inhibit P-glycoprotein function, such as spinosad or ketoconazole.

Historical Findings

- If ingestion is witnessed by the owner or packaging material is found, the owner may report that their pet ingested a macrocyclic lactone medication or pesticide.

Location and Circumstances of Poisoning

- Any area where the pet has access to either the medications (e.g., home, garage, barn, farm, etc.) or pesticides.
- Inadvertent overdose by a veterinarian (home/farm call or in the veterinary hospital setting).
- Access to areas where large animals recently treated with these medications defecate (e.g., fields, paddocks, barn, etc.).
- Use of large animal formulations to treat small animals.

Interactions with Drugs, Nutrients, or Environment

- Concurrent administration of drugs that decrease or inhibit the function of p-glycoprotein.
    - Spinosad
    - Ketoconazole
    - Verapamil
    - Tamoxifen
    - Cyclosporine

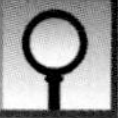

CLINICAL FEATURES

- Nervous – ataxia, weakness, disorientation, paddling, head pressing (seen in cats), tremors, seizures, coma.
- Ophthalmic – mydriasis, central blindness, retinal edema (may be multifocal), retinal folds, attenuated or extinguished ERG wave amplitude (measure of retinal function).
- Gastrointestinal – hypersalivation, vomiting.
- Respiratory – hypoventilation, poor chest excursions (e.g., intercostal breathing).
- Cardiovascular – hyperthermia, hypothermia, bradycardia, hypotension.

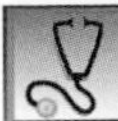

DIFFERENTIAL DIAGNOSIS

- Anticholinesterase insecticide ingestion
- Tremorgenic mycotoxin ingestion
- Ethylene glycol ingestion
- Benzodiazepine ingestion
- Barbiturate ingestion
- Opioid intoxication
- Lead toxicosis
- Metabolic disease – hepatic encephalopathy, portosystemic shunt, etc.
- Primary ophthalmic disease

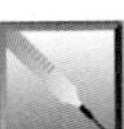

DIAGNOSTICS

- Depending on the patient's clinical status, diagnostics to assess the stability of the patient should take priority over confirmatory testing. Such emergency diagnostics may include the following.
  - Electrolytes, PCV/TS, blood glucose, BUN, creatinine
  - Blood pressure
  - Pulse oximetry
  - Arterial blood gas (to assess oxygenation and ventilation) or venous blood gas (to assess ventilation)
  - ECG
- Liquid chromatography mass spectroscopy to determine drug levels.
  - Can be performed on serum, adipose tissue, and liver samples.
  - If animal does not have an MDR1 mutation, serum levels correlate with clinical signs, as clinical signs are dependent on the concentration of the drug in the brain. The concentration of macrocyclic lactones in the brain of animals with dysfunctional P-glycoprotein will be much higher for any given serum concentration than in "normal" animals.
- MDR1 genotyping.
  - Should be considered in all susceptible breeds and mixed breed dogs as well as any canine patient whose clinical signs do not correlate with the amount of macrocyclic lactone ingested.
  - Requires either a cheek swab or EDTA blood sample sent to the Veterinary Clinical Pharmacology Laboratory, College of Veterinary Medicine, Washington State University, Pullman, WA 99164-6610 (www.vcpl.vetmed.wsu.edu).
  - Email the Veterinary Clinical Pharmacology Laboratory (vcpl@vetmed.wsu.edu) to inquire about MDR1 genotyping in cats.
- Fundoscopy.
  - Can be performed via direct or indirect ophthalmoscopy.
- ERG.
  - Allows for assessment of the neurosensory activity of the retina.
  - Requires specialized equipment and training.

Pathological Findings

- There are no characteristic gross or histopathological lesions.

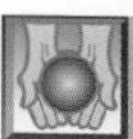

THERAPEUTICS

- Treatment entails decontamination, supportive care, and intensive monitoring.

Detoxification

- In neurologically appropriate patients, emesis should be induced as quickly and safely as possible.
- For neurologically inappropriate, symptomatic patients, initial treatment should be aimed at managing neurological signs, such as seizures. Sedation, intubation, and gastric lavage may also be considered.
- Due to enterohepatic recirculation, repeated doses of activated charcoal are indicated. Only the first dose should contain a cathartic. Administration of activated charcoal via a stomach tube for intubated patients may be necessary, with an inflated ETT to prevent secondary aspiration pneumonia.

Appropriate Health Care

- Seizures must be aggressively controlled to prevent cerebral edema, noncardiogenic pulmonary edema, and aspiration of GIT contents. Intubation may be necessary.
- Serum electrolytes (e.g., sodium, potassium, glucose) should be monitored and treated if needed for patients receiving multiple doses of activated charcoal, large amounts of IV fluids, and those with seizures.
- Frequent lung auscultation as well as serial measurement of blood oxygenation (e.g., pulse oximetry, arterial blood gas) should be performed in patients where aspiration pneumonia is a concern. Mechanical ventilation is indicated for patients with severe hypoxemia unresponsive to supplemental oxygen therapy.
- Ventilation should be closely monitored in patients with severe neurological impairment using venous or arterial (preferred) pCO_2 or end-tidal capnography. Mechanical ventilation is indicated for patients with hypoventilation.
- Continuous ECG can be used in patients with concerning bradycardia.

Drugs and Antidotes of Choice

- There is no antidote.
- For control of tremors or seizures, patients can be loaded with phenobarbital (2–4 mg/kg IV as needed to control seizures, up to 16 mg/kg) or levetiracetam (Keppra, 20 mg/kg IV q 8 hours). The lowest effect dose should be used, due to the risks of severe sedation.
- The authors have experience with using ILE to help treat dogs with ivermectin toxicosis. ILE is thought to create a lipid partition or "sink" within the intravascular space, which

helps to contain the lipophilic macrocyclic lactone in the vasculature, and therefore prevent penetration into the brain. There is also a published case report describing the use of ILE to treat a puppy with suspected moxidectin toxicosis. Unfortunately, ILE has not been helpful in treating macrocyclic lactone toxicosis in dogs with the MDR1 mutation (three cases described in the literature). The reader is encouraged to contact an established veterinary toxicology helpline or toxicologist if he or she wishes to use this therapy, as it is still considered experimental in veterinary medicine.

Precautions/Interactions

- Benzodiazepines (e.g., midazolam, diazepam) should be avoided for tremor or seizure management, as these drugs may potentiate the CNS toxicosis due to GABA binding leading to prolonged recovery.
- The use of physostigmine is not currently recommended.
- Picrotoxin is a GABA antagonist that has been used to treat a case of ivermectin toxicosis. However, it can cause seizures and is therefore not recommended.

Alternative Drugs

- If tremors or seizures do not respond to phenobarbital or levetiracetam, propofol (1–2 mg/kg IV bolus, 0.1–0.2 mg/kg/min CRI) or etomidate (0.5–4 mg/kg IV) may be used. Etomidate should not be used as a sole agent.

Nursing Care

- Intensive neurological monitoring (e.g., mentation, menace, visual ability, pupil size, PLR, ambulation, etc.) should be carried out every 2–4 hours, especially in patients with neurological impairment at presentation.
- Care should be provided for recumbent patients, including frequent turning, passive range of motion, bladder and colon care, and eye and oral care.
- Special attention should be given to patients with central blindness to protect their corneas with frequent lubrication and prevent trauma to the eyes since patients may not blink as a protective mechanism.
- For patients with seizures and any concerns for cerebral edema, a board under the head and neck, positioned at a 15–30° angle, should be used to help decrease ICP. Compression of the jugular veins (especially for venipuncture) and hyperthermia should be avoided in such patients. If tolerated, supplemental oxygen via a mask should be considered for all recumbent, neurological patients.
- Body temperature should be measured frequently. Heat support should be used for patients with hypothermia but should be discontinued when the body temperature has reached 99°F. In addition, gentle cooling measures, such as wetting of the fur and a fan, can be used for patients with hyperthermia. Cooling measures should be stopped once the patient's temperature has reached 103.5°F to prevent rebound hypothermia.

Follow-up

- Depending on the patient's clinical course, it is likely that follow-up care and monitoring will not be necessary after discharge.
- Patients that may require follow-up include those that develop aspiration pneumonia or severe seizures and neurological impairment.

Diet

- For patients with any neurological compromise, vomiting, regurgitation, or those that are sedated, oral food and water should be withheld until the patient is neurologically appropriate and any GIT signs have resolved.
- In patients with prolonged neurological compromise, recumbency, or those that require mechanical ventilation, parenteral nutrition may be necessary.

Activity

- Activity restriction is not necessary, as the patient's neurological status will likely determine its activity level.
- Patients with any visual impairment should be assisted and monitored closely when navigating unfamiliar surroundings.

Prevention

- Proper storage of antiparasitic medications (see Fig. 49.2).
- Ensuring correct dosage, particularly when large animal formulations are used.
- Preventing access to feces from large animals recently treated with these medications.
- Restrict animal's access to areas treated with macrocyclic lactone pesticides.
- MDR1 genotyping in all animals with toxicosis to rule out ABCB1 mutations.

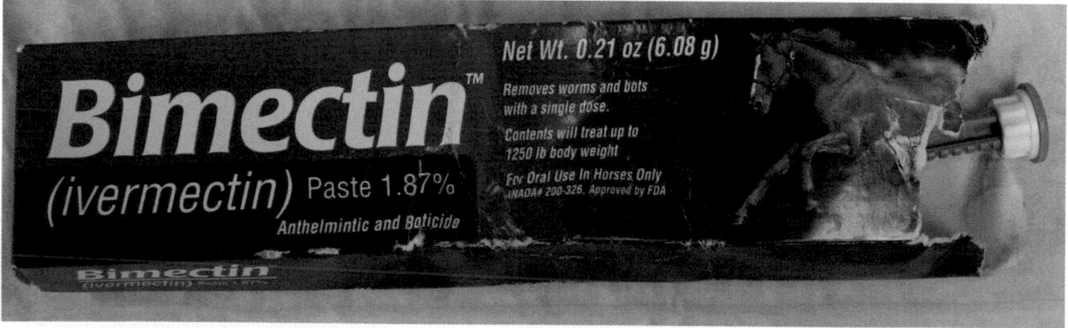

Fig. 49.2. A tube of equine ivermectin antihelmintic chewed by a dog. Ingestion of equine macrocyclic lactone antihelmintics is the most common cause of this toxicosis reported to the Pet Poison Helpline. Photo courtesy of Dana L. Clarke.

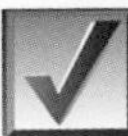

COMMENTS

Client Education

- Clients should be educated on the mechanism of action of toxicosis, as well as being given recommendations for safe storage and use options.
- Information should be provided about the gradual reintroduction of a bland diet, monitoring for ongoing GIT and neurological signs, and general observation instructions.
- For patients confirmed to be affected with the ABCB1 mutations, recommendations on other medications that must be avoided should be made (e.g., loperamide – see "Problem Drug" list at www.vcpl.vetmed.wsu.edu).

Possible Complications

- Aspiration pneumonia.
- Hypoventilation or hypoxemia requiring mechanical ventilation.

Expected Course and Prognosis

- The prognosis for recovery ingestion is largely dependent on dose and MDR1 genotype. Animals ingesting a larger dose, or those that lack functional P-glycoprotein at the BBB, are expected to require more intensive care and will likely have a more prolonged recovery.
- Duration to recovery can vary from days to weeks.
- Patients requiring more intensive care, especially mechanical ventilation, will also have increased costs associated with hospitalization, which may affect prognosis due to an owner's financial capabilities.
- Animals that recover usually have no long-term complications secondary to this toxicosis.

Synonyms

Ivermectin toxicosis/intoxication, milbemycin toxicosis/intoxication, moxidectin toxicosis/intoxication, macrolide toxicosis/intoxication

Abbreviations

See Appendix 1 for a complete list.

ABCB1 = ATP-binding cassette protein 1
BBB = blood–brain barrier
ERG = electroretinogram
ETT = endotracheal tube
GABA = gamma aminobutyric acid
ICP = intracranial pressure
ILE = intravenous lipid emulsion
MDR1 = multidrug resistance gene 1

Suggested Reading

Al-Azzam SI, Fleckstein L, Cheng K, et al. Comparison of the pharmacokinetics of moxidectin and ivermectin after oral administration to beagle dogs. Biopharm Drug Disposition 2007; 28:431–438.

Beal MW, Poppenga RH, Birdsall WJ, et al. Respiratory failure attributable to moxidectin intoxication in a dog. J Am Vet Med Assoc 1999; 215(12):1813–1817.

Crandell DE, Weinberg GL. Moxidectin toxicosis in a puppy successfully treated with intravenous lipids. J Vet Emerg Crit Care 2009; 19(2):181–186.

Hopper K, Aldrich J, Haskins SC. Ivermectin toxicity in 17 collies. J Vet Int Med 2002; 16:89–94.

Kenny PJ, Vernau KM, Puschner B, et al. Retinopathy associated with ivermectin toxicosis in two dogs. J Am Vet Med Assoc 2008; 233(2):279–284.

Mealey KL. Ivermectin: macrolide antiparasitic agents. In: Peterson ME, Talcott PA, eds. Small Animal Toxicology, 2nd edn. St Louis, MO: Elsevier, 2006.

Wright HM, Chen AV, Talcott PA, Poppenga RH, Mealey KL. Intravenous fat emulsion as treatment for ivermectin toxicosis in three dogs homozygous for the ABCB1-1D gene mutation. J Vet Emerg Crit Care 2011; 21(6):666–672.

Acknowledgment: The authors and editors acknowledge the prior contributions of Justine A. Lee, DVM, DACVECC, DABT, who co-authored this topic in the previous edition.

Authors: Katrina L. Mealey, DVM, PhD, DACVIM, DACVCP; Dana L. Clarke, VMD, DACVECC.
Consulting Editor: Ahna G. Brutlag, DVM, MS, DABT, DABVT

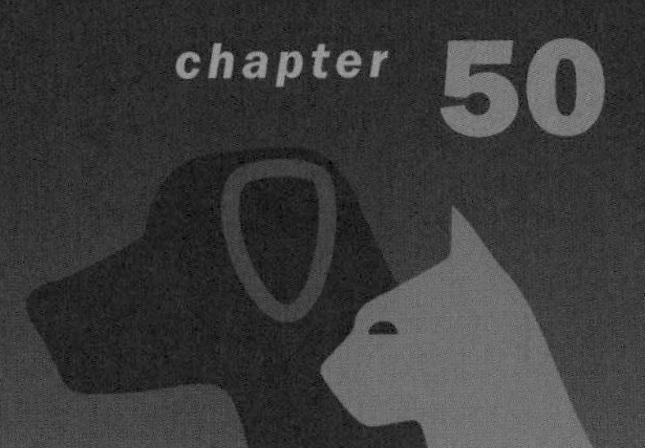

chapter 50

Phenylpropanolamine

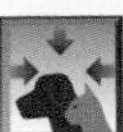

DEFINITION/OVERVIEW

- Phenylpropanolamine (PPA) is a sympathomimetic drug commonly used for the medical treatment of female urinary incontinence (urethral sphincter hypotonus).
- Overdoses are associated with tachycardia or reflex bradycardia, hypertension, agitation, excitability, tremors, urinary retention, and seizures.
- PPA is commonly available as flavored chewable tablets (Proin 25, 50, and 75 mg) and liquid (Proin drops 25 mg/mL), but multiple formulations are available through various manufacturers and compounding pharmacies.
- Intoxication is often due to animals ingesting large amounts of chewable medications.

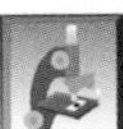

ETIOLOGY/PATHOPHYSIOLOGY

Mechanism of Action

- PPA is a sympathomimetic agent that primarily works via alpha-adrenergic receptor stimulation, which leads to its therapeutic effect of smooth muscle contraction in the urethra.
- The drug is also believed to increase norepinephrine release and have an effect on $beta_1$ receptors but has no reported effect on $beta_2$ receptors.

Pharmacokinetics – Absorption, Distribution, Metabolism, Excretion

- Absorption – well absorbed orally with good bioavailability, approximately 98%.
- Distribution – distributed widely throughout the body, including the CNS.
- Metabolism – partially metabolized by the liver into active metabolites; no enterohepatic recirculation.
- Excretion – 80–90% is excreted unchanged in urine within 24 hours. The half-life is generally within 3–4 hours.

Toxicity

- No known LD_{50} exists in veterinary medicine.

Blackwell's Five-Minute Veterinary Consult Clinical Companion: Small Animal Toxicology, Second Edition.
Lynn R. Hovda, Ahna G. Brutlag, Robert H. Poppenga, and Katherine L. Peterson.

Companion website: www.fiveminutevet.com/toxicology

- A recently published retrospective study reported clinical signs at doses as low as 1.9 mg/kg, just under the therapeutic dose (2 mg/kg PO 12 hours) but significant signs are not anticipated at this dose.
- Overdoses of 2–3 times the therapeutic dose should be decontaminated and monitored for at least 8 hours.

Systems Affected

- Cardiovascular – hypertension, tachycardia/tachyarrhythmias, reflex bradycardia, myocardial dysfunction.
- Gastrointestinal – anorexia, salivation and vomiting.
- Hemic – DIC (sequela to prolonged seizure activity and hyperthermia).
- Hepatobiliary – elevated liver enzymes.
- Musculoskeletal – tremors, rhabdomyolysis (sequela to prolonged seizure/tremors).
- Nervous – agitation, hyperactivity, hyperesthesia, tremors and occasionally seizures or coma.
- Ophthalmic – mydriasis (sympathomimetic stimulation), increased IOP.
- Renal/urological – urinary retention, myoglobinuria.
- Skin – piloerection, erythema.

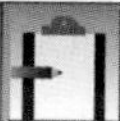

SIGNALMENT/HISTORY

- Although primarily prescribed for older spayed female dogs, any pet may ingest this medication.
- Dogs are the most common offenders.

Risk Factors

- Animals with preexisting cardiovascular disease (including hypertension), hyperthyroidism, or glaucoma may develop more severe clinical signs.
- Cats – PPA is rarely prescribed for cats as they may have signs of intoxication even at therapeutic doses.

Historical Findings

- History of accidental ingestion of medication (generally via dietary indiscretion but potentially through therapeutic error).
- Owners may report hiding, restlessness, CNS stimulation, excitability, vocalization, vomiting, anorexia, tremors, or seizures.

Interactions with Drugs, Nutrients, or Environment

- Concurrent treatment with MAOIs, SSRIs, TCAs, potentially amitraz (if inadvertent oral exposure occurs), NSAIDs, and other sympathomimetic agents.
- Benzodiazepines may exacerbate agitation.

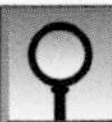

CLINICAL FEATURES

- Clinical signs noted as early as 30 minutes; typically noted within 8 hours after exposure.
- Agitation/hyperactivity.
- Piloerection.
- Erythema.
- Tachycardia.
- Bradycardia.
- Hyperthermia.
- Mydriasis.
- Hyphema/retinopathy.
- Ataxia.
- Tremors/twitching.
- Seizures.

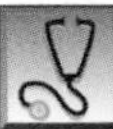

DIFFERENTIAL DIAGNOSIS

- Other intoxications that may result in similar symptoms include 5-HTP, albuterol, amphetamines/methamphetamines, anticholinergics, antihistamines, antipsychotics, benzodiazepines (paradoxical response), cocaine, hops, imidazoline, methylxanthines (caffeine, chocolate, etc.), marijuana, metaldehyde, methionine, mycotoxins, nicotine, pseudoephedrine, SSRIs, TCAs, thyroid medication (generally very large overdoses).
- Pheochromocytoma.
- Primary CNS lesion.
- Hyperthyroidism.

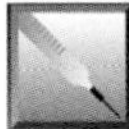

DIAGNOSTICS

- ECG – may see tachyarrhythmias or reflex bradycardia secondary to hypertension.
- Blood pressure monitoring for hypertension.
- Baseline chemistry – acute renal failure and elevated liver enzymes may be noted secondary to toxicosis.
- UA to evaluate renal function, check for tubular casts and monitor for pigmenturia and proteinuria.
- Serum CK to monitor for rhabdomyolysis.
- Coagulation panel if DIC is suspected.
- Cardiac troponin levels if suspicious for myocardial damage.
- Phenylpropanolamine levels can be detected in urine or blood via liquid and gas chromatography but this is rarely done.

Pathological Findings

- Myocardial infarction
- Pigmentary nephropathy and tubular damage
- Hemorrhagic stroke

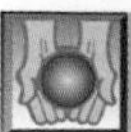

THERAPEUTICS

Detoxification

- Induce emesis within 2 hours of ingestion if the animal is asymptomatic.
- Activated charcoal with a cathartic at 1–2 g/kg PO once.

Appropriate Health Care

- Observation for 8 hours after exposure.
- IV fluids – rate will depend on blood pressure. High rates may exacerbate hypertension.
- Cooling measures as needed for hyperthermia. Stop cooling at 103.5°F.

Drugs and Antidotes of Choice

- No antidote available; provide symptomatic and supportive care for signs noted.
- Hyperactivity and hypertension – acepromazine 0.02–1.0 mg/kg IV, IM, SQ or chlorpromazine 0.5–1.0 mg/kg IV, IM as needed for sedation. Higher doses may be required. These drugs are preferred over other sedatives (see Precautions/Interactions).
- Hyperactivity – butorphanol 0.2–0.4 mg/kg IV, IM, SQ.
- Hypertension – hydralazine 0.5–3 mg/kg PO q 12 hours or nitroprusside 0.5–2 μg/kg/min IV, up to 10 μg/kg/min to effect.
- Tachycardia – propranolol 0.02–0.06 mg/kg IV slowly to effect.
- Seizures/tremors – phenobarbital 4 mg/kg IV to effect.

Precautions/Interactions

- Benzodiazepines (diazepam/midazolam) are not recommended in sympathomimetic overdoses as they may exacerbate clinical signs.
- Drugs used to treat bradycardia may exacerbate hypertension. Bradycardia is often reflexive and will resolve once hypertension is controlled.

Follow-up

- Uncomplicated cases do not require follow-up.
- Animals developing secondary complications such as cardiac dysfunction, rhabdomyolysis, DIC, or renal damage may require prolonged treatment.

Activity

- Patient should be kept in a quiet environment with minimal stimulation.

Prevention

- Secure all medications (especially chewable/flavored tablets) where they cannot be accessed by pets.

COMMENTS

Client Education

- Owner should be advised of the palatability of the tablets and about securing all medications, especially chewable/flavored tablets.
- Due to the potential for drug interactions with PPA, instruct clients not to administer other medications without veterinary approval.

Patient Monitoring

- Patient should be monitored (TPR, BP, CNS status) for 8 hours after an exposure.
- ECG and blood pressure monitoring should be frequent, ideally every 2–4 hours. Continuous ECG and blood pressure monitoring in serious cases.
- Symptomatic patients should be monitored closely for seizures.

Possible Complications

- Cardiac arrhythmias and myocardial dysfunction have been reported.
- Although not reported, myglobinuric renal failure and DIC may develop following prolonged seizures/tremors.
- Animals with preexisting renal or hepatic insufficiency may have decreased rate of drug clearance. These animals may require a longer and more aggressive course of treatment.

Expected Course and Prognosis

- Prognosis is generally good if treated early.
- Symptoms can persist for 24–72 hours depending on dose ingested.
- Animals exhibiting severe CNS symptoms or cardiac arrhythmias or developing DIC or myoglobinuria have guarded to poor prognosis.

Synonyms

PPA, Proin, Proin drops, Cystolamine, Propalin, Propalin syrup

See Also

Amphetamines
Decongestants (Pseudoephedrine, Phenylephrine)
Ephedra/Ma Huang
Methamphetamine

Abbreviations

See Appendix 1 for a complete list.

Suggested Reading

Bacon NJ, Oni O, White RAS. Treatment of the urethral sphincter mechanism incompetence in 11 bitches with a sustained-release formulation of phenylpropanolamine hydrochloride. Vet Rec 2002; 151:373–376.

Crandell JM, Ware WA. Cardiac toxicity from phenylpropanolamine overdose in a dog. J Am Anim Hosp Assoc 2005; 41:413–420.

Ginn JA, Bentley E, Stepien RL. Systemic hypertension and hypertensive retinopathy following PPA overdose in a dog. J Am Anim Hosp Assoc 2013; 49:46–53.

Peterson KL, Lee JA, Hovda LR. Phenylpropanolamine toxicosis in dogs: a review of 170 cases (2004–2009). J Am Vet Med Assoc 2011; 239:1463–1469.

Acknowledgment: The authors and editors acknowledge Nancy M. Gruber, DVM, for her previous contribution to this chapter.
Author: Katherine L. Peterson, DVM, DACVECC
Consulting Editor: Ahna G. Brutlag, DVM, MS, DABT, DABVT

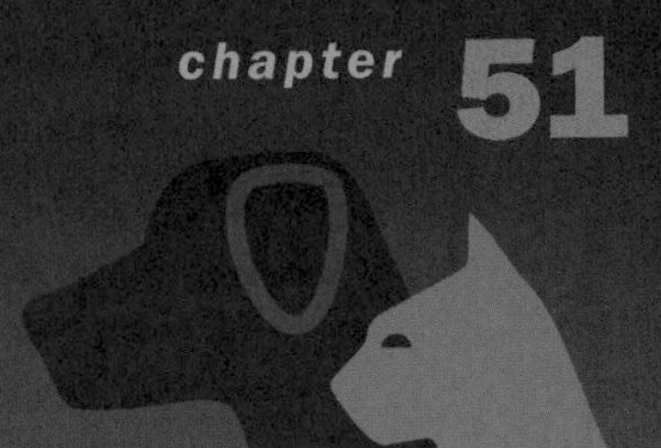

chapter 51

Pimobendan

DEFINITION/OVERVIEW

- Pimobendan is a drug used in management of canine congestive heart failure (CHF).
- The recommended dose in dogs is 0.4–0.6 mg/kg PO divided twice daily.

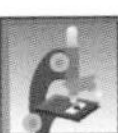

ETIOLOGY/PATHOPHYSIOLOGY

Mechanism of Action

- Pimobendan increases forward blood flow from the left ventricle.
- Pimobendan is an inodilator, with both calcium-sensitizing properties and phosphodiesterase III inhibition.
  - Inodilators have both positive inotropic (increased contractility) and vasodilating effects.
  - Pimobendan alters sensitivity of troponin C to calcium, resulting in greater actin–myosin interaction (positive inotropy).
  - Phosphodiesterase (PDE) III is expressed mainly in the heart and vascular smooth muscle. Inhibition of PDEIII causes increased contractility and vasodilation.

Pharmacokinetics – Absorption, Distribution, Metabolism, Excretion

- Pimobendan is absorbed rapidly when given orally and has a bioavailability of 60–65%.
- The onset of action is within 1 hour of administration.
- It is metabolized into its active form by the liver.
- The half-life of pimobendan in the blood is 0.4 hours and the half-life of its metabolite is 2 hours.
- Elimination is by excretion in the bile.
- Pimobendan is 90–95% bound to plasma proteins in circulation.

Toxicity

- Doses as low as 1 mg/kg have caused mild hypotension and tachycardia in dog cases reported to the ASPCA Animal Poison Control Center (APCC).

Blackwell's Five-Minute Veterinary Consult Clinical Companion: Small Animal Toxicology, Second Edition.
Lynn R. Hovda, Ahna G. Brutlag, Robert H. Poppenga, and Katherine L. Peterson.

Companion website: www.fiveminutevet.com/toxicology

- Doses up to 8 mg/kg in experimental dogs have failed to produce acute clinical signs.
- No studies have demonstrated an increased risk of sudden death or arrhythmias in dogs.
- Long-term studies have shown development of mitral valve pathology in dogs.
- Dogs receiving 10–30× the recommended dose developed myxomatous changes after 4 weeks.
    - Oral administration of clinically relevant doses for 2 years resulted in development of similar lesions in research dogs.
- Dogs receiving supraphysiological doses had elevations in alkaline phosphatase (ALP) without histological evidence of hepatotoxicity.
- One case study demonstrated a worsening of regurgitation in two dogs with mitral valve disease after pimobendan administration, which subsided upon withdrawal of the drug.
- In vitro evidence of platelet inhibition has failed to translate into clinical evidence of platelet inhibition or thrombocytopenia.
- Safety and efficacy have not been evaluated in cats. Anecdotal evidence suggests that the drug is well tolerated at doses similar to those in dogs.

Systems Affected

- Cardiovascular – possible hypotension, reflex tachycardia.
- Hepatobiliary – increased ALP.

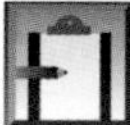

SIGNALMENT/HISTORY

Risk Factors

- Pimobendan is licensed for administration only to dogs with CHF secondary to mitral valve disease or dilated cardiomyopathy (DCM). Given the pathology of mitral and tricuspid valves with naturally occurring disease, administration of clinical doses of pimobendan is unlikely to cause additional valvular damage.
- Animals with hypertrophic cardiomyopathy (HCM), aortic stenosis, other outflow obstructions, or underlying arrhythmias may develop more severe clinical signs. However, studies of arrhythmogenesis with pimobendan have failed to demonstrate a significant proarrhythmic effect. No studies of the use of pimobendan in cats with HCM exist.
- Safety and efficacy have not been evaluated in cats. Anecdotal evidence suggests that the drug is well tolerated at doses similar to those in dogs.

Historical Findings

- Witnessed ingestion.
- Discovery of a spilled/chewed pill canister.

Location and Circumstances of Poisoning

- Usually unintended ingestion.

Interactions with Drugs, Nutrients, or Environment

- There are no known interactions with other cardiac medications. Clinical experience of combination therapy with digoxin, sildenafil, diuretics, ACE inhibitors, and antiarrhythmic agents has failed to demonstrate significant drug interactions.

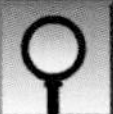

CLINICAL FEATURES

- Signs of intoxication would be expected to develop within 1–2 hours.
- Due to pimobendan's short half-life, signs would be expected to resolve in less than 6–8 hours. Hypertension seems to resolve in approximately 8 hours with little or no treatment.
- Vomiting can be seen at any dose.
- Hypotension and tachycardia are the most common signs following overdose. Doses as low as 1 mg/kg have caused mild hypotension and tachycardia in dog cases reported to the APCC.
- Hypertension was observed in about 3% of dog cases reported to the APCC. The lowest dose where hypertension was observed in a dog, without underlying cardiac disease, was 3.06 mg/kg.
- Massive overdoses may cause arrhythmias (atrial fibrillation with increased ventricular ectopic beats), syncope, and weak or irregular pulses.

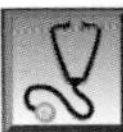

DIFFERENTIAL DIAGNOSIS

- Primary cardiac disease.
- Primary respiratory disease.
- Intoxication with other medications that cause hypotension, including other PDEIII inhibitors (amrinone, inamrinone, milrinone), erectile dysfunction drugs (sildenafil, tadalafil, vardenafil), nitroglycerin and other nitrites/nitrates, ACE inhibitors, alpha-adrenergic agents, beta-blockers, and angiotensin II blockers.

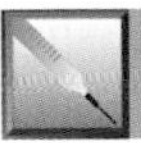

DIAGNOSTICS

- Monitor ECG, heart rate, and blood pressure for 6–8 hours.

Pathological Findings

- No changes expected acutely. In chronic dosing, cardiac histopathology can be performed but may be similar to changes seen in normal progression of heart failure.
- Chronic high-dose administration results in development of myxomatous changes of the mitral valve, consistent with changes seen with other potent inotropes (milrinone).

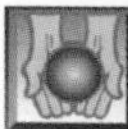

THERAPEUTICS

- Pimobendan has a wide margin of safety. It is important to note that observed clinical signs may be directly related to the animal's underlying cardiac disease rather than exposure to pimobendan.
- Preexisting cardiac disease must be taken into account when considering therapeutic intervention.

Detoxification

- With acute ingestion of large quantities of pimobendan, emesis is recommended within 1 hour, if the patient is asymptomatic.
- Activated charcoal, given early, may reduce the amount of systemically absorbed drug. Absorption is rapid.

Appropriate Health Care

- Treatment is symptomatic and supportive and based on clinical signs.

Antidotes

- There is no antidote for pimobendan toxicosis.

Drugs of Choice

- IV fluids (crystalloids and/or colloids) to control hypotension. Fluid therapy must be used judiciously in patients with underlying cardiac disease.
- Dopamine (1–3 µg/kg/min titrated up to 10 µg/kg/min IV CRI), dobutamine (5–15 µg/kg/min IV CRI), etc. may be needed for hypotension nonresponsive to IV fluids. Use with care in animals with preexisting heart disease.
- Tachycardia should resolve with control of blood pressure; beta-blockers if needed but use with care in animals with CHF or DCM.

Precautions/Interactions

- The effects of pimobendan may be attenuated by potent negative inotropes, vasoconstrictors, or calcium channel blockers.

COMMENTS

Patient Monitoring

- Monitor ECG, heart rate, and blood pressure for 6–8 hours.

Prevention/Avoidance

- Keep this and all medications in an inaccessible place away from animals.

Possible Complications

- None expected from acute overdose; chronic dosing may cause cardiac changes.

Expected Course and Prognosis

- Prognosis for acute pimobendan ingestion is good.

See Also

Angiotensin-Converting Enzyme (ACE) Inhibitors
Beta Receptor Antagonists (Beta-Blockers)
Calcium Channel Blockers

Abbreviations

See Appendix 1 for a complete list.

Suggested Reading

Chetboul V, Lefebvre HP, Sampedrano CC, et al. Comparative adverse cardiac effects of pimobendan and benazepril monotherapy in dogs with mild degenerative mitral valve disease: a prospective, controlled, blinded, and randomized study. J Vet Intern Med 2007; 21:742–753.

Häggström J, Boswood A, O'Grady M, et al. Effect of pimobendan or benazepril hydrochloride on survival times in dogs with congestive heart failure caused by naturally occurring myxomatous mitral valve disease: the QUEST study. J Vet Intern Med 2008; 22:1124–1135.

Smith PJ, French AT, van Israël N, et al. Efficacy and safety of pimobendan in canine heart failure caused by myxomatous mitral valve disease. J Small Anim Pract 2005; 46:121–130.

Tissier R, Chetboul V, Moraillon R, et al. Increased mitral valve regurgitation and myocardial hypertrophy in two dogs with long-term pimobendan therapy. Cardiovasc Toxicol 2005; 5:43–51.

Acknowledgment: The authors and editors acknowledge the prior contributions of Mark Rishniw, BVSc, MS, PhD, DACVIM, who authored this topic in the previous edition.
Author: Camille DeClementi, VMD, DABT, DABVT
Consulting Editor: Ahna G. Brutlag, DVM, MS, DABT, DABVT

chapter 52

Veterinary NSAIDs (Carprofen, Deracoxib, Firocoxib, Ketoprofen, Meloxicam, Robenacoxib, Tepoxalin)

DEFINITION/OVERVIEW

- NSAIDs are approved for use in small animals for the relief of pain and inflammation.
- They are inhibitors of COX-1, -2, and -3 as well as LOX enzymes, which decrease inflammation but can have adverse effects, most commonly on the GI tract and kidneys and at higher doses can have CNS effects. Hepatotoxicity has been reported but is suspected to be idiosyncratic.
- Veterinary NSAID drugs, formulations, and therapeutic doses.
    - Carprofen (e.g., Norocarp, Novocox, Quellin, Rimadyl, Vetprofen) is available in 25, 75, and 100 mg caplet and chewable tablets and injectable at 50 mg/mL and is approved for dogs only. Therapeutic dose: 4.4 mg/kg/day PO, IM, or SQ; can divide into q 12 dosing.
    - Deracoxib (Deramaxx) is available in chewable tablets in 25, 50, 75, 100 mg strength and is approved for dogs only. Therapeutic dose: 1–4 mg/kg PO q 24 hours.
    - Firocoxib (Previcox) is available in 57 and 227 mg chewable tablets and is approved for dogs only. An oral paste of 0.82% (8.2 mg/g) is available for use in horses. Therapeutic dog dose: 5 mg/kg PO q 24 hours.
    - Ketoprofen (Ketofen) is available in 100 mg/mL injectable multidose vials. There are oral forms approved in the UK and Canada. Ketoprofen is not approved for cats or dogs in the USA. Therapeutic dose: 0.25–2 mg/kg PO, IM, SQ, IV q 24 hours.
    - Meloxicam (e.g., Loxicom, Metacam, OroCAM) is available in oral suspension in 1.5 mg/mL, 5 mg/mL injectable. Tablets for human use (Mobic) are available in 7.5 mg and 15 mg. The injectable is approved for use in cats. Dog therapeutic dose: 0.2 mg/kg PO, IV, or SQ once then 0.1 mg/kg PO q 24 hours. Cat therapeutic dose: 0.3 mg/kg SQ once.
    - Robenacoxib (Onsior) is available in 6 mg tablets and is approved for use in cats in the United States and in dogs in Canada and other countries. Therapeutic cat dose: 1 mg/kg PO q 24 hours, for a maximum of 3 days.
    - Tepoxalin (Zubrin) is available in 30, 50, 100, and 200 mg strength and is approved for use in dogs. Therapeutic dose: 20 mg/kg PO once, then 10 mg/kg PO q 24 hours.

Blackwell's Five-Minute Veterinary Consult Clinical Companion: Small Animal Toxicology, Second Edition.
Lynn R. Hovda, Ahna G. Brutlag, Robert H. Poppenga, and Katherine L. Peterson.

Companion website: www.fiveminutevet.com/toxicology

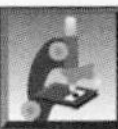

ETIOLOGY/PATHOPHYSIOLOGY

Mechanism of Action

- Carprofen, deracoxib, firocoxib, meloxicam, and robenacoxib are selective COX-2 inhibitors but may inhibit COX-1 at higher doses. Ketoprofen is a nonselective inhibitor of COX enzymes, and tepoxalin inhibits COX-1 and -2 as well as LOX enzymes.
- COX-1 enzymes serve constitutive functions in the body, which leads to the toxicity of these drugs at therapeutic doses and overdoses. COX-2 enzymes are associated with inflammation which leads to the therapeutic response.

Pharmacokinetics – Absorption, Distribution, Metabolism, Excretion

- All veterinary NSAIDs are well absorbed orally. Food will inhibit absorption of robenacoxib.
- They are highly protein bound and metabolized in the liver via glucuronidation and other hepatic metabolism.
- Enterohepatic recirculation: meloxicam (significant), carprofen (limited), ketoprofen (suspected), deracoxib (none), robenacoxib (none), tepoxalin (unknown). This will affect activated charcoal dosing during decontamination.
- Carprofen, deracoxib, firocoxib, meloxicam, robenacoxib, and tepoxalin are mainly excreted in the feces. A small amount is excreted in the urine. Ketoprofen is excreted in the urine.

Toxicity

- Dogs.
  - Acute – doses greater than five times the therapeutic dose of most veterinary NSAIDs can result in clinical signs and requires intervention.
  - Manufacturer safety data.
    - Carprofen – acute doses of 22 mg/kg resulted in GI signs.
    - Deracoxib – acute doses of >10 mg/kg resulted in GI ulceration. Doses up to 100 mg/kg did not show renal damage.
    - Firocoxib – acute doses of 50 mg/kg resulted in GI signs.
    - Meloxicam – acute doses up to five times therapeutic dose (0.1–0.5 mg/kg) resulted in some GI signs.
    - Tepoxalin – acute doses from 100 to 300 mg/kg may result in GI signs.
    - No company reported renal damage in their safety studies.
  - Manufacturer safety data may differ from postmarket experience as it is not necessarily reflective of animals with underlying medical conditions.
  - Chronic – therapeutic doses of all veterinary NSAIDs can result in clinical signs.
- Cats.
  - Manufacturer safety data.

    - ▫ Meloxicam – chronic doses of 0.3 mg/kg resulted in vomiting, diarrhea, anorexia. A black box warning for the drug states that repeated use of meloxicam in cats has been associated with acute renal failure and death.
    - ▫ Robenacoxib – chronic doses of 10 mg/kg result in vomiting, diarrhea, anorexia, and rear limb ataxia.
  - Acute and chronic doses of NSAIDs may cause toxicity, especially off-label use.

Systems affected

- Gastrointestinal – gastroenteritis, mucosal erosions, ulceration and perforation.
- Renal – tubular damage, azotemia, oliguric to anuric renal failure.
- Hemic/immune – blood loss anemia with platelet loss, platelet dysfunction, prolongation of clotting times.
- Nervous – agitation, depression, ataxia, seizures.

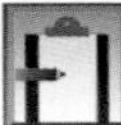

SIGNALMENT/HISTORY

- Older animals or those with underlying kidney or liver disease may be more susceptible to adverse effects. Younger pets may be more likely to retrieve medication bottles and chew on them.
- Chewable and flavored tablets pose a greater risk of massive ingestion due to palatability.
- Dogs
  - Although no specific breed or sex predilection has been proven, Labrador Retrievers may develop idiosyncratic liver toxicity from carprofen more often than other breeds.
- Cats
  - No sex or breed predilection reported.
  - More sensitive to NSAIDs than dogs due to decreased liver glucuronidation and longer elimination half-lives of most drugs.
  - Fewer products are approved for use in cats and off-label use is common.

Risk Factors

- Underlying GI, kidney, or liver disease and dehydration prior to use cause greater risk of intoxication.
- Concurrent use of steroids or other NSAIDs may contribute to GI ulceration and kidney damage.
- Chronic or off-label use may increase likelihood of developing clinical signs.

Historical Findings

- Owners may report anorexia, vomiting +/– hematemesis, diarrhea, melena or hematochezia, abdominal pain, polydipsia, and polyuria.

Location and Circumstances of Poisoning

- Most ingestions occur at home.
- Iatrogenic overdoses may occur, especially with injectable forms.

Interactions with Drugs, Nutrients, or Environment

- Toxicity may be enhanced in animals taking or concurrently ingesting:
  - ACE inhibitors, anticoagulants, aspirin, bisphosphonates, corticosteroids, ciclosporin, digoxin, fluconazole, furosemide, hepatic enzyme-inducing agents (e.g., phenobarbital), highly protein-bound drugs, methotrexate, nephrotoxic drugs, other NSAIDs, probenecid.

CLINICAL FEATURES

- Onset of clinical signs may occur within an hour after ingestion, but some signs such as renal failure or GI perforation may take 48–72 hours before they become evident.
- The most common signs will involve the GI tract and include vomiting, abdominal pain, melena, and diarrhea, which often causes secondary dehydration.
- Kidney damage will often manifest as increased drinking and urinating, anorexia, lethargy, and vomiting. Pale mucous membranes and tachycardia may occur after blood loss, hypovolemia, and poor perfusion develop.
- In severe toxicosis, CNS signs can develop, such as weakness, ataxia, and seizures; icterus may occur if liver damage is present.

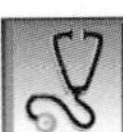

DIFFERENTIAL DIAGNOSIS

- Human NSAIDs may cause similar clinical signs but can result in a longer and more significant disease course due to prolonged half-life and differing metabolism in animals and should be ruled out. See chapter 45 (Human NSAIDs).
- Gastrointestinal – gastroenteritis, IBD, HGE, metabolic disease, foreign body, pancreatitis.
- Renal/urological – chronic kidney disease, pyelonephritis, dehydration, grape/raisin ingestion, ethylene glycol toxicity, ureteral obstruction, urethral obstruction.
  - Cats: Asiatic/Easter lily toxicity.
- Hepatic – xylitol or mushroom toxicity, hepatitis, pancreatitis, cholangiohepatitis.
- Neurological – epilepsy, other neurological toxins (mushroom, antidepressants), hypoglycemia.

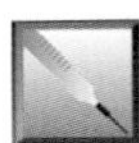

DIAGNOSTICS

- CBC – blood loss anemia, thrombocytopenia noted with blood loss, high or low WBC with GI perforation and sepsis.

- Serum chemistry profile – azotemia, liver enzyme/bilirubin elevations, elevated protein with dehydration, low albumin with liver failure, blood loss or sepsis.
- Urinalysis – isosthenuria, urinary casts with renal tubular damage.
- Clotting profile – typically unaffected; platelet function tests can be prolonged.
- Abdominocentesis or diagnostic peritoneal lavage – intracellular bacteria, glucose differential >20 mg/dL less in abdominal fluid versus peripheral glucose is consistent with a septic abdomen secondary to GI tract perforation.
- Abdominal radiograph – loss of abdominal detail, free gas in the abdomen.
- Abdominal ultrasound – complex free fluid, gastric ulceration, ileus.

Pathological Findings

- GI tract – erosions, ulceration and perforation of the stomach and small intestine.
- Kidney – multifocal renal tubular necrosis, renal tubular regeneration, membranoproliferative glomerulonephritis.
- Liver – hepatocellular necrosis.

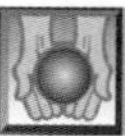

THERAPEUTICS

- Treatment is aimed at prevention and palliation of gastric erosion, ulceration, and perforation as well as prevention of renal failure.

Detoxification

- Induce emesis within 1 hour after ingestion; may be difficult to identify chewable tablets in the emesis.
- Activated charcoal with a cathartic 1–2 g/kg. Give multidose charcoal (without a cathartic) for drugs that undergo enterohepatic recirculation.

Appropriate Health Care

- IV fluids as needed to correct dehydration and hypovolemia. Continue IV fluids for 24–72 hours or as needed until clinical signs abate and to support kidney perfusion.
- A blood transfusion may be needed for significant blood loss associated with GI ulceration.

Drugs and Antidotes of Choice

- GI protectants – use an H_2 blocker, proton pump inhibitor, or misoprostol, and sucralfate for 5–10 days after ingestion or until clinical signs resolve. Use multiple drugs if clinical signs are severe.
    - H_2 blocker: famotidine 0.5–1 mg/kg PO, IV (slowly), IM, SQ q 12–24 hours.

- Proton pump inhibitor: pantoprazole 0.7–1 mg/kg IV over 15 minutes q 24 hours; omeprazole 0.5–1 mg/kg PO q 24 hours.
- Misoprostol 2–5 µg/kg PO q 8–12 hours.
- Sucralfate 0.25–1 g PO q 8 hours.

■ Antiemetic such as maropitant 1 mg/kg SQ or PO every 24 hours.

Precautions/Interactions

■ Discontinue use of other NSAIDs and steroids and use caution with drugs listed above that may have interactions with NSAIDs.

Alternative Drugs

■ Opioid pain medication to replace NSAID for postoperative pain control or arthritis pain, such as tramadol 1–4 mg/kg PO q 8–12 hours.
■ Hepatoprotective medications and antioxidants can be used prophylactically or if liver damage is noted (e.g., silymarin/milk thistle, SAMe).

Nursing Care

■ Keep animals clean and dry if having diarrhea.
■ Soft, comfortable bedding is important for animals with arthritis.

Diet

■ Bland diet or prescription GI diet can be considered in symptomatic animals.
■ Nutritional supplementation may be required for anorectic animals.

Surgical Considerations

■ Exploratory laparotomy may include repair of perforation as well as copious lavage of abdomen when a septic abdomen is identified. Standard postsurgical care as needed.

COMMENTS

Patient Monitoring

■ Monitor hydration, kidney values, urine output for patients with suspected kidney damage.
- Recheck kidney values every 24 hours until normal or at a steady state.

■ Animals can bleed into their GI tract without obvious melena or hematochezia. Monitor PCV/TP, CRT, heart rate, blood pressure, appetite, and stool quality where abnormalities can be early indicators of blood loss.

Prevention/Avoidance

- Discuss appropriate dosing of these medications and provide owners with symptoms to evaluate for at home so that signs can be addressed early before significant morbidity develops.
- Discuss palatability of chewable medication; keep medications out of reach so that animals are not tempted to ingest large amounts of tablets. Animals may take these medications out of purses or bags if left unattended.

Possible Complications

- Oliguria or anuria may develop and these patients need aggressive therapy and monitoring.
- Chronic renal failure may occur after ingestion and requires lifelong therapy.
- GI perforation can occur and surgery is required for these cases. A septic abdomen and surgery will complicate recovery and carry a poor prognosis.

Expected Course and Prognosis

- Clinical signs generally resolve in 48–72 hours.
- Prognosis is fair to good with acute and chronic ingestion with appropriate decontamination and therapy. Surgery for GI perforation may complicate recovery; multiple surgeries may be required. Owners should be informed of the prolonged hospitalization and expense associated with these cases.
- Renal tubules may be able to regenerate with time, but full recovery may not be possible. Oliguria or anuria carries a guarded to poor prognosis.

See Also

Aspirin
Human NSAIDs (Ibuprofen, Naproxen)

Abbreviations

See Appendix 1 for a complete list.

Suggested Reading

Carroll GC, Simonson SM. Recent developments in nonsteroidal anti-inflammatory drugs in cats. J Am Anim Hosp Assoc 2005; 41:347–354.

Enberg TB, Braun LD, Kuzme AB. Gastrointestinal perforation in five dogs associated with the administration of meloxicam. J Vet Emerg Crit Care 2006; 16:34–43.

Khan SA, McLean MK. Toxicology of frequently encountered nonsteroidal anti-inflammatory drugs in dogs and cats. Vet Clin Small Anim 2012; 42:289–306.

Lascelles BD, Blikslager AT, Fox SM, Reece D. Gastrointestinal tract perforation in dogs treated with a selective cyclooxygenase-2 inhibitor: 29 cases (2002–2003). J Am Vet Med Assoc 2005; 7:1112–1117.
Monteiro-Steagall BP, Steagall PVM, Lascelles BDX. Systemic review of nonsteroidal anti-inflammatory drug-induced adverse effects in dogs. J Vet Intern Med 2013; 27:1011–1019.

Author: Katherine L. Peterson, DVM, DACVECC
Consulting Editor: Ahna G. Brutlag, DVM, MS, DABT, DABVT

Envenomations

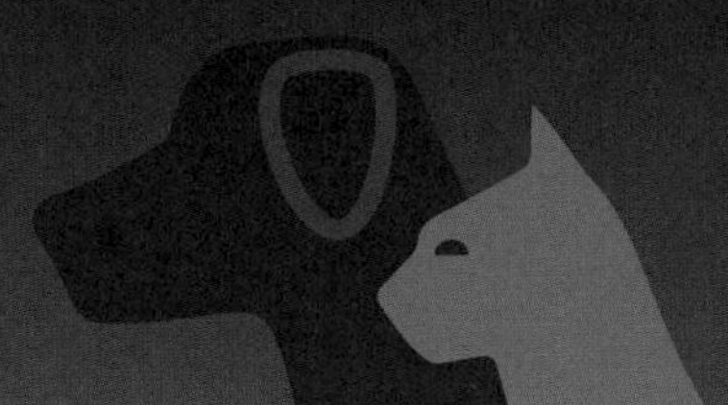

chapter 53

Black Widow Spiders

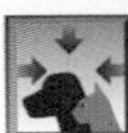

DEFINITION/OVERVIEW

- The black widow spider (*Latrodectus* spp.) is a black, shiny spider about 2–2.5 cm in length with a red or orange hourglass mark on the ventral abdomen. The immature female is brown with red to orange stripes that change into the hourglass shape as she darkens with age (Fig. 53.1). Males are brown, have no hourglass marks, and are generally thought to have fangs that are too small to penetrate the skin.
- Black widow spiders are found in every state except Alaska.

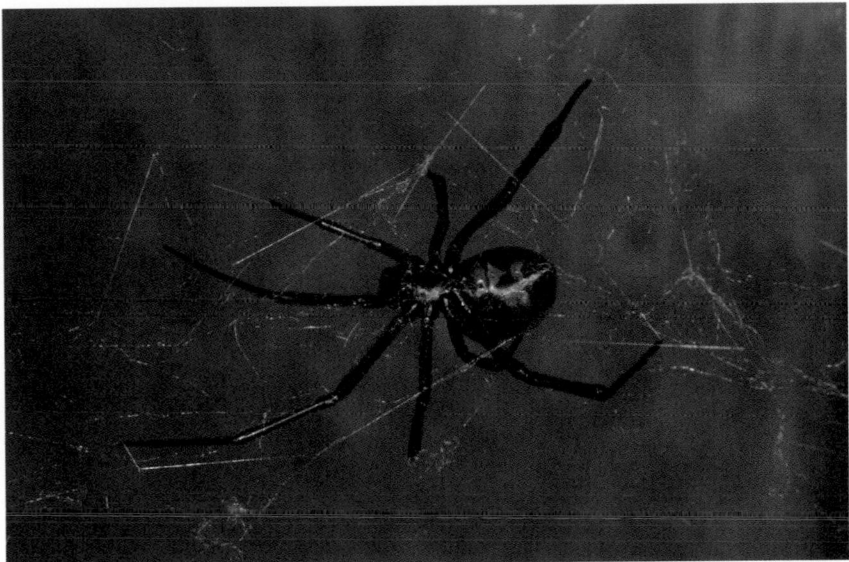

■ **Fig. 53.1.** Black widow spider (*Latrodectus* spp.). Photo courtesy of Richard Vetter, Department of Entomology, University of California–Riverside.

Blackwell's Five-Minute Veterinary Consult Clinical Companion: Small Animal Toxicology, Second Edition.
Lynn R. Hovda, Ahna G. Brutlag, Robert H. Poppenga, and Katherine L. Peterson.

Companion website: www.fiveminutevet.com/toxicology

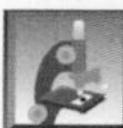

ETIOLOGY/PATHOPHYSIOLOGY

Mechanism of Action

- The venom contains alpha-latrotoxin, a potent neurotoxin that opens cation-selective channels at the presynaptic nerve terminal. This causes massive release and then depletion of acetylcholine and norepinephrine, resulting in sustained muscular spasms.
- Some proteolytic enzymes are also present, causing minimal localized tissue inflammation and pain.

Pharmacokinetics – Absorption, Distribution, Metabolism, Excretion

- After the venom is injected, it is taken up by the lymphatics, entering the bloodstream.
- In 30–120 minutes, muscle pain begins near the site of the bite.
- Within 2–3 hours, muscle pain and cramping spread to the muscles of the legs, abdomen, thorax, and back.
- Acute clinical signs generally resolve in 48–72 hours, but weakness and lethargy may continue for weeks to months.

Toxicity

- The neurotoxin is very potent.
  - LD_{50} in guinea pigs is 0.0075 mg/kg.
  - LD_{50} in mice is 0.9 mg/kg.
- Cats are particularly sensitive to the venom, and many do not survive evenomation. Muscle pain and cramping can proceed to muscle, ataxia, and paralysis.

Systems Affected

- Musculoskeletal – severe muscle pain and cramping.
- Nervous – in cats especially, ataxia, tremors, and paralysis.
- Cardiovascular – mild tachycardia and hypertension.
- Gastrointestinal – vomiting, diarrhea, hypersalivation.
- Respiratory – Cheyne–Stokes pattern prior to death.

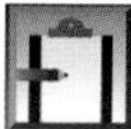

SIGNALMENT/HISTORY

- Diagnosis is based on history and clinical signs.

Risk Factors

- Geriatric animals or animals with cardiac compromise may be at greater risk of complications.

Historical Findings

- Owners have reported seeing the spider in the emesis of the animal.
- Clinical onset is usually acute but may be delayed by several days with mild envenomation.

Location and Circumstances of Poisoning

- Spiders are often found outside in leaf litter and debris or inside houses in dark areas under cabinets and in corners. Spiders are generally shy and will bite only if threatened by curious dogs and cats.

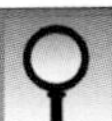

CLINICAL FEATURES

- Clinical signs usually develop within 30 minutes to 2 hours post exposure, and the duration of clinical signs is generally 48–72 hours.
- The most common signs are vomiting, diarrhea, vocalization, severe muscle spasms and cramping, pain, agitation, and restlessness.
- Examination may show abdominal rigidity without tenderness, hypertension, tachycardia, regional tenderness, and lymph node tenderness.

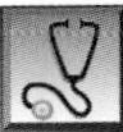

DIFFERENTIAL DIAGNOSIS

- Acute abdomen
- Acute injury (hit by car, falling downstairs, etc.)
- Back pain from invertebral disc disease

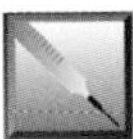

DIAGNOSTICS

- CBC – leukocytosis.
- Serum chemistry – elevated CK.

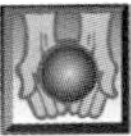

THERAPEUTICS

- Therapeutic goals are to provide symptomatic and supportive therapy to minimize pain, muscle tremors, and agitation. If obtainable, antivenom can be used to rapidly shorten clinical signs.

Detoxification

- None in particular.

Appropriate Health Care

- Monitor closely for signs of allergic reaction when giving antivenom.
- Monitor for signs of tachycardia and hypertension and treat appropriately.

Antidote

- Antivenom is the definitive antidote. It should be reserved for high-risk patients (pediatric, geriatric, metabolically compromised). In one case report, a cat was treated with antivenom 26 hours after becoming clinically compromised and quickly recovered neurological function.
    - Lycovac Antivenin Black Widow Spider (Human Antivenin, equine origin); Merck, West Point, PA.
        - One vial mixed with 100 mL crystalloid solution given IV slowly with monitoring of the ventral ear pinna for evidence of hyperemia (an indicator of allergic response).
        - One dose is usually sufficient with a response occurring within 30 minutes.
        - With proper use, reactions are rare. If an adverse reaction occurs, stop antivenin and administer diphenhydramine (2–4 mg/kg IM, lower dose in cats). Wait 5–10 minutes and restart the antivenin at a slower rate.
- A second antivenin (Aracmyn; Instituto Bioclon, Mexico) has completed human phase three trials but is not yet approved for human use. This is an equine-origin Fab2 antivenin product and may be less likely to trigger an allergic reaction.

Drugs of Choice

- Judicious use of IV fluids, especially if CK is elevated.
- Muscle rigidity and anxiety.
    - Methocarbamol 55–220 mg/kg/day slow IV. Do not exceed 330 mg/kg/day.
    - Diazepam 0.25–0.5 mg/kg IV as needed.
- Opioids may be used at the lowest effective dose to control pain without compromising respiratory function.
    - Buprenorphine 0.005–0.03 mg/kg IM, IV or SQ q 6–12 hours.
    - Tramadol 4–10 mg/kg PO q 8–12 hours in dogs; 1–2 mg/kg PO q 12 hours in cats. Extra-label use for both dogs and cats.
- Antiemetics.
    - Maropitant 1 mg/kg SQ q 24 hours.
    - Ondansetron 0.1–0.2mg/kg IV q 8–12 hours.

Nursing Care

- Thermoregulation.
- Frequent turning.
- Monitor vitals closely.
- Quiet environment.

Follow-up

- Weakness, fatigue, and insomnia may persist for weeks to months. Pets should be monitored closely.

Expected Course and Prognosis

- Clinical signs generally resolve within 48–72 hours.
- Prognosis is uncertain for days; envenomation in cats is usually fatal without antivenom administration.

Abbreviations

See Appendix 1 for a complete list.

Fab = fragment antigen binding

Suggested Reading

Gwaltney-Brant SM, Dunayer EK, Youssef HY. Terrestrial zootoxins. In: Gupta RC, ed. Veterinary Toxicology: Basic and Clinical Principles. New York: Elsevier, 2012; pp. 969–996.

Mebs D. Black widow spider. In: Mebs D, ed. Venomous and Poisonous Animals. Boca Raton, FL: CRC Press, 2002; pp. 184–187.

Peterson ME, McNally J. Spider envenomation: Black widow. In: Peterson ME, Talcott PA, eds. Small Animal Toxicology, 3rd edn. St Louis, MO: Saunders, 2006; pp. 817–821.

Twedt DC, Cuddon PA, Horn TW. Black widow spider envenomation in a cat. J Vet Intern Med 2008; 13:613–616.

Authors: Michael E. Peterson, DVM, MS; Catherine M. Adams, DVM
Consulting Editor: Lynn R. Hovda, RPh, DVM, MS, DACVIM

chapter 54

Brown Recluse Spiders

DEFINITION/OVERVIEW

- The brown recluse spider (*Loxosceles reclusa*) is 8–13 mm in length with comparatively long legs of 20–30 mm. Its color ranges in shades of brown; there is violin shape on the dorsal cephalothorax (Fig. 54.1).
- The spider is a hunter; the web is irregular and wispy.
- Various species of the *Loxosceles* spiders range over the temperate regions of Europe, Africa, and North and South America; however, most are found in the Americas. In the United States, the range is primarily in the southern Midwest, with certain species being found in the southern western states. It is a common misconception that they are more widespread (Fig. 54.2).

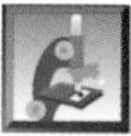

ETIOLOGY/PATHOPHYSIOLOGY

Mechanism of Action

- The venom is a mixture of proteases and phospholipases, causing local and systemic clinical signs.
- Sphingomyelinase D, present in the venom, causes platelet aggregation, complement cascade, cellular lysis, apoptosis, and an immune response that leads to dermonecrosis.
- There appears to be tremendous variability between species regarding the extent of the response and susceptibility to the venom.
  - Rabbits and humans had similar dermonecrotic lesions, but rabbit's lesions healed more quickly.
  - Dogs had a milder version of the dermonecrotic lesion with a similar dose of venom.

Pharmacokinetics – Absorption, Distribution, Metabolism, Excretion

- After venom injection, little or no pain may be felt initially.
- Within 3–8 hours after envenomation, the area develops pruritus, pain, swelling, and a target lesion. The center may form a vesicle that later becomes a black scab (eschar).

Blackwell's Five-Minute Veterinary Consult Clinical Companion: Small Animal Toxicology, Second Edition.
Lynn R. Hovda, Ahna G. Brutlag, Robert H. Poppenga, and Katherine L. Peterson.

Companion website: www.fiveminutevet.com/toxicology

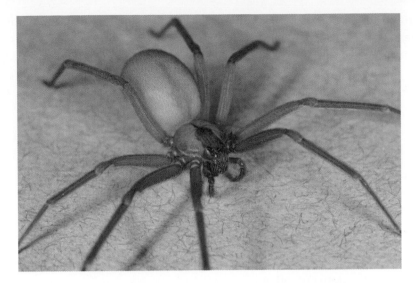

■ **Fig. 54.1.** Brown recluse spider (*Loxosceles reclusa*). Note the distinctive violin mark; it is often poorly demarcated in immature spiders or other species. Photo courtesy of Richard Vetter, Department of Entomology, University of California–Riverside.

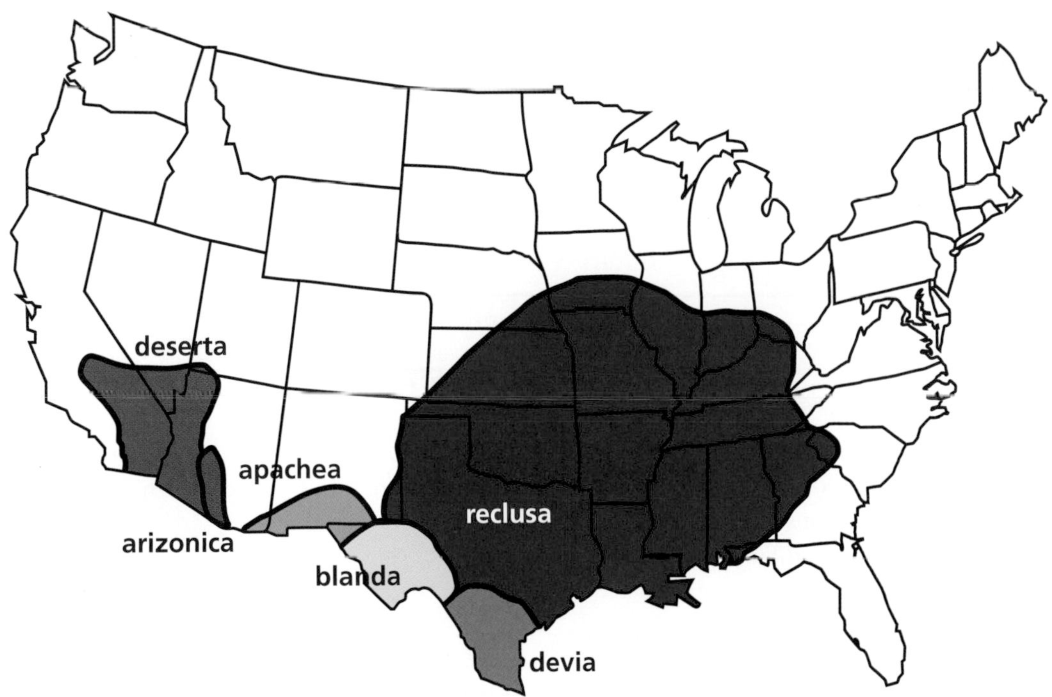

■ **Fig. 54.2.** North American distribution of the most widespread species of *Loxosceles* spiders. Map courtesy of Richard Vetter, Department of Entomology, University of California–Riverside.

- Tissue around the lesion, along with the scab, may slough after 2–5 weeks, leaving a deep, slowly healing ulcer that usually spares muscle tissue.
- Less commonly, hemolytic anemia with hemoglobinuria may occur within the first 24 hours.
- Other systemic signs (tachycardia, fever, vomiting, dyspnea, renal failure, coma) may develop 6–72 hours after envenomation.

Toxicity

- Severity of signs varies with the amount of venom injected and the victim's immune response, so even minute amounts can cause severe clinical signs.
    - Bites to fatty tissues are more severe.
- Very little research has been done, and since the clinical signs mimic many other rule-outs, the concern is that misdiagnosis of spider venom may prevent correct diagnosis of another illness with more serious consequences, such as MRSA, Lyme disease, corrosive injury, dermal infection, and others.
- Little animal-related scientific data is available. There have been only two in vivo studies done in dogs to determine the effects of envenomation and no studies in cats.

Systems Affected

- Skin/exocrine – localized pruritus, pain, swelling, classic target lesion, scabbing, ulceration.
- Hemic/lymphatic/immune – leukocytosis, hemolytic anemia, thrombocytopenia, prolonged coagulation times.
- Renal/urological – renal failure.
- Hepatobiliary – elevations in hepatic enzymes.
- Endocrine/metabolic – fever, lethargy.
- Gastrointestinal – vomiting.

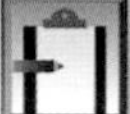

SIGNALMENT/HISTORY

- Diagnosis is based on history, clinical signs, and appropriate geographic environment.
    - In humans, over 60% of "recluse" bite diagnoses are made in areas with no endemic brown recluse spider populations (see Fig. 54.2).
- No breed or sex predilection.

Risk Factors

- Geriatric or pediatric patients may be at more risk of developing systemic effects.

Location and Circumstances of Poisoning

- The brown recluse spider is a shy, nocturnal creature that hides in dark areas under leaf litter, tree bark, or rocks. Inside houses, it hides in bedding, basements, under piles of clothes, and anywhere it will have protection.
- The spider will bite only if disturbed, attacking quickly and leaving immediately, making accurate identification difficult.

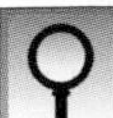

CLINICAL FEATURES

- Two distinct forms are seen in humans:
    - Cutaneous. After an initial mild edema or erythema, the bite area becomes necrotic. An eschar forms over the area, covering a deep ulcerating wound that heals very slowly. Secondary infection may occur.
    - Viscerocutaneous. Rare systemic reactions are more likely in pediatric or geriatric patients. Severe hemolytic anemia, with hemoglobinuria, hematuria, and thrombocytopenia, may occur within 6–24 hours. Renal failure may be a sequela.

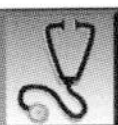

DIFFERENTIAL DIAGNOSIS

- In humans, the primary misdiagnosis is MRSA.
- Immune-mediated disease.
- Injury.
- Primary infections, including parasitic, fungal, bacterial, viral causes.
- Neoplastic cutaneous disease.
- Secondary cutaneous disease (diabetic ulcer, septic embolism).
- Vascular disease.

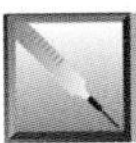

DIAGNOSTICS

- There are no specific tests for the disease.
- Other tests should be used to rule out other diseases (Lyme test, autoimmune tests, coagulation tests, chemistry panel, CBC, UA) and to predict treatment in the case.
- Baseline CBC with platelet count and serum chemistry in those animals with evidence of systemic disease.

Pathological Findings

- Pathological findings include dermal necrosis and ulceration with possible secondary infection.

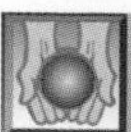

THERAPEUTICS

- The treatment goals are to provide symptomatic and supportive care (rest, antibiotics if needed, IV fluids, blood transfusion).
- There have been many suggested treatments, including surgical removal, dapsone, hyperbaric oxygen, anticoagulants, shock therapy, steroids, antihistamines, vitamin C, and meat tenderizer, but none has proven to be effective.

Detoxification

- None other than good wound care.

Appropriate Health Care

- Clean wound well with soap and water; prevent secondary infection.
- Cool compresses. Avoid application of heat.
- Elevation of area.

Antidote

- No specific antidote or antivenom is available.

Drugs of Choice

- IV fluids as needed for dehydration and cardiovascular support.
- Blood products as needed.
- Broad-spectrum antibiotics if wound becomes infected.
- Analgesics for pain.
  - NSAIDs.
    - Carprofen – dogs 2.2 mg/kg PO q 12–24 hours; cats: 1–2 mg/kg SQ q 24 hours. Limit dosing to 2 days.
  - Opioids.
    - Buprenorphine 0.005–0.02 mg/kg IM, IV or SQ q 6–12 hours.
    - Tramadol 4–10 mg/kg PO q 8–12 hours in dogs; 1–2 mg/kg PO q 12 hours in cats. Both are extra-label.
- Antiemetics.
  - Maropitant 1 mg/kg SQ q 24 hours.
  - Ondansetron 0.1–0.2 mg/kg IV q 8–12 hours.
- Antihistamines for pruritus.
  - Diphenhydramine 2–4 mg/kg IM or PO as needed.

Precautions/Interactions

- Heat treatment may exacerbate the condition.

Nursing Care

- Prolonged wound care may be necessary.

Surgical Considerations

- Wound debridement with Burrow's solution or dilute hydrogen peroxide followed by bandaging may be necessary.

Expected Course and Prognosis

- Full recovery may take weeks to months, but prognosis is good if systemic signs are not seen.

Abbreviations

See Appendix 1 for a complete list.

Suggested Reading

Gwaltney-Brant SM, Dunayer EK, Youssef HY. Terrestrial zootoxins. In: Gupta RC, ed. Veterinary Toxicology: Basic and Clinical Principles. New York: Elsevier, 2012; pp. 969–996.

Mebs D. Brown or fiddleback spiders. In: Mebs D, ed. Venomous and Poisonous Animals. Boca Raton, FL: CRC Press, 2002; pp. 188–189.

Pace L, Vetter R. Brown recluse spider (*Loxosceles recluse*) envenomation in small animals. J Vet Emerg Crit Care 2009; 19(4):329–336.

Peterson ME, McNally J. Spider envenomation: brown recluse. In: Peterson ME, Talcott PA, eds. Small Animal Toxicology, 3rd edn. St Louis, MO: Saunders, 2013; pp. 823–826.

Acknowledgment: The authors and editors acknowledge the prior contributions of Catherine M. Adams, DVM, who co-authored this topic in the previous edition.

Author: Michael E. Peterson, DVM, MS

Consulting Editor: Lynn R. Hovda, RPh, DVM, MS, DACVIM

chapter 55

Bufo Toads

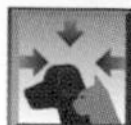

DEFINITION/OVERVIEW

- There are more than 200 species of "bufo" toads in the world.
- Two species in the family Bufonidae are of primary concern in the United States.
  - Colorado River toad (*Incilius alvarius*, formerly *Bufo alvarius*). Found primarily in parts of California and along the Colorado River between Arizona and California.
  - Marine toad (*Rhinella marina*, formerly *Bufo marinus*). Found primarily in Florida, Texas, Hawaii, and other tropical areas. Large toad that can grow up to 8 or 9 inches when mature (Fig. 55.1).

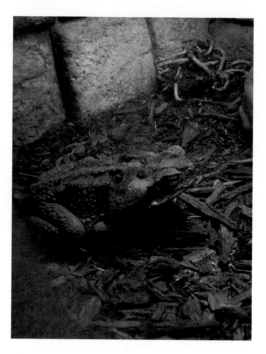

Fig. 55.1. Marine toad (*Rhinella marinus*). Photo courtesy of Tyne K. Hovda.

Blackwell's Five-Minute Veterinary Consult Clinical Companion: Small Animal Toxicology, Second Edition.
Lynn R. Hovda, Ahna G. Brutlag, Robert H. Poppenga, and Katherine L. Peterson.

Companion website: www.fiveminutevet.com/toxicology

- Marine toad is more toxic, and most exposed dogs will die if left untreated.
- Mouthing or ingestion of either can result in toxicity and death.
- Profuse salivation occurs within seconds of mouthing a toad.

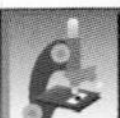

ETIOLOGY/PATHOPHYSIOLOGY

Mechanism of Action

- Venom is located in parotid glands and skin; released by contraction of periglandular muscles.
- Venom is rapidly absorbed across victim's mucous membranes.

Toxicity

- Venom contains several major components, including bufotenines (pressor agents similar to oxytocin that may be hallucinogenic), bufagenins, alternately referred to as bufadienolides (which act like digitalis cardiac glycosides), bufotoxins, and noncardiac sterols.
- Catecholamines, serotonin, and 5-hydroxytryptophan in bufotenines are responsible for some of the cardiovascular, neurological, and sympathetic effects.
- Limited information is available, but one rough estimate is that the contents of both parotid glands contain enough toxins to kill a 10–15 kg dog.
- Toads sitting in a water dish for several hours leave behind enough toxin to make an average-size dog ill after drinking the water.

Systems Affected

- Gastrointestinal – rapid onset of hypersalivation; occurs within seconds to minutes of mouthing or ingesting a toad; hyperemic mucous membranes.
- Respiratory – increased respiratory rate and difficulty in breathing in 15 minutes.
- Neurological – CNS stimulation ranging from ataxia to full seizures in 15–20 minutes.
- Cardiovascular – bradycardia or tachycardia with arrhythmias at any time.

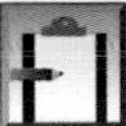

SIGNALMENT/HISTORY

- Primarily dogs; rarely, ferrets and cats.
- All ages can be affected.

Risk Factors

- Living in close proximity to toads. Toads are most active during periods of high humidity. Colorado River toads are especially active during the late summer monsoon season in the desert Southwest. Most encounters occur during the evening, night, or early morning hours.

CLINICAL FEATURES

- Onset is rapid, often occurring within a few minutes of exposure.
- Historical findings:
  - Crying and pawing at the mouth.
  - Ataxia or stiff gait.
  - Seizures.
- Physical examination findings:
  - Profuse hypersalivation within seconds to minutes.
  - Hyperexcitability with vocalization.
  - Vomiting and diarrhea.
  - Brick-red buccal mucous membranes.
  - Hyperthermia.
  - Recumbency, collapse.
  - Marked cardiac ventricular arrhythmia – less common with Colorado River toad intoxication.
  - Respiratory distress – dyspnea, tachypnea, cyanosis within 15 minutes.
  - Neurological signs (ataxia, nystagmus, seizures) within 15–20 minutes.

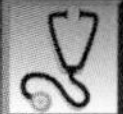

DIFFERENTIAL DIAGNOSIS

- Heat exhaustion.
- Infectious diseases resulting in cardiovascular compromise.
- Toxicants:
  - Caustic agents and oral irritants
  - Cardiac glycoside plants
  - Calcium channel blockers and beta-blockers
  - Digoxin
  - Organophosphate and carbamate insecticides
  - Metaldehyde
- Underlying cardiac disease.

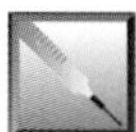

DIAGNOSTICS

- CBC, serum chemistry, and urinalysis are generally unrewarding; may see hyperkalemia and acid–base imbalances.
- Electrocardiogram may reveal ventricular arrhythmias.

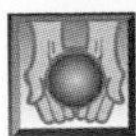

THERAPEUTICS

- Marine toad intoxication is a medical emergency and death is common.
- Rinsing the mouth with water is a first line of therapy and should be instituted at home and again in the veterinary hospital.

Detoxification

- Emesis and activated charcoal are not recommended due to rapid onset of neurological signs.
- Emesis or endoscopic removal will be needed in those dogs that have swallowed an intact toad.
- Flush mouth with copious quantities of water for 10–15 minutes. Use a garden hose for larger dogs and put smaller ones in the sink. Be careful not to drown to be overzealous and the animal.

Appropriate Health Care

- Rapid evaluation of cardiac activity is necessary as is treatment of hyperthermia. Rectal temperatures can go as high as 105°F (40.6°C).
- Treat hyperthermia with a cool bath, cooling vest, or other measures. As temperature falls below 103°F (39.4C), stop measures. Do not overcool.

Antidote

- No specific antidote is available.

Drugs of Choice

- IV fluids to treat hydration, electrolyte abnormalities, and hypotension.
- Atropine:
    - 0.04 mg/kg IM, SQ, IV as needed.
    - Reduces the amount of salivation and helps prevent aspiration.
    - Use with bradycardia, heart block, or other sinoatrial node alterations as a result of the digitalis-like effect of the toxin.
    - Heart rate and secretions should guide repeated dosing.
    - Not recommended if severe tachycardia present.
- Esmolol or propranolol for sinus tachycardia/tachyarrhythmias. Esmolol is very short acting and often used as a test dose. If the arrhythmia responds to treatment, propranolol should be used as the duration of action is much longer (hours).
    - Esmolol: 0.05–0.1 mg/kg IV every 5 minutes for a maximum dose of 0.5 mg/kg.
    - Propranolol: 0.02 mg/kg IV slowly over 2–3 minutes as needed up to a maximum dose of 1 mg/kg.

- Lidocaine for ventricular tachycardia in dogs.
  - 2 mg/kg IV slowly as a bolus; up to 8 mg/kg IV.
  - If response is good, switch to CRI at 25–100 µg/kg/min.
- Lidocaine in cats should be used judiciously. 0.25–0.5 mg/kg IV slowly as bolus; repeat 0.15–0.25 mg/kg IV in 5–20 minutes. If response is good, switch to CRI at 10–20 µg/kg/min.
- Antiemetics as needed.
- Diazepam or phenobarbital for seizures.
  - Diazepam 0.25–0.5 mg/kg IV.
  - Phenobarbital 3–5 mg/kg IV PRN.
- In severe cases, treatment with digoxin-specific Fab fragments may be indicated. Refer to chapter 3, Antidotes and Other Useful Drugs, for specific information.

Precautions/Interactions

- Cardiac disease or bronchial asthma – patient may not tolerate the use of beta-blockers such as esmolol and propranolol. Use test dose of esmolol (very short duration of action) and monitor closely before using propranolol (much longer duration of action).
- Barbiturates may depress function of an already compromised myocardium; use with caution.

COMMENTS

Patient Monitoring

- Continuous electrocardiographic monitoring is recommended until the patient is fully recovered.

Expected Course and Prognosis

- Colorado River toad *(I. alvarius)* intoxication.
  - Patients are usually normal within 30 minutes of onset of treatment.
  - Death is relatively uncommon if treated early.
  - Do not underestimate the risk of secondary heat stroke.
- Marine toad *(R. marinus)* intoxication is a true medical emergency and death is common.

Synonyms

Cane toad – Bufo toad, Dominican toad, giant toad, spring chicken toad
Colorado river toad – Sonoran desert toad

See Also

Beta Receptor Antagonists (Beta-Blockers)
Calcium Channel Blockers
Cardiac Glycosides

Abbreviations

See Appendix 1 for a complete list.

Suggested Reading

Gowda RM, Cohen RA, Khan IA. Toad venom poisoning: resemblance to digoxin toxicity and therapeutic implications. Heart 2003; 89(4):e14.

Palumbo NE, Perri S, Read G. Experimental induction and treatment of toad poisoning in the dog. J Am Vet Med Assoc 1975; 167:1000–1005.

Peterson ME, Roberts BK. Toads. In: Peterson ME, Talcott PA, eds. Small Animal Toxicology, 2nd edn. St Louis, MO: Saunders, 2006; pp. 833–839.

Reeves MP. A retrospective report of 90 dogs with suspected cane toad (*Bufo* marinus) toxicity. Aust Vet J 2008; 82(10):608–611.

Roberts BK, Aronsohn MG, Moses BL. *Bufo marinus* toxicity in dogs: 94 cases (1997–1998). J Am Vet Med Assoc 2000; 216:1941–1944.

Acknowledgment: The authors and editors acknowledge the prior contributions of Michael E. Peterson, DVM, MS, and Justine A. Lee, DVM, DACVEEC, DABT.
Author: Lynn R. Hovda, RPh, DVM, MS, DACVIM
Consulting Editor: Lynn R. Hovda, RPh, DVM, MS, DACVIM

chapter 56

Crotalids (Pit Vipers)

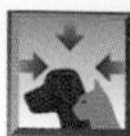

DEFINITION/OVERVIEW

- Local and systemic venom-induced toxicity may both occur following bites by snakes in the subfamily Crotalinae (pit vipers), which is composed of three genera: *Agkistrodon* (cottonmouths [water moccasins] and copperheads – Figs 56.1 and 56.2), and *Crotalus* and *Sistrurus* (rattlesnakes) in North America (Figs 56.3, 56.4, and 56.5).
- Identified by retractable fangs, heat-sensing pit between the nostril and eye (appearance of four nostrils), vertically elliptical pupils (live snakes in light), and a triangular-shaped head (Fig. 56.6).
- Venomous snakebite does not necessarily mean envenomation has occurred; in human beings, 25% of bites are "dry bites" with no venom injected.
- Typically signs are evident within 30–45 minutes of the bite. However, in some cases, the onset of clinical signs may be delayed up to 6 hours.
- Good emergency and supportive care coupled with antivenom therapy are key components for achieving an optimal outcome in cases of venomous snakebite.

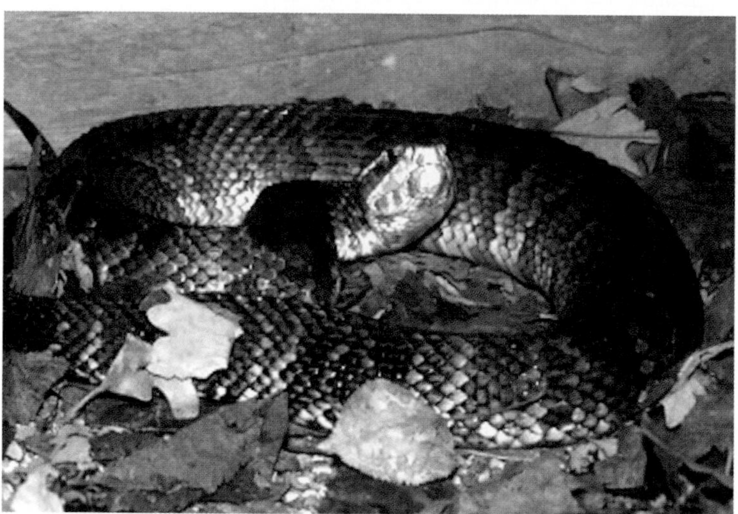

■ **Fig. 56.1.** Cottonmouth or water moccasin (*Agkistrodon piscivorus*). Photo courtesy of Dan Keyler.

Blackwell's Five-Minute Veterinary Consult Clinical Companion: Small Animal Toxicology, Second Edition.
Lynn R. Hovda, Ahna G. Brutlag, Robert H. Poppenga, and Katherine L. Peterson.

Companion website: www.fiveminutevet.com/toxicology

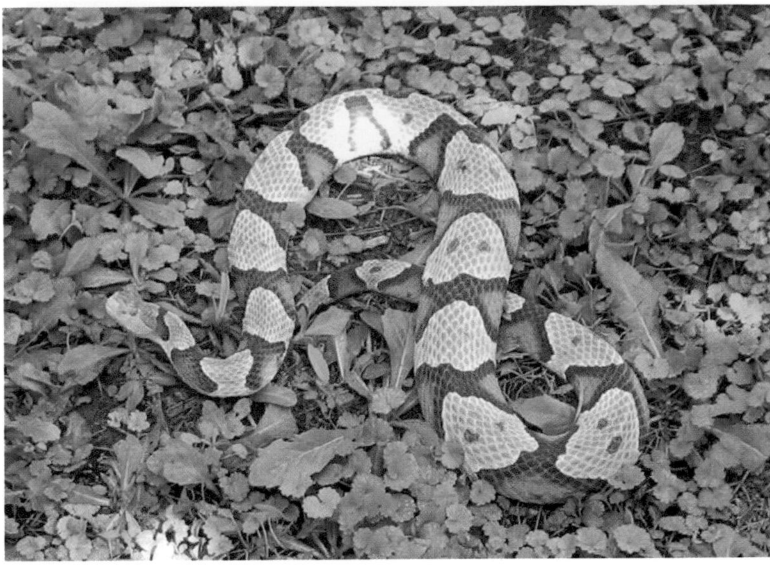

■ **Fig. 56.2.** Copperhead (*Agkistrodon contortrix*). Photo courtesy of Dan Keyler.

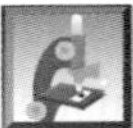

ETIOLOGY/PATHOPHYSIOLOGY

- Inquisitive companion animals living in regions where venomous snakes are indigenous (particularly the southeastern and southwestern regions of the US).
- Bites – frequently to face and front legs due to the curious nature of dogs and cats when they encounter a snake (see Fig. 56.7).
- Fang punctures may be evident but can be missed due to hair.

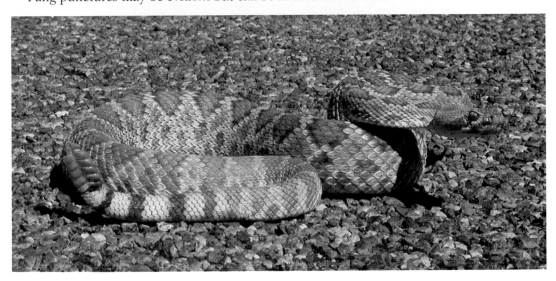

■ **Fig. 56.3.** Mohave rattlesnake (*Crotalus scutulatus*). Photo courtesy of Dan Keyler.

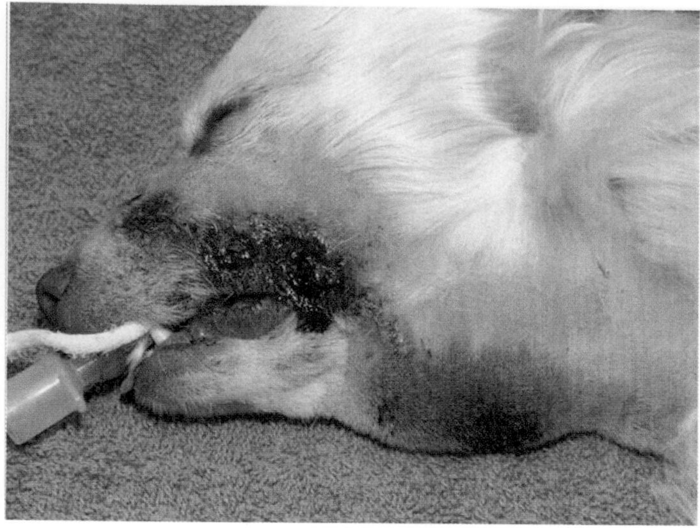

■ **Fig. 56.8.** Dog with airway compromise after bite from prairie rattlesnake. Photo courtesy of Barney Oldfield.

- Coagulopathy – typically occurs in cases of more severe envenomation.
- Edema, swelling, and wound necrosis should be monitored.

Mechanism of Action

- Pit viper venoms are primarily composed of numerous proteins (both enzymatic and non-enzymatic) and small peptides (neurotoxic components). These typically will work in concert to produce insults to blood clotting and tissue integrity, alter fluid (blood and serum) distribution, and in some cases (depending on the species of snake) affect central nervous system function.
- Envenomation frequently results in hypotension, due to fluid redistribution or hemorrhage resulting in central blood volume loss and consequent shock. Pooling of blood within the splanchnic (dogs) and pulmonary (cats) vessels may further compromise respiratory efforts.
- Blood clotting factors can be inhibited, and the function of fibrinogen and platelets may be compromised, potentially producing significant consumptive coagulopathy.
- Red blood cell morphology can be altered (echinocyte-like or burring appearance), rendering them dysfunctional, and RBCs may distributed to the extravascular space, further reducing function.

Pharmacokinetics – Absorption, Distribution, Metabolism, Excretion

- The multiple toxins that compose snake venom all have their own individual toxicokinetics but the toxins function collectively to enhance the absorption and distribution of specific toxins to target tissues and organs. Increased vascular permeability, third-spacing of fluids, and altered clotting system functions may result.

- The rate of distribution of venom toxins to target tissues and organs can be quite rapid in the case of intravenous bites, slower with intramuscular bites, and slowest with more superficial or subcutaneous bites (majority).
- Bites to the face and extremities generally have slower venom uptake than bites to the torso; peritoneal and tongue envenomations have rapid absorption.
- Metabolism and excretion kinetics are complex and, because of the multitoxin composition of venom, have not been well studied. However, some venom components or toxins may persist for weeks, and this is one reason why recurrent coagulopathy can occur.
- Toxins may remain depot at a bite site, disrupting local tissue integrity and resulting in a slower sustained-release systemic absorption. Toxins that penetrate deeper tissues may redistribute with time back into the systemic circulation, resulting in recurrent toxicity. This process of redistribution can occur days, and in some instances weeks, after the bite.

Toxicity

- General ranking of potential systemic venom toxicity: (1) rattlesnakes, (2) water moccasins, (3) copperheads.
- Several species of rattlesnakes have subpopulations with venom containing a potent neurotoxin.
    - Mohave rattlesnake – *Crotalus scutulatus* of southern Arizona.
    - Southern Pacific Rattlesnake – *Crotalus helleri* of California.
    - Timber/Canebrake rattlesnake – *Crotalus horridus* of South Carolina and Georgia.
- It is possible for a snake to have both neurotoxic and coagulopathic venom actions. Strictly neurotoxic venoms produce minimal or no evidence of coagulopathy.
- Venom delivery route influences the time to venom component-induced effects, and the level of systemic venom dosage (mg venom/kg BW).
- 85% of victims have altered laboratory values and clinically important swelling.
- Systemic toxic effects are greatest in highly perfused tissues, with certain organ systems being more susceptible to thrombocytopenia, hypofibrinogenemia (hyperfibrinogenemia, which is a result of volume depletion in the vascular circulation), and resultant coagulopathy.

Systems Affected

- Hemic/lymphatic/immune – coagulopathies and vascular hemorrhage.
- Respiratory – fluid shifts to lungs, respiratory compromise secondary to neuromuscular complications.
- Skin/exocrine – tissue destruction.
- Cardiovascular – shock.
- Renal/urological – renal failure.
- Gastrointestinal – vomiting and diarrhea.
- Neuromuscular – generalized weakness.

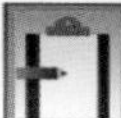

SIGNALMENT/HISTORY

- Cats and dogs of any age may encounter venomous snakes that are indigenous to their region.
- The veterinarian should be aware of the venomous snake species indigenous to the geographic area in which they practice.

Risk Factors

- Important factors include species of snake, size of snake, size of cat/dog, site of bite, age of cat/dog, venom quantity injected, and time to treatment.
- Smaller patients, those with predisposing health problems (cardiac, diabetic, renal), and older animals are at greater risk of more severe medical complications.
  - Smaller animals – venom dose (mg/kg BW of victim) may be quite large.
  - Geriatric animals lack resilience in their physiological systems.
- Animals receiving medications for existing medical problems.
  - NSAIDs may predispose to clotting anomalies.
  - Corticosteroids may decrease natural defenses.
  - Beta-blockers may mask the onset of anaphylaxis.
- Aggressiveness and motivation of snake.
  - Defensive strike – more likely to be "dry"; no venom injected.
  - Feeding strike – more venom injected.
  - Agonal bite – most of available venom injected.

Historical Findings

- If snake is not observed biting the animal, puncture wounds from fangs can frequently be observed; may require clipping hair in affected area.
- Owners should be questioned as to whether antivenom has ever been given in the past as prior antivenom treatment may increase the chances of allergic reaction.

Location and Circumstances of Poisoning

- Copperheads account for the majority of venomous snakebites in areas where they are endemic (eastern USA). Frequently found around human habitation.
- Owners may find their pet carrying around a snake that they have killed and chewed on. These patients should be checked carefully for multiple bite sites and are at high risk for agonal bites. If the snake has been killed (or photo available), it is useful in correct identification.

Interactions with Drugs, Nutrients, or Environment

- Because of the complex makeup of snake venom with numerous different toxins, there is the potential for interaction with many drugs. See Risk Factors.

- Environmental factors such as excessive heat and humidity may be additional burdens beyond the effects of snake venom alone. Careful and selective use of medications to maintain euthermia and homeostasis is key to optimal outcome.

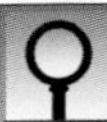

CLINICAL FEATURES

- Local signs may include:
  - Angioedema
  - Fang punctures – not always two, may be multiple, not always visible
  - Edema and swelling
  - Bleeding from the bite site
  - Erythema, ecchymosis
  - Lymphangitis
  - Necrosis.
- Systemic signs may include:
  - Hypotension
  - Respiratory changes (dyspnea)
  - Weakness/ataxia
  - Bleeding – epistaxis, gingival, hematuria, melena, retinal hemorrhage
  - Excessive salivation
  - Myokymia/fasciculations
  - Vomiting – hematemesis
  - Diarrhea
  - Oliguria – hematuria.

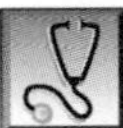

DIFFERENTIAL DIAGNOSIS

- Animal bites – nonsnake (e.g., scorpion, spider, rodents, shrews, etc.).
- Hymenoptera venom-induced angioedema. When touched, these swollen areas are generally not significantly painful in contrast to pit viper envenomation.
- Toxicants – brodifacoum or warfarin-based rodenticides, ethylene glycol.
- Trauma-induced puncture wounds (e.g., nails, barbed wire fence, etc.).
- Sepsis.

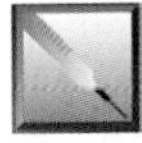

DIAGNOSTICS

- If snake (or photo) available, confirm identification – venomous or nonvenomous.
- Examine animal for fang marks, clip hair in affected area, examine for local tissue damage and ecchymosis.
- CBC, serum chemistry, UA, and coagulation profile – initial bloodwork sets a baseline reference for monitoring progression and resolution of envenomation syndrome.

  - CBC – if venom has been injected, 89% have echinocytosis (non-EDTA blood).
  - Creatine kinase (CK) elevation with intramuscular envenomation.
- Urinalysis – hemoglobinuria or myoglobinuria secondary to rhabdomyolysis.
- Coagulation parameters (INR, Plts, PT, PTT, Fib, FDP).
  - International normalized ratio (INR) –prolonged.
  - Prothrombin time (PT), partial thromboplastin time (PTT) – prolonged.
  - Platelets (Plts) – decreased.
  - Fibrinogen (Fib) – decreased.
  - Fibrinogen degradation products (FDP) – increased.
- ECG – ventricular arrhythmias may be detected in severely depressed patients.

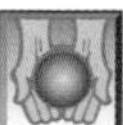

THERAPEUTICS

Detoxification

- Superficially wash wound area to remove any residual venom at bite site.
- Transport to animal care facility for treatment.
- Remove collars and other restrictive devices prior to transport.
- Clip and clean bite area.

Appropriate Health Care

- Minimize exercise/movement.
- Observe closely for airway obstruction and be prepared to intubate.
- Monitor cardiovascular system closely.
- Blood pressure (fluid replacement may be needed).

Antivenoms

- Antivenom is the definitive antidote for venomous snakebite. In the United States, there are potentially five antivenom products available for treating crotalid envenomation.
  - Two are licensed for veterinary use (available from most veterinary supply distributors).
  - One is licensed for human use in North America.
  - Two are licensed for human use in Mexico and Central America (usually maintained at zoos).
- In the absence of availability of the veterinary product, human antivenom products can be successfully used. Availability and economic factors (wide range of product costs to DVM) may determine whether antivenom therapy is an option.
- **The earlier antivenom is administered, the more effective it is**; one vial early is equal to several later.
- Antivenom has been used successfully in pregnant humans but specific studies in animals are lacking. Therapeutically, what is good for the mother should be good for the fetus. Consequences in the absence of antivenom therapy must be considered.

- Specifics of use (for further details refer to product package insert).
  - Lyophilized antivenin should be reconstituted with diluent and gently agitated or rolled between the hands to enhance solubility of lyophilized product. The vial can be gently flushed and swirled as significantly more antivenin can be withdrawn.
  - Dilute in 250 mL of crystalloids and administer IV slowly, looking for any sign of allergic reaction – pruritus, hyperemia of pinna, piloerection. If allergic-type reaction occurs, stop antivenin infusion.
  - Reaction is usually a complement-mediated anaphylactoid-type response to foreign proteins given too rapidly. Stop infusion, give diphenhydramine (2–4 mg/kg IM or PO), wait 5 minutes, and begin antivenin again at a slower rate. If problem persists, seek veterinary toxicology consult.
  - Anaphylactic reactions may also occur and the clinician should be prepared to respond. Epinephrine may be required for acute reactions.

Veterinary Antivenoms

Specific USDA-approved products available in the USA.

- Antivenin (Crotalidae) polyvalent (veterinary antivenin) – IgG (equine).
  - Boehringer-Ingelheim, Ridgefield, CT.
  - Dose varies from 1 to 5 vials IV depending on severity of symptoms.
  - 95% of cases controlled with a single vial.
- Lyophilized product, requires reconstitution.
- Venom Vet polyvalent crotalidae injectable antivenin solution – $(Fab')_2$ (equine).
  - MT Venom, LLC, Canoga Park, CA.
  - Ready to use, no reconstitution necessary.

Alternative Antivenoms (Human)

Doses not precisely determined for veterinary use.

- CroFab Crotalidae polyvalent immune Fab (ovine).
  - BTG International Inc., West Conshohocken, PA.
  - Supplied as a carton of two vials.
- Antivipmyn polyvalent equine antiviper serum – $(Fab')_2$ (equine).
  - Instituto Bioclon, Mexico.
  - Maintained by multiple zoos in United States.
  - Currently in veterinary trials.
- Costa Rican pit viper antivenin – polyvalent IgG (equine).
  - Instituto Clodomiro Picado, Costa Rica.
  - Maintained by multiple zoos in United States.

Drugs of Choice

- IV crystalloid fluids for volume resuscitation. The vast majority of cases are started on fluid therapy while antivenin is being prepared. Some envenomation syndromes can be controlled with IV fluids alone. Do not fluid overload.

- Blood products (FFP, whole blood) may be needed for animals with marked hypoproteinemia. Coagulopathies rarely corrected with blood products alone, and persistent defects require additional antivenom.
- Pain management.
  - Buprenorphine 0.005–0.03 mg/kg IM, IV or SQ q 6–12 hours.
  - Tramadol 4–10 mg/kg PO q 8–12 hours for dogs; 1–2 mg/kg PO q 12 hours for cats. Both are extra-label.
- Antiemetics for persistent vomiting.
  - Maropitant 1 mg/kg SQ q 24 hours.
  - Ondansetron 0.1–0.2 mg/kg IV q 8–12 hours.
- Antibiotics are not routinely needed in cases of snakebite unless localized tissue damage is severe and there is confirmed evidence of infection. Fluoroquinolone antimicrobials improved survival in one study, but wound infection was not assessed. No other antimicrobial agent had an effect on survival.

Precautions/Interactions

- Antivenom reactions.
  - Antibodies are foreign proteins and may precipitate allergic complications. This sometimes results from too rapid administration or when antivenom solution is too concentrated; appropriate dilution or simply slowing/stopping the infusion rate may reduce risk of this complication.
- Other drugs.
  - Corticosteroids have no documented value in the treatment of venomous snakebite; evidence suggests they may worsen the condition.
  - Colloids are avoided since they can alter coagulation and may pull fluids out of the extra- or intervascular space through damaged vessel walls.
  - DMSO enhances uptake and spread of venom.
  - Heparin should not be used as the coagulopathies induced by pit viper venoms work by a different mechanism. It has no clinical value and may worsen the condition.
  - Opiates (fentanyl, sufentanil, oxymorphone) may be used for pain. However, in cases of neurotoxic envenomation, they may confound the interpretation of symptoms. Morphine can cause histamine release reactions similar to early anaphylaxis.
  - NSAIDS should be avoided.
- Rattlesnake vaccine for dogs (Red Rock Biologics, Woodland, CA) – intended prophylaxis for western diamondback rattlesnake envenomation. Published documentation of efficacy unavailable. Efficacy evidence is anecdotal at this time.

COMMENTS

Patient Monitoring

- Baseline laboratory values should be obtained and repeated as necessary, particularly coagulation panel, packed cell volume, and total protein.

- Recurrence of clinical signs or coagulation abnormalities can occur with any antivenom. If patient has initial coagulopathy resolved with antivenom use, recurrence can occur usually within the next week (most commonly the next few days), although rarely as severe as initial defect. There have been no documented veterinary cases of clinical bleeding from subsequent coagulopathy; however, the clinician should be aware of the possibility.
- Renal complications may develop consequent to coagulopathy, and maintaining adequate renal function is important. Urinalysis and monitoring renal function are useful.

Expected Course and Prognosis

- Animals may also suffer recurrent symptoms following an apparent recovery. These may be both local and systemic, and as such warrant that animals are closely monitored for up to several weeks (as outpatients) following the snakebite and associated treatments.

See Also

Elapids (Coral Snakes)

Abbreviations

See Appendix 1 for a complete list.

Suggested Reading

Armentano RA, Shaer M. Overview and controversies in the medical management of pit viper envenomation in the dog. J Vet Emerg Crit Care 2011; 21:461–470.

Gilliam LL, Brunker J. North American snake envenomation in the dog and cat. Vet Clin Small Anim 2011; 41:1239–1259.

Hoggan SR, Carr A, Sausman KA. Mojave toxin-type ascending flaccid paralysis after envenomation by a Southern Pacific rattlesnake in a dog. J Vet Emerg Crit Care 2011; 21:558–564.

McCown JL, Cooke KL, Hanel R. Effect of antivenin dose on outcome from crotalid envenomation: 218 dogs (1988–2006). J Vet Emerg Crit Care 2009; 19(6):603–610.

Pashmakova MB, Bishop MA, Black DM, et al. Multicenter evaluation of the administration of crotalid antivenom in cats: 115 cases (2000–2011). J Am Vet Med Assoc 2013; 243:520–525.

Peterson ME, Matz, M, Seibold K, et al. A randomized multicenter trial of Crotalidae polvlent immune Fab antivenom for the treatment of rattlesnake envenomation in dogs. J Vet Emerg Crit Care 2011; 21:335–345.

Acknowledgment: The authors and editors acknowledge the prior contributions of Michael E. Peterson, DVM, MS, who co-authored this topic in the previous edition.
Author: Daniel E. Keyler, RPh, BS, Pharm D, FAACT
Consulting Editor: Lynn R. Hovda, RPh, DVM, MS, DACVIM

chapter 57

Elapids (Coral Snakes)

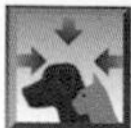

DEFINITION/OVERVIEW

- Elapidae family – frontal maxillary fixed fangs.
- Two genera in the United States (*Micrurus* and *Micruroides*).
- Three species in North America.
    - Eastern coral snake (*Micrurus fulvius*) – southeastern North Carolina and eastern South Carolina; southern Georgia, Alabama, and Mississippi; southeastern Louisiana; all of Florida (Fig. 57.1).
    - Texas coral snake (*Micrurus tener*) – west of Mississippi; southern Arkansas, western Louisiana, and southeastern half of Texas (Fig. 57.2).
    - Sonoran coral snake (*Micruroides euryxanthus*) – southern half of Arizona, and southwestern New Mexico (Fig. 57.3).
- Identification.
    - Brilliant glossy color pattern – red, yellow, and black bands (in this order) fully encircling the body (red and yellow colors touch each other; see Figs 57.1 and 57.2).

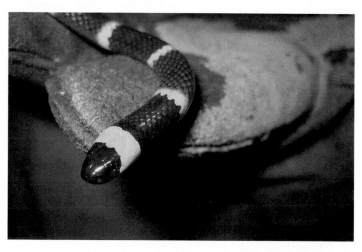

■ **Fig. 57.1.** Eastern coral snake (*Micrurus fulvius*); red and yellow bands touch each other; head is small with black snout. Photo courtesy of David Seerveld, AAAnimal Control, Orlando, Florida.

Blackwell's Five-Minute Veterinary Consult Clinical Companion: Small Animal Toxicology, Second Edition.
Lynn R. Hovda, Ahna G. Brutlag, Robert H. Poppenga, and Katherine L. Peterson.

Companion website: www.fiveminutevet.com/toxicology

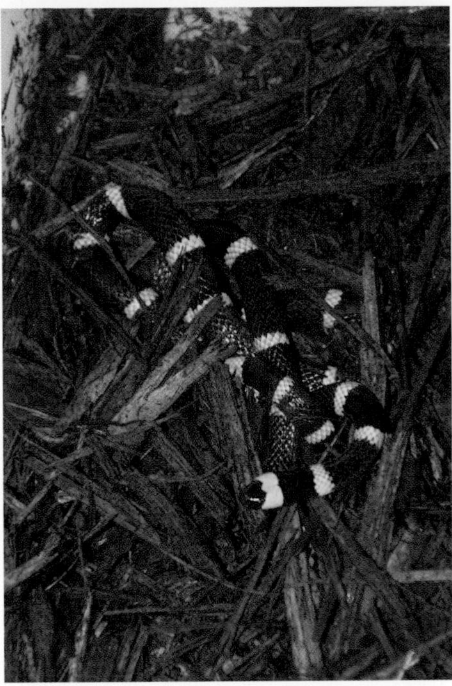

■ **Fig. 57.2.** Texas coral snake (*Micrurus tener*); red bands have more speckling compared to the Eastern Coral Snake. Photo courtesy of Dan Keyler.

- Same sequence pattern is observed in the Sonoran coral except colors are red, white, and indigo blue bands (see Fig. 57.3).
- Relatively small head – black-sock-snout that extends to behind the eyes, round pupils; no narrow demarcation between the head and neck.

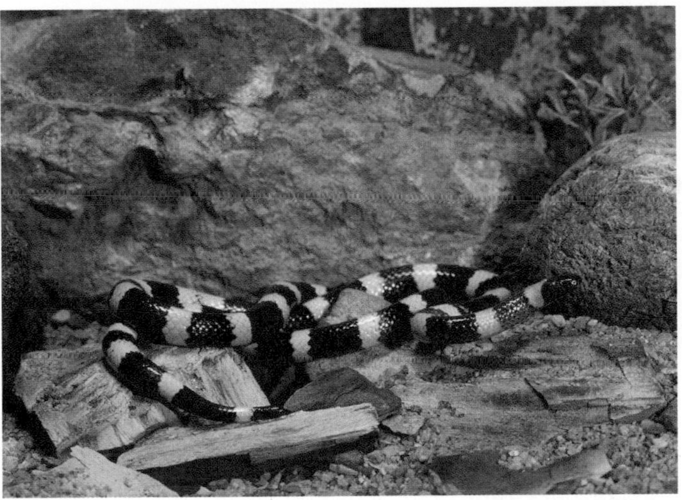

■ **Fig. 57.3.** Sonoran coral snake (*Micruroides euryxanthus*); red and white bands touch each other; head is small with black snout. Photo courtesy of Barney Oldfield.

- Non-venomous "mimic" species (similar color/size) and geographic range of eastern coral and Texas coral snakes.
  - Scarlet snake (*Cemophora coccinea*).
  - Scarlet king snake (*Lampropeltis triangulam elapsoides*).
  - Color pattern shows yellow bands with black bands on each side, yellow does not touch red.

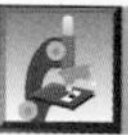

ETIOLOGY/PATHOPHYSIOLOGY

- Coral snakes – usually timid/nonaggressive; bites to animals usually occur because the animal is harassing the snake.
- Fixed small fangs – typically need to chew or hang on when biting to inject venom.
- Bites infrequent due to reclusive/fossorial behavior and nocturnal habits.
- Bites may occur in any month of the year.
- Early identification important.
  - Bite marks by non-venomous mimic species look similar to coral snake bite marks.
  - These snakes also chew when biting.

Mechanism of Action

- Bite wounds to soft tissues – primarily to lips, tongue, mouth (gums), and webbing of paws. Fang marks may or may not be distinctly observed, may appear as scratches.
- Envenomation usually associated with a protracted bite and puncture of skin.
- Venom is neurotoxic, causing muscle paralysis, CNS depression, and cardiovascular failure.
  - Primary site of action – neuromuscular junction. Presynaptic and postsynaptic blockade actions may occur. More rarely, cardiotoxin-like actions are observed.
  - Acetylcholinesterase inhibition is not a major action of coral snake venom.

Pharmacokinetics – Absorption, Distribution, Metabolism, Excretion

- Onset of clinical signs may be delayed several hours (up to 12–18 hours) after envenomation.
- Duration of venom effects may persist for days.

Toxicity

- Eastern coral snake envenomations – typically more severe and neurological in effect than the Texas coral snake.
- Sonoran coral snake bites quite rare; however, neurological venom effects have been reported to occur following envenomation.

Systems Affected

- Neuromuscular – depolarization in muscle fibers.
- Respiratory – respiratory depression.
- Cardiovascular – antagonism of acetylcholine receptors.

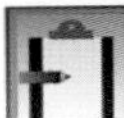

SIGNALMENT/HISTORY

- Dogs and cats – equally affected.
- Cats – more difficult time surviving if prolonged respiratory support needed.

Risk Factors

- Species of snake
- Size of snake
- Size of the cat/dog
- Site of the bite
- Age of the cat/dog
- Venom quantity injected
- Time to treatment

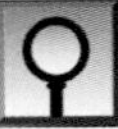

CLINICAL FEATURES

- Cats – primarily neurological: CNS depression, respiratory depression (erratic breathing), ascending flaccid quadriplegia, hypotension, anisocoria, hypothermia, reduced nociception, loss of spinal cutaneous trunci reflexes, vocalization, delayed pupillary light reflex.
- Dogs – CNS depression, generalized weakness/lethargic, shallow abdominal breathing (dyspnea/tachypnea), ptosis, hyperreflexia, tremor, sialorrhea, vomiting, bulbar paralysis affecting cranial motor nerves, delayed pupillary light reflex, acute flaccid quadriplegia, dysphoria, hypotension, ventricular tachycardia, hemolysis resulting in anemia and hemoglobinuria.
- Animals may appear ataxic/staggering, salivating excessively, and disoriented.
- Signs may appear within an hour of being bitten, but lack of signs does not mean envenomation has not occurred. Onset of signs may be delayed for up to 18 hours following a coral snake bite.

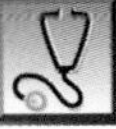

DIFFERENTIAL DIAGNOSIS

- Adverse drug reaction
- Botulism
- Myasthenia gravis

- Polyradiculoneuritis
- Spider bite (*Latrodectus* – widow spider species)
- Tick bite paralysis
- Toxicant-induced neuropathies
- Trauma puncture wounds, small, and not bite related

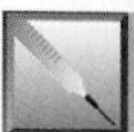

DIAGNOSTICS

- CBC.
- Serum chemistry.
  - ALP, AST, and CK (elevated), electrolyte abnormalities.
- Urinalysis.
  - Hemoglobinuria.
  - Myoglobinuria.
  - Hematuria (rarely).
- If snake or photo of offending snake is available, accurate identification is useful in confirmation of coral snake envenomation.
- Bite site – often difficult to determine if a bite has actually occurred. Fangs are very small. Use of magnifying glass and good lighting can aid in determination of skin penetration. Important to examine particularly facial soft tissue areas, tongue, and gums for bite/fang or scratch-like marks.
- Coagulopathy and pain are not typically observed.

Pathological Findings

- None specific.

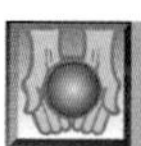

THERAPEUTICS

Detoxification

- Wash wound off with water to remove residual venom on skin surface.
- Minimize animal movement and transport immediately to nearest veterinary facility for antivenom administration and supportive care.
- Pressure-immobilization bandaging is a compression pressure wrap of the bitten limb with ace-type bandage to retard lymph flow and reduce systemic venom distribution.
  - May be of benefit for coral snake bites.
  - Should only be considered in cases where there is a long period of time before veterinary care can be reached.

Appropriate Health Care

- Do not wait for onset of clinical signs to initiate treatment.
- Treat signs as they develop.

- Hospitalize for a minimum of 48 hours.
- Clip and clean wound.
- Monitor respirations.
  - Be prepared to intubate.
  - If no antivenom, can provide mechanical ventilation (2-4 days may be required).
  - Aspiration pneumonia may occur secondary to loss of swallowing reflex.
- ECG monitor.
- Cardiopulmonary resuscitation as needed.
- Blood pressure monitoring for hypotension.
- Sequential neurological evaluations for 48 hours post envenomation.
- Maintain renal function with fluids – do not fluid overload.

Antivenoms

- North American coral snake antivenin (Wyeth, Antivenin *Micrurus fulvius*) (IgG equine origin) is of extremely limited availability, and primarily restricted for human use in the United States.
- Alternative coral snake antivenoms produced in other countries may sometimes be obtained from local zoos. Follow manufacturer's guidelines for preparation and administration.
- Protective cross-reactivity and para-specific coverage has been demonstrated with the following antivenoms.
  - Coralmyn, polvalent anti-coral fabotherapic (F(ab')2 equine origin); Instituto Bioclon, Mexico.
  - Anti-coral (elapid) antivenin (IgG equine origin), Costa Rican coral snake antivenin; Instituto Clodomiro Picado, Costa Rica.
  - Australian tiger snake (*Notechis scutatus*) antivenin; CSL Limited, Parkville, Victoria, Australia.
- Allergic reactions to antivenom are possible.
  - Anaphylaxis (type I hypersensitivity) should be treated with fluids and epinephrine.
  - Anaphylactoid reactions should be treated by stopping the antivenin administration, administering diphenhydramine (2–4 mg/kg PO or IM, lower dose for cats), waiting 5 minutes, and resuming antivenin administration more slowly.
  - Serum sickness-like reaction may occur 1–4 weeks after infusion and may be treated with corticosteroids and antihistamines.
- Pregnancy – antivenom has been used successfully in pregnant humans, and should be considered for use in pregnant dogs or cats if determined necessary.

Drugs of Choice

- IV crystalloids to prevent dehydration and treat myoglobinuria and hematuria. Do not fluid overload.
- Blood products if anemia is severe.
- Broad-spectrum antibiotics for 7–10 days may be needed if local tissue damage with infection has occurred.

- Pain management.
  - Buprenorphine 0.005–0.02 mg/kg IM, IV or SQ q 6–12 hours.
  - Tramadol 4–10 mg/kg PO q 8 hours for dogs;1–2 mg/kg PO q 12 hours for cats. Both are extra-label use.
- Further therapy is symptomatic and supportive.

Alternative Drugs

- Neostigmine – may be used if immediate restoration of neuromuscular transmission is needed until respiratory support can be implemented. This reversible cholinesterase inhibitor has been used successfully in human cases of coral snake envenomation. Will require repeated doses usually due to short half-life.

Nursing Care

- Frequent monitoring of vital signs.
- Wound care if local tissue damage evident (rare with coral snake envenomation).
- Frequent turning in cases of paresis.

COMMENTS

Expected Course and Prognosis

- Prognosis is reasonably good with early intervention.
- Aspiration pneumonia worsens the prognosis.
- Marked clinical signs may last 1–1.5 weeks.
- Full recovery may take months as receptors regenerate.

See Also

Crotalids (Pit Vipers)

Abbreviations

See Appendix 1 for a complete list.

Suggested Reading

Gilliam LL, Brunker J. North American snake envenomation in the dog and cat. Vet Clin Small Anim 2011; 41:1239–1259.

Morgan DL, Borys DJ, Stanford R, et al. Texas coral snake (Micrurus tener) bites. Southern Med J 2007; 100:152–156.

Perez ML, Fox K, Shaer M. A retrospective evaluation of coral snake envenomation in dogs and cats: 20 cases (1996–2011). J Vet Emerg Crit Care 2012; 22:682–689.

Sanchez EE, Lopez-Johnston JC, Rodriquez-Acosta, et al. Neutralization of two North American coral snake venoms with United States and Mexican antivenoms. Toxicon 2008; 51:297–303.

Wisniewski MS, Hill RE, Havey JM, et al. Australian tiger snake (Notechis scutatus) and Mexican coral snake (Micrurus species) antivenoms prevent death from United States coral snake (Micrurus fulvius fulvius) venom in a mouse model. J Clin Toxicol Clin Tox 2003; 41:7–10.

Acknowledgment: The authors and editors acknowledge the prior contributions of Michael E. Peterson, DVM, MS, who co-authored this topic in the previous edition.
Author: Daniel E. Keyler, RPh, BS, Pharm D, FAACT
Consulting Editor: Lynn R. Hovda, RPh, DVM, MS, DACVIM

chapter 58

Scorpions

DEFINITION/OVERVIEW

- Over 1500 species of scorpions are found in all parts of the world except Antarctica.
- Only one species in North America induces possibly life-threatening clinical signs after a venomous sting – the Arizona bark scorpion (*Centruroides exilicauda*, formerly *Centruroides sculpturatus*).
    - Natural range includes all counties of Arizona, part of western New Mexico, Southern Utah, and Southern Nevada.
    - This scorpion is light brown in color, nocturnal, ambushes its prey, and grows to about 8 cm (male) or 7 cm (female) (Fig. 58.1).

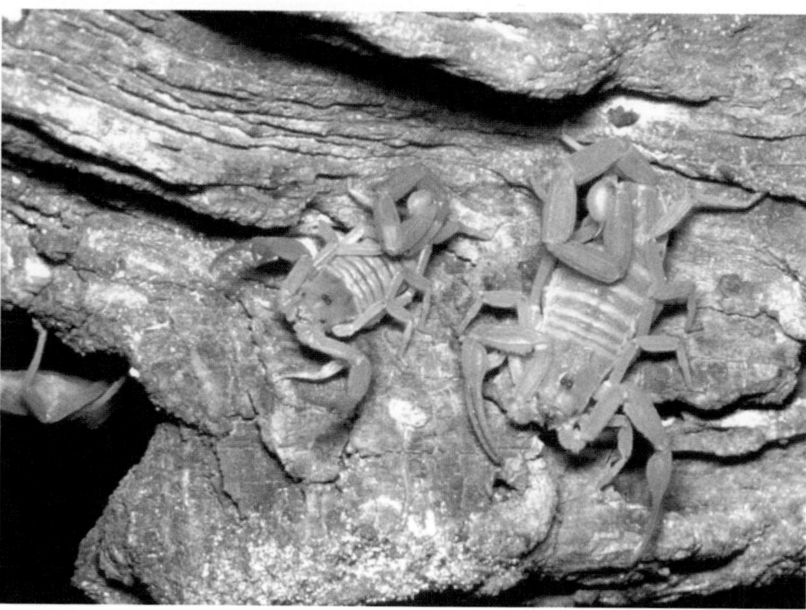

Fig. 58.1. Arizona bark scorpions (*Centruroides exilicauda*). Photo courtesy of Arizona Poison and Drug Information Center, Tucson.

Blackwell's Five-Minute Veterinary Consult Clinical Companion: Small Animal Toxicology, Second Edition.
Lynn R. Hovda, Ahna G. Brutlag, Robert H. Poppenga, and Katherine L. Peterson.

Companion website: www.fiveminutevet.com/toxicology

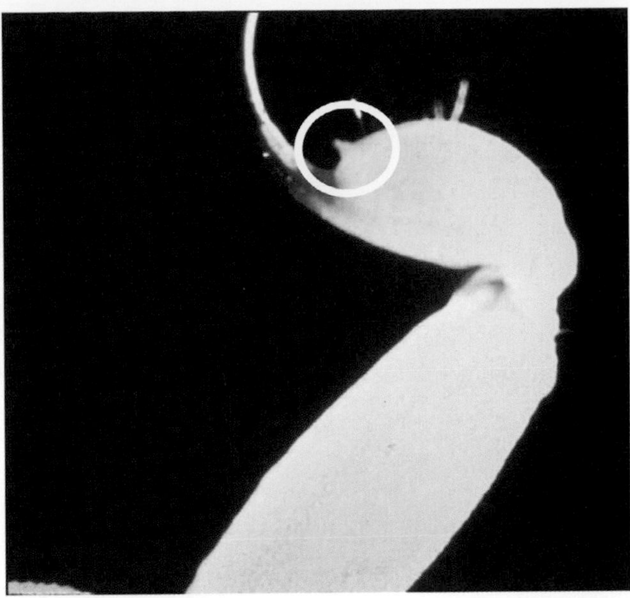

■ **Fig. 58.2.** The encircled tubercle located behind the stinger is characteristic of the bark scorpion. This tubercle may become less noticeable in some adults. Photo courtesy of Arizona Poison and Drug Information Center, Tucson.

  - It can be identified by the small tubercle under the stinger; magnification may be required to identify this (Fig. 58.2).
- The majority of stings result only in localized pain or pruritus and usually resolve within 24 hours.

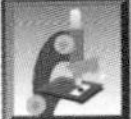

ETIOLOGY/PATHOPHYSIOLOGY

Mechanism of Action

- The venom is a complex mixture of polypeptides, proteins, and neurotoxins. The neurotoxins of the bark scorpion block or delay the opening of the sodium channels of cell membranes, inhibiting neuromuscular transmission.
- Envenomation causes release of neurotransmitters, both sympathetic (causing tachycardia, hypertension, mydriasis) and parasympathetic (causing hypersalivation, bradycardia, hypotension).

Pharmacokinetics – Absorption, Distribution, Metabolism, Excretion

- Animal studies involving other species of scorpions showed a distribution half-life of 4–7 minutes.
- Animal studies involving other species of scorpions showed an elimination half-life of 4.2–13.4 hours.

Toxicity

- There is very little data available in veterinary medicine. Anecdotal information documents pain and pruritus with the initial sting, followed by hypertension either associated with the toxins or secondary to the pain and distress.

Systems Affected

- Nervous – numbness at the site, paresthesia (human beings), tremors, ataxia.
- Cardiovascular – hypertension; tachycardia; possible hypotension, bradycardia.
- Endocrine/metabolic – hyperglycemia.
- Respiratory – rarely, pulmonary edema secondary to cardiovascular compromise.
- Ophthalmic – nystagmus.
- Gastrointestinal – salivation.

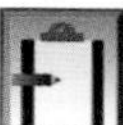

SIGNALMENT/HISTORY

- No particular breed predilection.
- Diagnosis is based on history, clinical signs, and appropriate geographic environment.
- No specific studies have been done on dogs and cats. Anecdotally, cats seem to be seldom, if ever, affected. They have been known to hunt the scorpions without consequence. There are, however, a few documented cases in Arizona where clinical signs in cats have occurred.

Risk Factors

- Geriatric or pediatric patients may be at higher risk of systemic involvement.

Location and Circumstances of Poisoning

- The bark scorpion is primarily nocturnal, hiding under rocks or in clothes or shoes during the day. It will attack if threatened by an inquisitive animal or when disturbed or crushed during movement of bedding, clothing, etc.

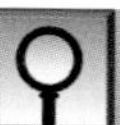

CLINICAL FEATURES

- Immediate pain at the site following the sting. Edema and pruritus may follow.
- Significant local tissue reaction rules out *C. exilicauda* envenomation.
- Hypertension may develop, especially in smaller animals. Whether this results from the venom itself or a pain response is unknown.
- Pulmonary edema may occur secondary to cardiovascular dysfunction.
- In humans, paresthesia and numbness have been documented at the site of the sting. Tremors and neuromuscular dysfunction were also noted.

- Other clinical features in dogs and cats reported by owners to the Arizona Poison and Drug Information Center (Tucson, AZ) include respiratory changes, gastrointestinal distress, CNS changes (restlessness and lethargy), sneezing, and a pain response as evidenced by vocalizing, limping, licking, pawing, and head shaking. Signs can persist for up to 24 hours but resolved on average at 8 hours.
  - It should be noted these data reflect owners calling into a poison center and the species of scorpion involved is unknown.
  - 71% of cats, 39% of dogs under 33 pounds, and only 13% of dogs over 33 pounds exhibited clinical signs, which is consistent with the human experience (smaller size, greater signs) with bark scorpion envenomation.
  - 72 of the 84 cases responded to follow-up; no fatalities were reported.
  - Anecdotally local veterinarians reported 100% fatalities in ferrets.
  - The key finding, as in humans, is that the smaller the patient, the higher the risk of mortality.

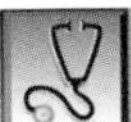

DIFFERENTIAL DIAGNOSIS

- Other venomous stings or bites (wasps, hornets, bees, spiders) causing pain or an allergic reaction.

DIAGNOSTICS

- No specific diagnostics tests are recommended.
- Hyperglycemia due to decreased insulin production has been documented occasionally in human medicine.
- Identification of the scorpion, if possible, is the best diagnostic tool.

Pathological Findings

- Rarely, the skin at the site of the envenomation may slough.

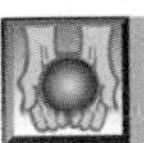

THERAPEUTICS

- The goal is to provide symptomatic and supportive care. This includes the use of analgesics or opioids for pain control, appropriate treatment for CNS and CV changes, careful monitoring of the skin at the envenomation site, and medications for allergic reaction to the venom should it occur.

Detoxification

- Wash the sting area well and apply cool compresses as needed.
- If available, bind venom components with antivenom until cleared from body.

Appropriate Health Care

- Monitor the sting site for evidence of infection or skin sloughing.
- Frequent vital signs for first 24 hours to monitor for hypertension.
- Observe for onset of pulmonary edema and be prepared to intubate and provide oxygen as needed.
- Watch closely for local and systemic signs associated with a rare allergic reaction to venom.

Antidotes and Drugs of Choice

- The use of scorpion antivenom (Anascorp®) is recommended in very small or geriatric patients with severe envenomation manifestations. The antivenom is very effective, but cost can be an issue. One vial should be sufficient.
- IV fluids as needed if hypotensive; caution required as many of these patients are hypertensive.
- Analgesics.
  - Carprofen.
    - Dogs 2.2 mg/kg PO q 12–24 hours.
    - Cats 1–2 mg/kg SQ q 24 hours. Limit dosing to 2 days.
  - Deracoxib 1–2 mg/kg PO q 24 hours (dogs).
  - Robenicoxib 1 mg/kg 2–24 hours (cats). Limit to < 6 days.
  - Buprenorphine 0.005–0.03 mg/kg IM, IV or SQ q 6–12 hours (dogs, cats).
  - Tramadol 4–10 mg/kg PO q 8–12 hours for dogs; 1–2 mg/kg PO q 12 hours for cats. Extra-label use for both species.
- Antihistamine.
  - Diphenhydramine 2–4 mg/kg IM or PO q 8–12 hours (dogs, cats).
- Hypertension – acepromazine 0.01–0.03 mg/kg IV, IM, SQ (dogs, cats).

Nursing Care

- Cool compresses or ice may alleviate some of the local pain and swelling.
- Nonstimulating environment.

Follow-up

- Monitor until clinical signs resolve.

COMMENTS

Patient Monitoring

- Monitor hydration, pain level, blood pressure, heart rate, temperature, and development of hyperglycemia as needed based on degree of clinical signs being experienced.

Prevention/Avoidance

- Keep clothes picked up, shake out shoes and blankets prior to use; monitor pets' activities and keep them away from suspicious areas.

Possible Complications

- Allergic reactions, pulmonary edema, CV collapse, coma, and death are rare complications.

Expected Course and Prognosis

- Clinical signs generally resolve within 24 hours with no sequelae.

Abbreviations

See Appendix 1 for a complete list.

Suggested Reading

Gwaltney-Brant SM, Dunayer EK, Youssef HY. Terrestrial zootoxins. In: Gupta RC, ed. Veterinary Toxicology: Basic and Clinical Principles, 2nd edn. New York: Elsevier, 2012; pp. 969–996.

Holzman D, Reilly L, McNally J, et al. Dogs and cats with scorpion stings. Venom Week, June 1–4, 2009; Albuquerque, NM (Abstract).

Mebs D. Scorpions. In: Mebs D, ed. Venomous and Poisonous Animals. Boca Raton, FL: CRC Press, 2002; pp. 172–178.

Acknowledgment: The authors and editors acknowledge the prior contributions of Catherine M. Adams, DVM, who authored this topic in the previous edition.
Author: Michael E. Peterson, DVM, MS
Consulting Editor: Lynn R. Hovda, RPh, DVM, MS, DACVIM

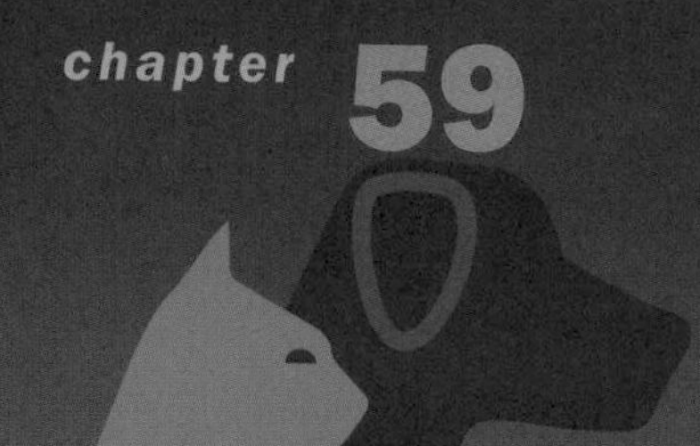

chapter 59

Venomous Lizards (*Heloderma*)

DEFINITION/OVERVIEW

- Local and systemic venom-induced toxicity may both occur following bites by the Gila monster (*Heloderma suspectum*) or the Mexican beaded lizard (*Heloderma horridum*).
  - Gila monster lizards are the only venomous lizard species native to North America and are geographically confined to the states of Arizona, New Mexico, extreme southern California and Utah, and southwestern Nevada (Fig. 59.1).

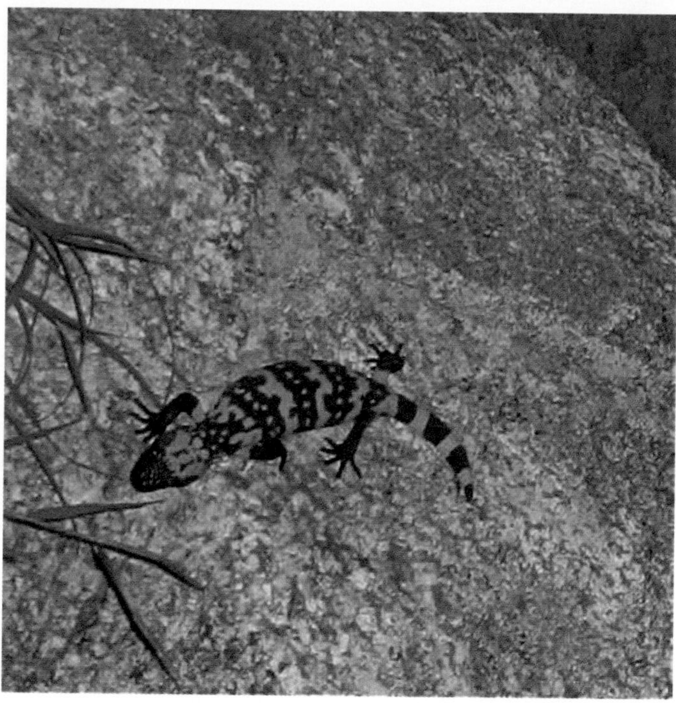

■ **Fig. 59.1.** Gila monster (*Heloderma suspectum*). Photo courtesy of Dan Keyler.

Blackwell's Five-Minute Veterinary Consult Clinical Companion: Small Animal Toxicology, Second Edition.
Lynn R. Hovda, Ahna G. Brutlag, Robert H. Poppenga, and Katherine L. Peterson.

Companion website: www.fiveminutevet.com/toxicology

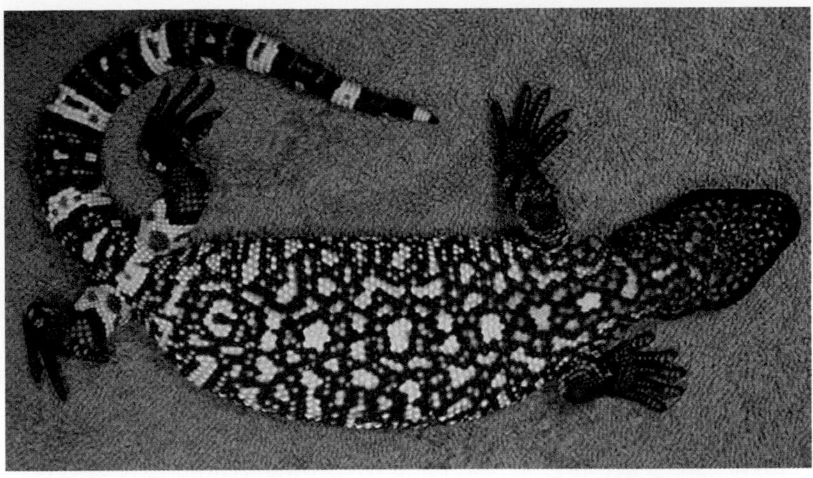

■ **Fig. 59.2.** Mexican beaded lizard (*Heloderma horridum*). Photo courtesy of Dan Keyler.

- The Mexican beaded lizard is geographically distributed along the west coast of Mexico and down to Guatemala (Fig. 59.2).
- Although documented cases of envenomation to animals is lacking, undocumented bites have likely occurred.

- Identifiable by their round-beaded, textured, multicolored skin (typically pink beads on black-bead background for *H. suspectum*, and yellow beads on a chocolate-bead background for *H. horridum*) covering their robust stout body. They are awkward, slow-moving lizards with a large blunt head. They range in size from 2 to 3 feet in length, with the beaded lizard attaining the greater length.
- Bites are typically tenacious and delivered with power, with the tendency being to clamp down and hold on. However, rapid slashing bites with quick release occur.
- Venom is released from secretory glands located in the mandibles, elaborated onto the grooved teeth, and introduced into the victim via mastication with the bite.
- Emergency and supportive care, along with good wound care, are the key components for achieving an optimal outcome.

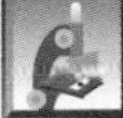

ETIOLOGY/PATHOPHYSIOLOGY

- Wound punctures are inflicted by small, solid, round peg-like teeth that have a small superficial groove.
  - Teeth are needle sharp and the bite itself usually results in significant trauma independent of venom delivery.
  - Unlike snakebite, the tooth puncture marks are typically more easily observed, and there may be more noticeable blood at the site of the bite.
- Venom quantity delivered with a bite is highly variable, and increased bite contact time results in more venom introduced with the bite.

- When envenomation has occurred, swelling, pain, ecchymosis, hypotension, and apnea follow.
- Hypotension may be significant and prolonged; renal complications are possible.

Mechanism of Action

- Protein and nonprotein substances comprise the venom, and include bradykinin-releasing substance, hyaluronidase, phospholipase A, proteases, and serotonin.
  - Phospholipase A_2, hyaluronidase, and proteases contribute to tissue destruction, allowing venom spread to tissues.
  - Endogenous hydrolases are activated and consequent third spacing of fluids and edema develop.
- A specific venom toxin referred to as gilatoxin is a serine protease that causes kallikrein-like and thrombin activating activities.
  - This toxin can cleave angiotensin I and trigger the hypotensive effects observed following envenomation. These combined pharmacological activities may result in significant hypotension.
  - Gilatoxin may also potentiate the effects of venom hemorrhagic toxins.

Pharmacokinetics – Absorption, Distribution, Metabolism, Excretion

- Toxins that compose Gila or Mexican beaded lizard venom all have their own individual toxicokinetics, but may act collectively to enhance the absorption and distribution of specific toxins.
  - Bites to extremities usually have slower venom uptake, while bites to highly vascularized areas such as the tongue and lips may result in more rapid absorption.
- Distribution of venom toxins can be quite rapid in the case of intravenous bites, but is generally slower with intradermal or intramuscular bites.
- Multitoxin venom component makes metabolism and elimination kinetics variable.

Toxicity

- Envenomation frequently results in hypotension due to the combined effects of fluid redistribution and gilatoxin-induced effects.
- Venom delivery route influences the time to effect (IV more rapid onset than IM which is more rapid than ID), and influences the level of systemic venom dosage (mg/kg BW).
- Teeth may be broken off in the process of biting or during lizard removal – check closely as X-rays may be needed.

Systems Affected

- Blood/lymphatic/immune – lymphangitis, coagulopathy (uncommon).
- Respiratory – fluid shift potentially to lungs.
- Dermal – erythema, edema, paresthesia, tissue destruction.

- Cardiovascular – hypotension, tachycardia, shock.
- Renal/urological – no reported effects.
- Gastrointestinal – vomiting and diarrhea.
- Neuromuscular – generalized weakness.

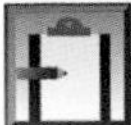

SIGNALMENT/HISTORY

- Cats and dogs of any age may encounter venomous lizards, particularly in geographic regions where the species are indigenous.
- Veterinarians should be aware of the geographic distribution of venomous lizards, which is highly restricted in the USA. However, Gila monster and beaded lizards may be present in any part of the country as they are frequently found in amateur collections.
- Bites to the face and front legs may occur due to the curious nature of dogs and cats.
- Removal of the lizard may be required. If the lizard is attached to a limb, it can be submerged in very warm water or very cold water for a brief period. Otherwise more aggressive measures may be used such as forcing the upper and lower jaws apart.

Risk Factors

- Smaller animals, those with predisposing health problems, and older animals may be at greater risk of severe complications.
  - In smaller animals, the venom dose (mg venom/kg BW) may be quite large.
  - Geriatric animals lack resilience in their physiological systems.
- Animals with cardiac, diabetic, renal, or other major physiological system compromise are also at increased risk of medical complications. These factors may necessitate intensive supportive veterinary medical management.
- Animals receiving medications for existing medical problems.
  - NSAIDs may predispose to clotting anomalies.
  - Corticosteroids may decrease natural defenses.
- Aggressiveness and motivation of lizard.
  - Rapid slashing bite delivers less venom.
  - Retracted bite delivers greater venom quantity.
  - Agonal bite – venom reservoirs may be depleted.

Historical Findings

- If the lizard is not observed biting the animal, puncture wounds from teeth can frequently be observed; may require clipping hair in affected area.

Location and Circumstances of Poisoning

- Helodermatids are not commonly encountered around human habitats.
- Owners may find their pet carrying around a lizard that they have killed and chewed on, or the lizard may be clamped onto a pet's appendages or mouth.

Interactions with Drugs, Nutrients, or Environment

- Because there are several pharmacologically active components in helodermatid venom, there is the potential for interaction with many drugs. See Risk Factors.
- Environmental factors such as excessive heat may be an additional burden beyond the effects of envenomation alone. Careful use of selective medications and the maintenance of euthermia and homeostasis are keys to an optimal outcome.

CLINICAL FEATURES

- Airway obstruction may occur with bites to the tongue, lips, or face.
- Various cardiovascular effects – ventricular arrhythmia and nonspecific ECG changes.

Local signs

- Angioedema
- Puncture wounds
- Edema and swelling
- Bleeding from the bite site
- Erythema, ecchymosis
- Lymphangitis

Systemic signs

- Hypotension
- Hypersalivation
- Respiratory changes (dyspnea)
- Weakness
- Bleeding – epistaxis, gingival, hematuria, melena, retinal hemorrhage
- Myokymia/fasciculations
- Vomiting – hematemesis
- Diarrhea
- Oliguria

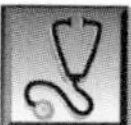

DIFFERENTIAL DIAGNOSIS

- Animal bites – snakes, cats, rodents, shrews, etc.
- Hymenoptera venom-induced angioedema. When touched, these swollen areas are generally not significantly painful, in contrast to lizard envenomation.
- Trauma-induced puncture wounds (e.g., nails, barbed wire fence, etc.).
- Sepsis.

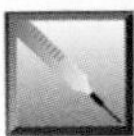

DIAGNOSTICS

- Obtain correct lizard identification.
- Examine for puncture wounds, clip hair in affected area, examine for local tissue damage and ecchymosis.
- CBC – leukocytosis.
- Coagulation parameters (INR, plts, PT, PTT, Fib) – typically not affected.
- ECG – ventricular arrhythmias may be detected in severely depressed patients.

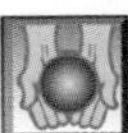

THERAPUETICS

Detoxification

- Gently wash wound area to remove any residual venom at the bite site.
- Transport to veterinary clinic immediately.
- Remove collars and other restrictive devices prior to transport.
- Clip and clean bite area with antiseptic.

Appropriate Health Care

- Minimize exercise/movement.
- Observe closely for airway obstruction and be prepared to intubate.
- Monitor cardiovascular system closely.
- Blood pressure monitor.

Antivenom

- Antivenom – no antivenom exists for treatment of lizard envenomation.

Drugs of Choice

- IV crystalloid fluids for volume resuscitation.
- Pain management.
    - Buprenorphine 0.005–0.02 mg/kg IM, IV, or SQ q 6–12 hours.
    - Tramadol 4–10 mg/kg PO q 8–12 hours for dogs; 1–2 mg/kg q 12 hours for cats. Both are extra label use.
- Antiemetics for persistent vomiting.
    - Maropitant 1 mg/kg SQ q 24 hours.
    - Ondansetron 0.1–0.2 mg/kg IV q 8–12 hours.
- Antibiotics are not routinely needed unless localized tissue damage is severe and there is confirmed evidence of infection.

Precautions/Interactions

- Other drugs.
  - Corticosteroids have no documented value in the treatment of venomous lizard envenomation.
  - DMSO may enhance uptake and spread of venom.
  - Heparin has no proven clinical value and may worsen the condition so should not be used.
  - Morphine can cause reactions similar to early anaphylaxis.

COMMENTS

Patient Monitoring

- Baseline laboratory values should be obtained and repeated as necessary. Coagulation panel is not routinely performed.

Expected Course and Prognosis

- Complete recovery should be anticipated.

See Also

Wasps, Hornets, and Bees

Abbreviations

See Appendix 1 for a complete list.

Suggested Reading

Ariano-Sanchez D. Envenomation by a wild Guatemalan Beaded Lizard Heloderma horridum charlesbogerti. Clin Tox 2008; 46:897–899.

Cantrell FL. Envenomation by the Mexican Beaded Lizard: a case report. J Tox Clin Tox 2003; 41:241–244.

Hooker KR, Caravati EM. Gila monster envenomation. Ann Emerg Med 1994; 24:731–735.

Preston CA. Hypotension, myocardial infarction, and coagulopathy following Gila Monster bite. J Emerg Med 1989; 7:37–40.

Author: Daniel E. Keyler, RPh, BS, Pharm D, FAACT
Consulting Editor: Lynn R. Hovda, RPh, DVM, MS, DACVIM

chapter 60

Wasps, Hornets, and Bees

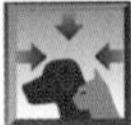

DEFINITION/OVERVIEW

- Two important families in the order Hymenoptera.
    - Vespoidea (wasps, hornets, and yellow jackets) (Fig. 60.1) and Apoidea (bees) (Figs 60.2 and 60.3).
- With the exception of killer bees, they are found worldwide.
    - Africanized killer bees/hybrid bees were introduced into Brazil and have made their way north. They are now found in Texas, Arizona, New Mexico, and southern California.
- Venom is injected through an adapted ovipositor.
    - Vespids do not have barbs on the stinger and are capable of stinging multiple times without dying.
    - Apids have a barbed stinger. After stinging, the barb and venom sac are left behind, allowing continued envenomation. This action is fatal to apids.

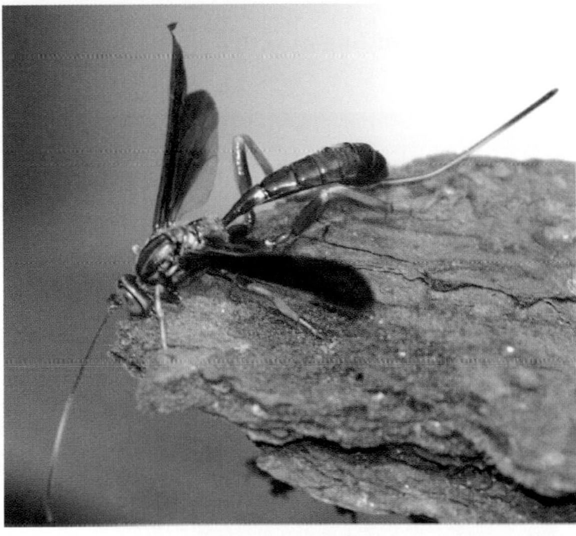

Fig. 60.1. Close-up of wasp. Photo courtesy of C. Morgan Wilson, Hollins University, Roanoke, VA.

Blackwell's Five-Minute Veterinary Consult Clinical Companion: Small Animal Toxicology, Second Edition.
Lynn R. Hovda, Ahna G. Brutlag, Robert H. Poppenga, and Katherine L. Peterson.

Companion website: www.fiveminutevet.com/toxicology

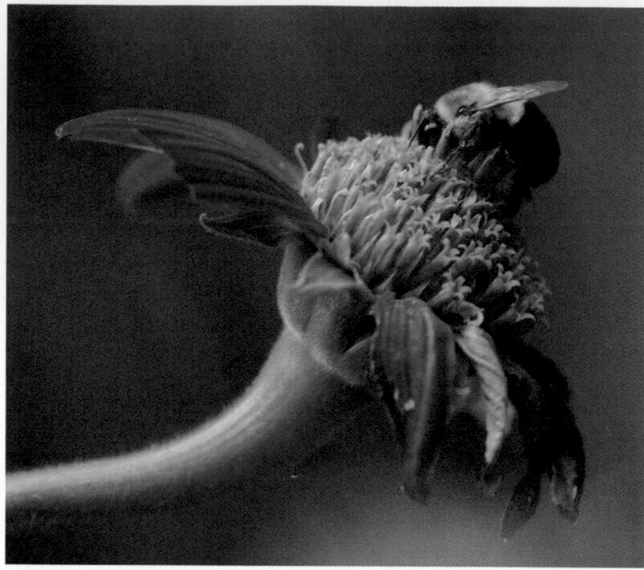

■ **Fig. 60.2.** Common Eastern bumble bee (*Bombus impatiens*). Photo courtesy of C. Morgan Wilson, Hollins University, Roanoke, VA.

- Hymenoptera venoms are composed mainly of proteins.
  - Potent biologically active compounds.
  - Some act directly.
  - Others act indirectly by converting to active substances from host substrates.

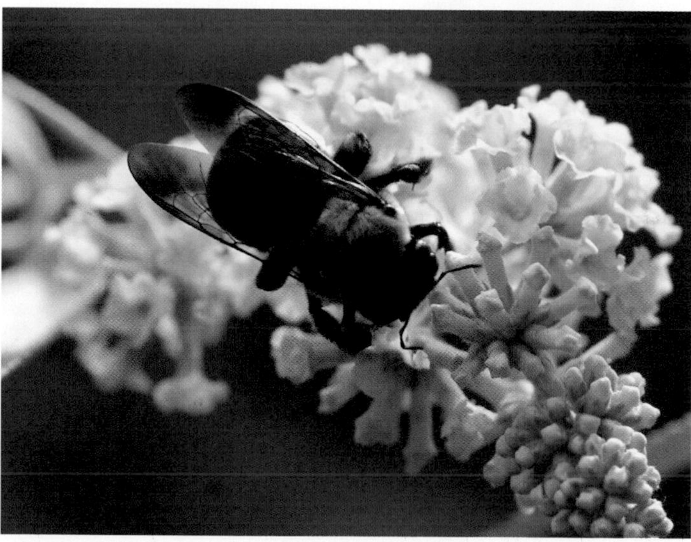

■ **Fig. 60.3.** Eastern carpenter bee (*Xylocopa virginica*). Photo courtesy of C. Morgan Wilson, Hollins University, Roanoke, VA.

- Stings cause a variety of acute clinical signs, including decreased heart rate, decreased arterial blood pressure, respiratory depression, and elevation of plasma cortisol. In severe cases, anaphylactic shock, hemolysis, acute renal failure, acute lung injury/acute respiratory distress syndrome, and death may occur.

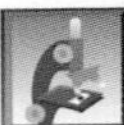

ETIOLOGY/PATHOPHYSIOLOGY

Mechanism of Action

- Vespid venom contains phospholipase A, hyaluronidase, biogenic amines, kinins, acid phosphatase, antigen 5, and mast cell degranulating peptide.
- Apid venom contains phospholipase A, hyaluronidase, mellitin, apamin, biogenic amines, acid phosphatase, mast cell degranulating peptide, and minimine.
  - Phospholipase A – disrupts cell membranes and causes release of pain-inducing agents.
  - Hyaluronidase – facilitates distribution and movement of the toxins through the tissues.
  - Mellitin – membrane-disrupting substance that increases a cell's susceptibility to attack by phospholipases. It also increases cell permeability and capillary blood flow, and causes pain and hemolysis. Most destructive part of Africanized bee venom.
  - Biogenic amines (histamine, serotonin, tyramine and catecholamines) – increase capillary permeability and induce itching and redness.
  - Kinins (bradykinin) – induce pain and cause smooth muscle contractions.
  - Mast cell degranulating peptide – release of biogenic amines.

Pharmacokinetics – Absorption, Distribution, Metabolism, Excretion

- Absorption is immediate; first manifested as intense pain due to vasoactive compounds.
- Regional reactions are mediated by allergic mechanisms.
- Anaphylaxis may occur within minutes of the sting.
- Delayed hypersensitivity reactions occur within 3–14 days.

Toxicity

- Most wasps inject about 17 µg of venom per sting.
- Africanized killer bees can inject 94 µg of venom per sting.
- Single stings may be toxic to susceptible animals but multiple stings result in serious consequences.
- Estimated lethal dose of honeybees in nonallergic mammals is 19 stings/kg.

Systems Affected

- Skin/exocrine – pain, erythema, swelling/edema, wheals, pruritus.
- Cardiovascular – tachycardia, collapse secondary to anaphylaxis.

- Hemic/lymphatic/immune – hemolysis, clotting disorders such as DIC, spherocytosis.
- Renal/urological – acute renal failure, systemic rhabdomyonecrosis and acute tubular necrosis (severe cases).
- Respiratory – acute lung injury/acute respiratory distress syndrome (severe cases).
- Neuromuscular – ataxia, neural dysfunction (severe cases).

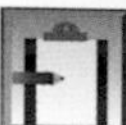

SIGNALMENT/HISTORY

- Diagnosis is based on history (if available) and clinical signs.
- Certain breeds (American Bull Terrier, American Staffordshire Terrier, Boxer) appear to have a higher rate of reaction to Hymenoptera venom.
- Envenomation occurs more frequently in dogs kept outside, particularly when not monitored and allowed to wander and disturb nests or swarms (Fig. 60.4).
- Stings are most common on the face (particularly around the muzzle, ears, eyes, and in the mouth), but can occur anywhere on the body (Fig. 60.5).

Risk Factors

- Pediatric, geriatric, and sensitive individuals are at increased risk for more serious clinical signs and complications that may take longer to resolve.

Historical Findings

- Owner may or may not report witnessing the event or seeing bees/wasps/hornets.

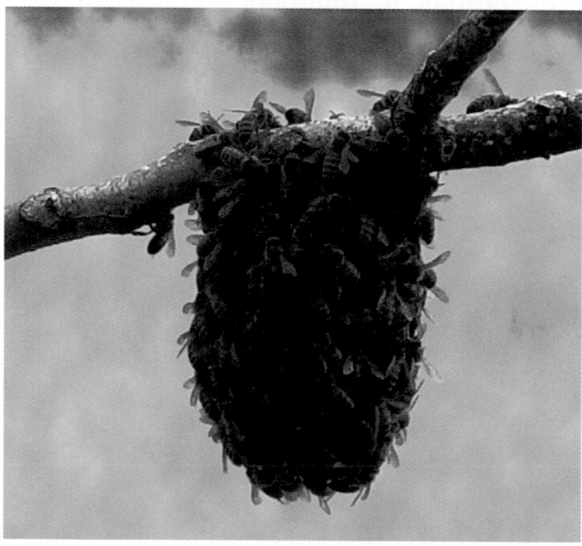

■ **Fig. 60.4.** Honeybee swarm. Photo courtesy of C. Morgan Wilson, Hollins University, Roanoke, VA.

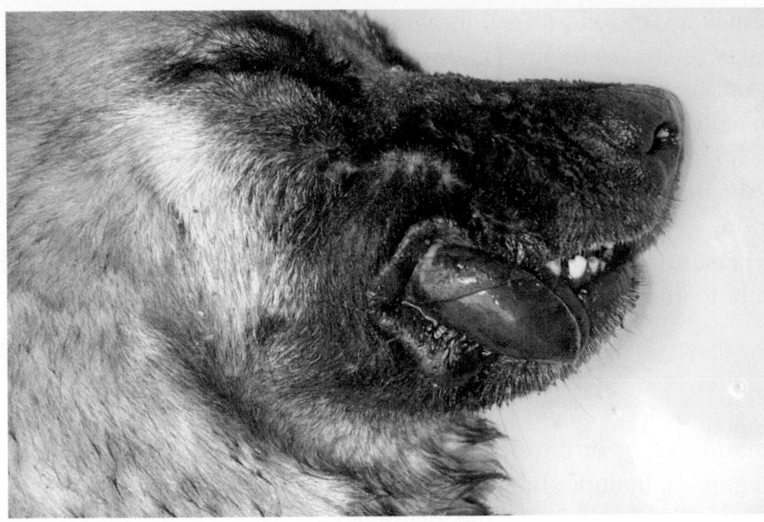

■ **Fig. 60.5.** Africanized killer bee strike in a dog. Note swollen face and tongue. Photo courtesy of David Driemiere, UFRGS, Porto Alegre, RS.

Location and Circumstances of Poisoning

- Hornets and wasps prefer to live in shrubs and trees, attacking when provoked and stinging multiple times.
- Yellow jackets are ground dwellers and are aggressive when aggravated. An attack may occur if the nest is accidentally stepped on or disturbed.
- Honeybees often build their hives in hollow trees and other cavities. They are not typically aggressive and only sting when provoked.
- Africanized killer bees are very aggressive when disturbed. This problem is compounded by the fact that they tend to travel in swarms.

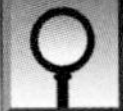

CLINICAL FEATURES

- There are four primary reactions seen after envenomation:
  - Local pain.
  - Regional reaction.
  - Anaphylactic response.
  - Skin rashes/serum sickness (unusual).
- Most stings simply result in localized edema and pain. The reaction is self-limiting and non-IgE mediated.
  - These cases tend to resolve within 24 hours.
- Regional reactions can take up to 24 hours to manifest. During this time, the mast cells are degranulating and cellulitis is forming.
- Systemic anaphylaxis usually occurs within minutes. If it hasn't started within 30 minutes, it is unlikely to happen.

    - Signs in dogs include urination, vomiting, defecation, urticaria, pruritus, muscular weakness, depressed respiration, angioedema, cardiovascular compromise, and seizures.
    - Signs in cats include pruritus, vocalization, hypersalivation, ataxia, and collapse.
- Fatalities usually occur within an hour of the stinging event.
- Severe cases involving massive envenomation will be febrile and markedly lethargic.
- Hemolytic anemia and immune-mediated thrombocytopenia (IMT) are reported with bee envenomation.
- Delayed hypersensitivity reactions include serum sickness, DIC, neuropathy, and renal damage, among others listed below in Possible Complications.

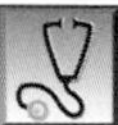

DIFFERENTIAL DIAGNOSIS

- Other venomous stings or bites. A third medically important family (Formicidae) of the order Hymenoptera includes fire ants which elicit similar clinical signs.
- Other causes of allergic reactions and anaphylaxis.

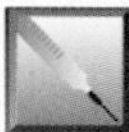

DIAGNOSTICS

- Laboratory analysis in severely affected animals should include a CBC, serum analysis, and coagulation tests as needed.
- Antiplatelet antibodies are the definitive diagnosis for IMT.

Pathological Findings

- No pathognomonic findings but stingers, insect parts, or entire bodies may be present at postmortem (Fig. 60.6).

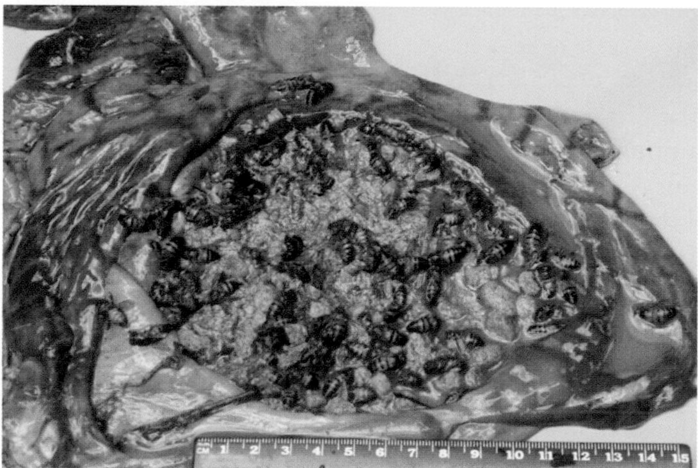

■ **Fig. 60.6.** Postmortem photo of dog's stomach filled with swallowed Africanized killer bees. Photo courtesy of David Driemiere, UFRGS, Porto Alegre, RS.

- The larynx is closely evaluated for evidence of hyperemia, edema, and hemorrhage.
- Findings consistent with anaphylaxis and DIC are supportive.

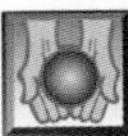

THERAPEUTICS

Detoxification

- Prompt removal of the bee stinger and venom sac.
- Cold compresses and basic wound care.

Appropriate Health Care

- Monitor for anaphylaxis and respiratory distress.
- In severe cases intubation and oxygen may be required.

Antidote

- No antidote available.

Drugs of Choice

- IV fluids may be necessary if the patient is hypotensive secondary to cardiovascular compromise and hypovolemia. If hypotension persists after aggressive IV therapy (including colloids) and if the animal is well hydrated, consider adding the following.
    - Dopamine: 5–20 µg/kg/min IV CRI.
    - Norepinephrine: 0.05–0.1 µg/kg/min IV CRI.
    - Epinephrine: 0.05–0.4 µg/kg/min IV CRI.
- Anaphylaxis.
    - Diphenhydramine 1–4 mg/kg IM or SQ; can be given IV but must be given very slowly and should be diluted.
    - Dexamethasone sodium phosphate 0.1–0.2 mg/kg IV q 12 hours.
    - Epinephrine 0.01–0.02 mg/kg IV, IM, SQ.
- Antiemetics if vomiting is severe or persists.
    - Maropitant 1 mg/kg SQ q 24 hours.
    - Ondansetron 0.1–0.2 mg/kg IV q 8–12 hours.
- Seizures.
    - Diazepam 0.25–0.5 mg/kg IV PRN.
    - Phenobarbital 3–5 mg/kg IV PRN.
- Analgesics.
    - Carprofen.
        - Dogs 2.2 mg/kg PO q 12–24 hours.
        - Cats 1–2 mg/kg SQ q 24 hours. Limit dosing to 2 days.
- Deracoxib 1–2 mg/kg PO q 24 hours (dogs).
- Robenacoxib 1 mg/kg PO q 24 hours (cats.)

- Buprenorphine 0.005–0.03 mg/kg IM, IV or SQ q 6–12 hours (dogs, cats).
- Tramadol 4–10 mg/kg PO q 8–12 hours for dogs; 1–2 mg/kg PO q 12 hours for cats. Extra-label for both.

Precautions/Interactions

- Animals should be monitored for at least 30–90 minutes due to the potential for an anaphylactic reaction.
- Beyond that, animals should be monitored at home by owners. Complications and delayed hypersensitivity reactions may occur.

Activity

- Patient should be kept quiet until clinical symptoms resolve.

COMMENTS

Client Education

- Owners with animals at risk for reactions should keep diphenhydramine available.
- Those with known reactions should have epinephrine readily available.

Patient Monitoring

- Monitor closely for signs of anaphylaxis and/or complications due to stings.
- Because of the risk of acute lung injury in severe cases, respiratory rate and effort should be monitored closely.

Prevention/Avoidance

- Avoid visible nests.
- Move away slowly if a nest is encountered when walking with a dog.

Possible Complications

- Severe envenomation – hemolysis, spherocytosis, neural dysfunction, acute lung injury/acute respiratory distress syndrome (ALI/ARDS), secondary immune-mediated hemolytic anemia, IMT, systemic rhabdomyonecrosis, acute tubular necrosis.

Expected Course and Prognosis

- Excellent in uncomplicated cases with only a localized reaction.
- Fair to good in severe cases with anaphylaxis and further complications.

Abbreviations

See Appendix 1 for a complete list.

Suggested Reading

Fitzgerald KT, Flood AA. Hymenoptera stings. Clin Tech Small Anim Prac 2006; 21(4):194–204.

Nakamura RK, Fenty RK, Bianco D. Presumptive immune-mediated thrombocytopenia secondary to massive Africanized bee envenomation in a dog. J Vet Emerg Crit Care 2013; 23(6):652–656.

Noble SJ, Armstrong PJ. Bee sting envenomation resulting in secondary immune-mediated hemolytic anemia in two dogs. J Am Vet Med Assoc 1999; 214(7):1026–1027.

Oliveira EC, Pedroso PMO, Meirelles EWB, et al. Pathological findings in dogs after multiple Africanized bee stings. Toxicon 2007; 49(8):1214–1218.

Reed HC, Landolt PJ. Ants, wasps, and bees (Hymenoptera). In: Mullen GR, Durden LA, eds. Medical and Veterinary Entomology, 2nd edn. London: Academic Press, 2009; pp. 371–396.

Shimada AT, Nakai T, Morita T, et al. Systemic rhabdomyonecrosis and acute tubular necrosis in a dog associated with wasp stings. Vet Rec 2005; 156(10):320–322.

Author: Sarah K. Jarosinski, BS, DVM elect 2016.
Consulting Editor: Lynn R. Hovda, RPh, DVM, MS, DACVIM

Foods

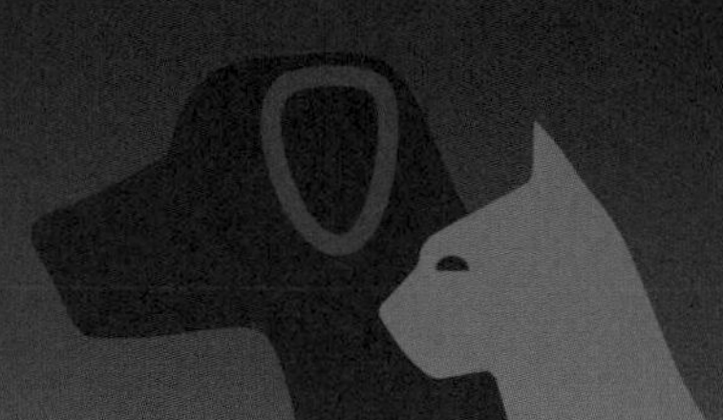

chapter 61

Bread Dough

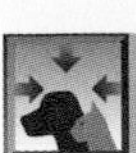

DEFINITION/OVERVIEW

- Bread dough toxicosis occurs when uncooked or unbaked bread, pizza dough, or roll products (including sourdough or starters) that contain live yeast are ingested during the process of rising.
- There are two main concerns following bread dough ingestion: ethanol toxicity and gastric distension leading to mechanical obstruction.

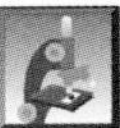

ETIOLOGY/PATHOPHYSIOLOGY

Mechanism of Action

- Live yeast within the dough produces ethanol when exposed to a moist, warm environment such as the stomach. Ethanol is rapidly absorbed and results in systemic alcohol intoxication.
- Metabolism of ethanol can result in metabolic acidosis.
- Hypoglycemia can be seen following ethanol toxicosis due to depletion of glucose stores and depressed gluconeogenesis.
- Uncooked dough expands and produces gas following ingestion. This leads to gastric distension, potential for gastric outflow obstruction, and severe gastric dilatation. This may lead to gastric rupture or volvulus (GDV).

Pharmacokinetics – Absorption, Distribution, Metabolism, Excretion

- Ethanol is rapidly absorbed from the stomach and small intestines.
- Metabolism occurs in the liver by the enzyme alcohol dehydrogenase forming acetaldehyde and acetic acid.
- Alcohol is distributed throughout the body, including the CNS.
- Alcohol is excreted through the lungs and kidneys.

Toxicity

- No known LD_{50} of bread dough exists in dogs and cats.

Blackwell's Five-Minute Veterinary Consult Clinical Companion: Small Animal Toxicology, Second Edition.
Lynn R. Hovda, Ahna G. Brutlag, Robert H. Poppenga, and Katherine L. Peterson.

Companion website: www.fiveminutevet.com/toxicology

Systems Affected

Signs due to bread dough expansion.

- Gastrointestinal – vomiting, nonproductive retching, gastric distension +/– volvulus.

Signs due to ethanol intoxication.

- Cardiovascular – hypotension, bradycardia, cardiovascular collapse.
- Endocrine – hypoglycemia.
- Nervous – altered mentation, ataxia, vocalization, blindness, coma.
- Respiratory – respiratory depression, respiratory arrest.

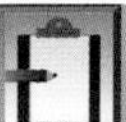

SIGNALMENT/HISTORY

- All reported cases of bread dough toxicosis have been in dogs but cats can be affected.
- Dogs that are highly food motivated may be more likely to ingest the dough.
- There may be a known history of dough ingestion prior to the onset of signs.
- Bread dough may be identified in emesis.

CLINICAL FEATURES

- Signs may be noted within 1 hour after exposure but can be delayed.
- Dogs may present with abdominal discomfort, gastric bloat, vomiting or unproductive retching.
- Ethanol toxicosis may result in abnormal mentation, ataxia, vocalization, and blindness. At high doses, it can cause cardiovascular collapse, respiratory arrest, coma, and death.

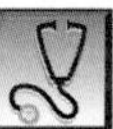

DIFFERENTIAL DIAGNOSIS

- Toxicities affecting the neurological system such as alcohol, ethylene glycol, marijuana, and barbiturates.
- Primary CNS disease.
- Metabolic disease – hepatic encephalopathy.
- Gastric dilatation or GDV.
- Food bloat.
- Foreign body obstruction.

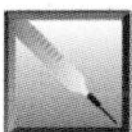

DIAGNOSTICS

- Quick assessment tests should be performed to assess patient stability.
  - Blood glucose levels.
  - Electrolytes.

  - PCV/TS.
  - Venous or arterial blood gas analysis to evaluate ventilation and acid–base status.
  - Pulse oximetry to evaluate oxygenation.
  - Blood pressure.
- Abdominal radiographs should be performed to assess the degree of gastric distension and verify correct positioning of the stomach.
- Blood ethanol levels can be obtained to help verify diagnosis and direct therapy.
  - Human or referral hospitals may have the ability to perform this analysis.
  - Blood alcohol levels at 2–4 mg/mL in adult dogs have produced signs ranging from ataxia to coma.

Pathological Findings

- The presence of bread dough in the stomach.
- Evidence of gastric necrosis, gastric rupture or GDV.
- Splenic congestion.

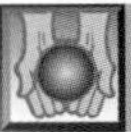

THERAPEUTICS

- Goals of treatment include decontamination, cardiovascular stabilization, and symptomatic/supportive care for ethanol toxicosis.

Detoxification

- Blood glucose should be checked prior to decontamination to ensure normoglycemia.
- If within 30 minutes of ingestion with no clinical signs, emesis with apomorphine can be performed.
- If neurological signs are present but patient is stable, place under general anesthesia with a cuffed endotracheal tube in place and pass a large-bore orogastric tube for cold water lavage and removal of dough.
  - Cold water gastric lavage may be effective at decreasing further yeast fermentation and ethanol production.
- Activated charcoal has been shown to be ineffective in alcohol poisoning and is not recommended.
- If neurological or cardiovascular signs are severe, consider referral for hemodialysis for ethanol removal.

Appropriate Health Care

- Dogs with mild symptoms can often be treated supportively with IV fluids and good nursing care.
- Heart rate/ECG, blood pressure, and blood gas analysis should be performed every 4–6 hours, depending on patient status.

- IV crystalloids to maintain hydration and perfusion.
- Vasopressors may be needed for hypotension unresponsive to fluid boluses.
- Hypoglycemia (BG <70 mg/dL) can be treated with 50% dextrose IV bolus of 1–2 mL/kg (0.5–1 g/kg) diluted 1:1 in saline followed by CRI of 2.5–5% dextrose as needed.
- Dogs with respiratory depression causing a venous or arterial CO_2 greater than 60 mmHg need to be intubated and ventilated.

Drugs of Choice

- Yohimbine 0.1 mg/kg IV can be considered for CNS stimulation in cases of ventilatory failure where mechanical ventilation is not available. If a positive response is observed, it can be administered q 2–3 hours.

Nursing Care

- Recumbent patients should be given clean, dry bedding and turned every 4 hours; urinary catheterization should be considered.
- Apply artificial tears every 6 hours to prevent corneal ulceration in patients that have a diminished blink response.

Diet

- Food and water should be withheld until neurological signs resolve. Once mentation is improved, patients can be offered small amounts of food and water every 4 hours. If signs persist for >24 hours and the patient cannot eat, nutritional support should be considered.

Surgical Considerations

- Surgery may be needed to remove bread dough if gastric lavage is not effective.
- If GDV is confirmed on right lateral radiograph, fluid resuscitation followed by surgery is necessary.
- Standard postoperative care should be provided with IV fluids, blood pressure support, GI protectants, and opioid analgesia.

COMMENTS

Prevention/Avoidance

- Inform owners of the toxicity associated with bread dough ingestion and keep pets out of the kitchen when the products are rising.

Possible Complications

- Monitor for aspiration pneumonia secondary to depressed mentation, vomiting/retching, and anesthesia.

Expected Course and Prognosis

- Dogs with mild-to-moderate neurological signs often improve with supportive care within 24 hours.
- Severe ethanol intoxication is an indication for referral for positive pressure ventilation and hemodialysis and carries a more guarded prognosis.
- Patients requiring surgery have a good prognosis but have a more prolonged recovery time.

See Also

Alcohols

Abbreviations

See Appendix 1 for a complete list.

Suggested Reading

Keno KA, Langston CE. Treatment of accidental ethanol intoxication with hemodialysis in a dog. J Vet Emerg Crit Care 2011; 21(4):363–368.

Means C. Bread dough toxicosis in dogs. J Vet Emerg Crit Care 2003; 13(1):39–41.

Smart L. Specialized gastrointestinal techniques. In: Burkitt Creedon JM, ed. Advanced Monitoring and Procedures for Small Animal Emergency and Critical Care. Chichester, UK: Wiley-Blackwell, 2012; pp. 457–474.

Suter RJ. Presumed ethanol intoxication in sheep dogs fed uncooked pizza dough. Aust Vet J 1992; 69(1):20.

Acknowledgment: The authors and editors acknowledge the prior contributions of Lisa L. Powell, DVM, DACVECC, who authored this topic in the previous edition.
Author: Jennifer M. Hall, DVM, MS, DACVECC
Consulting Editor: Katherine L. Peterson, DVM, DACVECC

Calcium Supplements

DEFINITION/OVERVIEW

- Calcium supplements come in a variety of formulations and concentrations (over the counter and prescription).
- Commonly available calcium salts include calcium carbonate, calcium gluconate, and calcium citrate.
- Calcium alone is generally poorly absorbed by the GI tract.
    - Many calcium supplements also contain vitamin D_3 which enhances calcium absorption and can increase risk of toxicity.

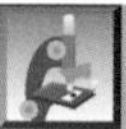

ETIOLOGY/PATHOPHYSIOLOGY

Mechanism of Action

- Ingestion of calcium salts (without vitamin D_3) typically only causes irritation to the GI tract (GIT).
- Ingestion of large quantities of calcium can result in transiently elevated blood calcium concentrations.
- Persistent hypercalcemia can lead to development of calcium deposits in the kidneys, cardiac vessels, and GIT.
- Deposition of calcium in the renal tubules causes mineralization and renal failure.
- Calcium carbonate can produce metabolic alkalosis by:
    - sodium excretion by the kidneys
    - volume depletion stimulating bicarbonate reabsorption
    - suppressing parathyroid hormone release, leading to further impairment of bicarbonate excretion.
- Hypercalcemia can lead to:
    - increasing the excitation threshold of nerve and muscle cells, causing cardiac arrhythmias, weakness, and lethargy
    - decreasing contractility of smooth muscle in GIT and potentially causing constipation

Blackwell's Five-Minute Veterinary Consult Clinical Companion: Small Animal Toxicology, Second Edition.
Lynn R. Hovda, Ahna G. Brutlag, Robert H. Poppenga, and Katherine L. Peterson.

Companion website: www.fiveminutevet.com/toxicology

- increasing gastrin secretion leading to increased hydrochloric acid secretion, which in turn causes GI irritation
- inhibiting ADH receptors in the renal tubules, leading to polyuria with compensatory polydypsia (secondary nephrogenic diabetes insipidus).

Pharmacokinetics – Absorption, Distribution, Metabolism, Excretion

- Calcium salts are poorly absorbed from the GI tract.
- Activated vitamin D_3 is necessary for calcium absorption.
- A small portion of calcium is distributed to the intracellular and extracellular fluid. The majority of calcium is taken up by bone.
- Calcium is excreted in the feces, with a small amount excreted by the kidneys.

Toxicity

- Acute ingestions of most calcium supplements do not typically result in clinical signs of hypercalcemia and toxicosis in healthy animals.
- Vitamin D_3 in the supplement increases risk for hypercalcemia to occur.

Systems Affected

- Cardiovascular – arrhythmias.
- Gastrointestinal – vomiting, diarrhea, anorexia, constipation.
- Endocrine/metabolic – transient hypercalcemia.
- Musculoskeletal – weakness.
- Nervous – depression.
- Renal/urological – PU/PD, rarely azotemia, oliguria, decreased GFR, renal mineralization, nephroliths, cystic calculi.

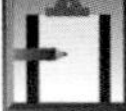

SIGNALMENT/HISTORY

- All breeds and species are susceptible to GI irritation.

Risk Factors

- Patients with renal impairment are at increased risk of complications associated with hypercalcemia.

Historical Findings

- Owners often report PU/PD, lethargy, vomiting, and anorexia.

Location and Circumstances of Poisoning

- Most ingestions will occur at home but iatrogenic calcium administration may occur within the hospital setting.

Interactions with Drugs, Nutrients, or Environment

- Vitamin D is necessary for calcium absorption. Supplements containing both calcium salts and vitamin D have increased risk of toxicity.
- Oral calcium may decrease the GI absorption of tetracyclines or phenytoin.
- The use of thiazide diuretics, vitamin A, or oral magnesium during treatment for calcium overdose may result in hypercalcemia.

Clinical Features

- Mild and self-limiting GI distress (vomiting, diarrhea) are the most likely clinical signs following an acute ingestion of calcium supplements.
- Though transient hypercalcemia may occur following ingestion, it is rarely clinically significant.
- If enough vitamin D_3 has been ingested in conjunction with the calcium ingestion, clinical signs of hypercalcemia could be expected (PU/PD, weakness, lethargy, nausea, vomiting, diarrhea, constipation). See chapter 113 Cholecalciferol for more information.

Differential Diagnosis

- Other causes of gastrointestinal upset.
  - Pancreatitis.
  - Dietary indiscretion.
  - GI obstruction.
  - Infectious or inflammatory GI diseases.
- Other causes of hypercalcemia.
  - Vitamin D ingestion.
  - Hypercalcemia of malignancy.
  - Hyperparathyroidism.
  - Fungal disease.
  - Feline idiopathic hypercalcemia.
  - Hypoadrenocorticism.
  - Renal disease.

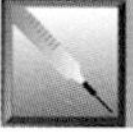

DIAGNOSTICS

- Acute ingestion of calcium supplements without vitamin D_3 is unlikely to result in biochemical abnormalities.
- Chemistry panel should be performed in sick patients and may identify the presence of hypercalcemia, hyperphosphatemia, azotemia.

Pathological Findings

- With acute ingestion of calcium supplements, GI irritation may be seen.
- With hypercalcemia, calcification in the kidneys, GIT walls, and cardiac vessels may be found.

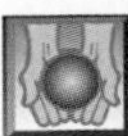

THERAPEUTICS

- The objectives of therapeutics are decontamination, evaluation for the presence of hypercalcemia, and treatment of the hypercalcemia if present.

Detoxification

- Induction of emesis can be performed with large number of tablet, or supplements ingested.
- In most cases of calcium supplement ingestion without vitamin D_3, no further intervention will be required.
- Unless toxic amounts of vitamin D_3 have been consumed along with the calcium supplement, no activated charcoal is required.

Appropriate Health Care

- If prolonged GI distress, symptomatic and supportive care can be provided with fluids (IV or SQ crystalloids depending on severity), antiemetics, antidiarrheals.

Drugs of Choice

- Antiemetic such as maropitant 1 mg/kg SQ q 24 hours.

Precautions/Interactions

- The concomitant ingestion of vitamin D along with calcium determines the degree of toxicity. Doses of vitamin D_3 >0.1 mg/kg BW may result in hypercalcemia (40,000 IU of vitamin D_3 = 1 mg vitamin D_3).

COMMENTS

Expected Course and Prognosis

- Clinical signs are typically mild and self-limiting in healthy patients and prognosis is good.
- If there is previous renal compromise, the prognosis will depend on the amount of the ingestion, the timing of intervention, and the degree of previous compromise.
- Concomitant vitamin D ingestion will require more aggressive treatment and may change prognosis.

See Also

Cholecalciferol

Abbreviations

See Appendix 1 for a complete list.

Suggested Reading

Green T, Chew DJ. Calcium disorders. In: Silverstein DC, Hopper K, eds. Small Animal Critical Care Medicine, 2nd edn. St Louis, MO: Saunders Elsevier, 2015; pp. 274–280.
McKnight K. Ingestion of over the counter calcium supplements. Vet Tech 2006; 7:446–448.
Messinger JS, Windham WR, Ward CR. Ionized hypercalcemia in dogs: a retrospective study of 109 cases (1998–2003). J Vet Intern Med 2009; 23(3):514–519.
Plumb DC. Calcium salts. In: Plumb's Veterinary Drug Handbook, 8th edn. Ames, IA: Wiley-Blackwell, 2015.

Acknowledgment: The authors and editors acknowledge the prior contributions of Catherine M. Adams, DVM, who authored this topic in the previous edition.
Author: Tracy Julius, DVM, DACVECC
Consulting Editor: Katherine L. Peterson, DVM, DACVECC

chapter 63

Chocolate and Caffeine

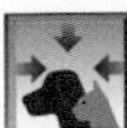

DEFINITION/OVERVIEW

- Methylated xanthine alkaloids (methylxanthines) include theobromine and caffeine.
- Onset of clinical signs is rapid and may include:
  - gastrointestinal upset (vomiting and diarrhea)
  - cardiovascular abnormalities (tachycardia, arrhythmias, and hypertension)
  - PU/PD and urinary incontinence
  - CNS abnormalities (ataxia, muscle tremors, seizure activity and hyperexcitability)
  - respiratory and circulatory collapse and death with high doses.
- Commonly ingested products include chocolate, coffee, caffeine tablets or, less commonly, cacao bean mulch.

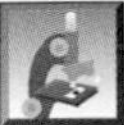

ETIOLOGY/PATHOPHYSIOLOGY

Mechanism of Action

- Methylxanthines increase contractility of cardiac and skeletal muscle through:
  - inhibition of cellular phosphodiesterases and adenosine leading to increased cAMP, causing an increase in free intracellular calcium
  - direct stimulation of release of catecholamines (epinephrine and norepinephrine) from the adrenal medulla.

Pharmacokinetics – Absorption, Distribution, Metabolism, Excretion

- Absorption.
  - Caffeine – rapid; peak plasma levels within 30–60 minutes.
  - Chocolate – delayed, with peak plasma levels up to 10 hours.
- High volume of distribution and crosses the blood–brain, blood–milk, and placental barriers.
- Metabolism is predominantly hepatic.
- Excretion is primarily biliary with enterohepatic recirculation. About 10% is renally excreted unchanged.

Blackwell's Five-Minute Veterinary Consult Clinical Companion: Small Animal Toxicology, Second Edition.
Lynn R. Hovda, Ahna G. Brutlag, Robert H. Poppenga, and Katherine L. Peterson.

Companion website: www.fiveminutevet.com/toxicology

- Excreted methylxanthines may be reabsorbed intact through the bladder wall.
- Half-life.
  - Caffeine is estimated to be 4.5 hours in the dog.
  - Chocolate is approximately 17.5 hours in the dog.

Toxicity

- The LD_{50} of caffeine is 140–150 mg/kg in dogs and 80–150 mg/kg in cats.
- The LD_{50} of theobromine is 250–500 mg/kg in dogs and 200 mg/kg in cats.
- Clinical signs are dose dependent.
- Chocolate products may contain both caffeine and theobromine together.
- Tables 63.1 and 63.2 provide the approximate amounts of caffeine and theobromine found in common products.

Systems Affected

- Gastrointestinal – nausea, vomiting/regurgitation, diarrhea.
- Cardiovascular – tachycardia, hypertension, VPCs, other tachyarrhythmias, bradycardia (rare).
- Nervous – hyperexcitability, ataxia, seizures.

TABLE 63.1. Caffeine content of common products.

Source	Caffeine content
OTC stimulants and diet pills (Vivarin tablets)	200 mg/tablet
Excedrin	65 mg/tablet
Tea	4–18 mg/oz
Chocolate-containing products	2–40 mg/oz, depending on type
Coffee beans	280–570 mg/oz
Regular coffee	6–18 mg/oz
Decaffeinated coffee	0.4–0.8 mg/oz
Cola beverages	5–7.5 mg/oz

TABLE 63.2. Theobromine content of common chocolate products.

Source	Theobromine content
Cacao beans	300–1500 mg/oz
Unsweetened baking chocolate	390–450 mg/oz
Dark chocolate (may vary by percentage)	135 mg/oz
Milk chocolate	44–60 mg/oz
White chocolate	0.25 mg/oz
Cocoa powder	400–737 mg/oz
Cacao bean mulch	56–900 mg/oz

- Musculoskeletal – muscle tremors.
- Renal/urological – PU/PD, urinary incontinence.
- Respiratory – tachypnea, respiratory failure (high doses).
- Endocrine/metabolic – hypokalemia.

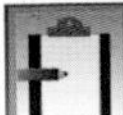

SIGNALMENT/HISTORY

- Any age or breed of dog can be affected.
- Cats are more sensitive but toxicosis is rare due to less indiscriminate eating habits.
- Toxicity has also been noted in pigs, chickens, and ducks when cacao bean shells were added to feeds.

Risk Factors

- Preexisting liver disease may slow metabolism.
- Preexisting heart disease may predispose patients to cardiac complications.

Historical Findings

- Ingestion of products containing caffeine or chocolate is often, but not always, witnessed.
- Chewed packages or wrappings are commonly reported.
- Owners may report PU/PD and emesis with chocolate in it.

Location and Circumstances of Poisoning

- Availability of products containing caffeine or chocolate in the environment should be assessed in dogs presenting with clinical signs of toxicity.
- Use of cacao bean mulch on the property may increase exposure.

CLINICAL FEATURES

- Initial clinical signs typically noted within 1–2 hours for caffeine toxicity and 2–4 hours for theobromine toxicity.
- Physical examination early after exposure (<1–2 hours) may be within normal limits.
- Restlessness and agitation/hyperactivity are typically noted on presentation.
- Cardiovascular signs including tachycardia, hypertension, and cardiac arrhythmias occur as dose ingested increases.
- Neurological signs of weakness, muscle tremors, ataxia, and seizures may occur as toxicity progresses.
- Hyperthermia is frequently noted due to hyperactivity and muscle tremors.
- In severe intoxications, death may occur secondary to respiratory failure, cardiac arrhythmias, or prolonged seizure activity.

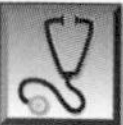

DIFFERENTIAL DIAGNOSIS

- Toxicities.
  - Cardiac stimulant medication ingestion (i.e., albuterol, theophylline, aminophylline).
  - Nicotine, amphetamines, or other illicit drugs.
  - Metaldehyde, strychnine, zinc phosphide, bromethalin.
  - Tremogenic mycotoxins.
  - Serotonin syndrome.
- Primary cardiac, CNS, or GI disease.

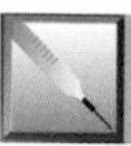

DIAGNOSTICS

- Evidence of chocolate may be seen or smelled from the vomitus or diarrhea.
- Routine blood work (CBC, serum chemistry profile, and urinalysis) is typically unremarkable. Mild hypokalemia and dilute urine may be noted.
- Although confirmatory tests are rarely needed, high-performance liquid chromatography can be performed on stomach contents, plasma, serum, urine, and liver for definitive diagnosis. These compounds are stable for 7 days at room temperature, 14 days if refrigerated, or 4 months if frozen.

Pathological Findings

- Products containing chocolate or caffeine may be found within the GIT on gross necropsy.
- There are no specific histopathological findings associated with caffeine or theobromine toxicosis.
- Findings consistent with gastroenteritis may be evident as well as postmortem congestion of other organs (liver, kidneys, spleen, thymus).

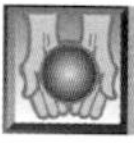

THERAPEUTICS

- Goals of treatment include decontamination, facilitation of toxin excretion, and supportive/symptomatic care for gastrointestinal, cardiac, and neurological symptoms.

Detoxification

- Emesis.
  - Consider patient status prior to emesis.
  - Caffeine emesis typically performed within 1–2 hours if asymptomatic.
  - Chocolate emesis can be performed within 6 hours after ingestion, especially with large ingestions or if patient appears visibly bloated.
- Gastric lavage should be considered with large-volume ingestion in symptomatic patients once stabilized.

- Activated charcoal is recommended 1–2 g/kg PO once with a cathartic (sorbitol) then q 6–8 hours without a cathartic for 24–48 hours.
  - Multidose activated charcoal may not be needed in all patients.
  - Use in symptomatic patients or those with large ingestions to help prevent further absorption of toxic compounds due to enterohepatic recirculation.
  - Repeated doses of charcoal can cause electrolyte abnormalities and dehydration.
- Urinary catheterization or frequent urination (q 2–4 hours) is recommended to decrease potential reabsorption of methylxanthines across the bladder wall.

Appropriate Health Care

- Intravenous fluid therapy is recommended to maintain hydration and perfusion and to promote urinary excretion of caffeine and theobromine. Potassium can be supplemented in IV fluids as needed.
- Continuous ECG and frequent blood pressure monitoring should be considered in symptomatic patients.

Antidote

- There is no known antidote for caffeine or theobromine toxicity.

Drugs of Choice

- For sedation.
  - Acepromazine 0.02–0.04 mg/kg IV, IM, SC, doses repeated/titrated to effect.
  - Butorphanol 0.1–0.5 mg/kg IV, IM, SC, q 2–4 hours.
- For seizures – diazepam or midazolam 0.25–0.5 mg/kg IV to effect; midazolam can be given IM.
- Continued seizures may necessitate treatment with barbiturates, levetiracetam, propofol or a CRI of anticonvulsants.
- Persistent sinus tachyarrhythmias (HR >180 bpm in dogs) or hypertension (systolic >180 mmHg) should be treated with a beta-blocker.
  - Propranolol 0.02–0.06 mg/kg IV q 6 hours to effect.
  - Esmolol 20 µg/kg/min IV CRI.
  - Metoprolol 0.2–0.4 mg/kg PO q 12 hours.
- For ventricular arrhythmias.
  - Lidocaine 1–2 mg/kg IV once, followed by a CRI of 25–75 µg/kg/min.

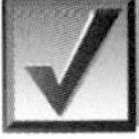

COMMENTS

Patient Monitoring

- Continuous ECG monitoring is recommended during hospitalization for patients with tachycardia, hypertension, or known high-dose exposure.

- Blood pressure, body temperature, and mental status monitoring every 4–6 hours for 12–24 hours post ingestion.

Prevention/Avoidance

- Educate clients on chocolate toxicity, particularly during the holidays (e.g., Easter, Halloween, Christmas).

Expected Course and Prognosis

- With appropriate decontamination and supportive care, the prognosis is generally good.
- For patients with more severe toxicosis and clinical signs such as cardiac arrhythmias or seizure activity unresponsive to therapy, the prognosis is guarded.
- Signs of toxicity generally last for 12–72 hours, with a longer clinical course associated with higher doses.

See Also

Amphetamines

SSRI and SNRI Antidepressants

Abbreviations

See Appendix 1 for a complete list.

Suggested Reading

Dolder LK. Methylxanthines: caffeine, theobromine, theophylline. In: Peterson ME, Talcott PA, eds. Small Animal Toxicology, 3rd edn. St Louis, MO: Elsevier, 2013; pp. 647–652.

Glauberg A, Blumenthal HP. Chocolate poisoning in the dog. J Am Anim Hosp Assoc 1983; 19:246–248.

Reddy BS, Reddy LV, Sivajothi S. Chocolate poisoning in a dog. Int J Vet Health Sci Res 2013; 1:401–403.

Theobromine content of common chocolate products available at: www.thehersheycompany.com/our-ingredients/what-we-believe/ingredient-i information/ingredient-topics/caffeine-theobromine.aspx

Acknowledgment: The authors and editors acknowledge the prior contributions of Elise M. Craft, DVM, and Lisa L. Powell, DVM, DACVECC, who authored this topic in the previous edition.
Author: Jayme E. Hoffberg, DVM, DACVECC
Contributing Editor: Katherine L. Peterson, DVM, DACVECC

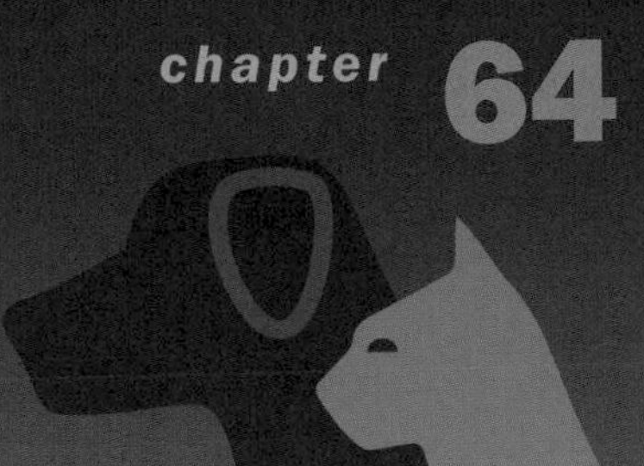

chapter 64

Grapes and Raisins

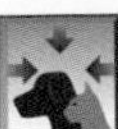

DEFINITION AND OVERVIEW

- Canine ingestion of fruit of the *Vitis* genus, including grapes, raisins, sultanas and currants, may cause a toxicity characterized by lethargy, anorexia, vomiting, diarrhea, ARF, hypercalcemia, hepatopathy, and possibly leading to death.
- The specific mechanism of toxicosis is currently unknown, including whether toxicity is idiosyncratic or dose related.
- Some dogs may show no adverse signs after ingestion of grapes or raisins while others develop acute renal failure.

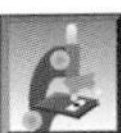

ETIOLOGY AND PATHOPHYSIOLOGY

Mechanism of Action

- The toxic component has not been identified and the mechanism of toxicity is unknown.
  - Proposed mechanisms include ochratoxins (a mycotoxin), pesticides, or components of the fruit that cannot be metabolized (tannins, monosaccharides).
- Organic, homegrown, seedless or seeded grapes have all been reported to be nephrotoxic.
- Acute renal failure occurs secondary to acute tubular necrosis and may lead to anuric renal failure and death.
- Grape seed extract has not been associated with nephrotoxicty. Toxicity of juice, wine, or cooked grapes is uncertain.

Pharmacokinetics – Absorption, Distribution, Metabolism, Excretion

- Grapes and raisins are not rapidly broken down in the gastrointestinal tract and may be found intact in vomitus or in feces several hours after ingestion.
- Metabolism and excretion are unknown but suspected to involve the kidneys.

Blackwell's Five-Minute Veterinary Consult Clinical Companion: Small Animal Toxicology, Second Edition.
Lynn R. Hovda, Ahna G. Brutlag, Robert H. Poppenga, and Katherine L. Peterson.

Companion website: www.fiveminutevet.com/toxicology

Toxicity

- There is no published LD_{50} for grapes and raisins.
- Currently, clinical signs are not thought to be dose dependent which indicates an idiosyncratic nature. This may explain the variation between individual dogs' sensitivity to development of ARF.
- Due to the idiosyncratic nature, appropriate decontamination and treatment should be recommended for all exposures.

Systems Affected

- Gastrointestinal – vomiting, diarrhea, abdominal pain, anorexia.
- Renal/urological – acute renal tubular necrosis and subsequent ARF including oliguric/anuric ARF.
- Hepatobiliary – mild elevations in liver enzymes (especially ALT).
- Endocrine/metabolic – hypercalcemia and hyperphosphatemia; metabolic acidosis due to the presence of uremic acids.
- Neuromuscular – weakness and ataxia (rare).

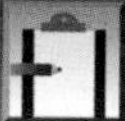

SIGNALMENT AND HISTORY

- Any age, sex, and breed of dog.
- Anecdotally reported ARF in two cats and the death of one ferret after suspected ingestion of *Vitis* spp.

Risk Factors

- Preexisting renal disease.

Historical Findings

- Witnessed ingestion of grapes or raisins.
- Suspected ingestion following discovery of chewed packages or trash that previously contained grapes or raisins (e.g., trail mix, granola, etc.).
- Emesis or stool/diarrhea containing fruit.

Location and Circumstances of Poisoning

- Availability of grapes or raisins in the animal's environment.

Interactions with Drugs, Nutrients, or Environment

- Nephrotoxic drugs should be avoided during treatment, such as NSAIDs or aminoglycosides.

CLINICAL FEATURES

- Physical exam findings will likely be normal in acute exposures.
- Vomiting is consistently the initial and most common clinical sign, often occurring between 2 and 24 hours post ingestion.
- Anorexia, lethargy, dehydration, and diarrhea follow within the next 12–24 hours.

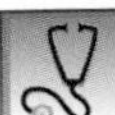

DIFFERENTIAL DIAGNOSIS

- Vomiting – dietary indiscretion, foreign body obstruction, intussusception, neoplasia, infectious disease, drug reaction, uremia, pancreatitis, hepatic disease, hypoadrenocorticism.
- Acute renal failure.
    - Toxicities – NSAID ingestion, aminoglycoside administration, ethylene glycol, cardiac medication ingestion.
    - Renal ischemia – hypovolemia, anesthetic procedures, trauma, heat stroke, sepsis/SIRS, pancreatitis.
    - Infectious and systemic disease – leptospirosis, pyelonephritis, myoglobinuria, hemoglobinuria, neoplasia.
- Hypercalcemia – hyperparathyroidism, hyperadrenocorticism, vitamin D toxicity, idiopathic, neoplasia.

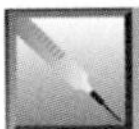

DIAGNOSTICS

- CBC – thrombocytopenia, mild anemia.
- Chemistry – elevations of BUN and creatinine; electrolyte derangements (hyponatremia, hyperkalemia, hypochloremia, hyperphosphatemia, hypercalcemia); decreases in HCO_3, elevations of liver enzymes (e.g., ALP, ALT), elevated amylase and lipase.
    - Serum creatinine and BUN elevation may be delayed 1–2 days post ingestion.
    - Hypercalcemia and hyperphosphatemia may be seen as early as 24 hours post exposure.
- Urinalysis – isosthenuria/hyposthenuria, proteinuria, glucosuria, hyaline or granular casts.
- Abdominal ultrasonography – renomegaly, hyperechoic renal cortices, or renal pelvic dilatation may be present.

Pathological Findings

- Moderate-to-severe renal tubular necrosis, with proximal tubules being more severely affected.
- Proteinaceous debris present within damaged renal tubular lumen.
- Intact basement membranes and evidence of renal epithelial regeneration in a majority of histopathological samples.

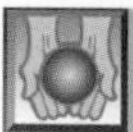

THERAPEUTICS

- Decontamination, supportive care, and monitoring are the objectives in the treatment of grape and raisin toxicosis. Treatment of all suspected intoxications is recommended.

Detoxification

- Emesis is recommended provided there are no contraindications to the procedure. Digestion and absorption of grapes and raisins are slow, and it may be beneficial to induce emesis up to 6 hours after exposure.
- One dose of activated charcoal with sorbitol is recommended. Repeated doses of AC are not currently recommended.

Appropriate Health Care

- Intravenous fluid therapy is recommended for at least 48 hours. Preemptive fluid diuresis allows for preservation of renal blood flow, decreasing tubule obstruction from necrosis, and potentially increasing the excretion of a nephrotoxic agent.
- If symptoms consistent with ARF occur, standard treatments and observations (e.g., aggressive intravenous fluid therapy, monitoring UOP, CVP, and blood pressure, etc.) should be instituted. Other possible interventions may include the use of CRI administration of dopamine, furosemide, and mannitol, antihypertensive therapy, and oral phosphate binder administration as indicated by the patient's clinical status.
- Critically ill patients (including those that are oliguric or anuric, volume overloaded, etc.) may require the use of peritoneal dialysis or hemodialysis.
- Gastric protectants and antiemetics should be administered to reduce vomiting and the severity of uremic gastritis.

Antidote

- There is no known antidote for grape and raisin toxicosis.

Drugs of Choice

- Maropitant 1 mg/kg SQ q 24 hours for vomiting.
- H_2 blocker such as famotidine 0.5 mg/kg PO, IM, SC, or IV q 12–24 hours.
- Proton pump inhibitor such as pantoprazole 0.7–1 mg/kg IV slowly q 24 hours or omeprazole 0.5–1 mg/kg PO q 24 hours.

Diet

- No specific diet change is needed. Bland diet can be considered if patient has GI symptoms.

- Patients that are treated for ARF following ingestion of grapes or raisins may benefit from a low-protein, low-phosphorus prescription veterinary diet until normal renal function is obtained.

Prevention

- Prevent patient access to all *Vitis* spp. fruits.
- Inform clients of the potential toxicity of these fruits.

COMMENTS

Patient Monitoring

- Blood pressure monitoring every 6–8 hours as dictated by the patient.
- Serial monitoring of renal values, electrolytes, serum calcium levels, serum phosphorus levels, and urine sediment should be performed every 12–24 hours to allow for early detection of nephrotoxicity.
- Blood work should be monitored for 48–72 hours post ingestion.

Possible Complications

- There is potential for long-term renal insufficiency and CRF following the ingestion of grapes and raisins.

Expected Course and Prognosis

- The prognosis for acute grape and raisin ingestion is good with appropriate decontamination and fluid therapy.
- More than 50% of dogs that ingest grapes or raisins will have no clinical signs.
- For patients that develop ARF, the prognosis may be poor to grave (particularly in anuric patients without access to peritoneal dialysis or hemodialysis). Survival is possible even with severe renal impairment if supportive care can be maintained until renal epithelial regeneration occurs but this may be weeks to months.

Abbreviations

See Appendix 1 for a complete list.

Suggested Reading

Eubig PA, Brady MS, Gwaltney-Brant SM, et al. Acute renal failure in dogs after the ingestion of grapes or raisins: a retrospective evaluation of 43 dogs (1992–2002). J Vet Intern Med 2005; 19:663–674.

Gwaltney-Brant SM, Holding JK, Donaldson CW, et al. Renal failure associated with ingestion grapes or raisins in dogs. J Am Vet Med Assoc 2001; 218:1555–1556.

Mazzaferro EM, Eubig PA, Hackett TB, et al. Acute renal failure associated with raisin or grape ingestion in 4 dogs. J Vet Emerg Crit Care 2004; 14:203–212.
Morrow CM, Valli VE, Volmer PA, et al. Canine renal pathology associated with grape or raisin ingestion: 10 cases. J Vet Diagn Invest 2005; 17:223–231.
Sutton NM, Bates N, Campbell A. Factors influencing outcome of Vitis vinifera (grapes, raisins, currants, and sultanas) intoxication in dogs. Vet Rec 2009; 164:430–431.

Acknowledgment: The authors and editors acknowledge the prior contributions of Elise M. Craft, DVM, and Justine A. Lee, DVM, DACVECC, who authored this topic in the previous edition.
Author: Jayme E. Hoffberg, DVM, DACVECC
Contributing Editor: Katherine L. Peterson, DVM, DACVECC

chapter 65

Hops

DEFINITION/OVERVIEW

- Hops, the common name of the flowers of the genus *Humulus lupulus* (Fig. 65.1), are commonly used during beer brewing to add flavor and prevent spoilage. Hops are also used as an ingredient in some herbal supplements.
- Hops (*Humulus lupulus*) should not be confused with wild hops (*Bryonia dioica*), which is a member of the gourd family.
- Toxicity can result from ingestion of either fresh or spent hops.
- Hops ingestion can result in malignant hyperthermia-like reactions in susceptible dogs. Common clinical signs include hyperthermia, panting, vomiting, and agitation.
- Toxicity can occur in any breed but susceptible dog breeds include the Greyhound, Labrador Retriever, Golden Retriever, Saint Bernard, Pointer, Doberman Pinscher, Border Collie, English Springer Spaniel, and northern breed dogs, such as Alaskan Malamutes and Siberian Huskies.

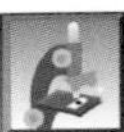

ETIOLOGY/PATHOPHYSIOLOGY

Mechanism of Action

- The mechanism of action is currently unknown. Toxicity is thought to occur from biologically active compounds found within the hops, which may uncouple oxidative phosphorylation, resulting in malignant hyperthermia.
- Hops contain the following biologically active compounds: resins, essential oils, nitrogenous constituents, and phenolic compounds.

Pharmacokinetics – Absorption, Distribution, Metabolism, Excretion

- The absorption, distribution, metabolism, and excretion of the toxic component of hops are currently unknown.

Blackwell's Five-Minute Veterinary Consult Clinical Companion: Small Animal Toxicology, Second Edition.
Lynn R. Hovda, Ahna G. Brutlag, Robert H. Poppenga, and Katherine L. Peterson.

Companion website: www.fiveminutevet.com/toxicology

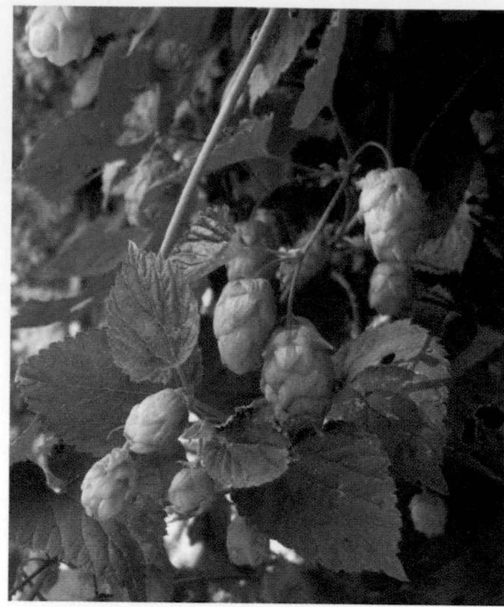

■ **Fig. 65.1.** Hops plant (*Humulus lupulus*). Photo courtesy of Tyne K. Hovda.

Toxicity

- No known LD_{50} exists in veterinary medicine.
- A 28 g plug of hops can expand into approximately 900 g of rehydrated plant material.

Systems Affected

- Cardiovascular – tachycardia.
- Endocrine/metabolic – hyperthermia; electrolyte abnormalities, including hyperkalemia, hypermagnesemia, hyperphosphatemia, hypercalcemia; metabolic acidosis; elevated creatine kinase.
- Gastrointestinal – vomiting, abdominal pain.
- Hemic/lymphatic/immune – disseminated intravascular coagulation (DIC).
- Musculoskeletal – myoglobinuria.
- Nervous – hyperesthesia, pain, restlessness, death.
- Respiratory – panting, tachypnea.

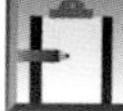

SIGNALMENT/HISTORY

- Any age and breed of dog can be affected.
- Breeds predisposed to malignant hyperthermia may be at higher risk of developing toxicity, including the Greyhound, Labrador Retriever, Golden Retriever, Saint Bernard, Pointer, Doberman Pinscher, Border Collie, English Springer Spaniel, and northern breed dogs, such as Alaskan Malamutes and Siberian Huskies.

Risk Factors

- Animals with a history of malignant hyperthermia or hyperthermia associated with anesthesia and breeds predisposed to malignant hyperthermia may be at higher risk of toxicity.

Historical Findings

- Witnessed ingestion of hops from a compost bin or brewing disposal area.
- Emesis with hops present.

Location and Circumstances of Poisoning

- Toxicity is typically seen in households with home beer brewers. Dogs may have access to composted or disposed hops during the brewing process.

CLINICAL FEATURES

- Clinical signs can develop rapidly within hours; fatality has been reported within 6 hours of ingestion.
- Initial clinical signs include hyperthermia, tachypnea, panting, tachycardia, pain, anxiety, and vomiting.

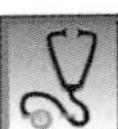

DIFFERENTIAL DIAGNOSIS

- Malignant hyperthermia.
- Hyperthermia – heat stroke, laryngeal paralysis, exogenous heat source.
- Fever – infectious, immune mediated, neoplasia, inflammatory.
- Drug related – anesthetic agents including amide local anesthetics, depolarizing skeletal muscle relaxants, and volatile inhalants.

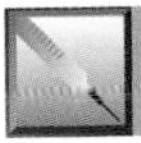

DIAGNOSTICS

- CBC – mild elevation in WBC (>18,000 × $10^3/\mu L$), thrombocytopenia if DIC develops.
- Chemistry – elevated CK, hyperkalemia, hypercalcemia, hyperphosphatemia, hypermagnesemia, elevated liver enzymes and azotemia secondary to hyperthermia injury.
- Venous blood gas analysis – metabolic acidosis, increased pCO_2, electrolyte imbalances.
- Urinalysis – pigmenturia, myoglobinuria.
- Coagulation testing – prolonged PT and PTT, elevated D-dimer levels may indicated DIC.
- Consider testing dogs for congenital malignant hyperthermia with erythrocyte osmotic fragility, caffeine muscle contracture tests, or halothane-succinylcholine challenge exposure test.

Pathological Findings

- Rapid onset of rigor mortis with death.
- Evidence of hops in GIT.

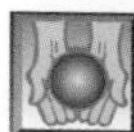

THERAPEUTICS

Detoxification

- Decontamination should be considered in cases when recent ingestion has occurred, especially if within 1–2 hours of ingestion.
- Emesis in asymptomatic patients can be performed.
- In symptomatic patients, gastric lavage with an inflated endotracheal tube placed with the patient under heavy sedation or general anesthesia should be performed to remove the hops from the stomach.
- Administration of a single dose of activated charcoal with a cathartic may prevent further absorption and decrease toxicity.
- Enemas may be performed to increase fecal expulsion.

Appropriate Health Care

- Initiate IV fluid therapy to lower body temperature, prevent myoglobin-induced ARF, and maintain perfusion.
- Cooling measures, such as cool water baths, IV fluids, use of fans on the patient, and alcohol on the paw pads may be helpful but should be stopped when a temperature of 103.5°F is reached to prevent hypothermia from developing.
- Sodium bicarbonate can be used with severe cases of metabolic acidosis (pH <7.0, BE >15 mmol/L, HCO_3 <11 mmol/L).
- Provide supportive care as needed, which may include antiemetics for vomiting, sedation if agitation is present, analgesia for pain.

Antidote

- Dantrolene sodium is a hydantoin derivative that is used for reversing malignant hyperthermia.
  - Dose: 2–3 mg/kg IV or 3.5 mg/kg PO once following development of clinical signs. Repeated doses can be administered at 100 mg PO q 12 hours for 3 days thereafter.

Drugs of Choice

- Maropitant 1 mg/kg SQ q 24 hours for vomiting.
- Acepromazine 0.02–0.04 mg/kg IV, IM, SC, q 4–6 hours for sedation; titrate sedation to effect.

Precautions/Interactions

- The use of dipyrone as an antipyretic is not recommended. Dipyrone works by inhibiting release of endogenous pyrogens. As malignant hyperthermia secondary to hops ingestion is not due to endogenous pyrogens, dipyrone is not thought to be effective.

- The administration of NSAIDs or steroids is not recommended as these drugs are not effective at normalizing the elevated temperatures caused by hops toxicity and can increase the risk of gastrointestinal signs, liver damage, and kidney toxicity, especially if shock is present.

Alternative Drugs

- Cyproheptadine has been helpful in treating some cases of hops toxicity, though it is not consistently as effective as dantrolene.
    - Dose (dogs): 1.1 mg/kg PO or rectally q 4–6 hours PRN.

Activity

- Keep the pet quiet and confined until the clinical signs subside. Exercise should be limited for 3–5 days after discharge to prevent additional myoglobinuria.

COMMENTS

Patient Monitoring

- Temperature should be monitored frequently, up to every 2–4 hours, depending on patient status; adjustments in thermoregulation should be based on temperature.
- Continuous or frequent HR/ECG monitoring and blood pressure monitoring should be done in symptomatic patients.
- Acid–base and electrolyte monitoring q 6–12 hours.

Prevention/Avoidance

- Prevent any access of pets to hops and educate clients, particularly those who are home brewers.

Possible Complications

- Hyperthermia may cause cellular injury leading to cardiac arrhythmias, renal failure, hepatic injury, DIC, and death.

Expected Course and Prognosis

- With early decontamination and appropriate supportive care, prognosis is good to fair.
- Severe clinical signs can develop requiring aggressive care and may worsen the prognosis.
- Clinical signs usually resolve within 24–72 hours.

Abbreviations

See Appendix 1 for a complete list.

Suggested Reading

Duncan KL, Hare WR, Buck WB. Malignant hyperthermia-like reaction secondary to ingestion of hops in five dogs. J Am Vet Med Assoc 1997; 210(1):51–53.
Hare WR. Hops. In: Plumlee KH, ed. Clinical Veterinary Toxicology. St Louis, MO: Mosby, 2004; pp. 430–431.
Nelson TE. Malignant hyperthermia in dogs. J Am Vet Med Assoc 1991; 198:989–994.

Acknowledgment: The authors and editors acknowledge the prior contributions of Justine A. Lee, DVM, DACVECC, who authored this topic in the previous edition.
Author: Charlotte Flint, DVM
Consulting Editor: Katherine L Peterson, DVM, DACVECC

chapter 66

Macadamia Nuts

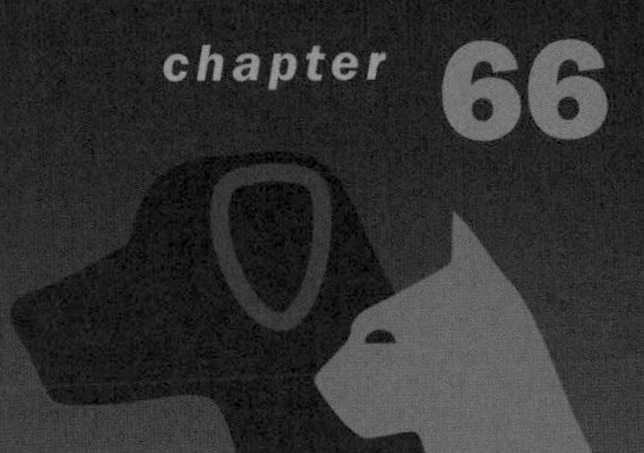

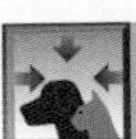

DEFINITION/OVERVIEW

- Macadamia nuts are popular snack foods and are often incorporated into candies, cakes, and cookies. They are harvested from *Macadamia integrifolia* and *Macadamia tetraphyalla* trees (family Proteaceae).
- Macadamia nuts contain 75% fat and 6–8% sugar.
- Macadamia nut toxicosis has only been reported in dogs.
- Ingestions as low as 0.7 g/kg of macadamia nuts have been associated with clinical signs, although signs are typically seen at doses greater than 2.2 g/kg.
- Common clinical signs include weakness, depression, vomiting, ataxia, pancreatitis, tremors, and hyperthermia.
- Prognosis for recovery is excellent with resolution of clinical signs within 24–48 hours.
- No fatalities have been reported to date with macadamia nut exposure.

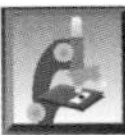

ETIOLOGY/PATHOPHYSIOLOGY

Mechanism of Action

- The mechanism of action is currently unknown.
- Toxicity may involve the constituents of the nut themselves, contaminants from processing, mycotoxins, or other unidentified causes.

Pharmacokinetics – Absorption, Distribution, Metabolism, Excretion

- No pharmacokinetic studies have been reported in dogs.
- In dogs experimentally dosed with macadamia nuts, serum triglyceride levels peaked in 3–6 hours, suggesting a relatively rapid absorption.

Toxicity

- Clinical signs have been reported at ingestions as low as 0.7 g/kg.
- Consistently toxicosis at greater than 2.2 g/kg.

Blackwell's Five-Minute Veterinary Consult Clinical Companion: Small Animal Toxicology, Second Edition.
Lynn R. Hovda, Ahna G. Brutlag, Robert H. Poppenga, and Katherine L. Peterson.

Companion website: www.fiveminutevet.com/toxicology

Systems affected

- Endocrine/metabolic – hyperthermia, pancreatitis.
- Gastrointestinal – vomiting, abdominal pain, diarrhea.
- Musculoskeletal – hindlimb weakness, joint pain, muscle pain, muscle tremors, reluctance to rise.
- Nervous – CNS depression, absent conscious proprioception, ataxia, tremors.

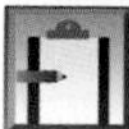

SIGNALMENT/HISTORY

- Any age or breed of dog may be affected.

Historical Findings

- Witnessed ingestion of nuts or baked goods containing nuts.

CLINICAL FEATURES

- Clinical signs have been reported as early as 1 hour after ingestion but generally develop within 6 hours of ingestion.
- Most common findings:
  - Weakness
  - Depression
  - Vomiting
  - Ataxia
  - Tremors
  - Hyperthermia
  - Joint/muscle pain
  - Inability to rise
- Clinical signs typically peak at 12 hours.
- Significant improvement in clinical signs expected within 24 hours with complete resolution in 48 hours.

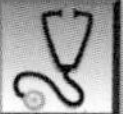

DIFFERENTIAL DIAGNOSES

- Weakness/depression with hyperthermia – bromethalin, metaldehyde, ionophore poisoning, hops.
- Ataxia/hindlimb weakness and joint pain – spinal cord lesion (IVDD, FCE, trauma, neoplasia), tick paralysis, tick-borne disease, polyradiculoneuritis, immune-mediated joint disease.

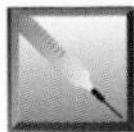

DIAGNOSTICS

- With known history of ingestion, no confirmatory tests or advanced diagnostics needed. If unknown exposure to macadamia nuts, may need to rule out other causes if lack of clinical improvement within 24–48 hours.
- Complete blood count – moderate increase in WBC (18,400–26,500), primarily characterized by a neutrophilia.
- Chemistry profile – elevations in serum lipase, triglycerides, and ALP, which are not clinically significant.

Pathological Findings

- No significant gross or histopathological lesions related to intoxication would be noted.

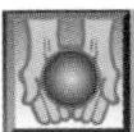

THERAPEUTICS

- Treatment is symptomatic and supportive.
- Dogs with mild clinical signs can typically be managed at home. Young or old dogs or those with significant preexisting health conditions may benefit from hospitalization and close monitoring.

Detoxification

- Consider induction of emesis in asymptomatic dogs with recent ingestion (within 1–2 hours).
- Activated charcoal with a cathartic, one dose, may be administered; efficacy of activated charcoal has not been established in this toxicity.

Appropriate Health Care

- IV crystalloids as needed for hydration, perfusion, and as a cooling measure.
- Additional cooling measures (cool water baths, IV fluids, use of fans on the patient, and alcohol on the paw pads) may need to be instituted for patients with significant hyperthermia.

Antidote

- No antidote.

Precautions/Interactions

- Dogs co ingesting chocolate may require treatment for methylxanthine toxicosis.

Nursing Care

- Recumbent patients should be given soft bedding and have their position switched every 4 hours.
- Patients may need assistance to stand to urinate and defecate; urinary catheterization may be needed.

Diet

- Avoid high-fat diet due to risk of pancreatitis following ingestion.

Activity

- Keep dogs quiet and confined until resolution of signs.

Follow-up

- No long-term complications have been reported.

COMMENTS

Patient Monitoring

- Symptomatic patients should be closely monitored for resolution of clinical signs for 24–48 hours.
- Body temperature should be measured every 4–8 hours and cooling measures instituted as needed.

Prevention/Avoidance

- Client education about the toxicity of macadamia nuts and preventing access of pets to macadamia nuts and baked goods containing the nuts.

Possible Complications

- Potential complications include pancreatitis, gastroenteritis, or intestinal obstruction (rare).

Expected Course/Prognosis

- Resolution of clinical signs expected in 24–48 hours with minimal veterinary intervention; prognosis is good.
- Dogs with preexisting diseases or those with co-ingestion of other toxicants may have slower recoveries.

Abbreviations

See Appendix 1 for a complete list

Suggested Reading

Botha CJ, Penrith ML. Potential plant poisonings in dogs and cats in Southern Africa. J S Afr Vet Assoc 2009; 80(2):63–74.
Gugler K, Piscitelli C, Dennis J. Hidden dangers in the kitchen: common foods toxic to dogs and cats. Compendium 2013; 35(7):E1–E6.
Gwaltney-Brandt SW. Macadamia nuts. In: PetersonM, TalcottP, eds. Small Animal Toxicology, 3rd edn. St Louis, MO: Saunders, 2013; pp. 625–628.
Hansen SR, Buck WB, Meerdink G, et al. Weakness, tremors, and depression associated with macadamia nuts in dogs. Vet Hum Toxicol 2000; 42:18–21.

Acknowledgment: The authors and editors acknowledge the prior contributions of Debra Liu, DVM, and Justine A. Lee, DVM, DACVECC, who authored this topic in the previous edition.
Author: Rebecca A. L. Walton, DVM
Consulting Editor: Katherine L. Peterson, DVM, DACVECC

chapter 67

Mycotoxins – Aflatoxin

DEFINITION/OVERVIEW

- Aflatoxin is produced by some species of *Aspergillus* (*A. flavus*, *A. paraciticus*, *A. nomius*), as well as a few *Penicillium* species.
- Contamination of food may occur prior to harvest (e.g., corn, cottonseed, peanuts, walnuts, pecans, potatoes) or in improperly stored foods after harvest and processing.
- Ingestion of other moldy foods (e.g., bread, garbage) or contaminated commercial pet food has also caused toxicosis.

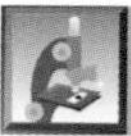

ETIOLOGY/PATHOPHYSIOLOGY

Mechanism of Action

- The active epoxide metabolite damages hepatocytes, resulting in cell necrosis, decreased liver function, fibrosis, and biliary hyperplasia.

Pharmacokinetics – Absorption, Distribution, Metabolism, Excretion

- Aflatoxin is absorbed rapidly from the intestinal tract into the portal circulation.
- Hepatic cytochrome P450 metabolism converts the toxin to an active epoxide, which then binds to DNA, RNA, and proteins in hepatocytes, interfering with cellular metabolism and protein synthesis.
- Secondary sites of metabolism include the small intestine and kidneys.
- Metabolites are present in milk and eggs.
- Excretion is through bile, feces, and urine.
- Variable rate of elimination, but usually within 24–72 hours post ingestion.

Toxicity

- Acute lethal exposure is not as common as chronic exposure.
- Oral LD_{50} in dogs has ranged from 0.5 to 1.8 mg/kg.

Blackwell's Five-Minute Veterinary Consult Clinical Companion: Small Animal Toxicology, Second Edition.
Lynn R. Hovda, Ahna G. Brutlag, Robert H. Poppenga, and Katherine L. Peterson.

Companion website: www.fiveminutevet.com/toxicology

- 60 ppb of aflatoxin in dog food and 6.7–15 ppm aflatoxin in moldy bread have been associated with canine aflatoxicosis.
- Experimental LD_{50} in cats is 0.55 mg/kg. No cases of natural exposure to aflatoxin in cats have been reported.

Systems Affected

- Gastrointestinal – anorexia, vomiting, diarrhea, GI hemorrhage.
- Hemic/immune/lymphatic – petechiae and ecchymosis, anemia, thrombocytopenia, neutrophilia, hypofibrinogenemia, elevated FDP, prolonged PT/PTT, decreased serum cholesterol and protein C.
- Hepatobiliary – jaundice, increased ALT, increased ALP, hyperbilirubinemia.
- Metabolic – fever.
- Musculoskeletal – weakness.
- Nervous – altered mentation, obtundation, coma.
- Renal – bilirubinuria, PU/PD.

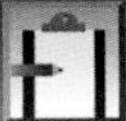

SIGNALMENT/HISTORY

- Toxicosis is rarely reported in small animals but has occurred sporadically in large outbreaks associated with contaminated pet foods.

Risk Factors

- Field and storage conditions predispose grain to aflatoxin contamination (i.e., hot, dry weather, insect damage to grain).
- Grain-based contaminated pet foods have been associated with outbreaks.

Historical Findings

- Lethargy, anorexia, vomiting, diarrhea, and weakness are commonly reported.
- Sudden death may occur.
- Dogs exposed to contaminated commercial foods may have a history of decreased willingness to consume the food due to altered palatability.
- More than one pet in the household is likely to be affected when pet food contamination is the cause.
- Diagnosis is based on history and clinical signs.

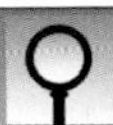

CLINICAL FEATURES

- Clinical signs may be delayed for 3 or more weeks post exposure.
- Acute clinical signs include anorexia, depression, vomiting, diarrhea (often with GI hemorrhage), fever, seizures, icterus, and death.

- Clinical signs of chronic ingestion include weight loss, decreased appetite, rough haircoat, icterus, depression, abdominal distension due to ascites, and PU/PD.

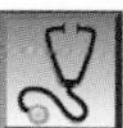

DIFFERENTIAL DIAGNOSIS

- Other causes of hepatic disease.
  - Inflammatory – hepatitis (chronic, active), copper storage disease.
  - Infectious – bacterial disease (leptospirosis), viral disease (adenovirus).
  - Neoplastic disease.
  - Other toxins – cyanobacteria, mushrooms, xylitol, acetaminophen, NSAIDs.
  - Congenital disease.
- Other causes of hemorrhage, especially intestinal.
  - NSAID toxicity.
  - Long-acting anticoagulant rodenticide toxicosis.
  - Parvoviral enteritis.

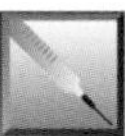

DIAGNOSTICS

- CBC – anemia, thrombocytopenia.
- Chemistry – hypoglycemia, hyperbilirubinemia, elevated ALT, variable elevations in GGT, AST, ALP, hypoalbuminemia, hypocholesterolemia.
- Coagulation panel – prolonged PT/PTT, elevated FDP, decreased serum protein C, hypofibrinogenemia.
- Blood work results within normal limits do not rule out possible aflatoxicosis.
- Abdominal ultrasound, liver aspirate/biopsy, and histopathology can be considered (see Pathological Findings).
- Assay of the suspected aflatoxin source, if available.
  - Available at many commercial and state veterinary diagnostic laboratories.
  - See www.aavld.org for a list of accredited laboratories.
  - Assay of affected food may be difficult if the whole bag has already been consumed by the time clinical signs have developed (which may be delayed for up to 3 weeks).
- Aflatoxin residues can be found in urine, liver, and kidney of recently exposed animals.
  - Due to relatively rapid aflatoxin excretion, absence of tissue residues does not rule out aflatoxicosis.

Pathological Findings

- Hepatomegaly with lipidosis.
- Icterus.
- Ascites.
- GI hemorrhage.
- Subserosal edema of the gallbladder.

- Multifocal petechiae, ecchymosis, and hemorrhage.
- Microvesicular fatty change in hepatocytes.
- Centrilobular hepatocellular necrosis, with evidence of regeneration possible.
- Canalicular cholestasis.
- Bridging portal fibrosis with proliferation of bile ducts.
- Renal proximal tubular necrosis.

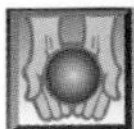

THERAPEUTICS

- The therapeutic goal is supportive care to limit hepatic and other organ damage. Hepatoprotective medications such as SAMe or N-acetylcysteine may minimize hepatic damage.

Detoxification

- Early emesis can be considered within 1–2 hours after exposure.
- One dose of activated charcoal with a cathartic may be beneficial for recent ingestion of moldy food.

Appropriate Health Care

- Monitor hydration, temperature, pulse, respiration, blood pressure, and urine output every 4–8 hours.
- IV crystalloid fluid therapy (may want to avoid LRS because of lactate metabolism) to correct dehydration and electrolyte disturbances associated with vomiting and diarrhea.
- Dextrose supplementation if hypoglycemia present.

Antidote

- No specific antidote is available for aflatoxicosis.

Drugs of Choice

- Antiemetics as needed for persistent vomiting or prior to oral N-acetylcysteine.
  - Maropitant 1 mg/kg SQ q 24 hours.
  - Ondansetron 0.1–0.4 mg/kg IV q 8–12 hours.
- GI protectants.
  - Famotidine 0.5–1 mg/kg PO, SC, IM, IV q 12 hours.
  - Omeprazole 0.5–1 mg/kg PO q 12–24 hours or pantoprazole 1 mg/kg IV q 24 hours.
  - Sucralfate 0.25–1 g PO q 8 hours.
- Coagulopathy – vitamin K_1 3–5 mg/kg PO or SQ daily; dose may be divided.
- Hepatic support.
  - SAMe 17–20 mg/kg q 24 hours or higher for dogs, 200 mg/day total daily dose for cats, given PO on an empty stomach.

- N-acetylcysteine (for severe acute toxicities) 140 mg/kg IV (through filter) once, then 70 mg/kg IV or PO q 6 hours for 7–17 doses. Dilution required prior to administration.

Precautions/Interactions

- Avoid drugs metabolized by the liver.
- Avoid pyrethroid insecticides, which may potentiate aflatoxicosis experimentally.

Alternative Drugs

- Silymarin/milk thistle (Marin) or silybin and SAMe (Denamarin) can be used alternatively to SAMe as a hepatoprotectant.

Prevention/Avoidance

- Report suspected cases associated with pet food to the manufacturer, FDA, and state regulatory agencies.
- Keep all food in clean containers in a cool, dry storage area.
- Keep garbage out of reach of pets.

COMMENTS

Patient Monitoring

- CBC and chemistry every 12–24 hours, and electrolytes every 8–12 hours and coagulation status as needed, depending on other findings.

Possible Complications

- None reported in surviving dogs and cats.
- Cirrhosis is a possible sequela.

Expected Course and Prognosis

- Prognosis is guarded to poor, even with treatment, once clinical signs are evident.

Abbreviations

See Appendix 1 for a complete list.

Suggested Reading

Bischoff K, Garland T. Aflatoxicosis in dogs. In: Bonagura JD, Twedt DC, eds. Kirk's Current Veterinary Therapy XIV. St Louis, MO: Saunders, 2009; pp. 156–159.

Dereszynski DM, Center SA, Randolph JF, et al. Clinical and clinicopathologic features of dogs that consumed foodborne hepatotoxic aflatoxins: 72 cases (2005–2006). J Am Vet Med Assoc 2008; 232(9):1329–1337.
Plumb DC. Plumb's Veterinary Drug Handbook, 8th edn. Ames, IA: Wiley-Blackwell, 2015.
Stenske KA, Smith JR, Newman SJ, et al. Aflatoxicosis in dogs and dealing with suspected contaminated commercial foods. J Am Vet Med Assoc 2006; 228(11):1686–1689.
Talcott PA. Mycotoxins. In: PetersonME, TalcottPA, eds. Small Animal Toxicology, 3rd edn. St Louis, MO: Saunders, 2013; pp. 677–682.

Acknowledgment: The authors and editors acknowledge the prior contributions of Catherine M. Adams, DVM, and Karyn Bischoff, DVM, MS, DABVT, who authored this topic in the previous edition.
Author: Tracy Julius, DVM, DACVECC
Consulting Editor: Katherine L. Peterson, DVM, DACVECC

chapter 68

Mycotoxins – Tremorgenic

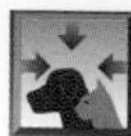

DEFINITION/OVERVIEW

- Penitrem A and roquefortine are tremorgenic mycotoxins responsible for producing toxicosis characterized by GI and neurological signs.
- Dogs and cats are most often exposed to tremorgenic mycotoxins through ingestion of moldy foods or after access to a compost pile.
- Although death can occur in severely affected animals, with early and aggressive treatment, prognosis is generally good.

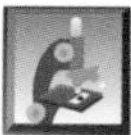

ETIOLOGY/PATHOPHYSIOLOGY

Mechanism of Action

- Mycotoxins are toxic metabolites produced by fungi. Effects vary based on chemical structure, concentration of the toxin in foods, and the species affected.
- Penitrem A and roquefortine are the tremorgenic mycotoxins reported to affect dogs and cats. Both are produced by *Penicillium* spp.
- Most commonly found in postharvest rot of crops, spoilage of moldy cheese, walnuts, dog food, bread, apples, and garbage.
- The exact pathophysiological mechanisms of toxicity are not well understood.
- Roquefortine – little is known about the mechanism of action.
- Penitrem A.
    - Inhibits calcium-regulated potassium channels and alters the spontaneous release of neurotransmitters such as glutamate, aspartic acid, and GABA in central and peripheral synapses.
    - In mice, penitrem A acts as an antagonist to the production of glycine which is an inhibitory neurotransmitter in the CNS. This action may facilitate transmission of impulses, leading to tremor activity.
    - In rats, may inhibit presynaptic transmission in the cerebellum and has been shown to cause widespread necrosis and loss of Purkinje neurons.

Blackwell's Five-Minute Veterinary Consult Clinical Companion: Small Animal Toxicology, Second Edition.
Lynn R. Hovda, Ahna G. Brutlag, Robert H. Poppenga, and Katherine L. Peterson.

Companion website: www.fiveminutevet.com/toxicology

Pharmacokinetics – Absorption, Distribution, Metabolism, Excretion

- Readily absorbed through the GI tract.
- Able to penetrate blood–brain barrier.
- Both toxins are metabolized in the liver and excreted in bile.

Toxicity

- The dose ingested is often difficult to determine and toxicity of mycotoxins varies depending on species and exact toxin present.
- Experimentally, penitrem A has elicited tremors at doses of 0.125 mg/kg and convulsions and death at 0.5 mg/kg administered intraperitoneally.

Systems Affected

- Cardiovascular – tachycardia.
- Gastrointestinal – hypersalivation, nausea, vomiting, diarrhea.
- Hemic/vascular – DIC secondary to prolonged muscle activity and hyperthermia.
- Hepatic – dose-related centrilobular hemorrhage and necrosis.
- Neuromuscular – generalized muscle tremors, ataxia, weakness, hyperesthesia, agitation, stiff gait, seizures, stupor to coma in severe intoxications.
- Ophthalmic – blepharospasm, mydriasis, nystagmus.
- Renal – pigmenturia if rhabdomyolysis occurs (uncommon).
- Respiratory – panting, tachypnea, aspiration pneumonia.

SIGNALMENT/HISTORY

- Dogs are most often affected due to their indiscriminate eating habits; cats may be affected by the toxins.
- No breed, sex, or age predilection.

Risk Factors

- Animals that are exposed to moldy foods, including human foods, food in garbage cans, and moldy dog food.
- Animals that have access to compost piles or are allowed access outside unsupervised.

Historical Findings

- Animals generally present for gastrointestinal (vomiting) or neuromuscular (tremors) signs.
- Owners may report that their dog is allowed to roam freely outdoors and may be unaware of toxin exposure.

- Dogs known to have indiscriminate eating habits who may have accessed trash, compost, or moldy food items.
- Feeding of dog food that has been exposed to moisture and may be moldy.

Location and Circumstances of Poisoning

- Exposure generally occurs in the home, yard, or on farms, especially unsupervised pets with access to moldy organic material or compost piles.

CLINICAL FEATURES

- Clinical signs typically develop within minutes to hours after toxin ingestion.
- Clinical signs include:
    - hypersalivation, vomiting and diarrhea
    - generalized muscle tremors, ataxia, weakness, hyperesthesia, agitation, stiff gait, seizure
    - hyperthermia
    - tachycardia, hyperemic mucous membranes, panting, tachypnea.

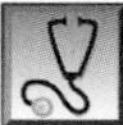

DIFFERENTIAL DIAGNOSIS

- Intoxications – strychnine, methylxanthines, bromethalin, amphetamines, SSRIs, organophosphates/carbamates, organochlorides, metaldehyde, macadamia nuts, pyrethroids, cocaine, nicotine, paintballs, ethylene glycol, ivermectin, heavy metals (lead), hexachloraphene.
- Metabolic – hypoglycemia, hypocalcemia, hypo- or hypernatremia, hypomagnesemia, severe uremia, hepatic encephalopathy.
- Primary neurological disease – idiopathic epilepsy, encephalitis (inflammatory and infectious), trauma, neoplasia, idiopathic cerebellar disorders, idiopathic white shaker dog syndrome.

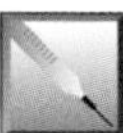

DIAGNOSTICS

- Diagnosis may be straightforward in cases of known exposure/ingestion with consistent clinical signs.
- In cases with an unknown exposure history, diagnosis may be suspected based on clinical signs, response to therapy, and ruling out other causes of neurological signs.
- Complete blood count, biochemical profile including electrolytes, and urinalysis to obtain baseline values, assess patient status and differentiate from other causes of neurological signs.
    - Mild elevations in ALP, ALT, and CK have been noted in penitrem A-intoxicated dogs.

- In cases with prolonged muscle activity and hyperthermia, potential sequelae include:
  - blood gas analysis – metabolic acidosis
  - chemistry – secondary organ dysfunction including azotemia, elevated liver enzymes, elevated CK
  - coagulation profile – DIC with prolonged PT/PTT, thrombocytopenia, increased FDPs, d-dimers.
- Abdominal radiographs to assess efficacy of decontamination, rule out other causes of vomiting, and evaluate for ingestion of other foreign substances.
- Thin-layer chromatography or high-pressure liquid chromatography analysis of vomitus or gastric contents for penitrem A or roquefortine analysis.

Pathological Findings

- Findings reported in dogs poisoned with penitrem A include:
  - hemorrhagic lungs and urinary bladder with engorgement of renal capsular vessels
  - hemorrhage and edema of the small and large intestinal serosa
  - hepatic congestion with evidence of fatty degeneration
  - microscopic findings include marked vascular centrilobular hepatic congestion.

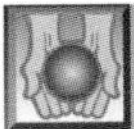

THERAPEUTICS

- The objectives of treatment are decontamination to prevent further toxin exposure, controlling tremors/seizures, and providing supportive care.

Detoxification

- Emesis can be performed in stable animals with low risk of aspiration.
- Gastric lavage should be considered in cases where emesis is ineffective, there is a large amount of material within the stomach, or in patients exhibiting clinical signs. These patients should be heavily sedated or anesthetized to allow placement of a cuffed endotracheal tube.
- Activated charcoal with a cathartic, one dose, can be administered orally in stable patients or via gastric tube after lavage has been performed.

Appropriate Health Care

- If animals present acutely after ingestion and are successfully decontaminated, outpatient treatment may be possible.
- For those animals demonstrating clinical signs, hospitalization is recommended to allow for appropriate treatment until the patient is asymptomatic and stable.
- In animals that are hyperthermic, active cooling measures can be instituted (tepid water bath, fan, intravenous fluids) but should cease once body temperature reaches 103°F so as not to induce hypothermia.

- Intravenous crystalloids may be necessary to correct dehydration, maintain perfusion, and aid in thermoregulation.
- Heart rate and blood pressure should be monitored every 4–8 hours.
- Respiratory rate and effort should be monitored frequently. In animals that are hypoxemic, oxygen supplementation may be necessary.
- Animals with severe respiratory compromise or those that are unresponsive/comatose may require mechanical ventilation.

Antidote

- There is no specific antidote available.

Drugs of Choice

- Methocarbamol 55–220 mg/kg IV administered at a rate of ≤2 mL/min to effect for muscle tremors; not to exceed 330 mg/kg/day.
- Seizures can be controlled with the following medications.
  - Diazepam 0.5–1 mg/kg IV; studies have shown that mycotoxin-induced seizures are less responsive to benzodiazepines.
  - Phenobarbital 2–4 mg/kg IV q 30 min loading to effect; not to exceed 18–20 mg/kg IV.
  - Levetiracetam 30–60 mg/kg IV slow bolus.
  - Propofol 2–8 mg/kg IV slow bolus, followed by CRI of 0.1–0.4 mg/kg/min.
- Antiemetics.
  - Maropitant 1 mg/kg SQ q 24 hours.
  - Ondansetron 0.1–0.3 mg/kg IV q 8–12 hours.
- For severe tachycardia unresponsive to fluids/sedation, use a beta-blocker such as propranolol 0.02–0.06 mg/kg IV to effect.

Precautions/Interactions

- Seizures may be unresponsive to benzodiazepines.
- Co-ingestion of other toxins (e.g., chocolate, medications, onions) is possible when getting into trash or compost.

Alternative Drugs

- If IV methocarbamol is unavailable, methocarbamol tablets can be given orally or crushed and administered rectally. Activated charcoal may bind methocarbamol depending on timing of administration.

Nursing Care

- Recumbent animals may require padded bedding, rotating body position, passive range of motion, and placement of an indwelling urinary catheter.

Diet

- Nutritional support (nasoesophageal tube, parenteral nutrition) may be necessary in patients requiring prolonged hospitalization that are unable to tolerate oral food/water.

COMMENTS

Patient Monitoring

- Symptomatic animals should be monitored for at least 12 hours after medication administration to ensure they remain asymptomatic.

Prevention/Avoidance

- Clients should be warned about the dangers of allowing their pets to roam freely unsupervised.
- Owners should be warned of the toxic potential of moldy foods and compost piles should be enclosed to restrict animal access.

Possible Complications

- If patients vomit, aspiration pneumonia may occur which alters treatment and prognosis.
    - Thoracic radiographs in animals with respiratory signs to evaluate for presence of aspiration pneumonia.
    - Pulse oximetry or arterial blood gas in tachypneic or dyspneic animals to determine oxygenation status.
- In cases with severe or prolonged hyperthermia, secondary organ dysfunction can occur (rhabdomyolysis, kidney injury, liver damage, DIC).
- Animals that develop complications (aspiration pneumonia, DIC) may require prolonged hospitalization and care.

Expected Course and Prognosis

- In cases of mild toxin exposure or those treated aggressively, signs generally resolve in 24–48 hours with no long-term effects.
- With severe intoxication or in cases where treatment has been delayed, clinical signs may persist for days.
- Patients suffering from toxicosis generally respond well to IV methocarbamol and supportive care. In patients that are unresponsive, persistent toxin in the stomach or other toxins should be considered.
- Rare reports of dogs with persistent neurological signs several months to years after toxin ingestion.
- Some cases can be fatal if large amounts of toxin are consumed before decontamination and treatment can be instituted.

Abbreviations

See Appendix 1 for a complete list.

Suggested Reading

Boysen SR, Rozanski EA, Chan DL, et al. Tremorgenic mycotoxicosis in four dogs from a single household. J Am Vet Med Assoc 2002; 221(10):1441–1444.

Eriksen GS, Jaderlund KH, Moldes-Anaya A, et al. Poisoning of dogs with tremorgenic Penicillium toxins. Med Mycol 2010; 48:188–196.

Munday JS, Thompson D, Finch SC, et al. Presumptive tremorgenic mycotoxicosis in a dog in New Zealand, after eating mouldy walnuts. N Zl Vet J 2008; 56(3):145–147.

Naude TW, O'Brien OM, Rundberget T, et al. Tremorgenic neuromycotoxicosis in 2 dogs ascribed to the ingestion of penitrem A and possibly roquefortine in rice contaminated with Penicillium crustosum. J S Afr Vet Assoc 2002; 73:211–215.

Walter SL. Acute penitrem A and roquefortine poisoning in a dog. Can Vet J 2002; 43:372–374.

Young KL, Villar D, Carson TL, et al. Tremorgenic mycotoxin intoxication with penitrem A and roquefortine in two dogs. J Am Vet Med Assoc 2003; 222:52–53.

Acknowledgment: The authors and editors acknowledge the prior contributions of Christy A. Klatt, DVM, and Stephen B. Hooser, DVM, PhD, DABVT, who authored this topic in the previous edition.

Author: Julie Schildt, DVM, DACVECC
Consulting Editor: Katherine L. Peterson, DVM, DACVECC

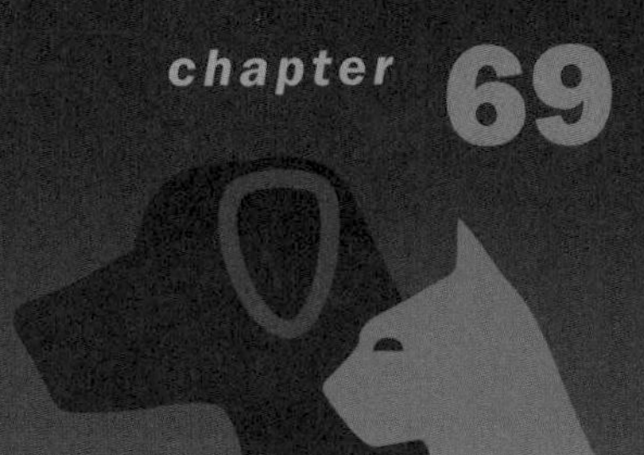

chapter 69

Onions and Garlic

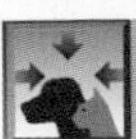

DEFINITION/OVERVIEW

- The genus *Allium* includes onions (*A. cepa*), leeks (*A. porrum*), garlic (*A. sativum*), and chives (*A. schoenoprasum*). Toxicosis occurs after oral ingestion of fresh or dried plant material, dietary supplements, or food preparations.
- The disulfides and thiosulfates in *Allium* spp. are metabolized to compounds that can cause oxidative damage to erythrocytes, leading to Heinz body production, methemoglobinemia, and hemolytic anemia.
- Treatment involves early decontamination and supportive care; prognosis is generally good.

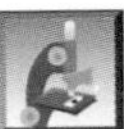

ETIOLOGY/PATHOPHYSIOLOGY

Mechanism of Action

- Several toxic compounds have been identified in *Allium* spp., including *n*-propyl disulfide and 3 sodium alk(en)yl thiosulfates (onion-induced toxicosis), and sodium *n*-propylthiosulfate (garlic-induced toxicosis).
- Metabolism of these compounds causes oxidative damage to hemoglobin, resulting in sulfhemoglobin and precipitation of hemoglobin (eccentrocytes), Heinz body formation, and oxidation of the heme ion (methemoglobinemia).
  - Sulfhemoglobin aggregates and forms Heinz bodies and eccentrocytes.
  - Heinz bodies and eccentrocytes increase RBC fragility and hemolysis may occur.
  - Direct oxidative damage to the cell membrane and sodium-potassium pump may contribute to cell lysis.
  - Methemoglobin may cause a left shift of the Hgb-oxygen dissociation curve, resulting in impaired oxygen delivery to tissues.
  - *n*-Propyl disulfide reduces glucose-6-phosphate dehydrogenase activity in RBCs, and interferes with reduced glutathione regeneration, which is needed to prevent oxidative denaturation of hemoglobin.

Blackwell's Five-Minute Veterinary Consult Clinical Companion: Small Animal Toxicology, Second Edition.
Lynn R. Hovda, Ahna G. Brutlag, Robert H. Poppenga, and Katherine L. Peterson.

Companion website: www.fiveminutevet.com/toxicology

- Allicin and ajoene, active agents in garlic, are cardiac and smooth muscle relaxants, vasodilators, antithrombotics, and hypotensive agents, and may exacerbate effects of anemia and impaired oxygen transportation.

Pharmacokinetics – Absorption, Distribution, Metabolism, Excretion

- Toxicosis most commonly occurs after oral consumption; rapidly absorbed from the GI tract.
- Metabolism occurs in the liver and red blood cells.
- Excretion is thought to occur through GI tract and kidneys.

Toxicity

- Fresh, cooked, boiled, dried, liquid, and dehydrated forms are all toxic.
- Acute LD_{50} values for dogs and cats have not been published.
- Dogs – hematological changes have been reported with ingestion of 15–30 g/kg of onions.
- Cats – toxicosis has been reported with ingestion of 5 g/kg of onions.
- Toxicosis consistently noted in animals that ingest >0.5% of body weight (kg) in onions.
- Cats fed a diet of 3% onion powder added to canned diet developed nearly 100% Heinz body anemia and a significant decrease in PCV within a week.
- Garlic can be up to five times more toxic than onions.

Systems Affected

- Cardiovascular – tachycardia secondary to anemia and methemoglobinemia, hypotension.
- Gastrointestinal – diarrhea, vomiting, abdominal pain, mucosal erosions.
- Hemic/lymphatic/immune – Heinz body anemia, methemoglobinemia.
- Renal/urological – hemoglobinuria, hemoglobin (possibly hemosiderin), urinary casts.
- Respiratory – tachypnea, hypoxemia secondary to anemia and methemoglobinemia.

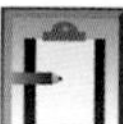

SIGNALMENT/HISTORY

- Dogs may present more often due to indiscriminate eating habits.
- Cats are more sensitive due to increased hemoglobin sulfhydryl groups and reduced methemoglobin reductase activity.
- Japanese breeds (Akita, Shiba Inu) or those with hereditary reduced glutathione and potassium concentrations have been shown to be more susceptible to oxidant injury.
- No age or sex predilections have been reported.

Risk Factors

- Animals fed homemade diets containing *Allium* spp.
- Animals with concurrent diseases causing oxidative stress (diabetic ketoacidosis, hepatic lipidosis) or preexisting anemia may manifest more severe toxicosis.

Historical Findings

- History of recent or chronic ingestion of *Allium* spp.
- Owners may note lethargy, weakness, anorexia, exercise intolerance, pale gums, diarrhea/vomiting, discolored urine.

Location and Circumstances of Poisoning

- Toxicosis most commonly occurs following oral consumption of a single large quantity of fresh plant material, juice, dietary supplements, powdered preparations, dehydrated material, or food preparations containing *Allium* spp.
- Chronic toxicosis may occur with long-term exposure when onions or garlic are added to the diet or treats.

Interactions with Drugs, Nutrients, or Environment

- Increased susceptibility with concurrent treatment with medications that induce erythrocyte oxidative injury (e.g., propofol, propylene glycol, dl-methionine, sulfonamides, high doses of vitamin K_3, sulfapyridine, benzocaine, acetaminophen).

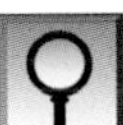

CLINICAL FEATURES

- Clinical signs of vomiting and diarrhea may appear within one day of consumption but typically signs associated with anemia lag by several days to a week.
- The toxic signs produced by onions/garlic mainly represent the effects on RBCs.
- Clinical signs and physical examination findings most commonly noted include the following.
    - Depressed mentation
    - Pale, icteric or cyanotic mucous membranes
    - Tachypnea
    - Tachycardia
    - Abdominal pain
    - Pigmenturia

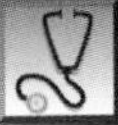

DIFFERENTIAL DIAGNOSIS

- Other toxicoses: brassicaceous vegetables, naphthalene, propylene glycol, acetaminophen, benzocaine, vitamin K_3, dl-methionine, zinc, and copper.
- Other causes of Heinz body formation in cats: diabetes mellitus, hepatic lipidosis, hyperthyroidism, neoplasia, repeated propofol infusions.
- Other causes of hemolytic anemia: primary IMHA, infectious agents (*Mycoplasma*, *Anaplasma*, *Babesia*), PK or PFK enzyme deficiencies, hypophosphatemia, neoplasia, envenomation.

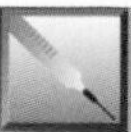

DIAGNOSTICS

- CBC and blood smear – regenerative anemia, decreased hemoglobin concentration, Heinz body formation, eccentrocytosis (common with garlic toxicity), leukocytosis.
- Biochemical profile – hyperbilirubinemia, elevated liver enzymes secondary to hypoxic injury, hemolytic or icteric serum.
- Urinalysis – hemoglobinuria, bilirubinuria, hemosiderin/hemoglobin casts.
- CO – oximeter analysis to assess methemoglobin concentration; typically performed at human hospital or veterinary specialty centers.
- Abdominal radiographs may be useful to help rule out other causes of hemolysis (zinc, neoplasia).
- Abdominal ultrasound may be normal or may reveal hepatomegaly or splenomegaly secondary to extramedullary hematopoiesis.

Pathological Findings

- Postmortem findings are consistent with hemolytic anemia and include hemosiderin deposition in liver, spleen, and renal tubular epithelium; renal tubular pigment necrosis; nephrotubular casts.

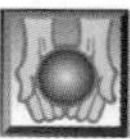

THERAPEUTICS

- Treatment objectives are decontamination to prevent further toxin exposure in those animals presenting acutely and in stable condition stabilization and aggressive supportive care in those patients exhibiting clinical signs.

Detoxification

- Induce emesis if recent ingestion (previous 1–2 hours) and asymptomatic.
- Administer a single dose of activated charcoal with a cathartic.

Appropriate Health Care

- Patients presenting after acute ingestion can be decontaminated and treated as outpatients.
    - Baseline blood work and PCV monitoring should be performed up to 1 week post ingestion.
- Animals presenting with clinical signs may require hospitalization and supportive care.
- Intravenous crystalloid fluid administration may be indicated in patients with vomiting/diarrhea, hemoglobinuria, or hypotension.
- Packed red blood cell transfusion should be considered if patients are showing clinical signs of anemia.

Antidote

- No antidote exists.

Drugs of Choice

- If vomiting present, consider:
    - famotidine 0.5–1 mg/kg IV, IM, SQ, PO q 12–24 hours
    - maropitant 1 mg/kg SQ q 24 hours
    - ondansetron 0.1–0.3 mg/kg IV q 8–12 hours.
- Antioxidants may be beneficial.
    - Vitamin C 30 mg/kg PO q 6–8 hours.
    - Vitamin E anecdotally used at 50–600 units PO once daily.
    - N-acetylcysteine – various dosing schedules exist. See drug handbooks for further recommendations.

Precautions/Interactions

- Avoid drugs that may induce erythrocyte oxidative injury (see earlier in this chapter).

Diet

- Avoid semi-moist diets that contain propylene glycol.
- Discontinue use of any diet containing *Allium* spp.

Activity

- Activity should be restricted in anemic animals until RBC count has returned to normal.

COMMENTS

Patient Monitoring

- Animals presenting after *Allium* spp. ingestion should have an initial CBC or minimally a PCV measured to obtain a baseline value. Recheck in 5–7 days as nadir may occur several days following ingestion.
- Clients should be educated about clinical signs to monitor at home (pale gums, weakness, inappetance, pigmenturia) and blood work should be evaluated immediately in any patient exhibiting these signs.

Prevention/Avoidance

- Clients should be educated about the toxicity of onions/garlic and should avoid feeding of all forms of *Allium* spp. to dogs and cats.

Possible Complications

- No long-term complications are anticipated.

Expected Course and Prognosis

- Prognosis is good with decontamination and supportive care.
- In patients presenting with anemia, hospitalization for several days may be necessary until clinical signs have resolved and anemia has stabilized.
- Prognosis is guarded for severely affected patients without aggressive care.

Abbreviations

See Appendix 1 for a complete list.

PFK = phosphofructokinase
PK = pyruvate kinase

Suggested Reading

Cope RB. Allium species poisoning in dogs and cats. Vet Med 2005; Aug:562–566.

Harvey JW, Rackear D. Experimental onion-induced hemolytic anemia in dogs. Vet Pathol 1985; 22:387–392.

Hill AS, O'Neill S, Rogers QR, et al. Antioxidant prevention of Heinz body formation and oxidative injury in cats. Am J Vet Res 2001; 62:370–374.

Lee K, Yamato O, Tajima M, et al. Hematologic changes associated with the appearance of eccentrocytes after intragastric administration of garlic extract to dogs. Am J Vet Res 2000; 11:1446–1450.

Tang X, Xia Z, Yu J. An experimental study of hemolysis induced by onion (*Allium cepa*) poisoning in dogs. J Vet Pharmacol Ther 2007; 31:143–149.

Yamato O, Kasai E, Katsura T, et al. Heinz body hemolytic anemia with eccentrocytosis from ingestion of Chinese chive (*Allium tuberosum*) and garlic (*Allium sativum*) in a dog. J Am Anim Hosp Assoc 2005; 41:68–73.

Acknowledgment: The authors and editors acknowledge the prior contributions of Catherine M. Adams, DVM, who authored this topic in the previous edition.
Authors: Kristin Smith, DVM; Julie Schildt, DVM, DACVECC
Consulting Editor: Katherine L. Peterson, DVM, DACVECC

Salt

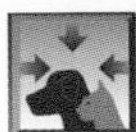

DEFINITION/OVERVIEW

- Sodium sources include table salt, homemade play dough (Fig. 70.1), rock salt used to de-ice roads, baking soda, sodium (Na) phosphate enemas, sea water, iatrogenic administration of Na-containing fluids such as Na bicarbonate and hypertonic saline, and ingestion of improperly mixed or formulated feeds (typically for large animals).

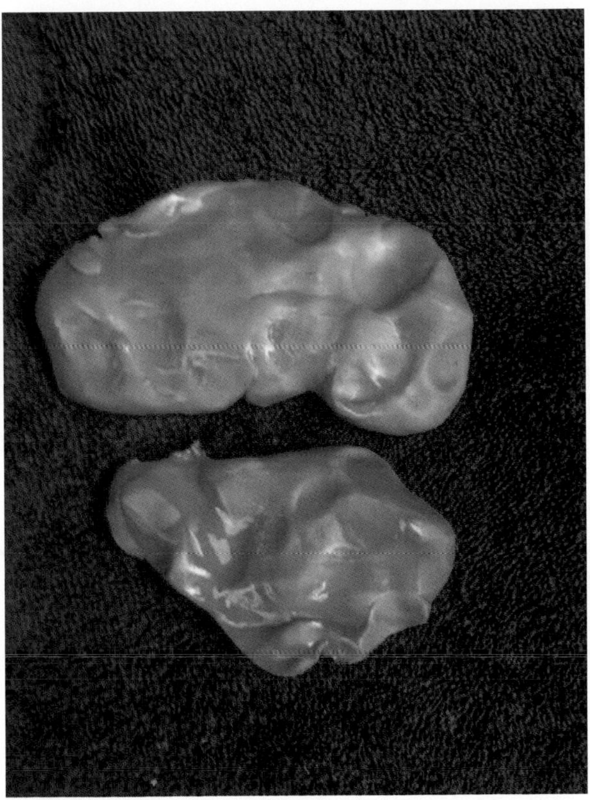

■ **Fig. 70.1.** Homemade play dough. Photo courtesy of Lynn R. Hovda.

Blackwell's Five-Minute Veterinary Consult Clinical Companion: Small Animal Toxicology, Second Edition.
Lynn R. Hovda, Ahna G. Brutlag, Robert H. Poppenga, and Katherine L. Peterson.

Companion website: www.fiveminutevet.com/toxicology

- Clinical signs of salt toxicosis have been reported to occur within 30 minutes after ingestion.
- Common clinical signs include GI signs (vomiting and diarrhea) and neurological signs (depression, lethargy, tremors, seizures, and coma).
- Treatment involves lowering the serum Na and symptomatic/supportive care.

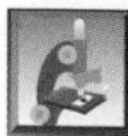

ETIOLOGY/PATHOPHYSIOLOGY

- Salt can have a direct irritant effect on the gastric mucosa.
- Neurological signs are due to rapid fluid shifts within the CNS, resulting in initial cell shrinkage, CNS intracellular hyperosmolality, and hemorrhage.

Mechanism of Action

- Hypernatremia is defined as serum Na levels >155 mEq/L in the dog or >158 mEq/L in the cat.
- The brain is affected by hypernatremia through two main mechanisms.
    - Sudden increases in serum Na and osmolality result in water shifting out of the cells and subsequent cellular dehydration.
    - Cerebral tissue dehydration causes shrinking of the brain mass, tearing of the fine meningeal vessels, and secondary hemorrhage/hematoma formation.
- Rapid increases in serum Na may also cause fluid shifts from the intracellular fluid compartment into the vasculature, resulting in hypervolemia.
- Treatment and lowering of the serum Na can result in fluid shifting back into the cells and subsequent cerebral edema by two theoretical mechanisms.
    - Rapid IV administration of free water (D5W) causes water to move from the vasculature into the CNS, resulting in cerebral edema.
    - Sodium passively diffuses from plasma to the CSF but transfer of Na back into plasma requires energy. Higher CSF Na levels (>145–185 mEq/L) result in decreased energy production, preventing transport of Na back into plasma and resulting in CSF hypernatremia. Water ingested or given IV (D5W) causes movement of water into the CNS, resulting in cerebral edema formation.

Pharmacokinetics – Absorption, Distribution, Metabolism, Excretion

- Sodium is absorbed rapidly from the GI tract.
- Sodium is distributed throughout the body and is the major cation in the extracellular space.
- Sodium and water balance is primarily regulated by the kidneys.
- Serum Na levels are controlled by the kidneys via the renin-angiotensin-aldosterone system and the hypothalamus via antidiuretic hormone and thirst.

Toxicity

- Signs of toxicosis are generally seen with serum Na concentrations ≥170 mEq/L; more severe signs are seen at a serum Na ≥180 mEq/L.

- Dogs ingesting 2–3 g/kg of sodium have shown signs of toxicity; 4 g/kg of sodium is reported to be a lethal dose in the dog.
- One tablespoon (15 g) of table salt contains approximately 17.85 g of NaCl; one cup contains 285.6 g of NaCl.
- Ingestion of 1.9 g/kg of homemade play dough can be toxic. Homemade play dough can contain 8 g of Na per tablespoon of dough, depending on the recipe.
- Sodium bicarbonate (baking soda) contains about 1/20th the Na content of table salt; 10–20 g/kg (2–4 teaspoonfuls/kg) can cause clinical signs.

Systems Affected

- Cardiovascular – tachycardia, arrhythmias.
- Endocrine/metabolic – hypernatremia, hyperchloremia, metabolic acidosis, hyperthermia, hyperosmolality.
- Gastrointestinal – vomiting, diarrhea, anorexia.
- Musculoskeletal – muscular rigidity and tremors, myoclonus, ataxia.
- Nervous – lethargy, depression, ataxia, tremors, seizures, coma.
- Respiratory – pulmonary edema or pleural effusion may develop from hypervolemia.
- Renal/urological – PU/PD, azotemia, acute tubular necrosis.

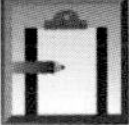

SIGNALMENT/HISTORY

- No known breed or sex predilection.

Risk Factors

- Lack of access to fresh water (e.g., water deprivation from a frozen water bowl) or unlimited access to water (after salt exposure) may exacerbate clinical signs.

Historical Findings

- Owners may report increased drinking and urinating, vomiting or diarrhea.
- Signs may occur as soon as 30 minutes but can be delayed up to 4 hours following ingestion.
- Neurological progression often follows the initial GI signs and includes ataxia, disorientation, tremors, seizures, and coma.
- A thorough history should be obtained in patients with hypernatremia. The sources of salt exposure (salt emetics, de-icers, homemade play dough or ornaments, salt water) and chronicity of signs may affect treatment.
- With unknown exposure, acute onset of vomiting followed by tremors or seizures with documented hypernatremia should raise suspicion for salt toxicity.

Location and Circumstances of Poisoning

- Exposure commonly occurs in the home with salt ingestion, in the clinic with hypertonic saline or at the beach with salt water ingestion.

CLINICAL FEATURES

- Clinical signs of salt toxicosis have been reported to occur within 30 minutes of exposure.
- The amount of salt ingested, water availability, duration of time since ingestion, and underlying health conditions of the patient all influence the clinical course and treatment.
- The most common initial clinical signs are vomiting, diarrhea, and anorexia.
- This may be followed by the development of neurological signs such as ataxia, tremors, seizures, and coma.
- On physical exam, the animal may appear dehydrated despite the presence of hypervolemia. They may be hyperthermic, tachypneic, tachycardic, or have the presence of arrhythmias with large exposures.

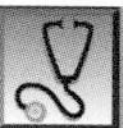

DIFFERENTIAL DIAGNOSIS

- Hypernatremia can also be caused by water losses (hypotonic or free water loss).
- Pure water losses.
    - Heat stroke
    - Diabetes insipidus (central or nephrogenic)
    - Fever
    - Inadequate access to water
    - Decreased water intake
    - Severe burns
- Hypotonic fluid losses.
    - Vomiting
    - Diarrhea
    - Chronic or acute renal failure
    - Diabetes mellitus
    - Diuretic administration
    - Paintball toxicosis
    - Activated charcoal, especially with a cathartic (sorbitol) and multidose administration.

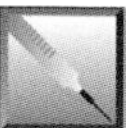

DIAGNOSTICS

- Measurement of the serum Na will confirm the presence of hypernatremia but not the inciting cause.
- Routine CBC, serum biochemistry profile, and UA should be performed to rule out other causes.
- Other confirmatory testing includes evaluation of CSF sodium levels with values >160 mEq/L being supportive (rarely performed).

Pathological Findings

- Gross pathological findings – hemorrhage to the GIT (stomach, small intestines, and colon), retraction of the brain from the calvarium, trauma to meningeal vessels, and hematoma formation.
- Microscopic changes – diffuse cerebral edema with widened extracellular spaces, blood vessel congestion, necrosis of vessel walls with extravasation of RBC and protein, renal necrosis, and hepatic necrosis.
- Postmortem cerebral tissue levels >1800 ppm are supportive of salt toxicity.

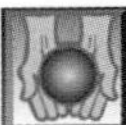

THERAPEUTICS

- The goal of therapy is to lower the serum Na concentration safely.
- Acute hypernatremia/exposure can be corrected more acutely until clinical signs abate.
- Chronic or unknown exposure with hypernatremia should be corrected slowly, no faster than 0.5 mEq/L/hour or 10–12 mEq/L/day.

Detoxification

- Emesis can be performed in asymptomatic patients within 1–2 hours.
- Gastric lavage may be helpful in symptomatic animals with evidence of material within the stomach (especially with play dough or ornaments).
- Activated charcoal is contraindicated and should not be administered.

Appropriate Health Care

- Asymptomatic patients should be monitored in the clinic for 8 hours with serum Na monitored every 4 hours.
    - If serum Na is normal after 8 hours, the patient can be discharge for at-home monitoring.
- Symptomatic patients should be hospitalized and monitored until serum Na is normalized and the patient is asymptomatic.
- IV balanced crystalloids may be used to correct dehydration in acute exposures.
    - To avoid rapid fluid shifts, especially with chronic hypernatremia, crystalloids can be made iso-osmotic to the patient (match serum sodium).
    - To do this, calculate the difference in Na between the patient and crystalloid fluid (patient Na – infusate fluid Na = mEq/L to add to bag).
    - Add the mEq of hypertonic saline to the crystalloid to match the patient's Na.
        - □ 23.4% hypertonic saline has 4 mEq NaCl per mL.
        - □ 7.5% hypertonic saline has 1.3 mEq NaCl per mL.
- Correct the free water deficit; water deficit needs to be calculated to help safely guide therapy.
    - Water deficit = $(0.6 \times BW_{kg}) \times [(\text{current serum Na}/\text{desired serum Na}) - 1]$.

  - Water replacement should occur over the appropriate time period to lower the serum sodium based on the chronicity and degree of elevation.
- Alternatively, the administration of 3.7 mL/kg/hour of D5W is estimated to lower the serum sodium level by 1 mEq/L/hour.
- Free water replacement can occur with oral or NE tube water, IV crystalloids, or IV D5W.
- Acute ingestion with neurological clinical signs – serum sodium can be lowered acutely until clinical signs abate.
- Intensive electrolyte monitoring is needed every 2–4 hours.
- Carefully monitor during treatment for clinical signs of cerebral edema, which can occur secondary to lowering the serum sodium.

Antidote

- No antidote for salt toxicity.

Drugs of Choice

- Antiemetics should be used in vomiting patients.
  - Maropitant 1 mg/kg, SQ q 24 hours, not labeled for cats.
  - Ondansetron 0.1–1.0 mg/kg, PO, IM, IV, SQ q 6–12 hours.
  - Metoclopramide 0.2–0.5 mg/kg, SQ, IM, IV, PO q 8 hours.
- Anticonvulsants.
  - Diazepam 0.5 mg/kg, IV to effect, followed by CRI at 0.5–1 mg/kg/hour, IV, to effect if needed.
  - Phenobarbital 4–16 mg/kg, IV to effect.
  - Propofol 1–8 mg/kg, IV to effect, followed by CRI dose of 0.1–0.6 mg/kg/min if uncontrolled seizures.
- Methocarbamol 55–220 mg/kg IV slowly to effect for tremors at a rate ≤2 mL/min and not to exceed 330 mg/kg/day.
- Furosemide 2.2–4.4 mg/kg, IV q 12–24 hours may aid in Na excretion in hypervolemic animals only, especially in those animals that have underlying cardiac or renal disease. Hydration status should be monitored closely.
- If neurologic signs worsen after treatment begins, recheck electrolytes immediately.
- If Na level decreases too quickly, cerebral edema may develop.
  - D5W should be slowed or stopped.
  - Treatment for cerebral edema initiated.
    - □ Head elevation for recumbent patients at 15–30° and minimize jugular restraint to prevent increased ICP.
    - □ Mannitol 0.5–2 g/kg, IV slow over 20–30 minutes to effect.
    - □ Furosemide 2.2–4.4 mg/kg, IV.

Precautions/Interactions

- If hypernatremia is chronic or slow in onset, idiogenic osmoles are produced by the CNS within 1–7 days from onset of hypernatremia.

- With chronic elevation, do not lower the serum sodium level faster than 0.5–1 mEq/L hour; too rapid a correction will result in cerebral edema formation.
- Patients with underlying renal or cardiac disease will need to be monitored closely for the development of pulmonary edema, as they may be less tolerant of the hypervolemia secondary to hypernatremia.

Nursing Care

- Careful fluid management with monitoring of hydration and perfusion is imperative.
- Intensive care (tremor and seizure monitoring, ECG and blood pressure monitoring, urinary catherization, etc.) may be needed, depending on the patient's neurological status.

Diet

- Due to the GI effects, a bland diet and soft foods may be indicated for 5–7 days.

COMMENTS

- Clinical signs in salt toxicosis are related to fluid shifts.
- Use caution when correcting the sodium level.

Patient Monitoring

- Monitor serum Na every 2–4 hours during fluid therapy. The fluid rate and type of fluid should be titrated based on the sodium level.
- Evaluation of the liver and kidney function in symptomatic animals should be repeated in 24–48 hours to evaluate for delayed injury.

Prevention/Avoidance

- Prevent ingestion of salt sources, including homemade play dough, table salt, and cold weather de-icing salt.
- Salt emetics are not recommended to induce vomiting.
- Ensure that pets have access to water.

Possible Complications

- Treatment can result in cerebral edema if the serum Na is dropped too quickly.
- Rare reports of renal and hepatic necrosis.

Expected Course and Prognosis

- Prognosis for acute exposure with mild signs is excellent. Signs typically resolve within 6–24 hours.
  Prognosis can be guarded depending on patient's Na level and clinical signs on presentation.

See Also

Paintballs

Abbreviations

See Appendix 1 for a complete list.

ECF = extracellular fluid
ICF = intracellular fluid
ICP = intracranial pressure

Suggested Reading

Ajito T, Suzuki K, Iwabuchi S. Effect of intravenous infusion of a 7.2% hypertonic saline solution on serum electrolytes and osmotic pressure in healthy beagles. J Vet Med Sci 1999; 61:637–641.

Barr JM, Safdar AK, McCullough SM, et al. Hypernatremia secondary to homemade play dough ingestion in dogs: a review of 14 cases from 1998 to 2001. J Vet Emerg Crit Care 2004; 14:196–202.

DiBartola SP. Disorders of sodium and water: hypernatremia and hyponatremia. In: DiBartola SP, ed. Fluid, Electrolyte, and Acid-Base Disorders in Small Animal Practice, 3rd edn. St Louis, MO: Elsevier Saunders, 2006.

Pouzot C, Descone-Junot C, Loup J, et al. Successful treatment of severe salt intoxication in a dog. J Vet Emerg Crit Care 2007; 17:294–298.

Tegzes JH. Sodium. In: Peterson ME, Talcott PA, eds. Small Animal Toxicology, 3rd edn. St Louis, MO: Saunders, 2013; pp. 807–810.

Author: Sarah L. Gray, DVM, DACVECC
Consulting Editor: Katherine L. Peterson, DVM, DACVECC

chapter 71

Xylitol

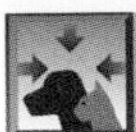

DEFINITION/OVERVIEW

- Xylitol is a naturally occurring, 5-carbon sugar alcohol commonly used as a sugar substitute in chewing gum, mints, candy, nicotine gum, toothpaste, vitamins, nutritional supplements and baked goods; it exists naturally in low levels in fruits and vegetables.
- Ingestion of xylitol can cause hypoglycemia and acute hepatic necrosis leading to vomiting, depression, diarrhea, weakness, ataxia, seizures, coagulopathy, and potentially death.
- Other sugar-free products (aspartame, acesulfame, malitol, sorbitol) are generally considered nontoxic.

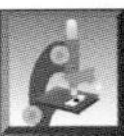

ETIOLOGY/PATHOPHYSIOLOGY

- Xylitol toxicity has two clinical manifestations: hypoglycemia and hepatic necrosis. The clinical syndrome typically depends on the amount of xylitol ingested.

Mechanism of Action

- Hypoglycemia occurs due to xylitol's direct stimulation of insulin secretion from the pancreas.
- The mechanism of hepatic necrosis is unknown. There are two proposed mechanisms.
    - Depletion of hepatic cellular ADP, ATP, and inorganic phosphorus molecules.
    - Production of reactive oxygen species during the metabolism of xylitol in the liver.

Pharmacokinetics – Absorption, Distribution, Metabolism, Excretion

- Rapidly absorbed after oral ingestion, with hypoglycemia seen within 10–15 minutes and peak plasma concentration within 30–60 minutes.
- The liver is the major organ of metabolism.

Blackwell's Five-Minute Veterinary Consult Clinical Companion: Small Animal Toxicology, Second Edition.
Lynn R. Hovda, Ahna G. Brutlag, Robert H. Poppenga, and Katherine L. Peterson.

Companion website: www.fiveminutevet.com/toxicology

Toxicity

- Hypoglycemia occurs at doses >0.1 g/kg.
- Hepatic failure has been reported at doses >0.5 g/kg.
- If listed as <2% of ingredients, xylitol amount can be approximated as 2% based on the weight of the product such as a piece of gum.
- Xylitol used for baking contains 190 g/cup.

Systems Affected

- Endocrine/metabolic – insulin secretion, hypoglycemia.
- Gastrointestinal – vomiting, diarrhea, melena.
- Hepatobiliary – acute hepatic necrosis, elevated liver enzymes, icterus, coagulopathy, hypoglycemia, hepatic encephalopathy.
- Nervous – behavioral changes, weakness, ataxia, tremors, seizures.

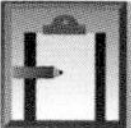

SIGNALMENT/HISTORY

- Any age and breed of dogs can be affected; cats and ferrets are also reportedly affected.

Risk Factors

- Preexisting liver diseases.
- Preexisting conditions predisposing to hypoglycemia (e.g., insulinoma, hepatoma, hepatocellular carcinoma, hunting dog hypoglycemia, diabetes mellitus with insulin administration).
- Availability of xylitol in the environment.

Historical Findings

- Acute onset of weakness, lethargy, vomiting, seizures.
- Witnessed ingestion.
- Discovery of chewed-up packages of xylitol products, baked goods or dental products. The owner may note the smell of gum from the pet's mouth or in the emesis.

Location and Circumstances of Poisoning

- Exposure typically occurs in the home. Pets often find gum or mints in purses or bags that are left unattended.

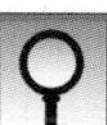

CLINICAL FEATURES

- Vomiting is usually the initial sign.
- Clinical signs of hypoglycemia (including weakness, depression, collapse, ataxia, tremors, or seizures) may occur within 10–60 minutes post ingestion.

- Hepatopathy may develop as early as 1-2 hours post ingestion although more typically 9–12 hours post ingestion; may be delayed up to 72 hours post ingestion. The patient may experience hepatic necrosis in the absence of initial hypoglycemia at presentation.
- Hepatic necrosis may lead to exacerbation of hypoglycemia. Depression, vomiting, icterus, melena, diarrhea, petechiae/ecchymosis, coagulopathy/DIC, and hepatic encephalopathy may be seen as the clinical condition progresses.
- Signs of muscle weakness may occur secondary to profound hypokalemia from endogenous insulin secretion.

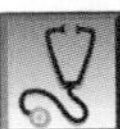

DIFFERENTIAL DIAGNOSIS

- Hypoglycemia – insulinoma, hypoadrenocorticism, juvenile hypoglycemia, hunting dog hypoglycemia, sepsis, drug administration or toxicosis (insulin overdose, glipizide), polycythemia.
- Liver failure.
    - Toxicities – sago palm (*Cycas revoluta*), acetaminophen, hepatotoxic mushrooms (*Amanita phalloides*), iron, aflatoxin, blue green algae, metaldehyde.
    - Infectious diseases – leptospirosis, mycoses, toxoplasmosis, infectious canine hepatitis.
    - Metabolic – cirrhosis, portosystemic shunt, microvascular dysplasia.
    - Neoplasia – hepatocellular carcinoma, lymphoma, etc.

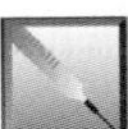

DIAGNOSTICS

- Blood glucose on presentation for all exposures.
- CBC – mild neutrophilic leukocytosis, hemoconcentration and thrombocytopenia with DIC.
- Chemistry – elevations of ALT, AST, ALP; hyperbilirubinemia; electrolyte derangements (hypokalemia, hypophosphatemia or hyperphosphatemia, and hypercalcemia).
- Clotting profile should be performed for patients with signs of liver enzyme elevations. May see prolonged coagulation tests (ACT, PTT, PT), thrombocytopenia, increased D-dimer or FDP.
- Abdominal ultrasound – with acute hepatic necrosis, the liver may be normal to increased in size. Echogenicity of the liver may be normal to hypoechoic or mottled.
- Cytology of the liver by fine needle aspirate may show degenerative changes such as non-lipid vacuolar changes, increased nuclear to cytoplasmic ratio, anisokaryosis, and lyzed cellular debris.
- Measurement of blood xylitol levels is not beneficial given the rapid metabolism by the liver.
- Insulin:glucose ratio can be performed to rule out insulinoma in cases with hypoglycemia and no known exposure to xylitol.

Pathological Findings

- Diffuse hepatic cell necrosis and organizational collapse may be seen as with other hepatotoxins.
- Widespread hemorrhage from DIC and icterus are common with acute hepatic necrosis.

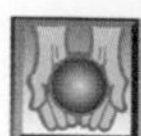

THERAPEUTICS

- Early decontamination, supportive care for hypoglycemia and hepatic injury, and monitoring are the mainstay of xylitol toxicity treatment.

Detoxification

- Check blood glucose prior to decontamination.
- Emesis induction for an asymptomatic patient if the ingestion is within 1–2 hours. Do not induce emesis if the patient has signs of hypoglycemia to avoid the risk of aspiration pneumonia and seizures.
    - With large ingestions, delayed emesis (within 6 hours) may still be beneficial, provided the patient's hypoglycemia has been treated appropriately, as xylitol products may aggregate in the stomach, delaying gastric emptying.
    - Activated charcoal is not recommended due to poor and unreliable binding to xylitol.

Appropriate Health Care

- Monitor BG every 1–4 hours for the first 6–8 hours. Adjust frequency based on the patient's clinical progression and degree of glucose supplementation.
- Dextrose boluses may be given if the patient develops hypoglycemia.
    - In hypoglycemic patients (BG <60 mg/dL), 0.5–1.5 mL/kg of 50% dextrose (diluted with saline) bolused IV over 1–2 minutes.
- Intravenous crystalloid fluids with 2.5–5% dextrose supplementation to maintain hydration and support blood glucose. Dextrose supplementation may also be hepatoprotective and may be recommended to prevent even if initial BG at presentation is normal.
- If the patient is not vomiting, small frequent meals should be fed to help prevent hypoglycemia.

Antidote

- There is no known antidote for xylitol.

Drugs of Choice

- Liver protectant/supportive medications are recommended, especially in cases of large dose ingestion (>0.5 g/kg).
    - S-adenosylmethionine (SAMe) 18 mg/kg PO q 24 hours and rounded to the closest tablet size or combination of sizes, given on an empty stomach.

- Silymarin (milk thistle) 5–10 mg/kg PO q 24 hours.
- Vitamin C 30 mg/kg PO, SQ q 6 hours.
- Vitamin E 50–600 units per dog PO q 24 hours.
- N-acetylcystine can be started with moderate liver enzyme elevations. 140 mg/kg IV (through filter) or PO once, then 70 mg/kg IV or PO q 6 hours for 7–17 doses depending on liver enzymes. Dilution required prior to administration.
- Vitamin K_1 3–5 mg/kg PO, SQ per day, dose can be divided.
- Fresh frozen plasma 10–20 mL/kg IV in the presence of DIC or coagulopathy.

■ Antiemetics as indicated for the patient's GI signs.
- Maropitant 1 mg/kg SQ q 24 hours.

Precautions/Interactions

■ Drugs which require hepatic metabolism should be avoided.

Diet

■ Consider small, frequent meals in nonvomiting patients.

COMMENTS

Patient Monitoring

■ Serial evaluation of clinical signs and blood glucose for 6–8 hours in asymptomatic patients; blood glucose should be normal for 2–4 hours after weaning IV dextrose.

■ Liver values should be monitored q 24 hours in symptomatic patients for at least 48–72 hours post ingestion.

■ Electrolytes should be checked q 6–12 hours depending on patient status.

Possible Complications

■ Long-term liver function abnormalities secondary to xylitol toxicity have not been investigated.

Expected Course and Prognosis

■ The prognosis for xylitol toxicity is good with lower doses ingested and prompt decontamination performed.

■ Prognosis for larger ingestion is fair to guarded even with prompt aggressive medical treatment. For patients that develop liver failure, the prognosis is guarded. Aggressive care may be needed for several days.

See Also

Acetaminophen
Blue-green Algae (Cyanobacteria)

Iron
Mushrooms
Sago Palm (Cycads)

Abbreviations

See Appendix 1 for a complete list.

Suggested Reading

Dunayer EK, Gwaltney-Brant SM. Acute hepatic failure and coagulopathy associated with xylitol ingestion in eight dogs. J Am Vet Med Assoc 2006; 229:1113–1117.
Peterson ME. Xylitol. Topics Compan Anim Med 2013; 28:18–20.
Todd JM, Powell LL. Xylitol intoxication associated with fulminant hepatic failure in a dog. J Vet Emerg Crit Care 2007; 17:286–289.
Xia Z, He Y, Yu J. Experimental acute toxicity of xylitol in dogs. J Vet Pharmacol Ther 2009; 32:465–469.

Acknowledgment: The authors and editors acknowledge the prior contributions of Ta-Ying Debra Liu, DVM, and Justine A. Lee, DVM, DACVECC, who authored this topic in the previous edition.
Author: Kelly M. Hall, DVM, MS, DACVECC
Consulting Editor: Katherine L. Peterson, DVM, DACVECC

Foreign Objects

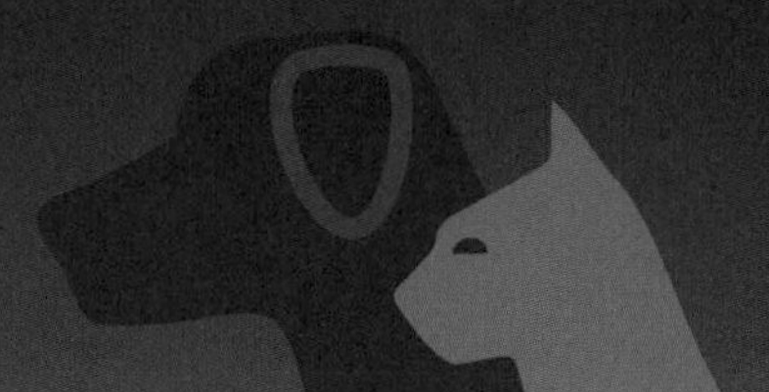

chapter 72

Foreign Objects

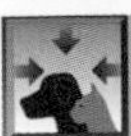

DEFINITION/OVERVIEW

- A foreign body is any object in an area of the body in which it does not belong. This broad term may include objects in the gastrointestinal tract, the respiratory system, subcutaneous/intramuscular tissues, etc.
- The most common foreign bodies in the dog and cat are GIT foreign bodies, those associated with a penetrating wound, and objects inhaled into the respiratory tree.

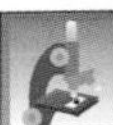

ETIOLOGY/PATHOPHYSIOLOGY

- GIT foreign bodies often lead to obstruction, which results in inappetance/anorexia, vomiting, electrolyte and acid–base abnormalities, and in severe cases, GIT perforation and death. Some can cause toxicity, such as metallic foreign bodies.
- Esophageal foreign bodies can cause acute onset of salivation, retching/gagging, pain, excessive swallowing, vomiting, and respiratory distress.
- Inhaled objects may result in airway irritation/inflammation, cough, hemoptysis, pneumonia, abscess, and respiratory distress.
- Penetrating foreign bodies result in local tissue damage/disruption, an inflammatory response, and possible abscess formation.
- For the purposes of this chapter, we will focus on gastrointestinal tract foreign bodies.

Toxicity

- The toxicity of foreign bodies is related to the composition of the material that was ingested.
- The majority of foreign bodies ingested (plastic, fabric, wood, rocks) are nontoxic but cause gastroenteritis and mechanical obstruction.
- Examples of toxic foreign bodies.
    - Zinc – vomiting, hemolytic anemia.
    - Lead – vomiting, neurological signs, red blood cell changes.
    - Homemade salt ornaments – hypernatremia, neurological signs.

Blackwell's Five-Minute Veterinary Consult Clinical Companion: Small Animal Toxicology, Second Edition.
Lynn R. Hovda, Ahna G. Brutlag, Robert H. Poppenga, and Katherine L. Peterson.

Companion website: www.fiveminutevet.com/toxicology

- Medication bezoars.
  - Certain medications, when ingested in large quantities, can form pharmacobezoars.
  - Medications reported to cause bezoars include aluminum hydroxide gel, enteric-coated aspirin, sucralfate, guar gum, cholestyramine, enteral feeding formulas, psyllium preparations, nifedipine XL, chewable iron supplements, and meprobamate.
  - Medications that are hygroscopic (absorb water) may also have an increased propensity to form pharmacobezoars.
  - Radiographic evidence – may see a large amount of radiopaque material within the stomach, often confused with kibble or metallic objects. If present, decontamination (e.g., emesis induction, gastric lavage) should be performed, followed by repeat radiographs to verify removal of all product.

Common Nontoxic Foreign Bodies

- Generally, decontamination and aggressive treatment is not necessary unless a massive ingestion has occurred. Radiographs should be performed and emesis or gastric lavage initiated if symptomatic and gastric foreign material is present, especially if there is risk for intestinal obstruction if material moves out of the stomach.
- Cat litter – clumping.
  - Small ingestions – loss of appetite, vomiting, and diarrhea.
  - With large ingestions, there is an increased risk of pyloric outflow obstruction, SI obstruction, or large intestinal obstruction.
  - Radiographic description – stippled, mineralized, foreign material.
- Charcoal/barbeque briquettes.
  - May contain charcoal and a combination of petroleum distillates, limestone, and sawdust. Used barbeque briquettes may have grill grease drippings dried on them, resulting in increased palatability and secondary gastroenteritis or pancreatitis.
  - Ingestion may result in loss of appetite, vomiting, diarrhea, and FBO.
  - Radiographic evidence – stippled material within the GIT, possible FBO.
- Crayons, markers, pens, pencils.
  - Check the package/label to verify nontoxicity.
  - Small ingestions typically do not result in clinical signs.
  - Large ingestions can cause clinical signs and illness, including loss of appetite, vomiting, diarrhea, and/or FBO.
  - May be difficult to identify radiographically.
- Silica gel packets.
  - Commonly found with newly purchased clothing, shoes, and other retail items.
  - Although inert, large ingestion can lead to expansion of the silica gel as it absorbs water, leading to GI signs such as diarrhea, vomiting, or even a gastric or intestinal FBO with massive ingestion (rare).
  - May be difficult to identify radiographically.

- Firestarter logs (e.g., Duraflame logs).
  - Constructed from sawdust, agricultural fibers, and nonpetroleum renewable waxes and oils.
  - Risk of gastroenteritis with small ingestion and FBO with a large ingestion.
- Wood glues (diisocyanate glues) – see chapter 9 for more information.
- Radiographic description – non-specific foreign material and FBO may be identified.

Systems affected

- Gastrointestinal – dehydration, vomiting, anorexia, local irritation/inflammation, perforation.
- Hematological – hemoconcentration.
- Hepatobiliary – bile duct obstruction and icterus (rare).
- Metabolic – hypochloremic metabolic alkalosis, lactic acidosis, compensatory respiratory acidosis.
- Respiratory – aspiration pneumonia, coughing.
- Renal – prerenal azotemia.

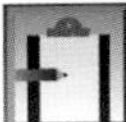

SIGNALMENT/HISTORY

- There is no breed or sex predilection for foreign bodies. Anecdotally, younger animals seem predisposed to ingesting foreign material, likely due to their curious and explorative nature.

Risk Factors

- Risk factors for the development of foreign bodies include foreign material in the environment while the pet is not being supervised and dogs with dietary indiscretion.
- Previous GI surgery (including enterotomy, resection and anastomosis) may predispose patients to reobstruction as the intestinal luminal diameter may be reduced from scar tissue.

Historical Findings

- This history may include known ingestion of a foreign body, eating garbage, or evidence of foreign material in the emesis or home.
- Owners may report vomiting, abdominal pain, and anorexia.

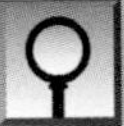

CLINICAL FEATURES

- The clinical course of dogs and cats with foreign bodies can be extremely variable.
- Onset of clinical signs may be very acute in esophageal or proximal small intestinal foreign bodies that are completely obstructive.
- The clinical course may be more mild and prolonged in cases of gastric, distal small intestinal, or large intestinal foreign bodies, or foreign bodies which are only partially obstructive.

- Animals with foreign bodies may present with:
  - lethargy
  - weight loss
  - diarrhea +/– hematochezia
  - vomiting, hematemesis, and regurgitation.
- Physical examination of the patient with a foreign body can be widely variable. Common abnormalities include:
  - abdominal pain
  - dehydration
  - palpable foreign object within the GI tract, bunching of the intestines (as in linear foreign bodies).
- Patients with esophageal foreign bodies may present with:
  - ptyalism
  - dysphagia
  - regurgitation
  - respiratory distress.
- Patients with partially obstructive foreign bodies are more likely to be in poor body condition with a more chronic history of illness.

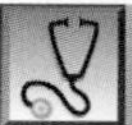

DIFFERENTIAL DIAGNOSIS

- Because the clinical signs associated with GIT foreign bodies are very nonspecific, a wide range of differential diagnoses exists.
- Primary GI disease – inflammatory bowel disease, gastroenteritis, dietary indiscretion, gastric dilatation and volvulus, mesenteric torsion, parvoviral enteritis, etc.
- Secondary GI disease/metabolic – kidney disease, liver disease, pancreatitis, hypoadrenocorticism, hyperthyroidism (cats), neoplasia, toxins/medications (NSAIDs, antibiotics, SSRIs/serotonin syndrome, irritants or corrosive substances, etc.).
- Generally, the history, physical exam findings, blood work, and radiographs will narrow down the differential list.

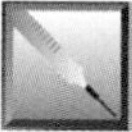

DIAGNOSTICS

- CBC – hemoconcentration, inflammatory leukogram.
- Biochemistry – hypochloremia, metabolic alkalosis (pH >7.4, increased bicarbonate), hypokalemia, hyponatremia, and hyperlactatemia. Prerenal azotemia, hyperbilirubinemia (if foreign body obstructs the common bile duct or in cases of pancreatitis and/or septic peritonitis).
- Radiography.
  - Abdominal radiographs (v/d, right lateral +/– left lateral) should be performed in all cases with a suspected GIT foreign body.

- Possible findings may include an obstructive pattern – gas accumulation and small intestinal dilation orad to the obstruction, bowel distension with two populations of bowel, visualization of the foreign material, plication of the small intestines.
- Evaluate for SI diameter.
  - Dog – SI diameter is not normally uniform, but on the lateral radiographic projection, the ratio of the maximal SI diameter to the height of the vertebral body of L_5 at its narrowest point should be less than 1.6.
  - Cat – SI diameter is normally more uniform and >12 mm diameter of SI on lateral or VD radiographic projection suggests FBO.
- Evaluate for the following.
  - Peritonitis – loss of abdominal detail.
  - Pneumoperitoneum – free gas in the abdominal cavity with visualization of gas opacity not contained in a viscus. This is typically found at the highest point of the peritoneal cavity on radiographs and is often superimposed on abdominal organs such as the liver or the GIT. Recent abdominal surgery, artificial insemination, and other benign causes for pneumoperitoneum should be ruled out.
- Thoracic and cervical radiographs are required for suspected esophageal foreign bodies. Direct visualization of the object, distension of the esophagus orad to the obstruction, as well as aspiration pneumonia/pneumonitis may be seen.

- Positive contrast studies – radiopaque contrast (typically barium) is administered orally at a dose of 10–12 mL/kg. Serial abdominal radiographs are taken after administration at time 0, 15, 30, 60, 90, 120, and 180 minutes to assess transit of the contrast through the SI. The study may be terminated early if all the contrast has left the SI. This functional study is very good at confirming a SI obstruction but is contraindicated in patients with protracted vomiting due to the risk of aspiration into the lungs.
- Abdominal ultrasound can be used to identify foreign material within the GI tract and may identify signs consistent with GIT obstruction; can be highly operator dependent.
- Abdominocentesis should be performed in all cases when abdominal effusion is present to evaluate for septic, suppurative inflammation, which may indicate GIT perforation. This information is useful for surgical planning as well as prognostication.

THERAPEUTICS

- Definitive treatment for obstructive foreign bodies usually includes general anesthesia and removal, either by gastric lavage, endoscopy, or surgery.
- Patients should be stabilized prior to anesthesia.
  - IV fluid therapy with an isotonic crystalloid to correct dehydration/hypovolemia and electrolyte abnormalities.
  - Opioid pain medication such as fentanyl or hydromorphone.
- In some cases where a small volume of foreign material is present, the material is nonobstructive, and there are no indications for immediate surgical intervention, foreign material may pass through the intestinal tract with supportive care (IV fluid therapy, antiemetics, pain control, GI protectants).

- Gastric foreign bodies may not require surgical intervention.
  - Emesis, gastric lavage, or endoscopy may successfully remove the FB.
  - Emesis should only be considered in stable patients and if the material ingested is not caustic or sharp; higher risk for further damage to the GI tract or aspiration pneumonia.
- Endoscopy can successfully remove a FB that is in the esophagus, stomach or very proximal small intestine. This procedure is very technical and operator dependent. General anesthesia is required.
- Obstructive foreign bodies in the small intestine or stomach that cannot be removed with endoscopy require surgical removal. A gastrotomy, enterotomy, or resection and anastomosis is performed depending on the location of the foreign body and the viability of the surrounding tissue.

Precautions/Interactions

- Antiemetics given prior to diagnosis may mask symptoms associated with an FBO.
- Patients with dehydration, gastroenteritis, and peritonitis should not be treated with NSAIDs as this may result in further gastroenteritis, ulceration, perforation or kidney damage.
- Owners should always be warned of the possibility of a “negative explore”, which occurs when no foreign material is identified in the GIT, whenever surgery is undertaken for a suspected foreign body and biopsies of the GI tract should be performed.

Nursing Care

- Incision should be monitored daily.
- E-collar should be worn at all times to prevent patients from licking their incision.
- Blood pressure, ECG, hydration, appetite should be monitored; frequency will depend on the stability of the patient.

Diet

- Bland diet should be considered in patients postoperatively.
- Nutritional support should be provided for patients with prolonged anorexia. A feeding tube can be placed during surgery if indicated.

Activity

- Patients should be encouraged to walk postoperatively to promote GI motility.
- Activity should be restricted for 14 days postoperatively to promote surgical site and incision healing.

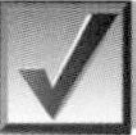

COMMENTS

Prevention/Avoidance

- Care should be taken to avoid leaving material in the pet’s environment that could be ingested, particularly if the pet has shown a predisposition for eating foreign objects. In some cases, this may include crate training when the pet is not being supervised.

Possible Complications

- Major complications associated with surgical removal include:
    - dehiscence of the surgical site and septic peritonitis; requires repeat surgery and broad-spectrum antibiotics, and carries a guarded to poor prognosis
    - strictures at the surgical site may develop during healing
    - vomiting pets and those requiring general anesthesia may develop aspiration pneumonia requiring antibiotics and oxygen supplementation and may affect prognosis.

Expected Course and Prognosis

- In general, the prognosis for GIT foreign bodies is good.
- Duration of clinical signs, presence of a linear foreign body, and the requirement for multiple intestinal procedures have been associated with a higher mortality rate.
- Patients with septic peritonitis from a FB perforation have a guarded to poor prognosis and require aggressive supportive care.

Abbreviations

See Appendix 1 for a complete list.

FB = foreign body
US = ultrasound

Suggested Reading

Beal MW. Approach to the acute abdomen. Vet Clin North Am Small Anim Pract 2005; 35(2):375–396.

Boag AK, Coe RJ, Martinez TA, et al. Acid-base and electrolyte abnormalities in dogs with gastrointestinal foreign bodies. J Vet Intern Med 2005; 19(6):816–821.

Hayes G. Gastrointestinal foreign bodies in dogs and cats: a retrospective study of 208 cases. J Small Anim Pract 2009; 50:576–583.

Sharma J, Thompson MS, Scrivani PV, et al. Comparison of radiography and ultrasonography for diagnosing small-intestinal mechanical obstruction in vomiting dogs. Vet Radiol Ultrasound 2011; 52(3):248–255.

Thompson HC, Cortes Y, Gannon K, et al. Esophageal foreign bodies in dogs: 34 cases (2004–2009). J Vet Emerg Crit Care 2012; 22(2):253–261.

Acknowledgment: The authors and editors acknowledge the prior contributions of Garret E. Pachtinger, VMD, and Kenneth J. Drobatz, DVM, MSCE, DACVIM, DACVECC, who authored this topic in the previous edition.

Author: Christopher M. McLaughlin, DVM
Consulting Editor: Katherine L. Peterson, DVM, DACVECC

Garden, Yard, and Farm Chemicals

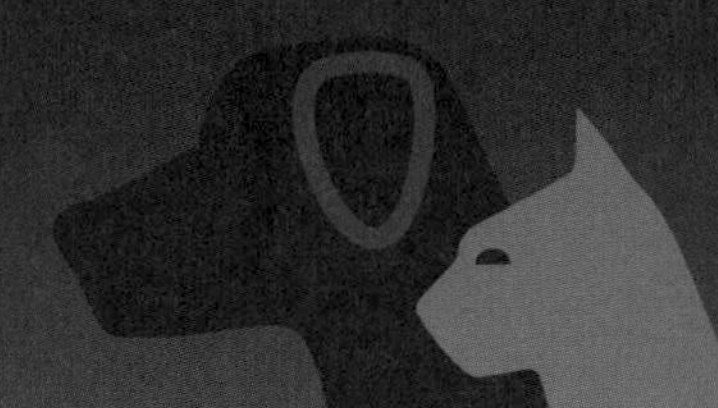

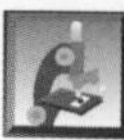

ETIOLOGY/PATHOPHYSIOLOGY

Mechanism of Action

- Direct irritation to the GI tract and potential for FBO.

Pharmacokinetics – Absorption, Distribution, Metabolism, Excretion

- Bone meal and blood meal are poorly absorbed through gastrointestinal and dermal routes.

Toxicity

- Bone meal and blood meal are generally considered low-level toxins.
- Large ingestions of bone meal or blood meal can congeal or solidify in the stomach, resulting in a gastric FBO.

Systems Affected

- Gastrointestinal – GI irritation (vomiting, diarrhea, drooling, anorexia, abdominal discomfort) FBO, and pancreatitis.

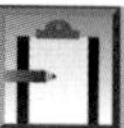

SIGNALMENT/HISTORY

- No breed or sex predilection.
- Outdoor dogs may have more opportunity for exposure and young dogs may be more prone to dietary indiscretion.

Historical Findings

- History of exposure to bone or blood meal.
- GIT signs with possible bone or blood meal, soil, or plant material in vomitus or feces.

Location and Circumstances of Poisoning

- Access to containers or spilled bone or blood meal in the garage, shed, or other storage facility.
- Access to recently fertilized crops, garden, or lawn.
- Use of organic lawn and gardening products may have increased exposure opportunities for animals.

Interactions with Drugs, Nutrients, or Environment

- Additives such as fungicides, insecticides, and herbicides may increase risk of toxicity (see appropriate chapters for more information).
- The scent of bone and blood meal may entice dogs to ingest newly planted toxic bulbs/plants as well.

CLINICAL FEATURES

- GIT signs including vomiting, diarrhea, anorexia, bloating, and abdominal discomfort.
- Blood meal ingestion can result in vomiting of partially digested blood and mucoid, foul-smelling diarrhea and melena.

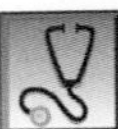

DIFFERENTIAL DIAGNOSIS

- GI irritants/gastroenteritis.
- Dietary indiscretion.
- Foreign body obstruction.
- Pancreatitis.
- Inflammatory bowel disease.
- Metabolic disease – liver or renal disease, Addison's disease.
- Other ingestions that cause GI signs.

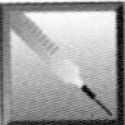

DIAGNOSTICS

- PCV/TS to monitor for dehydration, particularly if vomiting is persistent.
- Pancreatitis blood tests (e.g., amylase, lipase, canine pancreas-specific lipase [cPL], pancreatitis lipase immunoreactivity) or abdominal ultrasound if indicated by clinical signs.
- Abdominal radiographs to rule out FBO.

Pathological Findings

- Evidence of foreign material or FBO in GIT.

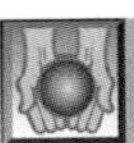

THERAPEUTICS

Detoxification

- Emesis within 2–4 hours if:
    - spontaneous emesis has not occurred
    - evidence of foreign material within the stomach
    - ingestion was a significant amount that could result in FBO or pancreatitis
    - patient is susceptible or has a prior history of pancreatitis.
- Unsuccessful emesis with large ingestion of blood meal – consider gastric lavage if no change in stomach contents with supportive care and time. Bone meal can be difficult to remove via gastric lavage.
- If medical management and gastric lavage are unsuccessful or evidence of FBO on radiographs, surgical intervention may be necessary.

Appropriate Health Care

- Antiemetics if vomiting is severe or persistent.
    - Maropitant 1 mg/kg SQ q 24 hours, not labeled for cats.
    - Ondansetron 0.1–0.5 mg/kg IV, IM, SQ, PO q 8–12 hours.
- Fluids – IV or SQ depending on patient status.
- GI protectants.
    - Famotidine 0.5 –1 mg/kg PO, SQ, IM, IV q 12 hours.
    - Omeprazole 0.5–1 mg/kg PO q 24 hours.
    - Sucralfate 0.25–1 g PO q 8 hours.

Antidote

- No antidote.

Diet

- Bland or low-fat diet until GI signs resolve.

Activity

- No change in activity is needed unless surgical intervention is required.

Surgical Considerations

- Surgical removal may be necessary for an FBO.

COMMENTS

Prevention/Avoidance

- Prevent access to bone and blood meal, especially to containers or other large quantities.

Expected Course and Prognosis

- Small exposures can typically be managed at home.
- Larger exposures may require supportive care but prognosis is good and clinical signs often resolve within 24 hours.

See Also

Fertilizers
Herbicides

Abbreviations

See Appendix 1 for a complete list.

Suggested Reading

Plumlee K. Clinical Veterinary Toxicology. Philadelphia, PA: Mosby, 2004; pp. 408–409.

Acknowledgment: The authors and editors acknowledge the prior contributions of Josephine L. Marshall, CVT, and Justine A. Lee, DVM, DACVECC, who authored this topic in the previous edition.
Author: Charlotte Flint, DVM
Consulting Editor: Katherine L. Peterson, DVM, DACVECC

Diquat and Paraquat

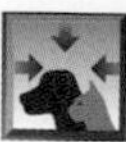

DEFINITION/OVERVIEW

Diquat (6,7-dihydrodipyrido[1,2-a:2′,1′-c] pyrazinediium dibromide; $C_{12}H_{12}Br_2N_2$) is a bipyridyl herbicide.

- General use nonselective herbicide, desiccant, and defoliant that is available as aqueous solutions (15–25% w/v) and as water soluble granules (2.5%) under many trade names.
- Moderately toxic but considerably less toxic than paraquat.
- Concentrated diquat is corrosive to the skin, eyes, and GI tract.
- Diquat typically causes GI signs but large exposures can cause more significant signs.

Paraquat (1,1′-dimethyl-4,4′-bipyridinium dichloride; $C_{12}H_{14}Cl_2N_2$) is an herbicide with use restricted to licensed applicators.

- Available in pressurized spray formulations that contain less than or equal to 0.44% paraquat bis (methyl sulfate) and liquid fertilizer formulations that contain no more than 0.04% paraquat dichloride.
- In the USA, it is often colored blue, has a noxious odor added to prevent accidental consumption and contains an emetic to induce vomiting if consumed.
- Paraquat is one of the most selective pulmonary toxins known.
- Toxicity can be severe and involve GI signs, respiratory distress, and multiorgan failure.

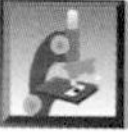

ETIOLOGY/PATHOPHYSIOLOGY

Mechanism of Action

Diquat

- Potent inducer of cyclic reduction-oxidation reactions, generates free radicals, and causes lipid peroxidation of cell membranes.

Paraquat

- Cyclic reduction-oxidation reactions in lung generate reactive oxygen species and free radicals and deplete antioxidants such as superoxide dismutase and NADPH.

Blackwell's Five-Minute Veterinary Consult Clinical Companion: Small Animal Toxicology, Second Edition.
Lynn R. Hovda, Ahna G. Brutlag, Robert H. Poppenga, and Katherine L. Peterson.

Companion website: www.fiveminutevet.com/toxicology

- Membrane damage, cellular incapacitation, and organ damage ensue. In the lungs, necrosis of type II pneumocytes occurs, denuding the alveolar basement membrane, leading to fibrosis.

Pharmacokinetics – Absorption, Distribution, Metabolism, Excretion

Diquat

- Absorption – poor cutaneous absorption; 10–20% absorbed within 6 hours after oral administration.
- Distribution – does not accumulate in the lungs; highest concentration found in the kidneys.
- Metabolized to mono- and dipyridones which are less toxic than the parent compound.
- Majority (85–90%) of ingested diquat excreted unchanged in the feces; monopyridone metabolite primarily excreted in the feces, dipyridone metabolite excreted in urine.
- Enterohepatic recirculation is minimal.
- Half-life of parent compound and metabolites is less than 24 hours.

Paraquat (Fig. 74.1)

- Absorption is incomplete (20–28%) after oral ingestion but is rapid, with peak plasma concentrations in 75 minutes.
- Absorption by inhalation or through skin causes a less severe reaction and is typically seen with chronic exposures.

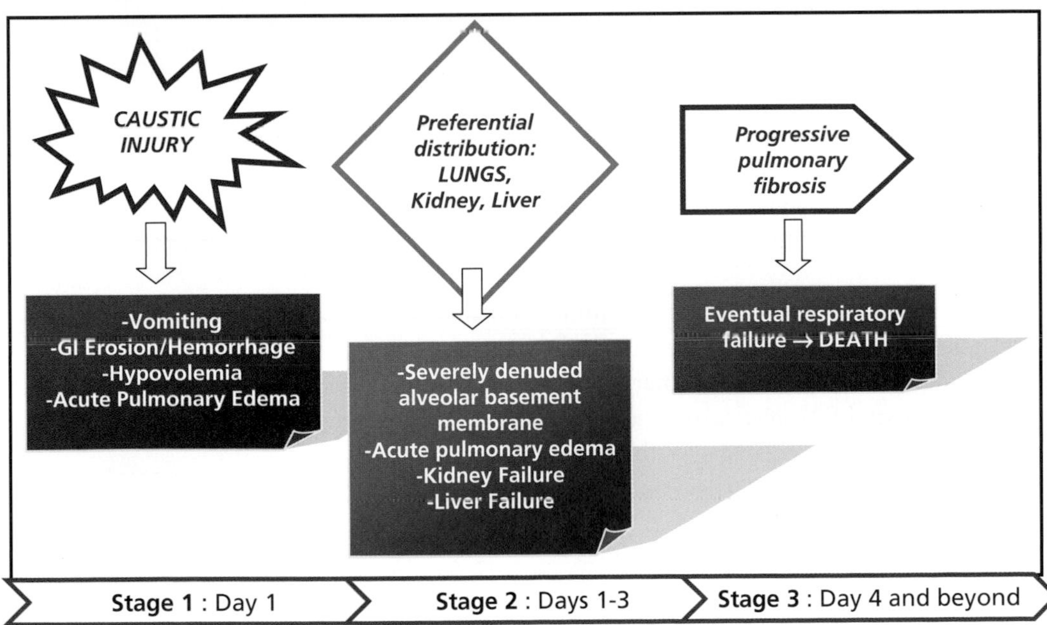

■ **Fig. 74.1.** Pathophysiology of paraquat toxicity.

- Distribution – selectively accumulates in lung alveolar type 1 and type 2 pneumocytes, and Clara cells as well as renal proximal tubule epithelium.
  - At 4 hours post exposure, concentration in lung is already 10× higher than at other sites; at 4–10 days post exposure, concentration in lung is 30–80× higher than plasma.
- Metabolism – extensive cyclic oxidation-reduction reactions in sequestering tissues but is excreted largely unchanged in the urine.
- Absorbed paraquat is rapidly excreted by the kidneys: 80–90% excreted within 6 hours, almost 100% by 24 hours (in the absence of paraquat-induced renal disease). Unabsorbed paraquat is excreted unchanged in the feces (detectable up to 7 days post exposure in rodents).
- As kidney damage worsens with toxicosis, the T½ increases dramatically from <12 hours to >120 hours.

Toxicity

- Diquat generally has a low level of toxicity with household use.
- Paraquat is highly toxic and often fatal.
  - LD_{50} varies by species (table 74.1).

TABLE 74.1. Comparative toxicity (oral LD_{50}) of paraquat in selected species.

	Dog	Cat	Human	Monkey	Cow	Sheep	Pig	Rat	Chicken	Turkey
LD_{50} (mg/kg)	25–50	35–50	25–75	50–70	35–50	8–10	75	100	110–360	290

Systems Affected

Diquat

- Gastrointestinal – vomiting, diarrhea, GI ulceration, GI hemorrhage, abdominal pain, paralytic ileus.
- Renal – azotemia, renal failure (rare).
- Respiratory – upper airway irritation, laryngeal edema, pulmonary edema, pneumonia, and ARDS.
- Cardiovascular – ventricular dysrhythmias and subendocardial hemorrhage (rare).
- Hepatic – mild liver enzyme elevations, hepatic necrosis (rare).
- Neurological – depression, lethargy, disorientation, diminished reflexes, collapse, nervousness, irritability, restlessness, decreased PLR, miotic pupils, coma, death (rare).
- Dermal – irritation, corrosive with concentrates.
- Ocular – eye irritation, corneal and conjunctival ulceration.

Paraquat

- Gastrointestinal – vomiting, diarrhea, aphagia, pain, esophageal or gastric ulceration.
- Respiratory – respiratory distress, pulmonary edema, ARDS, pulmonary fibrosis.

- Cardiovascular – hypertension, cor pulmonale, and cardiovascular collapse.
- Renal – azotemia (prerenal and renal), acute tubular necrosis, oliguria/anuria.
- Neurological (rare) – hyperexcitability, depression, ataxia, and seizures.
- Skin – irritation, ulceration, erythema, blistering.

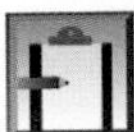

SIGNALMENT/HISTORY

- There is no breed, sex, or age predilection, as diquat and paraquat are toxic to all mammals.

Historical Findings

- Owners with high-risk jobs (pesticide industry, agriculture).
- Exposure to agricultural areas, where pesticides are used and recent spraying activity.
- Observed ingestion or finding malicious baits intended for pets.

Location and Circumstances of Poisoning

- Primarily accidental.
- Skin absorption from concentrated or prolonged exposure.
- Animals exposed to concentrates (agricultural centers, etc.).
- Paraquat has not been widely available since the 1960s but may still be stored in many places, including homes, garages, storage sheds, barns.

CLINICAL FEATURES

Diquat

- Mild-to-moderate toxicity – primarily gastrointestinal signs (oral/pharyngeal irritation/burning sensation, nausea, vomiting, abdominal pain, severe diarrhea), +/– renal impairment.
- Severe toxicity (rare) – GI ulceration, ileus, pulmonary edema, acute renal and hepatic failure, loss of consciousness, dysrhythmias, coma, death in 24–48 hours.
- Neurological signs can have progressive development over 72–96 hours in severe cases.

Paraquat

- Ptyalism, vomiting, diarrhea, and abdominal pain are usually the first presenting signs due to caustic nature of paraquat.
- Dose dependent and usually fatal.
- High-dose ingestion – rapid multisystem organ failure, massive pulmonary edema, ARF, liver damage, and death in 1–4 days.

- Moderate or subacute dose ingestion – slower onset of organ failure but eventual death from respiratory failure and pulmonary edema.
- Low and/or chronic exposure ingestion – death may not occur for several weeks and is usually secondary to pulmonary fibrosis and respiratory failure.
- Chronic exposure through the skin or inhalation – usually a less severe clinical presentation.
- Acute kidney failure can occur 1–3 days post injury.

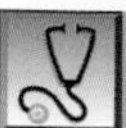

DIFFERENTIAL DIAGNOSIS

Diquat and Paraquat

- Gastrointestinal disease.
  - Ingestion of strongly alkaline or acidic compounds, zinc phosphide rodenticide, inorganic arsenic, zinc, mercury, or lead.
  - Infectious agents/gastroenteritis.
  - Pancreatitis.
- Primary renal or hepatic disease.

Paraquat only

- Primary cardiac disease.
- Primary or secondary pulmonary disease.
  - Pneumonia/pneumonitis.
  - Canine distemper.
  - Asthma/bronchitis.
  - *Pneumocystis* infection.
  - Pulmonary interstitial fibrosis.

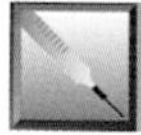

DIAGNOSTICS

Diquat

- Serum chemistry – azotemia, elevated liver enzymes.
- Urinalysis – isosthenuria.
- Thoracic radiographs – for patients with respiratory distress.
- Serum or urine diquat level (thin-layer or high-performance liquid chromatography, spectroscopy, spectrofluorometry) – not routinely available or done.
  - Store specimens for diquat analysis in plastic containers – diquat binds to glass.

Pathological Findings

- Oral, esophageal and/or gastric erosion, ulceration, hemorrhage.
- Upper airway irritation, laryngeal edema +/– pulmonary edema.
- Acute renal tubular necrosis.

Paraquat

- Chest radiographs should be performed for the first 1–3 days post ingestion.
- Serum chemistry – elevated lipase, azotemia, elevated liver enzymes.
- Urinalysis – isosthenuria, tubular casts.
- Arteriolar blood gas – hypoxemia.
- Dithionite spot test (1% aqueous sodium dithionite in 0.1 normal sodium hydroxide) may detect paraquat in urine (blue color) and tissues and is important for rapid diagnosis.
- Serum paraquat levels – this is most predictive of severity and prognosis but not readily available in veterinary laboratories; levels are quickly undetectable.
- Spectrometry and quantitative analysis of urine up to 48 hours after ingestion.
- Paraquat detection in stomach contents, vomitus, tissues, and organs (spectrophotometry, gas/liquid chromatography, radioimmunoassay).

Pathological Findings

- Gross pulmonary congestion, bullous emphysema, hemorrhage, bronchodilation, or atelectasis.
- Microscopic –necrosis of alveolar type II pneumocytes denuding alveolar basement membrane with severe pulmonary edema and/or fibroplasia.

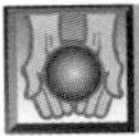

THERAPEUTICS

Detoxification

Diquat/Paraquat

- Emesis or gastric lavage as early as possible (<1 hour post ingestion).
    - Concentrated solutions are corrosive so emesis may not be advised.
- Activated charcoal with a cathartic (1 dose).
- Fuller's earth, bentonite or clay may provide some decrease in absorption.
- Paraquat – hemoperfusion through a charcoal filter or hemodialysis may be the most effective treatment at decreasing plasma concentrations; peritoneal dialysis is not useful.
- If ocular exposure has occurred, flush the eyes for at least 15 minutes, fluorescein stain, slit lamp examination, ophthalmology consult as needed.
- For dermal exposure, bathe in a mild liquid dish soap and rinse well (wear appropriate personal protective equipment).

Appropriate Health Care

- Treatment is supportive and symptomatic.
- IV fluid therapy – adjust therapy as indicated for dehydration and perfusion abnormalities.
- Antiemetics, GI protectants (H_2 blocker or proton pump inhibitor, sucralfate).
- Treat seizures with benzodiazepines, phenobarbital or propofol.
- Bronchospasm may require treatment with inhaled beta$_2$-adrenergic agonists and systemic corticosteroids.

Paraquat

- Early oxygen therapy is typically contraindicated because of oxidant damage. However, oxygen therapy may be useful for patient comfort secondary to respiratory compromise and progressive lung failure.
- Cautious IV crystalloid fluid therapy should be used but titrated to effect to prevent worsening of pulmonary edema.
- Antioxidant therapy with N-acetylcysteine (Mucomyst) and/or glutathione has been recommended (unknown benefit).
    - High-dose vitamin C (ascorbic acid) is not recommended based on findings of recent studies.
- In human medicine, treatment consists of gastric lavage, one dose of activated charcoal with a cathartic, hemoperfusion, hemodialysis, and pulse therapy (cyclophosphamide and steroids).

Drugs and Antidotes of Choice

- There is no antidote for diquat or paraquat.

Precautions/Interactions

- Emesis may further damage the esophagus or stomach if concentrated solutions are ingested.
- Paraquat – oxygen therapy early is typically contraindicated because it enhances oxidant damage (in human medicine, oxygen therapy is withheld until the PaO_2 is <50 mmHg).

COMMENTS

Patient Monitoring

- In symptomatic patients, monitor electrolytes renal and hepatic values q 24 hours; monitor urine output in patients with renal compromise.
- Severely affected patients should have ECG, BP, SpO_2 monitored.

Prevention/Avoidance

- Access to concentrated products or treated yards should be avoided.

Expected Course and Prognosis

Diquat

- Mild toxicity – prognosis is good with recovery expected within 24 hours with supportive care.
- Severe toxicity – prognosis can be guarded to poor with GI ulceration, cardiac arrhythmias, and organ damage.

Paraquat

- Prognosis is poor with resultant organ damage and respiratory failure within days of the exposure.

Abbreviations

See Appendix 1 for a complete list.

Suggested Reading

Bischoff K, Brizzee-Buxton B, Gatto N, et al. Malicious paraquat poisoning in Oklahoma dogs. Vet Hum Toxicol 1998; 40(3):151–153.

Cope RB. Toxicology brief: helping animals exposed to the herbicide paraquat. Vet Med 2004: 755–762.

Cope RB, Bildfell RJ, Valentine BA, et al. Fatal paraquat poisoning in seven Portland, Oregon, dogs. Vet Hum Toxicol 2004; 46(5):258–264.

Donaldson C. Paraquat, In: Talcott P, Peterson M, eds. Small Animal Toxicology, 3rd edn. St Louis, MO: Elsevier, 2013; pp. 731–739.

Gupta PK. Toxicity of herbicides. In: GuptaRC, ed. Veterinary Toxicology: Basic and Clinical Principles. New York: Elsevier, 2007; pp. 567–586.

Hampson EC, Effeney DJ, Pond SM. Efficacy of single or repeated hemoperfusion in a canine model of paraquat poisoning. J Pharmacol Exp Ther 1990; 254(2):732–740.

Acknowledgment: The authors and editors acknowledge the prior contributions of Carey L. Renken, MD, who authored this topic in the previous edition.
Author: Colleen M. Almgren, DVM, PhD, DABT, DABVT
Consulting Editor: Katherine L. Peterson, DVM, DACVECC

chapter 75

Fertilizers

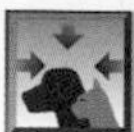

DEFINITION/OVERVIEW

- Fertilizers are soil amendment products used in agriculture, lawn and garden care, and indoor plant applications to enhance plant growth.
- Fertilizers are composed of organic and inorganic material containing varying percentages of nitrogen, phosphorus, and potassium (potash), as indicated by the three numbers on the packaging (e.g., 30-10-10).
- Fertilizers may also contain the following micronutrients: iron, sulfur, calcium, magnesium, copper, zinc, boron, manganese, and molybdenum.
- In general, fertilizer ingestions are of low-level toxicity and symptoms are primarily limited to gastrointestinal irritation. Iron-containing products, especially in large ingestions or concentrations, may cause iron toxicity.
- Ingestion of fertilizers containing Milorganite, a sewage-based fertilizer, carries increased risk of toxicity with potential for gastrointestinal signs, muscle pain, and stiffness.

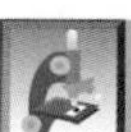

ETIOLOGY/PATHOPHYSIOLOGY

- The widespread use of lawn and garden fertilizers results in frequent exposure opportunities for animals.

Mechanism of Action

- Fertilizer exposure generally results in a low level of toxicity due to poor gastrointestinal and dermal absorption.
- Methemoglobinemia may occur if nitrates convert to nitrites in the intestine or colon, but this occurs rarely in dogs, cats, and other monogastric animals.
- Industrial fertilizers containing anhydrous ammonia have the potential to cause corrosive injury.
- The mechanism of action of toxicity with Milorganite fertilizer is unknown.
- Some fertilizers may also contain other additives such as fungicides, insecticides, and herbicides, which may produce an additive, synergistic, or even antagonist toxic effect.

Blackwell's Five-Minute Veterinary Consult Clinical Companion: Small Animal Toxicology, Second Edition.
Lynn R. Hovda, Ahna G. Brutlag, Robert H. Poppenga, and Katherine L. Peterson.

Companion website: www.fiveminutevet.com/toxicology

Pharmacokinetics – Absorption, Distribution, Metabolism, Excretion

- Fertilizers generally have poor gastrointestinal and dermal absorption.
- Metabolism is minimal except as indicated above for nitrates.

Toxicity

- Ingestion of appropriately diluted or ready-to-use fertilizers that have been applied according to labeled directions rarely results in toxicity beyond mild gastrointestinal irritation.
- Toxicity from ingestion of fertilizer is rare due to low concentrations of nitrogen, phosphorus, and potassium, combined with poor GIT absorption.
- Other ingredients (such as iron, herbicides, pesticides, and fungicides) may be added to fertilizers, increasing the risk of toxicity (see appropriate chapters for more information).
- Fertilizers containing iron in concentrations of ≥5% may result in iron toxicity with sufficient ingestion. Iron exposure of >60 mg/kg elemental iron can result in systemic iron toxicity.
- Stored, concentrated, and industrial products present greater risk of toxicity.
- For fertilizer applications, once applied and dried, there is little concern with ingestion or dermal exposure.

Systems Affected

- Gastrointestinal – vomiting, diarrhea, drooling, anorexia, and abdominal discomfort.
- Musculoskeletal – myalgia and stiffness with Milorganite ingestion.

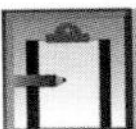

SIGNALMENT/HISTORY

- Any breed of dog and cat may be susceptible to ingestion and GI upset.

Risk Factors

- Outdoor or farm dogs may have more opportunity for exposure and young dogs may be more prone to dietary indiscretion.

Historical Findings

- History of exposure to fertilizer.
- GIT signs with possible fertilizer, soil, or plant material in vomitus or feces.

Location and Circumstances of Poisoning

- Access to garage, shed, or other storage facility containing fertilizer or spilled fertilizer.
- Access to recently fertilized crops, garden, or lawn.

Interactions with Drugs, Nutrients, or Environment

- Fertilizer additives such as fungicides, insecticides, and herbicides may increase risk of toxicity.
- Co-ingestion of toxic plants may increase risk of toxicity.
- Accidental ingestion of fertilizer may be increased with the addition of palatable soil additives like blood meal, bone meal, fish meal, and manure (see chapter 73).

CLINICAL FEATURES

- Clinical signs usually occur within 2–10 hours of ingestion.
- GIT signs including salivation, vomiting, diarrhea, abdominal discomfort, anorexia.
- Muscle pain and stiffness with Milorganite ingestion.
- Corrosive injury can occur with exposure to industrial fertilizers containing anhydrous ammonia.
- GIT symptoms generally resolve within 12–24 hours.

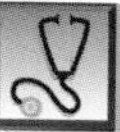

DIFFERENTIAL DIAGNOSIS

- Toxicosis from other GI irritants.
- Gastroenteritis.
- Foreign body obstruction.
- Pancreatitis.
- Inflammatory bowel disease.
- Metabolic disease – liver or renal disease.
- Orthopedic condition with Milorganite toxicity.

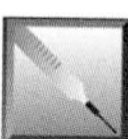

DIAGNOSTICS

- No specific or diagnostic features.
- Evaluation of hydration (based on PCV/TS) and electrolytes should be assessed if GIT signs are present.
- Abdominal radiographs and other advanced diagnostics may need to be performed to rule out other differential diagnoses.

Pathological Findings

- Evidence of fertilizer within the GIT.

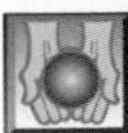

THERAPEUTICS

Detoxification

- Emesis within 2 hours if spontaneous emesis has not occurred and with large-volume ingestions.
  - Do not induce emesis with ingestion of corrosive fertilizers or liquid products containing xylene or toluene solvents.
- Activated charcoal is typically not needed.

Appropriate Health Care

- Antiemetics if vomiting is persistent.
  - Maropitant 1 mg/kg SQ q 24 hours.
  - Ondansetron 0.1–0.5 mg/kg IV q 8–12 hours.
- Fluids – IV or SQ depending on patient's level of dehydration.
- GI protectants as needed.
  - H_2 blockers.
    - Famotidine 0.5–1 mg/kg PO, SQ, IM, IV q 12 hours.
  - Omeprazole 0.5–1 mg/kg PO q 24 hours.
  - Sucralfate 0.25–1 g PO q 8 hours.
- Analgesics as needed for muscle soreness associated with Milorganite ingestions; may want to avoid NSAIDs if GI signs are present.

Antidote

- No antidote.

Precautions/Interactions

- Avoid use of NSAIDs if GI signs are present, especially with ingestion of corrosive fertilizers.

Diet

- Bland diet until GI signs resolve.

COMMENTS

Prevention/Avoidance

- Prevent access to stored, concentrated, and industrial fertilizers.

Expected Course and Prognosis

- Prognosis is good with minimal supportive treatment in most cases. Co-ingestions may cause additional toxicity requiring more aggressive treatment.

See Also

Bone and Blood Meal
Iron

Abbreviations

See Appendix 1 for a complete list.

Suggested Reading

Albretsen JC. Fertilizers. In: Plumlee KH, ed. Clinical Veterinary Toxicology. St Louis, MO: Mosby, 2004; pp. 154–155.

Campbell A, Chapman M. Handbook of Poisoning in Dogs and Cats. Ames, IA: Blackwell Science, 2000; pp. 133–134.

Gerken DF. Lawn care products. In: Bonuagura JD, ed. Kirk's Current Veterinary Therapy XII. Philadelphia, PA: WB Saunders, 1995; pp. 248–249.

Levengood JM, Beasley VR. Principles of ecotoxicology: environmental contaminants. In: Gutpa RC, ed. Veterinary Toxicology: Basics and Clinical Principles. New York: Elsevier, 2007; pp. 693–694.

Yeary RA. Oral intubation of dogs with combinations of fertilizers, herbicide and insecticide chemicals commonly used on lawns. Am J Vet Res 1984; 45:288–290.

Acknowledgment: The authors and editors acknowledge the prior contributions of Josephine L. Marshall, CVT, and Justine A. Lee, DVM, DACVECC, who authored this topic in the previous edition.

Author: Charlotte Flint, DVM
Consulting Editor: Katherine L. Peterson, DVM, DACVECC

chapter 76

Herbicides

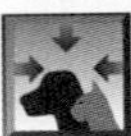

DEFINITION/OVERVIEW

- Herbicides are pesticides containing chemicals used to manipulate or control undesirable vegetation and are regulated by the Environmental Protection Agency (EPA) in the US.
  - Herbicide labels indicate the extent of toxicity by signal words (high-danger or poison; moderate-warning; low-caution).
- Products for home use have a low level of toxicity in animals.
- Chemicals frequently used in urban and suburban locations include:
  - phenoxy acid herbicides and their derivatives (2,4-D, MCPA, MCPP)
  - benzoic acids (dicamba)
  - dinitroanilines (trifluralin, pendimethalin, prodiamine)
  - phosphonomethyl amino acids (glyphosate, glufosinate)
  - older herbicides (arsenicals, dinitrophenols, chlorates) and paraquat are generally more toxic to animals than modern lawn and garden herbicides. See appropriate chapters for more information.
- Common signs include dermal or ocular irritation, vomiting, and diarrhea. Signs are typically self-limiting and require minimal symptomatic and supportive care.
- This chapter will cover the phenoxy acid herbicides (2,4-D, MCPA, and MCPP).

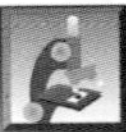

ETIOLOGY/PATHOPHYSIOLOGY

Mechanism of Action

- Depress ribonuclease synthesis, uncouple oxidative phosphorylation, and increase hepatic peroxisomes.
- In dogs, phenoxy acid herbicides affect muscle membranes and cause myotonia. The reported potential mechanism is increased paranitrophenyl phosphatase with increased potassium and compensatory chloride conductance at muscle membranes.
- Prolonged exposure is associated with mild-to-moderate reversible renal damage.

Blackwell's Five-Minute Veterinary Consult Clinical Companion: Small Animal Toxicology, Second Edition.
Lynn R. Hovda, Ahna G. Brutlag, Robert H. Poppenga, and Katherine L. Peterson.

Companion website: www.fiveminutevet.com/toxicology

Pharmacokinetics – Absorption, Distribution, Metabolism, Excretion

- 2,4-D is absorbed almost completely from GIT, skin, and lungs.
- Peak concentrations appear within 6 hours in blood, liver, kidney, lungs, and spleen.
- At high dosages, serum and kidney 2,4-D concentrations are approximately equal.
- Renal excretion is rapid with >80% excreted 2,4-D unchanged in the urine and a half-life of 10–20 hours.
- MCPA and MCPP kinetics are believed to be similar to 2,4-D but are less well described.

Toxicity

See table 76.1.1 for calculation and comparison of risk to small animals from grass treated with herbicides.

- Acute ingestion of 2,4-D has an LD_{50} in dogs of 100 mg/kg but dogs have survived ingestion up to 200 mg/kg.
  - Electromyograph changes occur at ≥8.8 mg/kg; vomiting and myotonia can occur at higher doses.
  - Dogs exposed to four times the recommended application on turfgrass for 7 days displayed no clinical signs or blood work abnormalities.
  - Chronic oral dosing may produce more significant clinical signs.
- MCPA canine no-effect dosage is 1 mg/kg. Dosages ≥20 mg/kg for 4 weeks caused only dry haircoat and mild changes in liver and kidney function.
- MCPP canine oral dosage of ≤16 mg/kg caused no effect; 64 mg/kg BW for 13 weeks caused decreased weight gains and anemia.

TABLE 76.1. Calculation and comparison of risk to small animals from grass treated with example herbicides.

Herbicide	Typical grass concentration (ppm)	Canine no-effect dietary concentration (ppm)	Ratio of dietary no-effect concentration to grass concentration (column 3 divided by column 2)
2,4-D	150	500	3.3
Dicamba	15–40	50	1.25–3.3
MCPA, MCPP	300–450	160	0.53–0.36*
Paraquat	75–150	34	0.45–0.23
Pendimethalin	80–120	500	6.25–4.2

*Ratio <1.0 suggests high risk. MCPA or MCPP and paraquat are available above the "no effect" concentration.

Systems Affected

- Gastrointestinal – nausea, vomiting, diarrhea, hematochezia.
- Musculoskeletal – reluctance to move, muscle rigidity, ataxia, and posterior weakness.
- Neurological – muscle tremors, opisthotonus, seizures (rare).
- Ophthalmic – irritation, conjunctivitis.

- Renal – azotemia, tubular degeneration.
- Skin/exocrine – irritation, erythema.

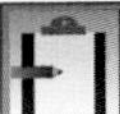

SIGNALMENT/HISTORY

- No breed, age, or sex predilections for this intoxication.

Risk Factors

- Pets on farms or those exposed to concentrates are at higher risk for toxicity.

Historical Findings

- Recent mixing, spraying, or other use of products; chemicals on property.
- History of pet gaining access to sprayed or treated areas, including nearby properties.
- Owner may report vomiting, diarrhea, depression.

Location and Circumstances of Poisoning

- Often reported after lawn treatment, especially with commercial applicator or concentrated use.
- Most incidents occur in the growing season, or during spring or fall treatments of lawns or gardens.

Interactions with Drugs, Nutrients, or Environment

- May affect other chemicals metabolized by hepatic mixed function oxidases.

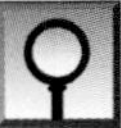

CLINICAL FEATURES

- Clinical signs likely to occur within a few hours of exposure.
- Vomiting, nausea, diarrhea, melena may be noted.
- Depression, muscle rigidity, posterior weakness, and ataxia at higher exposures; rarely progresses to seizures.
- Skin or eye irritation with dermal and ocular exposures.

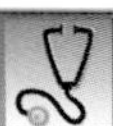

DIFFERENTIAL DIAGNOSIS

- Gastrointestinal – irritant or corrosive toxins, primary GI disease, metabolic disease.
- Muscular signs – nicotine, caffeine ingestion, macadamia nut toxicity, primary neuropathy, or myelopathy.

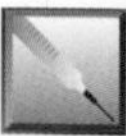

DIAGNOSTICS

- CBC, serum chemistry, and UA should be performed to rule out other causes.
- Serum chemistry – increased ALP, LDH, and CK.
- Serum/tissue assay – 2,4-D or other phenoxy herbicides in serum or renal tissue at 100–700 ppm confirm recent exposure to potentially toxic dosage.
- Electromyographic – increased insertional activity (harmonic change when electrode is inserted) at dosages lower than clinical toxicosis (rarely performed).

Pathological Findings

- Gastritis, oral ulceration, renal congestion, tubular necrosis, friable liver, hyperemia of lymph nodes.

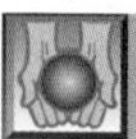

THERAPEUTICS

Therapy is typically minimal and is directed at decontamination and supportive care.

Detoxification

- For dermal exposure, bathe with warm water and a mild soap. Personnel should consider wearing personal protective equipment.
- For ocular exposure, flush eyes with isotonic saline or water for 10–15 minutes.
- With large oral exposures, consider emesis in asymptomatic animals with recent (<2 hours) ingestion, as long as there are no contraindications.
- Administer one dose of activated charcoal with a cathartic (1–2 g/kg BW) within 2 hours of ingestion, if exposure is significant.

Appropriate Health Care

- Supportive care as indicated if clinical signs are present.
- Fluids (oral, SQ, or IV) to maintain hydration.

Drugs and Antidotes of Choice

- No antidotes for herbicide exposure.
- Maropitant 1 mg/kg SQ q 24 hours as needed for persistent vomiting.

Precautions/Interactions

- Avoid acidification of urine, which will retard excretion of acidic agents such as phenoxy herbicides.

Diet

- Bland diet can be considered in pets with GI signs.

Activity

- Limit physical exertion for 2–3 days post recovery in symptomatic animals.

Precautions/Interactions

- Other ingredients, including fertilizers, insecticides, solvents or adjuvants added to improve herbicide performance may compound toxicity.

COMMENTS

Patient Monitoring

- In significantly symptomatic animals, kidney and liver values should be monitored q 24 hours until normal.

Prevention/Avoidance

- Keep pets off treated lawns and gardens for 24–48 hours or until product is dry.

Possible Complications

- Limited reports suggest association of phenoxy herbicides with lymphoma and urinary bladder transitional cell carcinoma in Scottish terriers. Subsequent studies have not confirmed early reports.

Expected Course and Prognosis

- The majority of exposures cause mild self-limiting GI signs that resolve with supportive care within 24 hours.
- Prognosis is generally good.

See Also

Fertilizers
Diquat and Paraquat

Abbreviations

See Appendix 1 for a complete list.

2,4-D = 2,4 dichlorophenoxyacetic acid
MCPA = 2-methyl-4-chlorophenoxyacetic acid
MCPP = 2-(4 chloro-methylphenoxy) propionic acid

Suggested Reading

Arnold EK, Lovell RA, Beasley VR, et al. 2,4-D toxicosis. III: an attempt to produce 2,4-D toxicosis in dogs on treated grass plots. Vet Hum Toxicol 1991; 33(5):457–461.

Beasley VR, Arnold EK, Lovell RA, et al. 2,4-D toxicosis. I: a pilot study of 2,4-dichlorphenoxyacetic acid and dicamba-induced myotonia in experimental dogs. Vet Hum Toxicol 1991; 33(5):435–440.

Gupta PK. Toxicity of herbicides. In: Gupta RC, ed. Veterinary Toxicology: Basic and Clinical Principles. New York: Elsevier, 2007; pp. 567–586.

Talcott PA. Miscellaneous herbicides, fungicides, and nematocides. In: PetersonME, TalcottPA, eds. Small Animal Toxicology, 3rd edn. St Louis, MO: Saunders, 2013; pp. 401–408.

Author: Sharon Welch, DVM, DABVT, DABT
Consulting Editor: Katherine L. Peterson, DVM, DACVECC

chapter 77

Methionine

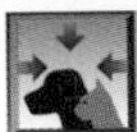

DEFINITION/OVERVIEW

- Methionine is an essential amino acid/nutrient, a urine acidifier, and treats fatty liver in choline deficiency.
- It is used in veterinary medicine for urine acidification, reduction of urine odor and is available OTC to decrease dog urine damage to lawns.
  - Therapeutic dose dogs 100 mg/kg PO q 12 hours.
  - Therapeutic dose cats 1000– 1500 mg/cat per day.
- May also be present in human dietary supplements.
- Clinical signs of toxicosis in dogs include gastrointestinal upset, neurological signs, and metabolic acidosis.
- Clinical signs of toxicosis in cats include gastrointestinal upset, methemoglobinemia, and Heinz body anemia.

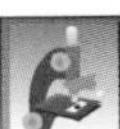

ETIOLOGY/PATHOPHYSIOLOGY

Mechanism of Action

- Unknown mechanism of action.
- Methionine overdose may cause the production of toxic mercaptans, including homocysteine, which have been demonstrated to act synergistically with ammonia to produce signs of hepatic encephalopathy.
- After methionine is metabolized, sulfate is excreted in the urine as sulfuric acid.
- Metabolites lead to the development of oxidative injury and subsequent development of Heinz body anemia and methemoglobinemia, especially in cats.

Pharmacokinetics – Absorption, Distribution, Metabolism, Excretion

- Pharmacokinetic data is limited in veterinary species.
- Methionine is absorbed from the intestinal tract.

Blackwell's Five-Minute Veterinary Consult Clinical Companion: Small Animal Toxicology, Second Edition.
Lynn R. Hovda, Ahna G. Brutlag, Robert H. Poppenga, and Katherine L. Peterson.

Companion website: www.fiveminutevet.com/toxicology

- Metabolism occurs in the liver and can follow two metabolic pathways.
  - Transsulfuration appears to be the primary route.
  - With high levels/toxicity, increased transamination occurs, leading to the production of mercaptans.

Toxicity

- Dogs.
  - Previously healthy dogs have experienced toxicity at doses greater than 25 g/dog.
  - Doses less than 200 mg/kg have been reported to cause mild, self-limiting gastrointestinal upset.
  - Doses greater than 400 mg/kg may results in signs of hepatic encephalopathy, especially in patients with underlying conditions (e.g., liver disease, kidney disease, pancreatitis).
- Cats.
  - Doses >0.5 g/kg/day or 0.75 g/cat have resulted in methemoglobinemia, increased Heinz body formation, cyanosis and hemolysis, especially in kittens.

Systems Affected

- Dogs.
  - Gastrointestinal – vomiting, salivation, diarrhea.
  - Renal/urological – aciduria.
  - Neurological – postural abnormalities/ataxia, hindlimb weakness, CNS depression/coma, seizures.
- Cats.
  - Gastrointestinal – anorexia, vomiting, diarrhea.
  - Hematological – methemoglobinemia, Heinz body anemia.
  - Neurological – ataxia.
  - Respiratory – cyanosis, tachypnea.

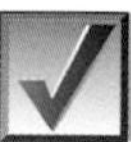

SIGNALMENT/HISTORY

- All species and breeds are affected.
- Dogs will more commonly ingest larger amounts of supplements.
- Kittens have been noted to be particularly sensitive and may develop signs at low doses.

Risk Factors

- Animals with documented liver disease, kidney disease, or pancreatitis may be more predisposed to toxicosis.

Historical Findings

- Recent exposure or administration.
- Owners may report vomiting with large exposures.

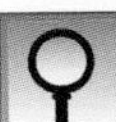

CLINICAL FEATURES

- Dogs.
  - Onset of signs typically develop within 3–4 hours of ingestion.
  - Gastrointestinal signs include drooling, vomiting, and abdominal pain.
  - Neurological signs include ataxia, posterior paresis, anxiety, hyperactivity, restlessness, panting, seizures.
- Cats.
  - Vomiting, anorexia, and ataxia.
  - Signs of hemolytic anemia secondary to Heinz body formation have been noted within days of administration: pale mucous membranes, tachycardia, tachypnea, weakness, lethargy.
  - Signs of methemoglobinemia may also be noted: muddy mucous membranes, cyanosis, tachypnea.

DIFFERENTIAL DIAGNOSES

- Heinz body anemia – onions/garlic, acetaminophen, zinc, naphthalene.
- Neurological disease – inflammatory, infectious, trauma, degenerative, structural disease, other neurological toxins.
- Metabolic disease – renal disease, liver disease, other causes of acidosis such as lactic acidosis, diabetic ketoacidosis, ethylene glycol toxicity, aspirin toxicity.
- Gastrointestinal disease – dietary indiscretion, gastroenteritis, pancreatitis, FBO.

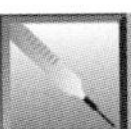

DIAGNOSTICS

- Complete blood count – Heinz body formation, regenerative anemia.
- Chemistry profile – increased liver enzymes, findings consistent with hepatic insufficiency.
- Serum ammonia – normal to elevated.
- Venous blood gas analysis – metabolic acidosis.
- Urinalysis – aciduria.

Pathological Findings

- Splenomegaly, splenic hemosiderosis.
- Erythrophagocytosis.

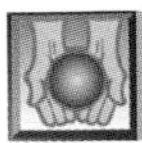

THERAPEUTICS

Detoxification

- Induction of emesis within 1–2 hours in asymptomatic patients.
- Administration of one dose of activated charcoal with a cathartic.

Appropriate Health Care

- Intravenous fluids for maintenance of hydration and perfusion.
- For severe metabolic acidosis (pH <7 or HCO_3 <10 mEq/L), consider sodium bicarbonate administration.
    - mEq bicarbonate = body weight (kg) × base deficit (mEq/L) × 0.3; administer 25% of this dose in intravenous fluids over 30 minutes and give the remainder over 4–6 hours.
    - Ensure appropriate patient ventilation prior to administration.

Antidote

- No specific antidote.

Drugs of choice

- Antiemetics as needed for vomiting.
    - Maropitant 1 mg/kg SQ q 24 hours.
    - Ondansetron 0.1–0.5 mg/kg IV slowly q 6–12 hours.
    - Metoclopramide 0.2–0.5 mg/kg IV, IM, or PO q 6–8 hours.
- GI protectants as needed.
    - Famotidine 0.5–1.0 mg/kg PO, IV, SQ or IM q 12 hours.
    - Pantoprazole 0.5–1 mg/kg IV q 24 hours.
- Seizure control as needed.
    - Diazepam 0.5 mg/kg IV.
    - Midazolam 0.1–0.25 mg/kg IV or IM.
    - Phenobarbital 10–20 mg/kg IV to effect.
- Control of agitation.
    - Acepromazine 0.02–0.1 mg/kg IM, IV or SQ PRN.
    - Trazodone 2–5 mg/kg PO for dogs PRN.
- Hematological support.
    - Patients with signs of severe cardiovascular collapse and anemia may require blood transfusions.
    - Oxygen therapy may be needed in severely affected patients.

Diet

- Discontinue supplementation.
- Bland diet until resolution of gastrointestinal upset.
- Protein-restricted diet in patients with evidence of hepatic insufficiency.

COMMENTS

Patient Monitoring

- Severely affected patients may need monitoring of BP, ECG, respiratory rate, and effort.
- Monitor complete blood count and chemistry profile q 24 hours for resolution of abnormalities.

Prevention/Avoidance

- Client education regarding the potential palatability of methionine supplements and preventing access of pets to methionine supplements.

Possible Complications

- No long-term complications are anticipated.

Expected Course and Prognosis

- Prognosis is good for most exposures, with full recovery within 24–48 hours.
- Dogs with preexisting conditions may have more severe clinical signs and a slower recovery.

Abbreviations

See Appendix 1 for a complete list.

Suggested Reading

Branam JE. Suspected methionine toxicosis associated with a portocaval shunt in a dog. J Am Vet Med Assoc 1982; 181:929–931.

Maede Y, Hoshino T, Inaba M, et al. Methionine toxicosis in cats. Am J Vet Res 1987; 48:289–292.

Plumb DC. Plumb's Veterinary Drug Handbook, 8th edn. Ames, IA: Wiley-Blackwell, 2015.

Villar D, Carson T, Osweiler G, et al. Overingestion of methionine tablets by a dog. Vet Hum Toxicol 2003; 45:311–312.

Acknowledgment: The authors and editors acknowledge the prior contributions of Katherine L. Peterson, DVM, DACVECC, who authored this topic in the previous edition.

Author: Rebecca A. L. Walton, DVM

Consulting Editor: Katherine L. Peterson, DVM, DACVECC

Herbals

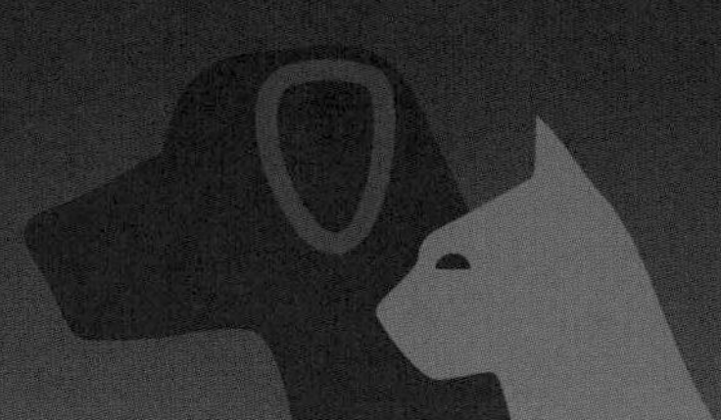

chapter 78

Ephedra/Ma Huang

DEFINITION/OVERVIEW

- *Ephedra sinica*, common name ma huang, is an herbal sympathomimetic used primarily as a weight loss aid, decongestant, and recreational drug known as herbal ecstasy.
- Overdoses cause hyperactivity, tachycardia, hypertension, tremors, seizures, hallucinations, and serotonin syndrome.
- The FDA banned dietary supplements containing ephedra from the market in 2004. Ephedra may still be obtained through various channels, including internet sales. Veterinarians should be aware that most products containing ephedra will not be manufactured with quality controls, standardization, or regard for purity and dosage. Some products will contain ingredients not listed on the label.

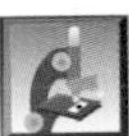

ETIOLOGY/PATHOPHYSIOLOGY

Mechanism of Action

- Ma huang contains ephedrine and pseudoephedrine. These alkaloids are structurally similar to amphetamines.
- Ma huang stimulates alpha- and beta-adrenergic receptors and releases endogenous catecholamines at synapses in the brain and heart. This results in peripheral vasoconstriction and cardiac stimulation.
- The clinical effects are increased blood pressure, tachycardia, mydriasis, ataxia, and restlessness. Central nervous system effects include tremors, seizures, agitation, and serotonin syndrome.
- Serotonin syndrome is the overstimulation of serotonin receptors in the nervous system, gastrointestinal tract, cardiovascular, and respiratory system. Clinical signs associated with serotonin syndrome seen in ma huang toxicity include tremors and seizures, hyperesthesia, hyperthermia, hypersalivation, and death.

Blackwell's Five-Minute Veterinary Consult Clinical Companion: Small Animal Toxicology, Second Edition.
Lynn R. Hovda, Ahna G. Brutlag, Robert H. Poppenga, and Katherine L. Peterson.

Companion website: www.fiveminutevet.com/toxicology

Pharmacokinetics – Absorption, Distribution, Metabolism, Excretion

- Ma huang is absorbed orally.
- It is metabolized in the liver and excreted in the urine.
- Ma huang excretion is enhanced if the urine is acidified.

Toxicity

- Clinical signs may be seen at 5–6 mg/kg.
- Death has been seen at 10–12 mg/kg.

Systems Affected

- Nervous – hyperactivity, hallucinations, tremors, seizures, head bobbing, serotonin syndrome.
- Cardiovascular – tachycardia, hypertension.
- Metabolic – hyperthermia.
- Musculoskeletal – rhabdomyolysis (sequela to prolonged seizure activity and hyperthermia).
- Hemic – DIC (sequela to prolonged seizure activity and hyperthermia).
- Renal – myoglobinuria.

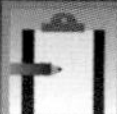

SIGNALMENT/HISTORY

- Dogs are the most common species to be affected by ma huang, although any species may develop toxicity if a sufficient dose is ingested.
- Younger dogs may be more likely to "counter-surf" or get into purses and thus have exposure to a supplement.
- Diagnosis is based on history and clinical signs.

Risk Factors

- Animals with preexisting cardiovascular disease (including hypertension) or seizure disorders may develop more severe clinical signs.

Historical Findings

- Witnessed ingestion.
- Access to herbal decongestants, diet products, and/or recreational drugs.
- Owners frequently report restlessness, pacing, vocalizing, hyperactivity, panting, apparent hallucinations, head bobbing, and tremors or seizures.

Location and Circumstances of Poisoning

- Most animals will ingest supplements in a home or car.

Interactions with Drugs, Nutrients, or Environment

- If ingested with other sympathomimetic agents (pseudoephedrine, phenylpropanolamine), methylxanthines (chocolate or caffeine), MAO inhibitors (seligiline), or tricyclic antidepressants, toxicity may be enhanced.

CLINICAL FEATURES

- Clinical signs can develop within 30 minutes to 8 hours post exposure.
- The duration of clinical signs is 24–72 hours.
- The most common signs are mydriasis, hyperactivity, panting, hyperthermia, nervousness, and tachycardia, followed by collapse.
- Hypertension, muscle tremors, and/or seizures may be noted on exam.
- Head bobbing has been associated with increased mortality.
- Death is usually due to cardiovascular collapse.

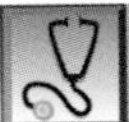

DIFFERENTIAL DIAGNOSIS

- Clinical signs are similar to the ingestion of pseudoephedrine found in cold and sinus medications, as well as amphetamine ingestion (attention deficit disorder drugs such as methylphenidate and dextroamphetamine) and illicit substances.

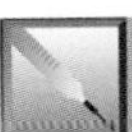

DIAGNOSTICS

- Clinical pathology – hyperglycemia and hypokalemia may be noted.
- OTC drug tests will test positive for amphetamines if ma huang is ingested. Most OTC tests require urine.

Pathological Findings

- No specific gross or histopathological findings have been reported.

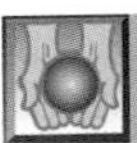

THERAPEUTICS

- The treatment plan goals are to prevent further absorption, stabilize the cardiovascular system, control CNS signs, and provide supportive care.

Detoxification

- Induce emesis only in asymptomatic animals within 1 hour of ingestion.
- Activated charcoal may be given within 4 hours of ingestion in an asymptomatic animal.

Appropriate Health Care

- IV fluids as needed for supportive care in symptomatic animals.

Drugs and Antidotes of Choice

- Acepromazine, 0.05–1.0 mg/kg IM or IV, to control restlessness and agitation. Start at low end of range and increase as needed.
- Propranolol, 0.02–0.06 mg/kg, slow IV to effect, for tachycardia. Propranolol also is a serotonin antagonist and may help reduce some clinical signs associated with serotonin syndrome.
- Cyproheptadine, 1.1 mg/kg q 6–12 hours for dogs, 2–4 mg/cat q 6–12 hours, for serotonin syndrome. Cyproheptadine is a specific serotonin antagonist. Cyproheptadine should only be given if appropriate clinical signs of serotonin syndrome are present.

Precautions/Interactions

- Diazepam can potentially cause increased CNS excitation resulting in crying, head bobbing, and death.

Alternative Drugs

- If propranolol is unavailable, or if an animal is hypertensive and tachycardic, a specific $beta_1$ antagonist may be preferred.
    - Esmolol 0.05–0.1 mg/kg IV boluses up to 0.5 mg/kg, or an infusion of 50–200 µg (0.05–0.2 mg)/kg/min in dogs. A loading dose of 200–500 µg/kg IV over 1 minute followed by a CRI of 10–200 µg/kg/min can be used in cats.
    - Atenolol 0.2–1 mg/kg PO q 12–24 hours for dogs, 2 mg/kg or 6.25–12.5 mg PO q 24 hours for cats.
    - Metoprolol 0.2 mg/kg PO q 12 hours for dogs, 2–15 mg PO q 8 hours for cats.
- If acid–base status can be monitored, administer ammonium chloride, 200 mg/kg/day, divided 4 times daily orally, or ascorbic acid/vitamin C, 20–30 mg/kg IM or IV q 8 hours, to acidify the urine.

Nursing Care

- Thermoregulation.
- Minimize sensory stimulation.

Follow-up

- Animal should be monitored until clinical signs resolve, generally in 1–3 days.

COMMENTS

Client Education

- Make sure the environment is safe for the pet before releasing to go home. Owners should check crates, blankets, under beds, etc. to make sure all pills or capsules have been removed.

Patient Monitoring

- Hydration.
- Electrolytes.
- Heart rate.
- Blood pressure.
- Heart rhythm (ECG).
- Body temperature
- Frequency of monitoring will vary with severity of clinical syndrome.

Prevention/Avoidance

- Owners should be educated about keeping medications out of reach of pets.
- Discuss "counter-surfing," keeping purses, briefcases, etc. out of pet's reach. Discuss use of training aids like scat mats for pets constantly getting items off counters.

Possible Complications

- DIC, rhabdomyolysis, and myoglobinuria (with subsequent renal failure) are possible if prolonged, untreated tremors/seizures or hyperthermia present.

Expected Course and Prognosis

- Clinical signs generally resolve within 24–72 hours.
- Prognosis is generally good.
- If head bobbing, myoglobinuria, or DIC present, prognosis is poor.

Synonyms

- Ma huang is also known as yellow horse or sea grape.
- There are several *Ephedra* species, but *Ephedra sinica* is the plant used in manufacturing of supplements.
- *Sida cordifolia*, also known as Indian common mallow, is another plant containing pseudoephedrine and ephedrine alkaloids sometimes used in herbal supplements.

See Also

Amphetamines
Decongestants (Pseudoephedrine, Phenylephrine)
Methamphetamine

Abbreviations

See Appendix 1 for a complete list.

CRI = constant rate infusion
DIC = disseminated intravascular coagulation
MAO = monamine oxidase
OTC = over the counter

Suggested Reading

DerMarderosian A, Beutler JA. The Review of Natural Products, 3rd edn. St Louis, MO: Facts and Comparisons, 2002; pp. 265–266.

Fugh-Berman A. The 5-minute Herb and Dietary Supplement Consult. Philadelphia, PA: Lippincott Williams & Wilkins, 2003; pp. 116–117.

Means C. Selected herbal toxicities. Vet Clin North Am Small Anim Pract 2002; 32:367–382.

Ooms TG, Khan SA, Means C. Suspected caffeine and ephedrine toxicosis resulting from ingestion of an herbal supplement containing guarana and ma huang in dogs: 47 cases (1997–1999). J Am Ved Med Assoc 2001; 218:225–229.

Author: Charlotte Means, DVM, MLIS, ABVT, ABT
Contributing Editor: Ahna G. Brutlag, DVM, MS, DABT, DABVT

Essential Oils/ Liquid Potpourri

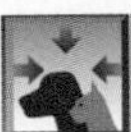

DEFINITION/OVERVIEW

- Essential oils are the volatile, organic components of plants that contribute to plant fragrance and taste. They are extracted from plants generally via distillation or, more rarely, via cold pressing.
- Essential oils are utilized in a variety of ways: insecticides, aromatherapies, personal care products (e.g., antibacterials), flavorings, herbal remedies, and liquid potpourri.
- A number of essential oils are not recommended for use on animals due to their potential for intoxication (e.g., pennyroyal oil, bitter almond, wormwood, concentrated melaleuca/tea tree oil – see chapter 80).

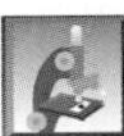

ETIOLOGY/PATHOPHYSIOLOGY

Mechanism of Action

- There is limited data with regard to specific pathophysiological mechanisms for many essential oils.

Pharmacokinetics – Absorption, Distribution, Metabolism, Excretion

- Essential oils are lipophilic and are well absorbed through mucous membranes and the skin.
- Specific pharmacokinetic data for cats or dogs is generally lacking and mostly derived from laboratory animal and human studies.
- Because of differences in detoxification pathways, some essential oil constituents are more toxic to cats than dogs (e.g., oil of wintergreen 98% methylsalicylate when hydrolyzed, and essential oils with terpene metabolites undergo glucuronidation prior to elimination).
- Pulegone, the main constituent in pennyroyal oil, is bioactivated to a hepatotoxic metabolite called menthofuran.

Blackwell's Five-Minute Veterinary Consult Clinical Companion: Small Animal Toxicology, Second Edition.
Lynn R. Hovda, Ahna G. Brutlag, Robert H. Poppenga, and Katherine L. Peterson.

Companion website: www.fiveminutevet.com/toxicology

Toxicity

- Toxicity varies considerably (reported LD_{50}s range from 0.4 g/kg for pennyroyal oil to 1.90 g/kg for melaleuca/tea tree oil).
- Toxicity data specific to cats and dogs is limited; most data are derived from laboratory animal studies.
- Liquid potpourri also contains cationic surfactants, which can cause some of the reported clinical signs. Small ingestions (2–3 licks) and dermal exposures may result in corrosive injury. See Chapter 88 for more information.

Systems Affected

- Affected systems vary depending on the specific essential oil.
  - Pennyroyal oil – hepatobiliary.
  - Clove oil – hepatobiliary.
  - Citrus oil/d-limonene – gastrointestinal, musculoskeletal, nervous.
  - Peppermint oil – gastrointestinal, nervous.
  - Cinnamon oil – gastrointestinal.
  - Oil of wintergreen – gastrointestinal, hemic, hepatobiliary, respiratory.
- Many essential oils and cationic surfactants in liquid potpourri are irritating (and potentially corrosive) to the skin and mucous membranes.

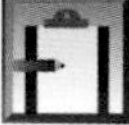

SIGNALMENT/HISTORY

Risk Factors

- Cats are more severely affected by liquid potpourri than dogs.
- Cats are more likely to be exposed to liquid potpourri due to the placement of containers on countertops or tables.
- Cats may develop oral exposures secondary to grooming of dermal exposures.
- Animals with underlying liver disease may be more severely affected.

Historical Findings

- History of use on or in animals (especially for external parasite control).
- Access to essential oils or products containing essential oils (e.g., liquid potpourri).
- Discovery of spilled essential oils or disturbed liquid potpourri simmer pots.
- Characteristic smell on haircoat, skin, breath, or in vomitus.

Location and Circumstances of Poisoning

- Typically occurs in the household (e.g., liquid potpourri simmer pots or spills).
- Following direct application to skin or mucous membranes (e.g., often for external parasite control).

Interaction with Drugs, Nutrients, or Environment

- Limited data is available.
- Essential oils contain high concentrations of terpenes, which are metabolized by the liver. Thus, the co-ingestion of other chemicals undergoing significant hepatic metabolism can potentially cause interactions.

CLINICAL FEATURES

- Clinical features are variable depending on the essential oil.
  - Pennyroyal oil – dog (and presumably other species as well): acute hepatic failure.
  - Citrus oil – cat: hypersalivation, muscle tremors, ataxia, lateral recumbency, coma, death.
  - Liquid potpourri – cat and dog: gastrointestinal, dermal, and mucosal irritation or caustic injury; CNS depression; hyperthermia; ocular exposure can cause mild to severe corneal injury.
- Ingestion of cationic surfactants (occasionally found in potpourri) can cause systemic effects such as emesis, dyspnea secondary to pulmonary edema, hypotension, metabolic acidosis, and CNS depression.

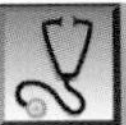

DIFFERENTIAL DIAGNOSIS

- Pennyroyal oil – hepatotoxins such as microcystins, amanitins, aflatoxins, phenolic compounds (cats), acetaminophen, cycads, acute or chronic copper intoxication, xylitol. Also, idiosyncratic drug reactions, leptospirosis, infectious canine hepatitis, toxoplasmosis, rickettsial disease, acute necrotizing pancreatitis.
- Citrus oil – CNS-depressant drug overdose, hypoglycemia, hypotension, ethylene glycol, head trauma, and many etiologies associated with trembling, stupor, or coma.
- Liquid potpourri – many etiologies associated with gastrointestinal upset, other acid or alkaline corrosives, ethylene glycol, paraquat, and digoxin intoxications.

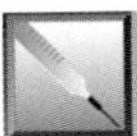

DIAGNOSTICS

- Pennyroyal oil –serum ALT, AST, ALP, CK, total bilirubin, coagulation profile, abdominal imaging, liver needle biopsy.
- Liquid potpourri – endoscopy will assist in determining the degree of damage to upper GI tract if exposure to cationic surfactant-containing potpourri has occurred.
- Citrus oils – no specific diagnostics.

Pathological Findings

- Limited information is available.
    - Pennyroyal oil – severe hepatic necrosis.
    - Other essential oils or liquid potpourri formulations – dermal, ocular, or mucosal irritation or caustic injury.

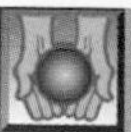

THERAPEUTICS

Detoxification

- Bathe thoroughly if dermal exposure using a mild hand-dishwashing detergent or noninsecticidal pet shampoo.
- Irrigate eyes copiously with tepid tap water, eye wash solution, or physiological saline for 15–20 minutes if ocular exposure occurred.
- Oral exposures.
    - For noncaustic exposures, induction of emesis in asymptomatic patients within 1 hour might be useful followed by administration of activated charcoal. Be alert for CNS depression.
    - For caustic exposures, dilution with milk or water is recommended. Do not induce emesis or give activated charcoal as this may cause vomiting.

Appropriate Health Care

- Treatment is largely symptomatic and supportive (and empirical).
- For severe oral irritation or caustic damage, provide adequate hydration via IV fluids and nutritional support.
- If caustic damage.
    - Buprenorphine 0.005–0.03 mg/kg, IM, IV, SQ or PO (transmucosally) q 6–8 hours.
    - Sucralfate 0.25–1 g, PO q 8 hours as a slurry, for oral, esophageal, gastric, or duodenal ulcers.
    - H_2 blocker such as famotidine 0.5–1 mg/kg IV, IM, SQ or PO.
    - Corticosteroids such as prednisone, 0.5–1 mg/kg IV, for one dose. Note, this is controversial. While one dose may be beneficial, there is limited evidence to support this.
- Antiemetics.
    - Metoclopramide 1–2 mg/kg/day, IV as a CRI for mild or infrequent emesis.
    - Maropitant 1 mg/kg, SQ q 24 hours.
    - Ondansetron 0.1–0.2 mg/kg, IV q 8–12 hours.
- Hepatoprotectants (consider use of one or all).
    - Silymarin (milk thistle).
        - Dose: 20–50 mg/kg PO q 24 hours.
        - Silymarin is composed of three flavonoids (silybin, silydianin, and silychristin).
        - Serious adverse effects have not been observed.

   - N-acetylcysteine, loading dose at 140 mg/kg IV or PO; if using the oral formulation IV, dilute to a 5% solution in saline and administer via 0.2 μm nonpyrogenic filter, followed by 70 mg/kg q 6–12 hours.
   - SAM-e, loading dose at 40 mg/kg PO, followed by 18–20 mg/kg PO q 24 hours.
- Corneal burns should be treated with ophthalmic lubricant ointments and antibiotics such as gentamicin sulfate or tobramycin 4+ times per day.
- Antibiotics if needed (e.g., severe ulceration or hepatic failure).
   - Metoclopramide 1–2 mg/kg/day, IV as a CRI for mild or infrequent emesis.
- Fresh whole blood or fresh frozen plasma if needed for coagulopathies.

Drugs and Antidotes of Choice

- No antidotes are available for any essential oil or cationic surfactants-containing liquid potpourri. See Appropriate Health Care.

Precautions/Interactions

- If significant liver damage is present, use drugs metabolized by the liver cautiously.

Nursing Care

- IV fluids to maintain hydration and tissue perfusion.
- Maintain body temperature as needed.
- Provide pain control (e.g., buprenorphine, fentanyl as needed) if caustic damage.

Follow-Up

- If hepatic damage, monitor liver function every 2–3 days until improvement.

Diet

- Feed a soft or easily digestible diet if there is GI irritation or caustic damage.

Surgical Considerations

- For severe oral irritation or caustic damage, a feeding tube might be necessary to provide adequate nutrition.
- For severe ocular exposure and corneal damage, conjunctival flaps might be warranted.

COMMENTS

Patient Monitoring

- Pennyroyal oil – monitoring of hepatic function.
- Caustic damage due to cationic surfactant exposure – follow-up endoscopy to assess healing or residual damage (strictures due to scar tissue).

Possible Complications

- Pennyroyal oil – hypoglycemia, DIC, hepatic encephalopathy, chronic hepatic insufficiency.
- Liquid potpourri – scarring and stricture formation if significant caustic damage to upper GI tract.

Prevention/Avoidance

- Owner should be educated about the risks associated with specific essential oils or use of liquid potpourri.

Expected Course and Prognosis

- Variable depending on specific exposure.
    - Pennyroyal oil – guarded to poor.
    - Liquid potpourri – good.
    - Others – good to guarded.

See Also

Phenols and Pine Oils
Soaps, Detergents, Fabric Softeners, Enzymatic Cleaners, and Deodorizers
Tea Tree Oil/Melaleuca Oil

Abbreviations

See Appendix 1 for a complete list.

DIC = disseminated intravascular coagulation
LD = lethal dose

Suggested Reading

Genovese AG, McLean MK, Khan SA. Adverse reactions from essential oil-containing natural flea products exempted from Environmental Protection Agency regulations in dogs and cats. J Vet Emerg Crit Care 2012; 22(4):470–475.

Hooser SB, Beasley VR, Everitt JI. Effects of an insecticidal dip containing D-limonene in the cat. J Am Vet Med Assoc 1986; 189:905–908.

Schildt JC, Jutkowitz LA, Beal MW. Potpourri oil toxicity in cats: 6 cases (2000–2007). J Vet Emerg Crit Care 2008; 18(5):511–516.

Sudekum M, Poppenga RH, Raju N, et al. Pennyroyal oil toxicosis in a dog. J Am Vet Med Assoc 1992; 200:817–818.
Woolf A. Essential oil poisoning. Clin Toxicol 1999; 37(6):721–727.

Acknowledgment: The authors and editors acknowledge the prior contributions of Robert H. Poppenga, DVM, PhD, DABVT, who authored this topic in the previous edition.
Author: Sarah Alpert, DVM
Consulting Editor: Ahna G. Brutlag, DVM, MS, DABT, DABVT

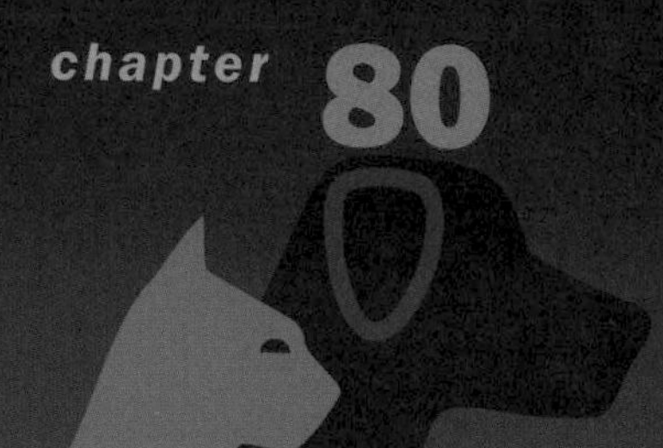

chapter 80

Tea Tree Oil/ Melaleuca Oil

DEFINITION/OVERVIEW

- An essential oil produced from the Australian tea tree, *Melaleuca alternifolia.*
- Tea tree oil is also known as melaleuca oil.
- Known antibacterial and antifungal properties; possible antipruritic and antiinflammatory properties.
- Found in gels and body lotions, shampoos, conditioners, toothpastes, balms, insect repellants, and other household cleaning products, ranging from <1% to 100% oil.
    - Marketed for use on dogs, cats, ferrets, and horses.
- Intoxication commonly results from 100% oil applied as external parasite repellant.
    - As little as seven drops of 100% oil have caused clinical toxicosis.
    - Toxicosis generally produces CNS dysfunction, muscular tremors, and hypothermia. May also result in hepatic injury.

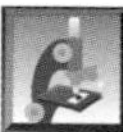

ETIOLOGY/PATHOPHYSIOLOGY

- Toxicosis results from dermal application or oral ingestion.
- Prevalence of intoxication may increase as pet owners' interest in "natural" therapies grows.
- Toxicosis is similar to other essential oils, such as pine oil, eucalyptus, and d-limonene.
- Composed of 50–60% terpenes, 6–8% cineole, and other alcohols.
- Terpinen-4-ol is the main antimicrobial and antifungal agent.
- Cineole produces irritation of mucous membranes and skin.

Mechanism of Action

- Exact mechanism of action is unknown. Presumed similar to turpentine and other essential oil toxicities.

Pharmacokinetics – Absorption, Distribution, Metabolism, Excretion

- Dermal and GI absorption is rapid due to highly lipophilic nature.
- Terpene metabolism is largely hepatic.

Blackwell's Five-Minute Veterinary Consult Clinical Companion: Small Animal Toxicology, Second Edition.
Lynn R. Hovda, Ahna G. Brutlag, Robert H. Poppenga, and Katherine L. Peterson.

Companion website: www.fiveminutevet.com/toxicology

- Phase I and phase II biotranformation via cytochrome P450 enzymes.
- Conjugated to glycine or glucuronide in the liver.
- Undergoes enterohepatic recirculation.
- Urinary excretion of metabolites takes 2–3 days; small amount via fecal elimination.

Toxicity

- Exact toxic doses are not established.
- Oral LD_{50} (various species) = 1.9–5 g/kg or 1.9–2.6 mL/kg.
- Poisoning is most often seen with direct application of 100% oil. Products with low concentrations (i.e., shampoo, conditioner, toothpaste) are generally not considered toxic.
- Clinical toxicosis with 7–8 drops of 100% oil applied to the skin.
- Applications of approximately 10 mL of 100% oil has resulted in toxicosis in cats and dogs.
- Three cats with dermal flea bite lesions received 20 mL each of concentrated oil and suffered severe toxicosis (3) and death (1).

Systems Affected

- Nervous – target system of toxicity resulting in CNS depression/coma (similar to other terpenes).
- Hepatobiliary – elevated liver enzymes secondary to induction of microsomal P450.
- Skin – possible contact irritation, especially of the mucous membranes.
- Musculoskeletal – unknown MOA; possible direct affect of toxic metabolites.
- Cardiovascular – peripheral vasodilation following all routes of absorption.
- Respiratory – primary or secondary affects due to CNS depression.
- Gastrointestinal – vomiting and/or ptyalism likely from oral irritation, secondary from hepatic effects, shock.

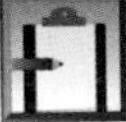

SIGNALMENT/HISTORY

- There are no reported breed, sex, or age predilections.
- Cats may be more sensitive due to metabolism (glucuronidation).

Risk Factors

- Animals with underlying CNS or hepatic disease may exhibit more severe clinical signs or suffer toxicity at lower doses.
- Juveniles and smaller animals may be more sensitive due to poor metabolism and lower body surface area.

Historical Findings

- Well-intentioned but misinformed owners may admit to administering tea tree oil directly to the pet.

- There may be a characteristic and strong odor (minty) associated with the pet.
- Oily/greasy fur on the neck/back from topical application.
- Owners may report CNS depression, unresponsiveness, difficulty or inability to walk, shaking or tremors.
- Witnessed ingestions/discovery of chewed tea tree oil containers.

Location and Circumstances of Poisoning

- Given the heightened interest in "natural remedies," the incidence of misuse may increase.

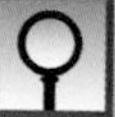

CLINICAL FEATURES

- Onset of clinical signs is 1–2 hours after application (up to 12 hours).
- Signs slowly resolve over 2–4 days. Mild cases may resolve within hours.
- The most common clinical signs are mild-to-moderate hypothermia, weakness, CNS depression, ataxia, and generalized muscle tremors.
- Less common signs include skin/mucous membrane irritation, vomiting, salivation, bradypnea, bradycardia, hypotension secondary to shock or CNS depression, unresponsive pupils, paralysis, and coma.

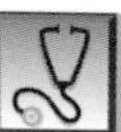

DIFFERENTIAL DIAGNOSIS

- Cardiovascular – shock (sepsis, hypovolemia, hemorrhagic), primary cardiac disease, other toxins (e.g., narcotics, benzodiazepine overdose).
- Neuromuscular – focal or diffuse primary CNS disease (e.g., neoplasia, distemper, other infectious disease), ethylene glycol, hypocalcemia, hepatic or uremic encephalopathy, IVDD, FCE, other neurotoxins.
- Respiratory – primary respiratory disease (e.g., allergic and parasitic airway disease, fungal or bacterial pneumonia), congestive heart failure, pain, sedative/narcotic overdose.
- Integument – drug eruption/reaction, sunburn, thermal burn, vasculitis, contact dermatitis, pyoderma, insect/arthropod bite, parasitic, other primary skin disease may be suspected based upon location of lesion.
- Gastrointestinal – primary gastrointestinal disease (e.g., parasite, foreign body, infectious, inflammatory), other toxin, primary neuropathy, secondary gastrointestinal (neoplasia, pancreatitis, hepatobiliary disease, renal disease, endocrinopathy).

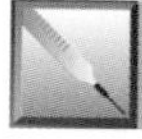

DIAGNOSTICS

- Confirmation of terpinen-4-ol in urine by GC-MS (concentration will decrease with IV fluid therapy, so pretreatment samples should be obtained).
- Chemistry profile— possible increase in AST, ALP, and ALT.

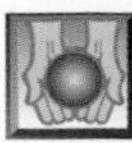

THERAPEUTICS

Detoxification

- Bathe with liquid dishwashing detergent to remove excess oils and reduce dermal absorption.
- Induce emesis only if asymptomatic and the ingestion was within 15–30 minutes. Due to rapid GI absorption, emesis is unlikely to prevent toxicity.
- Repeated doses of activated charcoal (PO q 6–8 hours over 24 hours) due to enterohepatic recirculation.
- If mucous membrane/oral irritation is present, consider flushing the oral cavity.

Appropriate Health Care

- Supportive treatments.
  - IV fluid therapy to maintain hydration and tissue perfusion. The use of colloid therapy for persistent hypotension may be necessary (i.e., Hetastarch). Vasopressors (i.e., dopamine 2–10 mg/kg/min IV CRI) for persistent hypotension.
  - Body temperature regulation and heat support PRN, as hypothermia is common.
  - Atropine, 0.02–0.04 mg/kg IV, IM, or SC as needed, for severe bradycardia.
  - Other supportive measures are largely related to nursing care dependent upon the CNS status of the patient (see Nursing Care).
  - With severe CNS depression, intubation and mechanical ventilation may be needed.

Drugs and Antidotes of Choice

- No antidote available.
- Hepatoprotectants if indicated based on lab results (e.g., SAMe, loading dose 40 mg/kg q 24 hours × 2–4 days, maintenance dose 18–20 mg/kg PO q 24 hours × 2–3 weeks).
- Methocarbamol 25–250 mg/kg, IV, as needed; administer slowly, to effect; may be administered as a constant rate infusion (cats).
- Diazepam 0.5–1 mg/kg, IV or rectally, as needed.
- Maropitant 1 mg/kg, SC q 24 hours, if needed for vomiting or prior to activated charcoal.

Precautions/Interactions

- Do not administer oral medications/activated charcoal to animals with CNS depression unless the airway is protected.

Nursing Care

- Monitor during use of warming therapies to prevent hyperthermia or burns.
- If severe CNS signs:
  - Monitor TPR every 5–15 minutes until stable

- Rotate body position to prevent atelectasis or thermal burns
- Monitor blood pressure closely until stable.

Follow-up

- With mild signs and no liver enzyme elevation, follow-up is generally not necessary (see Patient Monitoring).

Diet

- Typically, no changes are needed.
- With severe CNS depression, withhold feeding until stable.

Activity

- Restricted until neurological signs are minor or resolved.

COMMENTS

- Specific and thorough history and PE are of utmost importance.

Client Education

- Provide appropriate client education on the use of herbal or "natural" remedies.
- Urge clients to consult with veterinarian prior to use of any alternative therapies.
- Appropriate dilutions of tea tree oil can be used, but clients should consult with veterinarian prior to use; the use of 100% oil is never recommended.
- Owners should be aware that concentrated tea tree oil is toxic to humans if ingested. Poisoning has been reported in children and adults.

Patient Monitoring

- Daily renal values should be evaluated while in hospital until normal.
- Hepatic values may not normalize and appropriate short-term monitoring is needed.
    - Recheck liver enzymes q 5–7 days until clinical signs and liver enzymes return to normal.
    - PRN monitoring of vital parameters until stabilized, then 3–4 times daily.

Prevention/Avoidance

- Veterinary consultation prior to administering alternative/home therapies (see Client Education).

Possible Complications

- Severe and unresponsive CNS depression leading to bradycardia, hypoperfusion, and coma.

Expected Course and Prognosis

- Good with appropriate treatment and no underlying health problems.

Synonyms

Tea tree oil is also called melaleuca oil (from *Melaleuca alternifolia*, the tea tree).

See Also

Essential Oils/Liquid Potpourri
Phenols and Pine Oils

Abbreviations

See Appendix 1 for a complete list.

FCE = fibrocartilaginous emboli
GC-MS = gas chromatography-mass spectrometry
IVDD = intervertebral disk disease
SAMe = s-adenosyl-methionine

Suggested Reading

Bischoff K, Fessesswork G. Australian tea tree (Melaleuca alternifolia) oil poisoning in three purebred cats. J Vet Diagn Invest 1998; 10:208–210.

Khan SA, McLean MK, Slater MR. Concentrated tea tree oil toxicosis in dogs and cats: 443 cases (2002–2012). J Am Vet Med Assoc 2014; 244:95–99.

Villar D, Knight M, Hansen S, Buck W. Toxicity of melaleuca oil and related essential oils applied topically on dogs and cats. Vet Hum Toxicol 1994; 36:139–142.

Author: Seth L. Cohen, DVM
Consulting Editor: Ahna G. Brutlag, DVM, MS, DABT, DABVT

Home Care and Recreational Products

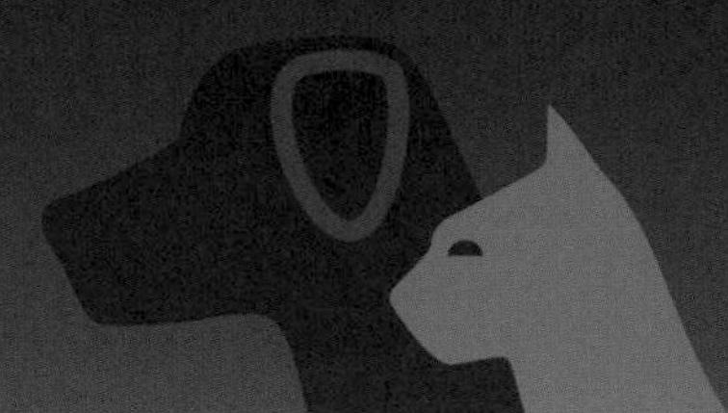

chapter 81

Acids

DEFINITION/OVERVIEW

- Acids have a pH <7, are proton donors, and have a sour taste.
- Tissue injury from acids depends on the pH, specific acid, concentration, volume, and duration of tissue contact time.
- Common household products containing acids:
  - Automobile battery fluid – sulfuric acid (25–30%).
  - Drain cleaners – sulfuric acid (95–99%).
  - Engraver's acid – nitric acid (63%).
  - Hair wave neutralizers – acetic acid (6–40%).
  - Lemon juice – citric acid (2–8%).
  - Metal cleaners and antirust compounds – phosphoric acid (5–90%), oxalic acid (1%), hydrochloric acid (5–25%), sulfamic acid (5–10%), sulfuric acid (10–20%), chromic acid (5–20%).
  - Toilet bowl cleaners – hydrochloric acid (9–25%), oxalic acid (2%), sodium bisulfate forms sulfuric acid upon contact with water (70–100%), sulfuric acid (up to 80%).
  - Vinegar – acetic acid (4–6%).
- Exposure to weak (pH 2–4) or dilute acids may cause mild tissue irritation.
- Exposure to strong (pH <2) or concentrated acids may cause corrosive injury (see Toxicology).
  - Products likely to cause corrosive injury include toilet bowl and drain cleaners, calcium/rust/lime-removing compounds, swimming pool sanitizers, automotive batteries, and gun barrel cleaners.
  - Many US household products containing corrosive agents will display the signal word *Danger* clearly on the packaging.
- Treatment following exposure to acids is focused on the prevention/management of corrosive injury, including analgesia and nutritional support.
- Serious complications include severe corrosive injury followed by systemic infection, stricture formation, GIT perforation, and septic peritonitis.

Blackwell's Five-Minute Veterinary Consult Clinical Companion: Small Animal Toxicology, Second Edition.
Lynn R. Hovda, Ahna G. Brutlag, Robert H. Poppenga, and Katherine L. Peterson.

Companion website: www.fiveminutevet.com/toxicology

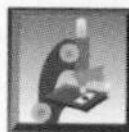

ETIOLOGY/PATHOPHYSIOLOGY

- Exposure in animals generally occurs following accidental ingestion or dermal contact.
- Small ingestions/tastes of corrosive acids are unlikely to result in severe tissue damage.
- Strong acids have a sour taste and typically cause immediate pain upon tissue contact. Thus, large ingestions of strong acids are very rare.

Mechanism of Action

- Acids cause rapid surface protein coagulation (leading to coagulation necrosis) followed by the formation of a thick eschar.
- Theoretically, the eschar may limit tissue penetration and damage.
- Significant tissue damage from corrosive injury may result in stricture formation.

Pharmacokinetics – Absorption, Distribution, Metabolism, Excretion

- Systemic absorption of acids is not typically a concern (except hydrofluoric acid – see chapter 11).
- Rarely, acidemia may result from systemic absorption through injured tissue.
- Ions such as hydrogen, chloride (hydrochloric acid), or sulfate (sulfuric acid), if systemically absorbed, are well distributed and may disrupt normal metabolic function.

Toxicity

- Tissue damage of most acids is directly related to pH and concentration.
    - pH 2–4: agents cause mild-to-moderate tissue irritation.
    - pH <2: agents are extremely corrosive.
- Specific acids:
    - Weak irritants.
        - Acetic acid 5–10%
        - Aluminum sulfate 5–20%
        - Hydrochloric acid <5%
        - Phosphoric acid 15–35%
    - Strong irritants.
        - Acetic acid 10–50%
        - Aluminum sulfate 20%
        - Glycolic acid 0.5–10%
        - Hydrochloric acid 5–10%
        - Oxalic acid <10%
        - Phosphoric acid 35–60%
        - Sulfuric acid <10%
    - Corrosive.
        - Acetic acid >50%

- Aluminum sulfate >20%
- Glycolic acid >10%
- Hydrochloric acid >10%
- Oxalic acid >10%
- Phosphoric acid >60%
- Sulfamic acid >10%
- Sulfuric acid >10%

Systems Affected

- Organs having direct contact with acid (GIT, skin, eyes, and lungs) are most at risk.
- Gastrointestinal – ingestion causes mild tissue irritation to significant ulceration of the oral cavity, esophagus, stomach, and duodenum. The GIT is most often involved in life-threatening exposures.
- Skin – mild irritation to severe corrosive injury of the superficial layers of the skin followed by eschar formation.
- Ophthalmic – mild irritation to severe corrosive injury of the cornea and conjunctiva with ocular exposure.
- Respiratory – inhalation of powdered acids/fumes may cause irritation (common) or pulmonary edema, shock, or corrosive injury (very rare).
- Hemic/lymphatic/immune – sepsis may result following severe corrosive injury.

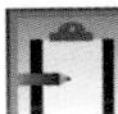

SIGNALMENT/HISTORY

- There are no species, breed, or sex predilections.
- Animals with known dietary indiscretion may be at higher risk of accidental exposure.

Risk Factors

- Animals with preexisting dermal or upper GI disease may have an increased risk of developing tissue injury.

Historical Findings

- Witnessed ingestion or discovery of chewed acid-containing cleaners or products.
- If acid is ingested, owners may report excessive salivation, vomiting, oral lesions, stridor, and abnormal behavior (due to pain) such as pawing at the mouth or hiding, refusal of food/water, and vocalization.
- If animal is dermally exposed, owners may report red, irritated skin, excessive licking at the skin, “burned” or damaged hair, or open sores.

Location and Circumstances of Poisoning

- Often in areas where acids are kept: bathroom, utility/hobby room, garage, workshop, etc.

CLINICAL FEATURES

- Evidence of irritation or corrosive injury to the exposed tissues is often immediate.
- In cases of severe corrosive injury, ulcerations may persist for weeks to months.
- Oral cavity – corrosive lesions typically progress from white/gray to black and wrinkled (eschar).
  - Up to 37% of patients with esophageal damage will NOT exhibit oral lesions (human data).
- Upper GI – ptyalism, dysphagia, vomiting/regurgitation, hematemesis, abdominal pain.
- Dermal – hyperemia, irritated or abraded skin, damaged hair.
- Ocular – conjunctivitis, blepharospasm, ± grossly visible corneal damage.
- Respiratory – stridor (laryngeal/epiglottic edema), tachypnea (pain), coughing.

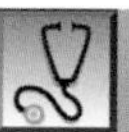

DIFFERENTIAL DIAGNOSIS

- Toxicities:
  - Tissue injury caused by alkalis or neutral corrosive agents (e.g., phenol). See chapters 87 and 88.
  - Oral injury secondary to chewing on electrical cords.
  - GI erosion/ulceration secondary to NSAID intoxication. See chapters 45 and 52.
- Primary or secondary esophageal or GI disease resulting in esophagitis, esophageal stricture, gastric ulceration, or gastric outflow obstruction.

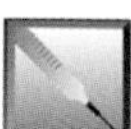

DIAGNOSTICS

- Endoscopy – cautious examination of the esophagus, stomach (especially pyloric region), and duodenum to determine the extent and severity of injury.
  - Ideally, use a flexible endoscope with minimal insufflation.
  - Endoscopy is recommended in all cases involving the following:
    - ☐ The ingestion of large volumes of acid.
    - ☐ The ingestion of a corrosive agent.
    - ☐ The ingestion of agents with a pH <4.
    - ☐ If clinical signs have not resolved in <12–24 hours.
- CBC or PCV/TS – blood loss anemia, WBC changes with GI perforation and sepsis.
- Chemistry panel – monitor electrolytes, BUN, and creatinine in cases of corrosive injury.
- Acid–base – monitor for acidemia in cases of severe corrosive injury/large ingestions (rare).
- Abdominocentesis – increased WBCs, protein, and fibrinogen levels, bacteria, and amorphous cellular debris are consistent with GI perforation and a septic abdomen.
- Radiographs of the neck, thorax, and abdomen for evidence of perforation.
- Positive contrast barium esophagogram to look for strictures/evaluate motility.
- Abdominal ultrasound – complex free fluid, evidence of perforation.
- Fluoroscopy to evaluate esophageal motility/strictures.

Pathological Findings

- Gross – evidence of partial- or full-thickness corrosive injury.
- Histopathological findings will be consistent with coagulation necrosis, including evidence of edema, acute inflammation (polymorphonuclear leukocyte infiltrate), and granulation tissue. Damage may extend through multiple tissue layers.

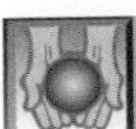

THERAPEUTICS

- Initial management following corrosive ingestions involves rapidly evaluating the airway and obtaining vital signs.
- Once stable, treatment focuses on the prevention or management of corrosive injury, including gastroprotection, analgesia, and nutritional supplementation.

Detoxification

- Immediately flush exposed skin or oral membranes with large volumes of water or saline for 20 minutes (should be started at home if possible). Eye wash products or tap water are preferred for ocular irrigation.
- Decontamination of the GIT is very limited (see Precautions/Interactions).
    - The induction of emesis is contraindicated.
    - Activated charcoal is contraindicated.
    - Neutralizing ingested acids with alkalis is not recommended.
    - Dilution with water can be attempted but has not been proven effective.

Appropriate Health Care

- Use injectable instead of oral drug formulations in the event of corrosive injury.
- Manage corrosive injury.
    - Gastroprotection (treat for weeks to months, depending on extent of injury).
        - Sucralfate liquid (0.25–1.0 g PO q 6–8 hours).
        - H_2 blockers (e.g., famotidine 0.5 mg/kg PO, IV, SQ q 12 hours).
        - Proton pump inhibitors (e.g., pantoprazole 0.7–1 mg/kg, IV over 15 minutes q 24 hours).
    - IV fluids – use a balanced electrolyte crystalloid to maintain euvolemia, hydration, and renal perfusion.
    - Analgesia – powerful analgesics may be warranted.
    - Nutritional support – patients with corrosive injury become hypercatabolic and require substantial nutritional support, including total parenteral nutrition, gastrostomy, or jejunostomy. See Diet and Surgical Considerations.
    - Corticosteroids – use remains controversial.
        - Unlikely to benefit in cases of minor injury.

    - If significant injury and stricture formation is very likely, antiinflammatory doses may be of slight benefit.
    - Must be accompanied by antibiotics due to the increased risk of infection.
- Antibiotics – prophylactic use remains controversial.
    - In cases of known infection, parenteral use is advised.
    - Broad-spectrum coverage is recommended (e.g., enrofloxacin with ampicillin).
- If hypoproteinemia results, artificial colloid therapy (e.g., Hetastarch at 1–2 mL/kg/hour) should be considered to maintain colloid osmotic pressure.
- Blood transfusion with pRBCs as needed to maintain PCV ≥15–20% if gastric hemorrhage is noted.
- In cases of shock/loss of consciousness (very rare), intubation with mechanical ventilation if necessary.

Drugs and Antidotes of Choice

- No antidote exists.
- Sucralfate liquid, 0.25–1 g PO immediately upon ingestion, may be beneficial.
- See Appropriate Health Care.

Precautions/Interactions

- Neutralization of the exposed tissue by adding an alkali is not recommended as exothermic reactions may result (thermal burns).
- The induction of emesis or gastric lavage is contraindicated due to the increased risk of aspiration, reexposure injury, and GIT perforation.
- Activated charcoal does not bind to corrosive agents and is contraindicated.
- The use of oral NSAIDs is not typically recommended due to the compromised GIT.

Follow-up

- Esophageal and gastric ulcerations may persist for weeks to months.
- Esophageal strictures may not form until weeks to months after the initial injury.

Diet

- Depending on the extent and severity of injury, a soft or liquid diet or parenteral nutrition may be needed. See Surgical Considerations.

Surgical Considerations

- A feeding tube placed distal to GIT ulcerations may be needed to maintain nutritional support (e.g., gastrostomy or jejunostomy tubes).
- Strictures in the GIT may necessitate surgical attention (bougienage, balloon dilation, resection, etc.).

COMMENTS

Client Education

- Inform clients that esophageal strictures may not form until weeks to months after the initial injury.
- Alert clients to common household items that may cause corrosive injury (toilet bowl, metal, drain, and metal cleaners; calcium/lime/rust removers; and pool sanitizers).

Prevention/Avoidance

- Potentially corrosive cleaners and products should be stored in original containers and kept in pet/child-proof areas.

Possible Complications

- Esophageal strictures (may form weeks to months after the initial injury).
- Gastric stricture, pyloric stenosis, or GIT perforations with septic peritonitis.
- Long-term esophageal dysmotility.
- Esophageal carcinomas (human data).

Expected Course and Prognosis

- Most acid ingestions will be small and are unlikely to result in corrosive injury. In such cases, the prognosis is excellent.
- In cases involving corrosive injury, the prognosis is dependent on the extent and severity of injury. Prognosis is grave in cases of severe injury and no medical management and fair in cases of severe injury with aggressive management.

See Also

Alkalis
Aspirin
Batteries
Essential Oils/Liquid Potpourri
Hydrofluoric Acid
Phenols and Pine Oils
Soaps, Detergents, Fabric Softeners, Enzymatic Cleaners, and Deodorizers

Abbreviations

See Appendix 1 for a complete list.

Suggested Reading

Gwaltney-Brant SM. Miscellaneous indoor toxicants. In: Peterson ME, Talcott PA, eds. Small Animal Toxicology, 3rd edn. St Louis, MO: Saunders, 2013; pp. 291–308.

Rella JG, Hoffman RS. Acids and bases. In: Brent J, Wallace KL, Burkhart KK, et al., eds. Critical Care Toxicology: Diagnosis and Management of the Critically Poisoned Patient. Philadelphia, PA: Mosby, 2005; pp. 1035–1043.

Tohda G, Sugawa C, Gayer C, et al. Clinical evaluation and management of caustic injury in the upper gastrointestinal tract in 95 adult patients in an urban medical center. Surg Endosc 2008; 22:1119–1125.

Author: Ahna G. Brutlag, DVM, MS, DABT, DABVT
Consulting Editor: Lynn R. Hovda, RPh, DVM, MS, DACVIM

chapter 82

Alkalis

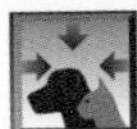

DEFINITION/OVERVIEW

- Alkaline substances (also called bases) have a pH >7, produce hydroxide ions upon contact with water, and are proton acceptors.
- Tissue injury from alkaline agents depends on the pH, specific agent, concentration, volume, and duration of contact.
    - Exposure to weak (pH 10–11) or dilute alkalis may cause mild tissue irritation.
    - Exposure to strong (pH greater than 11–12) or concentrated alkalis may cause corrosive injury (see Toxicology). The term "corrosive" is synonymous with "caustic" which is conventionally used to describe corrosive injury resulting from alkalis. Both terms are used in this chapter.
    - Many US household products containing corrosive agents will display the signal word *Danger* clearly on the packaging.
- The most common household alkaline agent is regular-strength chlorine bleach.
    - Sodium hypochlorite, 4–6%; typical pH = 11–12.
    - Regular bleach is typically irritating to tissues, not corrosive (see Toxicology).
- Common household products containing potential alkaline corrosives.
    - Automatic dishwasher detergents.
    - Batteries (dry cell such as AA, C, D).
    - Bleach – nonchlorine ("Color Safe," "Oxy," and "Ultra") formulations may be corrosive in large amounts or with prolonged tissue contact. They contain sodium percarbonate, sodium perborate, sodium carbonate, and sodium metasilicate.
    - Cement – when mixed with water, becomes corrosive (60–65% calcium oxide).
    - Dairy and industrial pipeline cleaners.
    - Drain cleaners.
    - Hair relaxers.
    - Lye (sodium or potassium hydroxide).
    - Oven cleaners.

Blackwell's Five-Minute Veterinary Consult Clinical Companion: Small Animal Toxicology, Second Edition.
Lynn R. Hovda, Ahna G. Brutlag, Robert H. Poppenga, and Katherine L. Peterson.

Companion website: www.fiveminutevet.com/toxicology

- Treatment following exposure to alkaline agents is focused on the prevention/management of caustic injury, including analgesia and nutritional support.
- Serious complications include severe caustic injury followed by systemic infection, stricture formation, GIT perforation, and septic peritonitis.

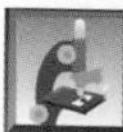

ETIOLOGY/PATHOPHYSIOLOGY

- Exposure in animals generally occurs from accidental ingestion or dermal contact.
- Small ingestions/tastes of alkaline corrosives are unlikely to result in severe tissue damage.
- Alkaline products typically have little odor or taste; thus, larger ingestions may occur. Bittering agents may be added to deter ingestion.
- Pain, though common, is not always evident immediately upon contact.

Mechanism of Action

- Alkaline corrosives cause liquefaction necrosis with resulting edema and inflammation and rapidly penetrate deeply into tissues, often involving multiple tissue layers (transmural necrosis).
- Triglycerides in cell membranes become saponified by hydroxyl ions, resulting in membrane lysis. Proteins become denatured, resulting in functional loss of transport proteins and enzymes. Cell death, reduced mechanical strength, and impaired repair mechanisms are the cellular end result.
- Thrombosis occurs in arterioles and venules.
- Tissues release heat and gases upon contact with caustic alkalis.
- Significant tissue damage from caustic injury may result in stricture formation.

Pharmacokinetics – Absorption, Distribution, Metabolism, Excretion

- Systemic absorption of alkalis is not typically concerning, and systemic alkalosis is not expected.
  - Exception: large ingestions of chlorine bleach may cause hyperchloremic acidosis and hypernatremia.

Toxicology

- Corrosive injury occurs rapidly, within seconds of tissue contact.
- Exposures to large volumes and high concentrations cause more severe injury.
- For most alkaline agents, serious burns are less likely if the pH is <11.5–12.
- Experimental cat model: 1 mL of 30% sodium hydroxide (lye) = transesophageal necrosis.
- Toxicity of household bleach (sodium hypochlorite, 4–6%).
  - Typical pH = 11–12; corrosive if pH >12–12.5.
  - Expect corrosive injury with ingestions >5 mL/kg or concentrations >10%.
  - When mixed with a strong acid, chlorine gas is released.

- When mixed with ammonia, chloramine gas is released.
  - Gases irritate the nasal and oral mucosa, respiratory tract, eyes, etc.
  - In significant exposures, the gas may cause corrosive damage to mucosal membranes.
- Toxicity of specific alkaline chemicals.
  - Irritants (mild to moderate).
    - Sodium hydroxide <2%.
    - Sodium hypochlorite <10%.
  - Corrosives.
    - Sodium carbonate >15%.
    - Sodium hydroxide >2%.
    - Sodium hypochlorite >10%.
    - Sodium metasilicate >0.5%.
    - Sodium silicate >20–40%.
  - Sodium percarbonate, on contact with water, breaks down into hydrogen peroxide and sodium carbonate. Depending on concentration, may irritate or corrode tissue.

Systems Affected

- Organs having direct contact with the product are most at risk (GIT, skin, eyes, and lungs).
- Gastrointestinal – ingestion causes mild tissue irritation to significant ulceration of the oral cavity, esophagus, stomach, and duodenum. The GIT is most often involved in life-threatening exposures.
- Skin – mild irritation to severe caustic injury.
- Ophthalmic – mild irritation to severe caustic injury of the cornea and conjunctiva with ocular exposure.
- Respiratory – inhalation or aspiration of powdered alkaline agents/gaseous by-products may cause irritation (common) or pulmonary edema, shock, or caustic injury (very rare).
- Hemic/lymphatic/immune – sepsis may result following severe caustic injury.
- Endocrine/metabolic – large ingestions of chlorine bleach may cause hyperchloremic acidosis and hypernatremia.

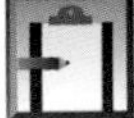

SIGNALMENT/HISTORY

- There are no species, breed, or sex predilections.
- Animals with known dietary indiscretion or "chewers" may be at higher risk of accidental exposure.

Risk Factors

- Animals with preexisting dermal, upper GI, or respiratory disease may have an increased risk of developing tissue injury or clinical signs.

Historical Findings

- Witnessed ingestion or discovery of chewed alkaline-containing products.
- If an alkaline is ingested, owners may report excessive salivation, vomiting, oral lesions, stridor, and abnormal behavior (due to pain) such as pawing at the mouth or hiding, refusal of food/water, and vocalization.
- If the animal is dermally exposed, owners may report red, irritated skin, excessive licking at the skin, "burned" or damaged hair, or open sores.

Location and Circumstances of Poisoning

- Often in areas where alkaline agents are kept: bathroom, utility/hobby room, garage, workshop, etc.

Interactions with Drugs, Nutrients, or Environment

- Chlorine bleach, when mixed with strong acid or ammonia, produces chlorine and chloramines gases, respectively (see Toxicology).

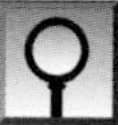

CLINICAL FEATURES

- Evidence of irritation or corrosive injury is often immediate although pain may be delayed.
- In cases of severe caustic injury, ulcerations may persist for weeks to months.
- Oral cavity – tissue irritation or ulceration.
  - Up to 37% of patients with esophageal damage will NOT exhibit oral lesions (human data).
- GI – ptyalism, dysphagia, vomiting/regurgitation, hematemesis, abdominal pain, diarrhea.
- Dermal – hyperemia, irritated or abraded skin, damaged hair.
- Ocular – blepharospasm, eyelid edema, chemosis, conjunctival hyperemia and/or ischemia, whitish haze of corneal stroma, mild corneal edema, uveitis, ± grossly visible corneal damage.
- Respiratory – stridor (laryngeal/epiglottic edema), tachypnea (pain), coughing.

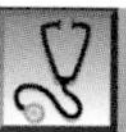

DIFFERENTIAL DIAGNOSIS

- Toxicities.
  - Tissue injury caused by acids or neutral caustic agents (e.g., phenols or quaternary ammonium cationic surfactants – see Chapters 87 and 88).
  - Oral injury secondary to chewing on electrical cords.
  - GI erosion/ulceration secondary to NSAID or aspirin toxicosis (see Chapters 42, 45, and 52).
- Primary or secondary esophageal or GI disease resulting in esophagitis, esophageal stricture, gastric ulceration, or gastric outflow obstruction.

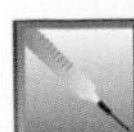

DIAGNOSTICS

- Endoscopy – cautious examination of the esophagus, stomach, and duodenum to determine the extent and severity of injury.
  - Ideally, use a flexible endoscope with minimal insufflation.
  - Endoscopy is recommended in all cases involving the following:
    - The ingestion of large volumes of any alkaline agent (>5 mL/kg).
    - Ingestion of a known corrosive agent.
    - Ingestion of agents with a pH >11.5.
    - If clinical signs have not resolved in <12–24 hours.
  - Endoscopic evaluation of lesions aids in prediction of stricture formation.
- CBC or PCV/TS – blood loss anemia, WBC changes with GI perforation and sepsis.
- Chemistry panel – monitor electrolytes, BUN, and creatinine in cases of caustic injury. Large ingestion of chlorine bleach may cause hyperchloremic acidosis and hypernatremia.
- Acid–base – monitor for acidosis if a large volume of chlorine bleach was ingested.
- Abdominocentesis – increased WBCs, protein and fibrinogen levels, intracellular bacteria, and amorphous cellular debris are consistent with GI perforation and a septic abdomen.
- Radiographs of the neck, thorax, and abdomen for evidence of perforation. Positive contrast barium esophagogram to look for strictures/evaluate motility.
- Abdominal ultrasound – complex free fluid, evidence of perforation.
- Fluoroscopy to evaluate esophageal motility/strictures.

Pathological Findings

- Gross – evidence of partial- or full-thickness caustic injury (involving the mucosal, serosal, submucosal, and muscular layers).
- Histopathological findings will be consistent with liquefaction necrosis, including evidence of edema, acute inflammation, and granulation tissue. Damage may extend through multiple tissue layers.

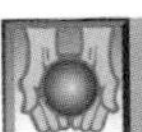

THERAPEUTICS

- Initial management following caustic ingestions involves rapidly evaluating the airway and obtaining vital signs.
- Once stable, treatment focuses on the prevention or management of caustic injury, including gastroprotection, analgesia, and nutritional supplementation.

Detoxification

- Immediately flush exposed skin or oral membranes with large volumes of water or saline for 20 minutes. Eye wash products or tap water are preferred for ocular irrigation.

- Decontamination of the GIT is very limited (see Precautions/Interactions).
  - The induction of emesis is contraindicated.
  - Activated charcoal is contraindicated.
  - Neutralizing ingested alkaline agents with acids is not recommended.
  - Dilution with water can be attempted but is often ineffective due to the massive volumes required to effectively reduce the pH.

Appropriate Health Care

- Use injectable drug formulations (when possible) in the event of caustic injury.
- Manage caustic injury.
  - Gastroprotection (treat for weeks to months, depending on extent of injury).
    - Sucralfate liquid (0.25–1.0 g PO q 6–8 h) binds to damaged tissue.
    - H_2 blockers (e.g., famotidine 0.5 mg/kg PO, IV, SC q 12 hours).
    - Proton pump inhibitors (e.g., pantoprazole 0.7–1 mg/kg, IV over 15 minutes q 24 h).
  - IV fluids – use a balanced electrolyte crystalloid to maintain euvolemia, hydration, and renal perfusion.
  - Analgesia – powerful analgesics may be warranted (see Precautions/Interactions).
  - Nutritional support – patients with caustic injury become hypercatabolic and require substantial nutritional support, including total parenteral nutrition, a gastrostomy, or jejunostomy. See Diet and Surgical Considerations.
  - Corticosteroids – use remains controversial.
    - Unlikely to benefit in cases of minor injury.
    - If significant injury and stricture formation are very likely, antiinflammatory doses may be of slight benefit.
    - Must be accompanied by antibiotics due to the increased risk of infection.
  - Antibiotics – prophylactic use remains controversial.
    - In cases of known infection, parenteral use is advised.
    - Broad-spectrum coverage is recommended.
  - If hypoproteinemia results, artificial colloid therapy (e.g., Hetastarch at 1–2 mL/kg/hour) should be considered to maintain colloid osmotic pressure.
  - Blood transfusion with pRBCs as needed to maintain PCV ≥15–20% if gastric hemorrhage is noted.
  - In cases of shock/loss of consciousness (very rare), intubation ± mechanical ventilation if necessary.

Drugs and Antidotes of Choice

- No antidote exists.
- See Appropriate Health Care.

Precautions/Interactions

- Neutralization of the exposed tissue by adding an acid is not recommended as exothermic reactions may result (thermal burns).

- The induction of emesis or gastric lavage is contraindicated due to the increased risk of aspiration, reexposure injury, and GIT perforation.
- Activated charcoal does not bind to caustic agents and is contraindicated.
- The use of oral NSAIDs is not typically recommended due to the compromised GIT.

Follow-up

- Esophageal and gastric ulcerations may persist for weeks to months.
- Esophageal strictures may not form until weeks to months after the initial injury.

Diet

- Depending on the extent and severity of injury, a soft or liquid diet or parenteral nutrition may be needed. See Surgical Considerations.

Surgical Considerations

- A feeding tube placed distal to GIT ulcerations may be needed to maintain nutritional support (e.g., gastrostomy or jejunostomy tubes).
- Strictures in the GIT may necessitate surgical attention (bougienage, balloon dilation, resection, etc.).

COMMENTS

Client Education

- Inform clients that esophageal strictures may form weeks to months after the initial injury.
- Alert clients to common household items that may cause caustic injury (drain and toilet bowl cleaners, dry cell batteries, concentrated bleach, lye, hair relaxers, wet cement).

Prevention/Avoidance

- Caustic cleaners and products should be stored in original containers and kept in pet/child-proof areas.

Possible Complications

- Esophageal strictures (may form weeks to months after the initial injury).
- Gastric stricture, pyloric stenosis, or GIT perforations with septic peritonitis.
- Long-term esophageal dysmotility.
- Esophageal carcinomas (human data).

Expected Course and Prognosis

- Most ingestions will be small and are unlikely to result in caustic injury. In such cases, the prognosis is excellent.

- In cases involving caustic injury, the prognosis is dependent on the extent and severity of injury. Prognosis is grave in cases of severe injury and no medical management, and fair in cases of severe injury with aggressive management.

See Also

Acids
Batteries
Essential Oils/Liquid Potpourri
Hydrofluoric Acid
Phenols and Pine Oils
Soaps, Detergents, Fabric Softeners, Enzymatic Cleaners, and Deodorizers

Abbreviations

See Appendix 1 for a complete list.

Suggested Reading

Busse C, Hartley C, Kafarnik C, Pivetta M. Ocular alkaline injury in four dogs – presentation, treatment, and follow-up – a case series. Vet Ophthalmol 2015; 18(2):127–134.
Farrell M, Dunn A, Marchevsky A. Surgical reconstruction of canine footpads burned by sodium hypochlorite drain cleaner. Compend Contin Educ Vet 2011; 33(7):E1–8.
Gwaltney-Brant SM. Miscellaneous indoor toxicants. In: Peterson ME, Talcott PA, eds. Small Animal Toxicology, 3rd edn. St Louis, MO: Elsevier, 2013; pp. 291–308.

Author: Ahna G. Brutlag, DVM, MS, DABT, DABVT
Consulting Editor: Lynn R. Hovda, RPh, DVM, MS, DACVIM

chapter 83

Batteries

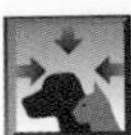 DEFINITION/OVERVIEW

- When the casing of a battery is ruptured, alkaline or acidic material can leak from the battery and ulcerate exposed tissues.
- The design of button- or disk-shaped batteries allows an electric current to be passed to the tissues of the GIT. This current causes necrosis and possible GIT perforation, tracheoesophageal fistulas, fistulization into major vessels, and massive hemorrhage/exsanguination.
- The greatest damage occurs from lithium disk batteries. One 3-volt battery can cause esophageal necrosis with 15 minutes of contact.
    - In children, the most serious outcomes and greatest number of deaths have been reported with larger-diameter lithium cell batteries (≥20 mm). Death is often due to exsanguination after fistulization into major vessels (following esophageal entrapment).
- Batteries may also contain the metals lead, mercury, zinc, cobalt, nickel, or cadmium. Heavy metal toxicosis may occur if batteries are retained in the GIT for more than 2–3 days.

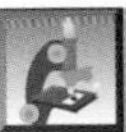 ETIOLOGY/PATHOPHYSIOLOGY

Mechanism of Action

- Lithium disk batteries: contain no corrosive compounds, but the esophagus becomes increasingly alkaline on the cathode side and acidic on the anode side as the current passes through the battery. This results in severe tissue damage/possible perforation.
- Dry cell batteries.
    - Acid dry cells usually contain ammonium chloride or manganese dioxide. When either component comes in contact with mucosa, it causes coagulation necrosis.
    - Alkaline dry cells (the majority of household batteries) contain potassium hydroxide or sodium hydroxide. When the compounds come in contact with tissue, liquefaction necrosis occurs, resulting in deeply penetrating ulcers.

Blackwell's Five-Minute Veterinary Consult Clinical Companion: Small Animal Toxicology, Second Edition.
Lynn R. Hovda, Ahna G. Brutlag, Robert H. Poppenga, and Katherine L. Peterson.

Companion website: www.fiveminutevet.com/toxicology

Pharmacokinetics – Absorption, Distribution, Metabolism, Excretion

- Lithium disk/button batteries: significant systemic absorption of lithium rarely occurs. Stomach acid does not significantly alter the battery casing. The battery is passed unchanged in the feces.
- Dry cell batteries: the alkaline or acidic component can leak if the casing is ruptured. This may occur before ingestion or within the stomach as the casing is further degraded. As the acid or alkaline contents react with local tissues, the contents become nonreactive and systemic absorption does not typically occur. If the battery remains lodged in the gastrointestinal tract for a prolonged period, the heavy metals in the casing (lead, mercury, zinc, cobalt, cadmium) may cause toxicosis.

Systems Affected

- Gastrointestinal – ulcerations in the oral cavity, esophagus, stomach, and small intestine are possible. Ulceration may lead to GIT perforation, secondary peritonitis, and tracheo-esophageal fistulas.
- Skin – ulceration and irritation if exposed to battery contents.
- Respiratory – stridor from pharyngeal or esophageal ulceration. Dyspnea from airway obstruction. Pleuritis, dyspnea, or fever if esophageal perforation occurs and ingesta leaks into pleural cavity. Chemical pneumonitis if corrosive material inhaled.
- Hemic – ulceration of the GIT may lead to fistulization into major vessels, and massive hemorrhage/exsanguination. Intravascular hemolysis may develop secondary to heavy metal toxicosis if batteries are retained in the GIT (see chapters 95–97 and Appendix 3 on metallic toxicants).
- Hepatobiliary – hepatic damage may occur secondary to heavy metal toxicosis if batteries are retained in the GIT (see chapters 95–97 and Appendix 3 on metallic toxicants).
- Nervous – CNS abnormalities may occur secondary to heavy metal toxicosis if batteries are retained in the GIT (see chapters 95–97 and Appendix 3 on metallic toxicants).

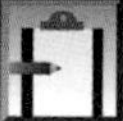

SIGNALMENT/HISTORY

- No breed, age or sex predilections exist.

Risk Factors

- Use of toys or bedding with batteries in them; chewing on remote controls, hearing aids, or other battery-operated devices.

Historical Findings

- Owner often reports having witnessed the ingestion or finding the partially ingested battery or battery-containing device. With an unwitnessed ingestion, owners may report hypersalivation, pawing at the mouth, anorexia, or vomiting. Signs typically begin 2–12 hours after ingestion.

Location and Circumstances of Poisoning

- Ingestion usually occurs within the home. The holiday season has been anecdotally associated with a greater number of ingestions (battery-containing gifts and decor).

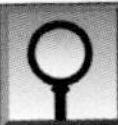

CLINICAL FEATURES

- Physical examination should begin with evaluation of the oral cavity. Look for erythema and ulceration of the gums, tongue, and laryngeal/pharyngeal area. Occlusal surfaces of the teeth may be discolored (black or gray) from exposure to dry cell battery contents.
- Signs of nausea such as hypersalivation and frequent swallowing.
- Abdominal palpation may reveal pain, free abdominal fluid, or distension.
- Other clinical signs (e.g., evidence of hemolysis) may develop if sufficient time has passed for heavy metal toxicosis to develop (see chapters 95–97 and Appendix 3 on metallic toxicants).
- In children, serious outcomes and death from tracheoesophageal fistulas, fistulization into major vessels, and massive hemorrhage/exsanguination have been reported.

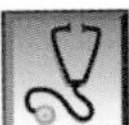

DIFFERENTIAL DIAGNOSIS

- There are multiple other conditions that can cause acute gastroenteritis with ulceration and possible perforation. NSAID toxicity, foreign body ingestion, pancreatitis, corrosive chemical ingestion, and endotoxemia ("garbage gut") can all present with very similar clinical signs.

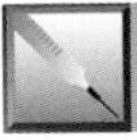

DIAGNOSTICS

- Radiograph the GIT to look for a retained battery. This should include the back of the mouth, the esophagus, stomach, and small and large intestine.
    - Disc batteries can easily be mistaken for coins on radiographs.
- PCV/TS or CBC – to assess blood loss, hydration, inflammation or infection.
- Endoscopy to characterize ulcerations and potentially remove lodged batteries from the esophagus or stomach.

Pathological Findings

- Ulceration, necrosis, and perforation anywhere along the GIT with hemorrhage and adjacent tissue injury; edema and ulceration of the larynx, trachea, and lower airways from inhalation of caustic battery components.

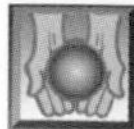

THERAPEUTICS

- Do not induce vomiting. See Detoxification.
- Initial therapy should include dilution of caustic components, removal of retained batteries, treatment for corrosive injury, pain management, and infection control.

Detoxification

- The induction of emesis is not often advised due to the potential for corrosive injury or esophageal entrapment of the battery.
- Activated charcoal is not recommended as it will not bind to battery contents and increases the risk of vomiting.
- Dilution.
  - Give small amounts of tepid tap water every 10–15 minutes until evaluation can be completed. Rinse the oral cavity and any exposed skin for 10–15 minutes with water to remove or dilute any remaining caustic material.
- Battery removal.
  - Once radiographs reveal the location of a battery, a method of removal should be selected.
    - □ Esophagus – immediate endoscopic removal is ideal. If the battery is leaking, care should be taken to minimize further damage.
    - □ Stomach – surgical removal is appropriate to protect the esophagus as endoscopic removal of a punctured battery or disk battery may cause ulcerations. Small, nonpunctured dry cell batteries *may* pass through the GIT without causing further damage. Repeated GI radiographs are needed to ensure passage of the battery/casing. Retention may lead to heavy metal toxicity and leakage of caustic contents.
    - □ Small intestine – immediate surgical removal if the battery is punctured/leaking. Monitor (radiographs, examination of stool) for GI passage if the battery is not leaking.

Appropriate Health Care

- Depending on the extent of corrosive injury, patients may have discomfort when eating and drinking. Placement of a gastrostomy (PEG) tube may be necessary to ensure adequate nutrition, reduce the likelihood of infection, allow earlier release from the hospital, and improve patient comfort. PEG tubes may be placed at the time of battery removal.

Drugs and Antidotes of Choice

- GI protectants and antacids to allow ulceration to heal rapidly with less discomfort.
  - H_2 blockers (e.g., famotidine 0.5 mg/kg IV, IM, or PO q 12 hours).
  - Proton pump inhibitors (e.g., omeprazole 0.5–1 mg/kg PO q 24 hours).
  - Sucralfate 0.25–1 g PO q 8 hours, on an empty stomach.

- Antimicrobials if necessary.
  - Cefazolin 10–30 mg/kg IV q 8 hours and enrofloxacin 5–20 mg/kg IV q 12–24 hours (dogs).
  - Metronidazole 15 mg/kg PO q 12 hours.
- Analgesics (see Precautions/Interactions).
  - Buprenorphine 0.005–0.01 mg/kg IV, IM, SQ or sublingual q 8 hours.
  - Tramadol 1–4 mg/kg PO q 8 hours.

Precautions/Interactions

- Avoid early use of NSAIDs as prostaglandin inhibition will reduce the protective lining of the stomach.

Alternative Drugs

- H_2 blockers – cimetidine and ranitidine are also excellent choices.
- Analgesics – other opioid analgesics can be used, such as hydromorphone, morphine, oxymorphone, or butorphanol.
- Antimicrobials – any broad-spectrum antibiotic can be used to prevent infection.

Follow-up

- Follow-up endoscopy may be needed to evaluate the esophagus for stricture formation. Consider balloon therapy to relieve a stricture.

Diet

- Keep pet NPO for 12–24 hours after exposure if any tissue damage is suspected.
- Consider placing a feeding tube to bypass the most severely affected areas (see Appropriate Health Care).

Surgical Considerations

- Standard anesthetic protocols are appropriate as long as the patient has no underlying medical conditions
- Surgical versus endoscopic removal of battery material should be carefully considered (see Detoxification).
- Efforts need to be focused around preventing esophageal damage and rapid removal of the material.

Prevention/Avoidance

- Do not give pets toys or bedding containing batteries. Prevent access to batteries by removing old batteries from the environment.

Public Health

- Owner can sustain injuries from touching a ruptured battery and should use protection to prevent damage to their skin.
- In children, the most serious outcomes and greatest number of deaths have been reported with larger diameter lithium cell batteries (≥20 mm). Death is often due to exsanguination after fistulization into major vessels (following esophageal entrapment).

Environmental Issues

- Consult your local recycling service before disposing of used batteries.

COMMENTS

Client Education

- The owner will need to monitor closely for evidence of esophageal strictures, including anorexia, hypersalivation, and regurgitation.

Patient Monitoring

- Patients who initially have mild lesions can be monitored based on resolution of clinical signs. Those with more severe lesions should have an endoscopy performed in 7–14 days to determine progression and look for esophageal stricture or diverticulum.

Possible Complications

- Long-term esophagitis, esophageal stricture, or esophageal diverticulum.

Expected Course and Prognosis

- Lithium disk battery in the esophagus.
  - With rapid removal, expect short-term esophagitis with complete recovery. Risk for stricture is low.
  - With delayed removal or no removal, expect extensive tissue damage. Risk for esophageal perforation is high. Long-term esophageal malformation is likely.
- Lithium disk battery in the stomach.
  - With rapid surgical removal, expect mild-to-moderate gastritis with possible stomach ulceration. Complete recovery expected in 7–10 days (with appropriate care).
  - With delayed or no removal, expect extensive tissue damage. The risk of perforation is high. If perforation is prevented, long-term effects are unlikely. If perforation occurs, septic peritonitis will likely result and immediate surgical intervention is needed to correct the perforation.
- Dry cell battery that is intact.
  - No ulcerations in the oral cavity or esophagus are expected. If the battery is removed from the stomach, recovery is expected to be uneventful.

- If the battery is not removed from the stomach, it may pass uneventfully or it may become trapped in the stomach, causing symptoms of a pyloric obstruction. Over time, the casing will corrode, leading to content leakage, stomach ulceration, and heavy metal toxicity.

- Dry cell battery that is ruptured/leaking.
  - Mild-to-severe ulcerations of the oral cavity, esophagus, and stomach are expected. Esophageal damage may result in long-term esophageal malformation or may heal normally.
  - With delayed or no removal, expect extensive tissue damage. The risk of perforation is high. If perforation is prevented, long-term effects are unlikely. If perforation occurs, septic peritonitis will likely result and immediate surgical intervention is needed to correct the perforation.

Synonyms

Dry cell battery, lithium ion battery, button battery, disk battery, alkaline battery, acid battery, nickel-cadmium battery

See Also

Acids
Alkalis
Metallic Toxicants (Appendix 3)

Abbreviations

See Appendix 1 for a complete list.

PEG = percutaneous endoscopic gastrostomy

Suggested Reading

Litovitz, T, Whitaker N, Clark L, White NC, Marsolek M. Preventing battery ingestion: an analysis of 8648 cases. Pediatrics 2010; 125:1178–1183.

Rebdandl W, Steffan I, Schramel P, et al. Release of toxic metals from button batteries retained in the stomac: an in vitro study. J Pediatr Surg 2002; 37:87–92.

Tanaka J, Yamashita M, Yamashita M, et al. Effects of tap water on esophageal burns in dogs from button lithium batteries. Vet Hum Toxicol 1999; 41:279–282.

Wormald PJ, Wilson DAB. Battery acid burns of the upper gastro-intestinal tract. Clin Otolaryngol Allied Sci 2007; 18:112–114.

Yoshikawa T, Asai S, Takekawa, Kida A, Ishikawa K. Experimental investigation of battery-induced esophageal burn injury in rabbits. Crit Care Med 1997; 25:2039–2044.

Author: Catherine Angle, DVM, MPH
Consulting Editor: Ahna G. Brutlag, DVM, MS, DABT, DABVT

Matches and Fireworks

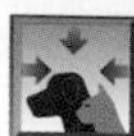

DEFINITION/OVERVIEW

- Most match ingestions only cause GI signs, while serious toxicosis can result with firework ingestions.
- Poisoning by matches and fireworks is not common.
- Matches contain potassium chlorate and possibly phosphorus sesquisulfide. The chlorates are the biggest concern for toxicosis. Animals exposed to chlorates can develop methemoglobinemia.
- In fireworks, chlorates and barium are the toxins of most concern. They can cause methemoglobinemia, cardiovascular effects, and renal failure (see table 84.1 for other possible ingredients). Used fireworks can have a different composition from unused, and the kinetics and toxicity can vary (increased or decreased bioavailability).

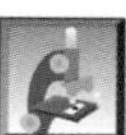

ETIOLOGY/PATHOPHYSIOLOGY

Mechanism of Action

- Barium: causes severe systemic hypokalemia by blocking the exit channel for potassium in skeletal muscle cells. Barium also stimulates skeletal, smooth, and cardiac muscle, causing violent peristalsis, arterial hypertension, and arrhythmias.
- Chlorates: locally irritating and potent oxidizing agents. The irritation leads to vomiting and diarrhea while oxidation of red blood cells causes hemolysis and methemoglobin formation. Chlorates are directly toxic to the proximal renal tubules, producing cellular necrosis and renal vasoconstriction. Hemoglobinemia and methemoglobin catalysis also contribute to the renal effects.

Pharmacokinetics – Absorption, Distribution, Metabolism, Excretion

- Barium: oral absorption of barium is generally rapid but depends on the solubility of the particular barium salt. Peak serum concentrations are reached within 2 hours after ingestion. Barium is distributed into the bone, with an estimated half-life of 50 days. The main route of excretion of barium is fecal (less than 3% is excreted renally).

Blackwell's Five-Minute Veterinary Consult Clinical Companion: Small Animal Toxicology, Second Edition.
Lynn R. Hovda, Ahna G. Brutlag, Robert H. Poppenga, and Katherine L. Peterson.

Companion website: www.fiveminutevet.com/toxicology

TABLE 84.1. Toxicological information on the ingredients commonly found in fireworks.

Ingredient	Fireworks usage/toxicity information
Aluminum	Silver and white flames and sparks (common in sparklers) Poor oral absorption; little risk of toxicity
Antimony (antimony sulfide)	Glitter effects Poor oral absorption; poisoning is very rare
Barium (barium chlorate, barium nitrate)	Green colors and can help stabilize other volatile elements
Beryllium	White sparks Poor oral absorption; inhalation can cause lung cancer
Calcium (calcium chlorate)	Orange coloring and used to deepen other colors
Cesium (cesium nitrate)	Indigo colors Toxicity is of minor importance
Chlorine	Component of many oxidizers in fireworks
Copper (copper chloride, copper halides)	Blue colors Copper salts are locally corrosive
Iron	Gold sparks (see chapter 95, Iron)
Lithium (lithium carbonate)	Red color
Magnesium	White sparks and improves brilliance
Phosphorus	Glow-in-the-dark effects and may be a component of the fuel Red phosphorus (safety matches) is an insoluble substance that is nontoxic in oral ingestions. White phosphorus (fireworks) can cause severe gastroenteritis and cardiotoxic effects
Potassium (potassium nitrate, potassium perchlorate)	Violet color, black powder explosive and used to oxidize firework mixtures Animals with normal renal function have minimal toxicity consisting of GI signs
Rubidium (rubidium nitrate)	Violet color
Sodium (sodium nitrate)	Gold or yellow colors
Strontium (strontium carbonate)	Red color and used to stabilize firework mixtures
Sulfur (sulfur dioxide)	Component of black powder Vomiting and diarrhea are common following sulfur ingestion
Titanium	Silver sparks Poor oral absorption; heavy dust exposures can cause coughing and dyspnea
Zinc	Smoke effects

- Chlorates: chlorates are well absorbed orally and are slowly excreted unchanged by the kidney.

Toxicity

- Barium: LD_{LO} (oral) human = 11 mg/kg; LD_{50} (oral) human = 1 g.
- Barium chloride: LD_{50} (oral) rat = 220 mg/kg.
- Chlorates: LD_{50} (oral) dog = 1000 mg/kg.

- Potassium chlorate: LD_{50} (oral) rat = 1870 mg/kg.
- Sodium chlorate: LD_{50} (oral) mouse = 596 mg/kg; rat = 1200 mg/kg.

Systems Affected

- Gastrointestinal – vomiting (possibly bloody), diarrhea, hypersalivation.
- Skin – dermal burns.
- Nervous – lethargy.
- Hemic – hemolysis, methemoglobinemia.
- Cardiovascular – arrhythmias, hypertension.
- Respiratory – tachypnea, dyspnea.
- Endocrine/metabolic – hyperkalemia (chlorates), hypokalemia (barium).
- Renal – renal failure (rare, chlorates).
- Musculoskeletal – weakness, paresis (rare, barium).

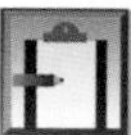

SIGNALMENT/HISTORY

Risk Factors

- Animals that ingest wooden matches are at risk for developing a GI foreign body.

Historical Findings

- Vomiting, lethargy, diarrhea, bloody diarrhea.
- Owners may report matches or fireworks in vomitus.

CLINICAL FEATURES

- Vomiting, lethargy, diarrhea, hypersalivation, and hematemesis are most common.
- Tachycardia, hemolysis, hyperkalemia, methemoglobinemia, and nephropathy have also been reported.
- Barium: ingestion can cause vomiting, diarrhea, salivation, cyanosis, bradycardia, and dyspnea within 10–60 minutes after exposure. Later signs (2–3 hours) include tremors, seizures, paralysis, mydriasis, severe hypokalemia, hypertension, arrhythmias, tachypnea, respiratory failure, and cardiac shock. If no signs within 6–8 hours, none are expected to develop.
- Chlorates: vomiting, tachycardia, hemolysis, hyperkalemia, methemoglobinemia, and nephropathy can be seen in sodium chlorate toxicosis. Methemoglobinemia may not develop for 1–10 hours after exposure.

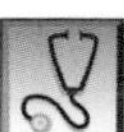

DIFFERENTIAL DIAGNOSIS

- Methemoglobinemia – acetaminophen, 3-chloro-p-toluidine hydrochloride (Starlicide®), phenols (cats), garlic, onions, aniline dyes, naphthalene, phenazopyridine.
- Hemorrhagic gastroenteritis – arsenic, parvoviral enteritis, HGE.

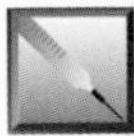

DIAGNOSTICS

- CBC: methemoglobin level (chlorates), hematocrit (chlorates).
- Chemistry panel and electrolytes.
    - Renal panel (chlorates).
    - Potassium (barium, chlorates).
- Urinalysis: hemoglobinuria (chlorates).
- Blood gases (barium).
- ECG: QRS or QTc interval changes (barium).
- Special tests: contact lab for most appropriate sample and volume required.
- Chlorate levels: blood or urine.

Pathological Findings

- Chocolate-colored blood and tissues (methemoglobinemia), dark kidneys, renal tubular necrosis (chlorates).
- Oral, esophageal, GI ulcers (corrosive salts).

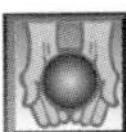

THERAPEUTICS

- Objectives of treatment include decontamination if asymptomatic, administration of an antidote (if appropriate), and supportive care.
- With firework ingestion, it is common that the exact composition is unknown and treatment is tailored to the clinical signs.

Detoxification

- Emesis if asymptomatic and only if noncorrosive agents were ingested.
- Dilution with milk or water with corrosive agents.
- Gastric lavage: only if noncorrosive agents ingested and large amount of material.
- Barium: magnesium sulfate will precipitate barium in the GI tract and prevent further absorption.
- Chlorates: mineral oil gastric lavage may prevent further GI absorption of chlorates and help speed unabsorbed chlorate through the intestinal tract. It may be mixed with 1% sodium thiosulfate for increased efficacy.

Appropriate Health Care

- Intravenous fluids to maintain normal blood pressure and urine production.

Drugs and Antidotes of Choice

- Oxygen if cyanotic.
- Saline diuresis to increase excretion (barium).
- Silver sulfadiazine topically for burns.

- Gastroprotectants.
  - Sucralfate (0.25–1 g PO q 6–8 hours) for gastric irritation (corrosive salts).
  - Famotidine (0.5–1 mg/kg PO, SQ, IM, IV q 12–24 hours) or other H_2 blocker for gastric irritation (corrosive salts).
  - Omeprazole (0.5–1 mg/kg PO q 24 hours) or other proton pump inhibitor.
- Sodium bicarbonate (1–2 mEq/kg IV, titrate up as needed) to shift potassium intracellularly (chlorates).
- Potassium chloride (do not exceed 0.5 mEq/kg/hour IV) to correct hypokalemia, cardiac arrhythmias and diarrhea (barium).
- Methylene blue (10 mg/kg IV, as a 2–4% solution) to convert methemoglobin to hemoglobin (chlorates).
- Sodium thiosulfate (2–5 g in 200 mL of 5% sodium bicarbonate, PO or IV) to inactivate chlorate ions.

Precautions/Interactions

- Activated charcoal does not bind to chlorate or heavy metals and, with the risk of aspiration, it should be avoided. Activated charcoal should also not be given if corrosive agents were ingested.

Alternative Drugs

- Ascorbic acid (10–20 mg/kg IV, SQ, PO q 4 hours) to aid in the conversion of methemoglobin to hemoglobin (chlorates).

Diet

- NPO while symptomatic; may need an esophagostomy or gastrostomy tube if severe oral or esophageal burns are evident.

Activity

- Cage rest while symptomatic.

COMMENTS

Patient Monitoring

- Monitor SPO_2 to evaluate oxygenation (initially, monitor continuously).
- Liver and renal function – baseline, 24, 48, and 72 hours.
- Urine output – daily.

Expected Course and Prognosis

- Most animals will recover within 24–72 hours with supportive care. Barium and chlorate ingestion carries a more guarded prognosis.

See Also

Metallic Toxicants (Appendix 3)
Iron
Smoke Inhalation
Zinc

Abbreviations

See Appendix 1 for a complete list.

HGE = hemorrhagic gastroenteritis
LD_{50} = median lethal dose
LD_{LO} = lowest lethal dose

Suggested Reading

DiBartola SP. Fluid Therapy in Small Animal Practice, 2nd edn. New York: W.B. Saunders, 2000.
Gahagan P, Wismer T. Toxicology of explosives and fireworks in small animals. Vet Clin North Am Small Anim Pract 2012; 42(2):361–373.
Sheahan BJ, Pugh DM, Winstanley EW. Experimental sodium chlorate poisoning in dogs. Res Vet Sci 1971; 12:387–389.

Author: Tina Wismer, DVM, DABVT, DABT, MS
Consulting Editor: Ahna G. Brutlag, DVM, MS, DABT, DABVT

chapter 85

Mothballs

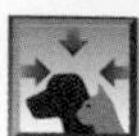

DEFINITION/OVERVIEW

- Moth repellants are composed of two major toxic ingredients: naphthalene or paradichlorobenzene (PDB). Camphor is also used in some countries.
- Moth repellants are sold as flakes, crystals, cakes, scales, powder, cubes, and spheres ("mothballs").
- Naphthalene is a dry, white, solid crystalline material with a classic "mothball odor."
  - Historically, naphthalene has been used as an antiseptic, expectorant, anthelmintic and insecticide (in dusting powders), and as a treatment for intestinal and dermal diseases.
- PDB is an organochlorine insecticide.
  - Found in deodorizers for diaper pails, urinals, and bathrooms.
  - PDB is considered less toxic than naphthalene.
- Routes of exposure include inhalation, ingestion, and transdermal absorption.
- Mothballs may take several days to completely dissolve in the GIT.
- GI signs are most common.
- Hepatic, renal, and neurological signs have also been reported.

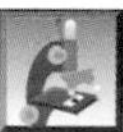

ETIOLOGY/PATHOPHYSIOLOGY

- Ingestion, inhalation, and dermal contact with mothballs can lead to toxicity.
- Majority of cases are due to ingestion.

Mechanism of Action

- Depletes cellular glutathione, impeding ability to counteract oxidative damage.
- GI, dermal, and ocular effects are likely secondary to irritant properties.

Blackwell's Five-Minute Veterinary Consult Clinical Companion: Small Animal Toxicology, Second Edition.
Lynn R. Hovda, Ahna G. Brutlag, Robert H. Poppenga, and Katherine L. Peterson.

Companion website: www.fiveminutevet.com/toxicology

Pharmacokinetics – Absorption, Distribution, Metabolism, Excretion

- Absorption.
  - Readily soluble in oils and fats. Dermal absorption is increased if oils/lotions have been applied or if ingested with fatty meals.
  - Rapid uptake by the lungs with inhalational exposure.
  - GI absorption can be delayed as mothballs may be slow to dissolve in the GIT.
- Distribution.
  - Greatest affinity for adipose tissue. High concentrations also found in lungs, kidneys, and liver.
  - Can enter placental blood supply and affect the fetus.
- Metabolism.
  - Naphthalene is metabolized in the liver by microsomal P450 enzymes and conjugated to glutathione, glucuronide, sulfate, or mercapturate.
  - PDB's major metabolite is 2,5-dichlorophenol, which can cause oxidative damage to liver, kidneys, lungs, and CNS. PDB is oxidized to phenolic compounds prior to conjugation with sulfate and glucuronide.
  - Detoxification depends on glucuronide conjugation in the liver.
  - Glutathione depletion may result secondary to oxidative damage.
  - Metabolite oxidation of Hb to MetHb. Results in Heinz body formation and erythrolysis.
- Excretion.
  - Excreted almost exclusively via the kidneys (up to 91–97%). PDB is eliminated via the urine in 5 days.
  - Small amounts may be eliminated in bile/stool and breast milk.
  - Half-life of naphthalene in guinea pig blood is 10.4 hours and decay is biphasic in other tissues.

Toxicity

- PDB is less toxic than naphthalene (approximately by one-half).
- PDB.
  - Rat oral LD_{50} = 3.8 g/kg.
  - Dogs ingesting 1.5 g/kg developed no clinical signs.
  - Rats receiving 770–1200 mg/kg for 5 days showed CNS signs.
- Naphthalene.
  - Rat oral LD_{50} = 1.8 g/kg.
  - Hemolytic anemia reported in 1 dog from single 1.525 g/kg dose.
  - Hemolytic anemia reported in 1 dog from 263 mg/kg/day over 7 days.
  - Lowest reported canine oral lethal dose = 400 mg/kg.
- Mothballs typically weigh 2.7– 4 g; rarely 5 g/mothball.

Systems Affected

- Gastrointestinal – vomiting, diarrhea due to irritant properties.
- Neuromuscular – CNS stimulation followed by depression (with PDB).

- Hemic/lymphatic/immune – oxidation of Hb to MetHb; depletion of glutathione.
- Hepatobiliary – direct injury via oxidative damage; secondary to hemolysis or metabolism of toxin.
- Respiratory – cellular damage via direct inhalation or secondary to anemia.
- Skin – local irritation if absorbed/contacted.
- Renal – primary or secondary damage, likely secondary to hemolysis. With chronic toxicity of PDB, kidney is primary organ injured.
- Ophthalmic – metabolized in the lens causing free radical damage.
- Cardiovascular – secondary to hematological effects/hemorrhagic shock.

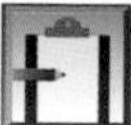

SIGNALMENT/HISTORY

Risk Factors

- Cats may be more sensitive to toxic effects based on metabolism (glucuronidation).
- There is no known breed, age, or sex predilection.

Historical Findings

- Witnessed ingestion, inhalation or contact with substance.
- Discovery of ingested material in the emesis.
- Mothball-scented breath.
- Owner may notice signs of toxicity from mothballs, including vomiting, lethargy, trembling, depression, weakness, anorexia, seizures.

Location and Circumstances of Poisoning

- Exposure will often occur in the home or yard (some people may use mothballs to repel outdoor pests).
- Not confined to mothballs – active ingredients are found in cake deodorizers used in diaper pails, urinals, and bathrooms.
- Pet owner may find cat playing with mothballs.

Interactions with Drugs, Nutrients, or Environment

- GI and dermal absorption is enhanced by fat, oil, or lotion.

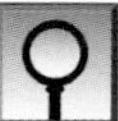

CLINICAL FEATURES

- Clinical signs typically begin within minutes to hours of exposure.
- Duration of signs is based on effect and dose (may last for days).
- GI – dehydration, nausea/hypersalivation, anorexia, vomiting, abdominal pain.
- CNS – depression, trembling, tremors, ataxia, seizures, stimulation.

- Cardiovascular – mucous membrane pallor/icterus/brown discoloration, tachypnea, tachycardia, weakness, hypotension.
- Respiratory – tachypnea, dyspnea, hypoxemia.
- Integument – dermal abrasions/irritation if contacted, jaundice.

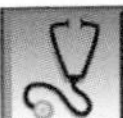

DIFFERENTIAL DIAGNOSIS

- Gastrointestinal signs.
  - Primary GI diseases.
  - Secondary GI disease.
  - Toxicities – NSAIDs, aspirin, iron, soaps/detergents, etc.
- Neurological signs.
  - Primary CNS disease – inflammatory, infectious, neoplasia, epilepsy.
- Anemia.
  - Blood loss – melena, neoplasia, coagulopathy, DIC, cavital bleed, anticoagulant rodenticide toxicity.
  - Lack of production – bone marrow disease, aplastic anemia, drug/toxin.
  - Destruction – immune- and nonimmune-mediated disease/causes for hemolysis, zinc toxicity, toxins such as zinc, acetaminophen, Heinz body anemia.
- Primary metabolic disease – renal, hepatic, hypoadrenocorticism, hypoglycemia; other hepatic toxicities – acetaminophen, *Amanita* mushroom, blue-green algae (cyanobacteria), xylitol.
- Dermatological signs.
  - Infectious – pyoderma, insect/arthropod bite, parasitic.
  - Inflammatory – drug eruption/reaction, vasculitis.
- Other – sunburn, thermal burn, contact dermatitis.

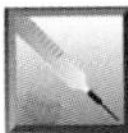

DIAGNOSTICS

- To help differentiate naphthalene from PBD mothballs, float mothballs in plain water and a saturated salt solution.
  - To make a saturated salt solution, mix 4 ounces tepid water with 3 heaping tablespoons of table salt. Stir vigorously (at least 45 seconds) until salt will not dissolve further.
  - Naphthalene mothballs sink in water and float in salt solution.
  - PDB mothballs sink in both.
  - Camphor sinks in both.
- Alternative method to differentiate naphthalene from PBD mothballs.
  - Using 100 mL of 50% dextrose – naphthalene floats, PDB sinks.
- CBC – anemia, Heinz bodies, evidence of hemolysis.
- Chemistry – azotemia, liver enzyme elevation, hyperbilirubinemia.
- Venous blood gas analysis – metabolic acidosis, electrolyte abnormalities from vomiting.

- Urinalysis – pigmenturia, hemoglobinuria, isosthenuria if underlying renal injury.
  - Urine can be submitted to a laboratory for isolation of naphthalene and metabolites using TLC or HPLC and identification using GC-MS.
- Radiographs – PDB mothballs are densely radiopaque; naphthalene mothballs are radiolucent or faintly radiopaque.

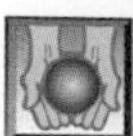

THERAPEUTICS

Detoxification

- Stabilize symptomatic animals prior to decontamination.
- Induce emesis in asymptomatic patients (due to slow dissolution, emesis may be effective many hours after ingestion).
- Emesis is contraindicated in animals exhibiting CNS signs (i.e., depression, ataxia, tremors, seizures).
- Gastric lavage if emesis is nonproductive or in cases of massive ingestions.
- Activated charcoal with a cathartic may be given once within 24 hours of ingestion.
- Decontaminate dermal exposures by bathing the area (see chapter 1, Decontamination and Detoxification of the Poisoned Patient).
- Irrigate exposed eyes with isotonic saline or water for 10–15 minutes.
- Animals exposed to naphthalene fumes should be removed from the source of exposure.

Appropriate Health Care

- Immediate patient assessment and stabilization are extremely important.
- Treatments are supportive and symptomatic, based upon the clinical signs of the patient.
- Dyspneic patients should receive supplemental oxygen if needed.
- Patients with signs of hemorrhagic shock (i.e., hypotension, tachycardia, anemia, severe hemolysis or MetHg) should be volume resuscitated and transfused, if needed.

Drugs and Antidotes of Choice

- IV fluid therapy with a balanced, isotonic crystalloid should be used for all symptomatic animals.
- GI signs may be treated with the following.
  - Antiemetics.
    - Maropitant 1 mg/kg, SQ q 24 hours.
    - Metoclopramide 0.2–0.5 mg/kg, PO, IM, SQ q 8 hours; 1–2 mg/kg/day CRI IV.
  - Sucralfate 0.25–1 g, PO q 8 hours.
  - H_2 antagonist (e.g., famotidine 0.5–1.0 mg/kg, PO, SQ, IM, or IV q 12–24 hours).
  - Proton pump inhibitor (e.g., omeprazaole, 0.5–1.0 mg/kg PO q 24 hours in dogs and 0.7 mg/kg, PO q 24 hours in cats).
- Anticonvulsant therapy.
  - Diazepam, 0.5–1 mg/kg, IV to effect.

    - Phenobarbital 4 mg/kg, IV q 4–6 hours × 4 doses. Use higher doses if needed. If refractory, may add diazepam CRI IV at 0.25–0.5 mg/kg/hour.
- MetHb can be treated with ascorbic acid and/or methylene blue.
    - Ascorbic acid reduces MetHb to Hb, but is a slow conversion.
        - □ 20 mg/kg, PO, IM, SQ q 6 hours.
    - Methylene blue converts to leukomethylene blue to rapidly reduce MetHb to Hb.
        - □ Dogs – 1–4 mg/kg IV, slow infusion given once.
        - □ Cats – 1–1.5 mg/kg IV, slow infusion given once. This drug can also cause Heinz body anemia in cats so should be used cautiously.

Precautions/Interactions

- Methylene blue can induce further MetHb.
- Cats are at greater risk for adverse effects from methylene blue.

Alternative Drugs

- N-acetylcysteine (NAC) may be useful to maintain glutathione and sulfate concentrations.
    - 10% or 20% solutions should be diluted to a 5% solution prior to IV administration.
    - Initial loading dose of 140 mg/kg, then 70 mg/kg PO every 6 hours for 7–17 treatments.
    - Oral formation may be given IV (off-label) slowly over 15–20 minutes through a 0.2 micron, bacteriostatic filter.
- S-adenosyl-methionine (SAMe), 18–20 mg/kg, PO q 24 hours on an empty stomach, may help with glutathione production and maintenance.

Nursing Care

- Proper monitoring and nursing care should be provided accordingly as it pertains to symptoms of each patient (TPR, oxygenation).
- Patients with CNS depression and/or sedated from anticonvulsants should have appropriate nursing care and be monitored carefully.

Follow-up

- CBC and chemistry values should be monitored to ensure return to normal.

COMMENTS

Client Education

- Clients should be made aware of the potential for mothball toxicity and advised to use them in secure locations in/around the home/yard.

Patient Monitoring

- PCV should be assessed minimum twice daily in anemic patients.
- Hepatic and/or renal values should be monitored daily in affected patients.
- Blood assessment for resolving MetHb or presence of hemolysis as needed.

Expected Course and Prognosis

- Good, provided treatment is initiated early and no underlying hepatic or renal impairment.

See Also

Essential Oils/Liquid Potpourri
Phenols and Pine Oils

Abbreviations

See Appendix 1 for a complete list.

Hb = hemoglobin
MetHb = methemoglobin
NAC = N-acetylcysteine
PDB = paradichlorobenzene

Suggested Reading

DeClementi C. Moth repellant toxicosis. Vet Med 2005; 100:24.

Desnoyers M, Hebert P. Heinz body anemia in a dog following naphthalene ingestion. Vet Clin Path 1995; 24(4):124–125.

Gwaltney-Brant SM. Miscellaneous indoor toxicants. In: Peterson ME, Talcott PA, eds. Small Animal Toxicology, 3rd edn. St Louis, MO: Saunders, 2013; p. 304.

Tang KY, Chan CK, Lau FL. Dextrose 50% as a better substitute for saturated salt solution in mothball float test. Clin Toxicol 2010; 48:750–751.

Author: Seth L. Cohen, DVM
Consulting Editor: Ahna G. Brutlag, DVM, MS, DABT, DABVT

chapter 86

Paintballs

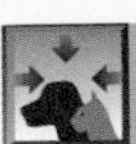

DEFINITION/OVERVIEW

- Paintball toxicosis in dogs and, rarely, cats and ferrets is uncommon. While the ingredients within paintballs are technically nontoxic, the components are osmotically active which can draw free water into the GIT, causing diarrhea and electrolyte abnormalities.
- Common components of paintballs include glycerol, glycerin, polyethylene glycol (PEG), sorbitol, gelatin, propylene glycol, wax, mineral oil, and dye. The exact ingredients vary by manufacturer.
- Common clinical signs include vomiting, diarrhea, ataxia, and tremors.
- Treatment includes decontamination of the GIT, management of hypernatremia and neurological complications, and supportive care.
- Though clinical reports detailing paintball toxicosis are very limited in veterinary medicine, the prognosis appears to be good with appropriate supportive care and monitoring.

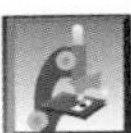

ETIOLOGY/PATHOPHYSIOLOGY

Mechanism of Action

- The ingredients in paintballs are nontoxic (see Definition/Overview).
- After the paintballs are ingested, the osmotically active ingredients (e.g., sorbitol, glycerol, propylene glycol, and PEG) draw water from the interstitial fluid compartment into the GIT. The result is an overall loss of free water, which causes increase in plasma osmolality and hypernatremia. Neurological effects are secondary changes in osmolality and serum sodium concentrations due to loss of water from the CNS tissues.
- Large volumes of free water within the GIT, in addition to the osmotically active ingredients of the paintballs themselves, can cause vomiting and diarrhea.

Blackwell's Five-Minute Veterinary Consult Clinical Companion: Small Animal Toxicology, Second Edition.
Lynn R. Hovda, Ahna G. Brutlag, Robert H. Poppenga, and Katherine L. Peterson.

Companion website: www.fiveminutevet.com/toxicology

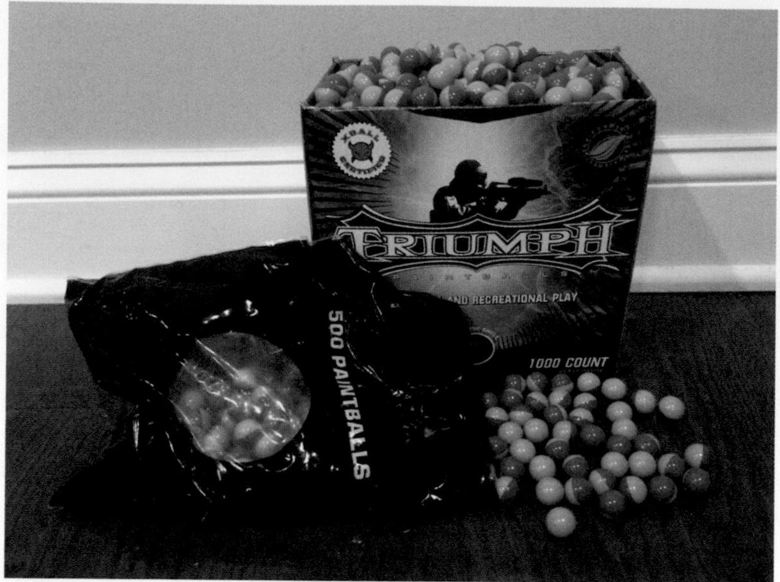

■ **Fig. 86.1.** An example of commercially available paintballs, size and appearance, and original packaging.

Pharmacokinetics – Absorption, Distribution, Metabolism, Excretion

- The osmotically active ingredients within paintballs remain in the GIT until the patient vomits or they are excreted through the feces. They are not absorbed from the GIT or metabolized by other organs.

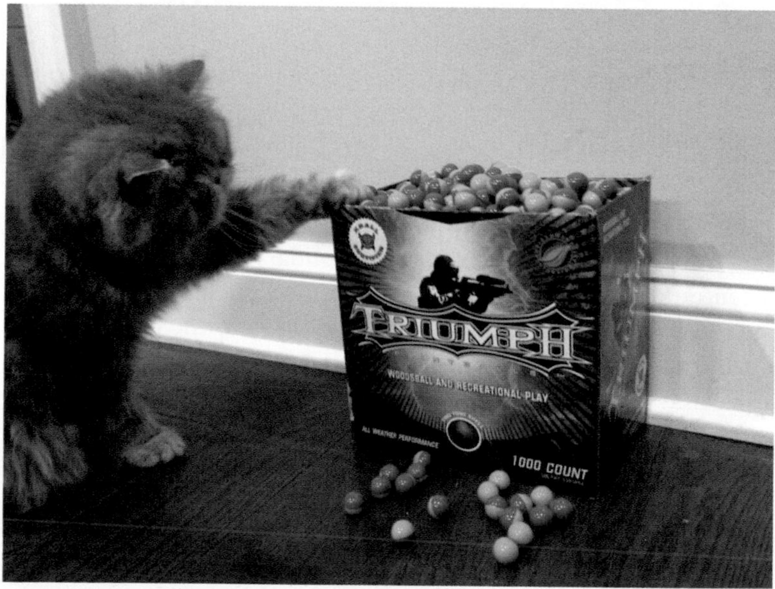

■ **Fig. 86.2.** The author's own cat, who was very interested in playing with the paintballs being photographed.

Toxicity

- None of the commonly used components of paintballs are toxic. Toxicosis is a secondary complication that results from the fluid and electrolyte shifts due to the osmotically active nature of many of the ingredients used.
- As few as 5–10 paintballs have caused symptoms in a 30 kg dog.

Systems Affected

- Gastrointestinal.
  - Direct irritation of the esophageal or gastric mucosa may cause vomiting.
  - Free water movement into the stomach (with secondary fluid distension of the stomach) and intestines may result in vomiting and diarrhea.
  - Polydipsia may occur as a consequence of hypernatremia and stimulation of central osmoreceptors.
- Nervous.
  - Movement of free water into the GIT leads to increased serum osmolality via hypernatremia and hyperchloremia.
  - Acute increases in serum sodium result in increased serum osmolality, which causes dehydration, free water shifts, and eventually leads to cerebral cellular dehydration and cell shrinkage. Cerebral and meningeal vessels may tear with cellular shrinkage and lead to cerebral and subarachnoid hemorrhage, which may exacerbate neurological signs.
- Renal/urological.
  - Prerenal azotemia secondary to dehydration may result.
- Endocrine/metabolic.
  - Antidiuretic hormone (ADH) may be released secondary to significant free water shifts/loss.
  - Metabolic acidosis can result from hyperchloremia (secondary to free water loss), bicarbonate loss through diarrhea, prerenal azotemia, and lactic acidosis if perfusion is compromised.
- Cardiovascular.
  - Hypovolemia may occur secondary to significant fluid losses, resulting in tachycardia (compensatory), decreased pulse quality, poor perfusion, and hypotension.
- Neuromuscular.
  - Weakness may occur secondary to electrolyte imbalances, dehydration, hypovolemia, and neurological impairment.
- Ophthalmic.
  - Cerebral cellular shrinkage may cause central blindness.

SIGNALMENT/HISTORY

- There are no breed, sex, or age predilections.
- Paintball toxicosis has been reported in dogs, cats, and ferrets; however, dogs represent the majority of animals affected.

- No mean age has been reported. Younger animals are more frequently affected due to their increased incidence of ingesting foreign objects (Fig. 86.2).

Risk Factors

- Animals living in homes or areas where paintballs are stored.
- Animals that have access to outdoor areas where paintballs are fired.
- Animals with underlying diseases that cause increased water loss (such as renal, metabolic, or gastrointestinal disease) could be at increased risk of more severe consequences with paintball ingestion.

Historical Findings

- Witnessed ingestion.
- Discovery of damaged/chewed packaging or spilled paintballs.
- Owners may see paint on the pet's coat or face and may witness vomiting (which may or may not contain paint or paintball pieces), diarrhea (+/- paint), and CNS changes.

Location and Circumstances of Poisoning

- Pets with access to paintballs, either indoors or outdoors, are those that could ingest these objects.

CLINICAL FEATURES

- The onset of clinical signs can occur quickly (within 1 hour) due to rapid shifting of free water from the interstitial space into the GIT.
- The severity of clinical signs is dependent upon the number of paintballs consumed and any underlying disease process predisposing to fluid loss (see earlier). Since packages may contain up to 2000 paintballs and the exact amount ingested is often unknown, it can be difficult to predict the severity of signs that will result (Fig. 86.1).
  - Gastrointestinal – hypersalivation, vomiting, diarrhea, gastric distension.
  - Renal/urological – polydipsia, polyuria.
  - Nervous – depression, ataxia, stupor, coma, hyperexcitability, seizures.
  - Cardiovascular – tachycardia, poor pulse quality, hypotension.
  - Neuromuscular – weakness.
  - Ophthalmic – central blindness.
  - Skin/exocrine – paint on the skin or haircoat.

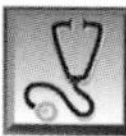

DIFFERENTIAL DIAGNOSIS

- Diabetes insipidus.
- Salt toxicosis (e.g., sea water ingestion, homemade play dough, salt emetic).

- Ethanol ingestion.
- Ethylene glycol toxicosis.
    - The early clinical signs of ethylene glycol toxicosis are similar to those seen with paintball toxicosis. In addition, several common paintball components, including sorbitol, glycerol, and propylene glycol, can react with the chemicals used in blood ethylene glycol tests to produce false-positive results. For more information on ethylene glycol toxicosis, see chapter 7.

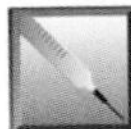

DIAGNOSTICS

- There are no specific diagnostic tests.
- Serum sodium concentration and other electrolytes should be determined at presentation and monitored frequently during treatment (q 2–4 hours during hospitalization).
- To distinguish true ethylene glycol toxicosis from other chemicals that cross-react with ethylene glycol tests, high-performance liquid chromatography is needed.

Pathological Findings

- There are no characteristic gross or histopathological lesions.
- Gross necropsy findings may include paintball paint and remnants within the alimentary tract, edema of the intestinal wall, and increased fluid content within the GIT. If hypernatremic patients have a necropsy performed prior to fluid therapy, there may be gross signs of brain shrinkage and retraction of the meninges and attachments to the calvarium. If necropsy is performed after aggressive fluid therapy for hypernatremia, there may be signs of cerebral edema such as herniation of the cerebellum or brainstem.
- Histopathology may reveal edema of the mucosa and submucosa of the GIT, cerebral cellular shrinkage, torn meninges and meningeal vessels, or cerebral cellular swelling.

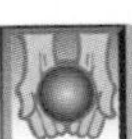

THERAPEUTICS

- Treatment includes aggressive decontamination if the patient is presented soon after ingestion, electrolyte and neurological monitoring, fluid therapy, and supportive care.
- The use of activated charcoal is contraindicated.

Detoxification

- In asymptomatic animals, emesis should be induced as quickly and as safely as possible.
- The use of activated charcoal is contraindicated (see Precautions/Interactions).
- For neurologically inappropriate patients, initial treatment should be aimed at managing neurological signs, such as seizure control. Appropriate sedation, intubation (to protect the airway), and gastric lavage should be considered. Emesis should not be induced in neurologically inappropriate patients.

- Warm water enemas (2–4 mL/kg) may be considered to help evacuate the osmotically active paintball remnants from the large intestine and to help decrease free water loss into the GIT. The frequency will depend on the patient's serum sodium concentration and clinical signs. Given the large absorptive capacity of the colon for water, the enemas may provide an additional source of free water. However, it is important to continue to closely monitor serum sodium concentrations since colonic absorption may be unpredictable, resulting in rapid sodium concentration changes.

Appropriate Health Care

- Acute hypernatremia (<18 hours) may be treated aggressively to normalize the sodium level, and sodium levels can be dropped relatively quickly with IV fluids with *acute* toxicosis.
- Chronic hypernatremia (>18 hours) must be treated slowly and sodium should not be altered more than 0.5 mEq/L per hour (12 mE/L per day).
- Serum electrolytes (e.g., sodium, potassium, chloride), PCV/TS, and blood glucose should be obtained at presentation and monitored at least every 2–4 hours initially, depending on the extent of electrolyte derangements. Once electrolyte derangements have stabilized, monitor every 4–6 hours.
- Aggressive fluid therapy may be necessary, given the large volumes of free water that may be lost into the GIT. Careful monitoring of hydration parameters (e.g., patient weight, physical exam, UOP, urine specific gravity, PCV/TS) should be performed.
- When managing hypernatremia, the chronicity or duration of time for which the electrolyte was increased is imperative information. If this information cannot be ascertained from the patient's history and clinical course, hypernatremia must be assumed to be chronic and therefore treated as such (slowly).
    - For patients with both acute and chronic hypernatremia that require fluid boluses, 0.9% NaCl should be used, as this isotonic crystalloid will have the least impact on serum sodium concentration when compared with other crystalloids. Hypertonic saline (7.5%) should be avoided for the management of hypovolemia, as this will perpetuate interstitial dehydration and hypernatremia. Hypovolemia should be treated prior to attempting to safely manage dehydration and hypernatremia.
    - For patients with **chronic** (>18 hour) duration of hypernatremia, serum sodium should be decreased by no more than 0.5 mEq/L/hour, due to the presence of idiogenic osmoles and their ability to osmotically draw fluid into cerebral cells. The isotonic crystalloid's sodium content should be selected so that it is closest to the patient's current serum sodium concentration.
    - Once hydration is restored, D5W (5% dextrose in sterile water) or 0.45% NaCl may be used to provide free water to compensate for GIT losses and manage hypernatremia. This therapy should be used with caution in patients with chronic or unknown duration of hypernatremia, as rapid decreases in serum sodium concentration may result. D5W and 0.45% NaCl are hypotonic fluids and should **never** be administered as a bolus.
    - Serum sodium levels should be monitored every 2–4 hours to ensure safe, gradual decreases in serum sodium concentration.

  - For patients with chronic hypernatremia who have a rapid decrease in serum sodium and develop signs of depressed mentation, decreased PLR, decreased responsiveness, or seizures, cerebral edema should be suspected and treated appropriately.
  - For patients with **acute** (<18 hour) duration of hypernatremia, serum sodium concentration can be decreased more rapidly, as idiogenic osmoles will not yet have formed and there is little risk of cerebral edema developing secondary to changes in serum sodium concentration.
- For patients that develop seizures secondary to fluid shifts from paintball toxicosis, as well as iatrogenically from fluid therapy and rapid serum sodium concentration decrease, seizures should be controlled with diazepam (0.5–1 mg/kg IV) or midazolam (0.2–0.5 mg/kg IV). Mannitol (0.25–2g/kg) may be considered for management of cerebral edema but should be used with caution due to concerns for worsening of free water losses via osmotic diuresis.
- Seizures must be aggressively controlled to prevent cerebral edema, noncardiogenic pulmonary edema, and aspiration of GIT contents. Any patient for whom the ability to protect their airway is questionable should be intubated.
- In neurologically impaired patients, serum potassium and blood glucose should be monitored and appropriately supplemented as needed. Hyperglycemia should be avoided.
- Antiemetic therapy should be used in any nauseated or vomiting patient to prevent further fluid losses, electrolyte derangements, and to decrease the risk of aspiration pneumonia. Options for antiemetic therapy include:
  - Ondansetron 0.1–0.2 mg/kg IV q 8–12 hours
  - Dolasetron 0.6–1 mg/kg IV/SQ q 24 hours
  - Metoclopramide CRI 1–2 mg/kg/day
  - Maropitant 1.0 mg/kg IV/SQ q 24 hours.

Drugs and Antidotes of Choice

- There are no specific antidotes for paintball toxicosis.
- If there is any concern that a patient's neurological signs could be secondary to ethylene glycol ingestion, then treatment for this fatal toxicosis must take priority. See chapter 7 for specific information on the treatment and management of patients with ethylene glycol toxicosis.

Precautions/Interactions

- Treatment with activated charcoal with a cathartic, such as sorbitol, is contraindicated, as the cathartic will exacerbate fluid flux into the GIT and could further contribute to hypernatremia.
- Since none of the components of paintballs are themselves toxic, administration of activated charcoal is of little value, especially in patients with altered mentation or neurological status, which have an increased risk of aspiration.
- Warm water enemas are contraindicated in patients with chronic hypernatremia due to unpredictability of rate of water absorption and changes in serum sodium concentration.

Nursing Care

- Intensive nursing care and neurological monitoring should be performed every 2–4 hours.
- Care for recumbent patients should be provided, including frequent turning, passive range of motion, bladder and colon care, and eye and oral care.
- For patients with seizures and concerns for cerebral edema, a board under the head and neck, positioned at a 15–30° angle, should be used to help decrease intracranial pressure. Compression of the jugular veins (especially for venipuncture), sneezing, coughing, and hyperthermia should be avoided in such patients. Mannitol (0.25–2 g/kg, IV, to effect) can also be considered but may contribute to hyperosmolality and should be used judiciously.

Follow-up

- It is likely that follow-up care and monitoring will not be necessary after discharge, provided the sodium levels have normalized and the patient's neurological signs have stabilized.

Diet

- For patients with neurological compromise, vomiting, regurgitation, or those that are sedated, oral food and water should be withheld until the patient is neurologically appropriate and GIT signs have resolved.
- Due to gastric irritation from vomiting, a bland diet should be implemented for 3–5 days before gradual transition back to the normal diet over another 3–5 days.

Activity

- Activity restriction is not necessary, as the patient's neurological status will likely determine its activity level.

Prevention/Avoidance

- Proper storage of paintballs in an area inaccessible to pets will help prevent exposure. Those involved with paintball sports should be advised of the risks to pets, and pets should not be allowed access to areas where paintball games are played. Any paintball remnants in the environment should be disposed of properly.

COMMENTS

Client Education

- Clients should be educated on the mechanism of action of paintball toxicosis, as well as being given recommendations for safe storage and use.
- Information about the gradual reintroduction of a bland diet, monitoring for ongoing GIT and neurological signs, and general observation instructions should be provided to the client upon discharge.

Patient Monitoring

- See Appropriate Health Care.

Possible Complications

- In most patients, a full recovery is made after appropriate monitoring and supportive care.

Expected Course and Prognosis

- Since a toxic dose of ingested paintballs is not known, every exposure should be managed aggressively.
- Between 2012 and mid-2015, Pet Poison Helpline and the ASPCA Animal Poison Control Center received nearly 700 calls for paintball ingestion by dogs, cats, and ferrets. Euthanasia or death was uncommon. For the vast majority of pets exposed, complete recovery often occurred within 24 hours. The overall prognosis for paintball toxicosis is good to excellent with appropriate monitoring and treatment.

Synonyms

- Paintball ingestion, paintball toxicity, paintball toxicosis

See Also

Diuretics
Ethylene Glycol and Diethylene Glycol

Abbreviations

See Appendix 1 for a complete list.

ADH = antidiuretic hormone
D5W = dextrose in water
PEG = polyethylene glycol

Suggested Reading

DiBartola SP. Disorders of sodium and water: hypernatremia and hyponatremia. In: DiBartola SP, ed. Fluid, Electrolyte, and Acid-Base Disorders in Small Animal Practice, 4th edn. St Louis, MO: Elsevier, 2012.
Donaldson CW. Paintball toxicosis in dogs. Vet Med 2003; 98(12):995–998.
Howard J. Paintball toxicosis. Vet Tech 2007; 28(5):336–337, 340.
King JB, Grant DC. Paintball intoxication in a pug. J Vet Emerg Crit Care 2007; 17(3):290–293.

Acknowledgment: The authors and editors acknowledge the prior contributions of Justine A. Lee, DVM, DACVECC, DABT, who co-authored this topic in the previous edition.
Author: Dana L. Clarke, VMD, DACVCC
Contributing Editor: Ahna G. Brutlag, DVM, MS, DABT, DABVT

chapter 87 Phenols and Pine Oils

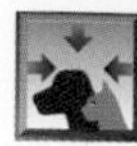 DEFINITION/OVERVIEW

- Phenol, phenolic compounds, and pine oil are used in household cleaning products, disinfectants, medicated shampoos, scents, and, rarely, insecticides.
- **Phenol** is an aromatic alcohol originally derived from coal tar.
  - Phenols are highly corrosive in all species and can cause neurological, renal, and liver disease.
- **Phenolic derivatives** include creosote, creosol, hexachlorophene (Phisohex), phenylphenol, chlorophenol, dinitrophenol, alkyl phenols, phenolic resins and epoxy (bisphenol A), and others (see Synonyms).
  - Phenolic disinfectants may contain chlorophenols (3–8%), phenyl phenol (2–10%) or pure phenol (20–50%).
  - Phenolic derivatives are generally less corrosive than phenol.
- **Pine oil** is an essential oil derived from pine trees. Pine oil contains alpha-terpineol, terpene ethers, and phenolic compounds.
  - Pine Sol, a popular home cleaning product, contains up to 20% pine oil.
  - Pine oil is a gastric irritant for most species, but when ingested in large amounts, in high concentrations, or by cats, it can cause GI signs followed by changes in mentation, respiratory depression, ataxia, anemia, and nephritis.
- Cats are very sensitive to these chemicals due to their limited glucuronide transferase activity and develop toxicosis at lower doses than dogs.
- Toxicosis can follow all routes of exposure (dermal, inhalation, ingestion, etc.).

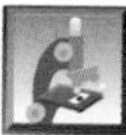 ETIOLOGY/PATHOPHYSIOLOGY

Mechanism of Action

- **Pine oils** are a direct irritant to the mucous membranes. The mode of action is poorly understood.
- **Phenols** are corrosive to the skin and mucous membranes. The true mode of action is unknown, but theories include a cardiac sodium channel blockade, a direct toxic effect

Blackwell's Five-Minute Veterinary Consult Clinical Companion: Small Animal Toxicology, Second Edition.
Lynn R. Hovda, Ahna G. Brutlag, Robert H. Poppenga, and Katherine L. Peterson.

Companion website: www.fiveminutevet.com/toxicology

on the CNS and the myocardium, or CNS stimulation from an increased acetylcholine release.

- **Phenolic derivatives** have a similar MOA as phenols but are less corrosive.

Pharmacokinetics – Absorption, Distribution, Metabolism, Excretion

- Pine oil.
  - Dermal and GIT absorption occurs (extent varies).
  - Well distributed with highest concentrations in the brain, lungs, and kidneys.
  - Metabolized via epoxide pathway, then oxidized in the liver by cytochrome P450 and conjugated with glucuronic acid.
  - Excreted in the urine.
- Phenol and phenolic derivatives.
  - Rapidly absorbed following oral, dermal, or inhalation exposures. Absorption begins within 5 minutes and is complete within a few hours.
  - Distributed to all tissues with peak concentration within 1 hour of ingestion and 6–10 hours of dermal exposure. The highest concentrations are found in the liver.
  - Metabolized by glucuronyl- and sulfotransferases. The metabolites are excreted via the kidneys in 24–72 hours.

Toxicity

- Toxicity is dependent upon the concentration, the volume ingested/applied, and the amount of exposed body surface area.
- Cats are more sensitive than dogs (limited glucuronide transferase activity).
- Pine oil.
  - LD_{50} = 1–2.5 mL/kg.
  - Severe toxicosis develops at much lower doses.
  - One cat ingesting 100 mL of undiluted Pine Sol died within 12 hours.
  - 0.5 oz of pure oil fatal in a child; 8 oz fatal in an adult human being (ingestion).
- Phenol.
  - Cat LD_{50} (unknown route) = 80 mg/kg.
  - Dog LD_{50} (oral) = 500 mg/kg.
  - Mouse and rat LD_{50} (oral) = 270–317 mg/kg.
  - Rat LD_{50} (dermal) = 669 mg/kg.
  - Concentrations 1–5%: expect tissue irritation. May result in dermal burns.
  - Concentrations 5–10%: dermal burns possible. May result in oral/GI burns.
  - Concentrations >10%: expect corrosive damage to all tissues.
- Hexachlorophene.
  - Concentrations above 3% can cause severe dermal damage.
  - Rat and mouse LD_{50} (oral) = 56–67 mg/kg.
  - Mice LD_{50} (dermal) = 270 mg/kg.
  - Rate LD_{50} (dermal) = 1840 mg/kg.

Systems Affected

- Gastrointestinal – irritation at low concentration and ulcerations at high concentrations. Salivation, emesis, diarrhea, laryngeal edema, and esophageal strictures may result.
- Skin/exocrine – deep caustic burns to the dermis with prolonged exposure. Burns may not be painful initially due to local anesthetic properties of some phenols.
- Nervous – ataxia, tremors, CNS stimulation or depression, seizures, or coma.
- Hepatobiliary – hepatic failure as early as 12 hours post exposure.
- Renal – renal failure as early as 12 hours post exposure.
- Respiratory – respiratory depression and panting (in dogs) followed by pulmonary edema and cardiac muscle damage. Aspiration pneumonia.
- Cardiovascular – prolonged CRT with pale to muddy mucous membranes.
- Hemic – methemoglobinemia, hemoglobinemia, and Heinz body anemia (especially cats).
- Ophthalmic – ulcers with direct exposure to the cornea.

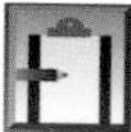

SIGNALMENT/HISTORY

Risk Factors

- Compared to dogs, cats develop toxicosis at lower doses due to their limited glucuronide transferase activity.

Historical Findings

- Witnessed ingestion of pine oil/phenol-based products (most common).
- Drooling, gagging, or emesis are typically reported by the owner.
- Chewed mop heads after phenol-based cleaners were used. (Water evaporates faster than phenols, resulting in a potentially corrosive concentration of phenols.)
- History of chewing on pine needles/cones.
- Pine oil/phenol products applied directly to pets (often by children).
- Animals enclosed in a garage/utility room without other water sources.

Location and Circumstances of Poisoning

- Exposure usually occurs within the home and is rarely intentional.

CLINICAL FEATURES

- All chemicals may create deep, penetrating ulcers.
    - Phenols have anesthetic properties that may render the injury initially painless.
- Common clinical signs following oral exposure include drooling, gagging, or vomiting.
- Inhalation may cause tissue irritation/damage leading to dyspnea, panting, and increased respiratory effort.

- CNS abnormalities may develop within 5 minutes of ingestion and 1 hour of dermal exposure.
    - Ataxia, mydriasis, muscle tremors, CNS stimulation or depression, seizures, or coma.
    - Convulsions, coma, or death are most common in the following.
        - Significant dermal exposures (>25% body surface area).
        - Exposures to highly concentrated products (see Toxicology).
- Hepatic or renal failure may develop within 12–24 hours.
- Animals that remain asymptomatic for 6 hours or more following exposure are not expected to develop clinical signs.

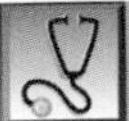

DIFFERENTIAL DIAGNOSIS

- Corrosive injury from acid or alkaline products.
- Dermal or GI exposures to other essential oils/liquid potpourri.
- Ethylene glycol toxicosis.
- Primary renal failure.

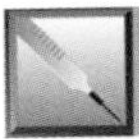

DIAGNOSTICS

- Diagnosis is usually made based on the history, an odor of the animal's breath or coat, or postmortem evaluation of the liver, kidneys, or GIT.
- A CBC, UA, chemistry panel, and acid–base analysis should be performed upon presentation and again 12–24 hours after the exposure (in symptomatic animals).
    - CBC –hemolysis, Heinz body formation, hemolytic anemia, methemoglobinemia, thrombocytopenia, and Döhle bodies in neutrophils.
    - UA – the urine may have a dark green to black discoloration from the passage of phenolic intermediates or due to methemoglobinemia, hematuria, albuminuria, and casts.
    - Chemistry panel – used to establish a baseline (liver, kidneys). Elevation of liver enzymes, BUN, and creatinine may develop 12–24 hours after exposure. The chemistry may show multiple changes such as elevations in CPK, Mg, or K.
    - Acid–base status – metabolic acidosis or a respiratory alkalosis.
- Cautious endoscopic examination of the esophagus and stomach to evaluate for ulceration or stricture.
- If ocular or respiratory exposure occurred, further diagnostics may include corneal stain/slit lamp examination, thoracic radiographs, arterial blood gas, or bronchoscopy.

Pathological Findings

- Necropsy may reveal an enlarged, congested, and friable liver with hepatocellular necrosis; severe renal proximal tubular and cortical necrosis; pulmonary edema and congestion; a hyperemic gastrointestinal tract; or edema of the cerebral cortices.

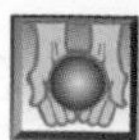

THERAPEUTICS

- The primary goals of therapy include decontamination, stabilization, correction of laboratory abnormalities, liver and kidney support, and the treatment of corrosive injury.

Detoxification

- Protect human caregivers: Gloves and other protective equipment should be worn to prevent dermal contact.
- Dermal.
    - Blot visible material.
    - Use polyethylene glycol (PEG) 300 or 400 to initially dilute and remove the product. (*Water may increase dermal absorption and is not recommended.*) Follow this by washing the animal with a mild liquid dishwashing detergent and then rinse with water.
    - If PEG is not available, isopropyl alcohol can be used on small areas. Alternatively, use liquid dishwashing detergents and copious amounts of water.
        - Lavage the skin until the smell of the product has gone away.
        - Multiple reapplications of soap and water will be needed.
        - Monitor body temperature.
- GI.
    - Do not induce emesis (risk of corrosive injury and aspiration).
    - Activated charcoal – not proven to bind pine oil but may have some benefit against phenols. It is not often recommended because of the risk of vomiting.
    - Pine oil – if the pet is presented within 1 hour of a large ingestion, gastric lavage with an inflated endotracheal tube is recommended, provided no tissue damage is present.
    - Phenol – because phenols are highly corrosive, gastric lavage could increase the risk of ulceration and stricture. The decision to lavage should be based on the amount ingested and the concentration of that product. If gastric lavage is not indicated, dilute the product with water or saline and prevent emesis.
    - Some sources recommend oral mineral oil (10 mL/kg lavage) to dilute (vs water).
- Ocular – flush the eye for 20 minutes with tepid water or saline.

Appropriate Health Care

- Stabilize.
    - If hydration or tissue perfusion is inadequate, provide a balanced electrolyte solution IV.
    - Evaluate neurological activity. For seizures, give diazepam 0.25–1 mg/kg IV or phenobarbital 2–5 mg/kg IV (increase if needed).
    - Evaluate body temperature. Slowly return to normal using standard methods.

- Address blood work abnormalities.
  - Correct acid–base imbalances. Metabolic acidosis should be alleviated with sodium bicarbonate administration if pH is less than 7.2.
  - Methemoglobinemia.
    - □ Methylene blue 1–4 mg/kg slowly IV in dogs or 1.5 mg/kg slowly IV in cats one time. Use cautiously.
    - □ Ascorbic acid 20–50 mg/kg PO in dogs or 20 mg/kg PO in cats.
- Support the liver and kidney.
  - Intravenous fluids – since metabolic acidosis is common, consider a nonacidic fluid such as saline or Normasol-R.
  - Supportive medications for the liver have been tried with varying success.
    - □ SAMe – loading dose of 40 mg/kg PO q 24 hours 2–4 days, then 20 mg/kg PO q 24 hours. Give on an empty stomach.
    - □ N-acetylcysteine – loading dose of 140 mg/kg PO or IV as a 5% solution, then 70 mg/kg q 4–6 hours.
- Treat ulcerations.
  - Topical therapy (triple antibiotic ointment or silver sulfadiazine cream) and bandaging (bandages to prevent soiling or wet to dry bandages pending severity).
  - Antibiotics for gastrointestinal or dermal lesions.
    - □ Metronidazole 15 mg/kg PO or IV q 12 hours.
    - □ Cephalexin 22 mg/kg PO q 8 hours or cefazolin 22 mg/kg IV q 8 hours.
  - GI ulcerations.
    - □ H_2 blockers (e.g., famotidine 0.5 mg/kg IV, IM, or SQ q 12 hours).
    - □ Sucralfate 0.25–1 g PO on an empty stomach q 8 hours.
  - Consider antiinflammatory therapy, but use cautiously and weigh against risk of worsening GI ulcerations.
    - □ Carprofen 2.2 mg/kg PO or SQ q 12 hours.
    - □ Prednisone 0.5 mg/kg PO or dexamethasone equivalent SQ or IV. Use is controversial.
  - Analgesia. Although these chemicals often have an initial anesthetic effect, it is short-lived, and discomfort from oral, gastric, or dermal ulceration should be controlled with opiate therapy.
    - □ Buprenorphine 0.005 mg/kg IV, IM, or SQ q 8–12 hours.
    - □ Tramadol 1–4 mg/kg PO q 8 hours.

Drug(s) and Antidotes of Choice

- No antidote exists.
- See Appropriate Health Care

Precautions/Interactions

- Methylene blue – may affect accuracy of urinalysis due to green/blue discoloration of urine. May also increase Heinz body formation. Use is controversial.

Nursing Care

- The patient must be kept clean to prevent infection of dermal ulcerations.
- Body temperature should be monitored closely, especially after bathing.

Follow-up

- Patient will require regular evaluation of skin ulcerations until healed. Recheck initial ulcerations 2–5 days after flushing, then as needed pending progression.
- Continue to recheck liver and kidney values q 24–48 hours while hospitalized or until they return to normal and the patient is stable.
- Esophageal ulcers may take weeks to heal. Also, it takes weeks to months before clinical evidence of a stricture may be noted. Repeated esophageal endoscopy is recommended to follow progress.

Diet

- NPO for up to 72 hours after ingestion if oropharyngeal damage is severe and patient can tolerate fasting. Obese cats should not be fasted for greater than 24 hours. Consider feeding a liquid diet while ulcerations heal. Consider stomach tube placement if eating is painful. Diet modification may be needed if renal or liver failure develops.

Activity

- No changes needed.

Surgical Considerations

- Endoscopy may be needed to determine the full extent of gastrointestinal damage or to remove pinecones or pine needles lodged in the stomach. Careful consideration of anesthetic protocol, coupled with recent renal and liver chemistry evaluation, is needed.
- Endoscopy should be done carefully as tissues may be fragile and risk of perforation is high.
- Surgical correction of gastrointestinal perforation may be needed.

Prevention/Avoidance

- Do not prescribe pine oil-based insecticides to cats, and caution owners not to use canine products on cats.
- See Client Education.

Public Health

- Humans can absorb these chemicals from the skin, eyes, and gastrointestinal tract. Protect caregivers from accidental exposure to contaminated vomit or skin. If an exposure does occur, clean the area immediately, flush with PEG solution or water, and contact a human poison control center for further recommendations.

- Death has occurred in children following accidental ingestion of pine oil, phenol, and phenolic derivatives.

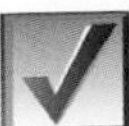

COMMENTS

- Animals that remain asymptomatic for 6 hours or more following exposure are not expected to develop clinical signs. Their prognosis is excellent.

Client Education

- Do not allow pets to have access to products that contain phenol or pine oil.
- Secure used mops or mop water out of the reach of children and pets. Rinse mops well before drying.
- Even if pet makes a full recovery, subclinical damage may have been done to the liver or kidneys.

Patient Monitoring

- If liver or renal disease, methemoglobinemia, or metabolic acidosis occurs, hospitalization until resolution is recommended.
- Chemistry panel and CBC should be checked every 24–48 hours pending the severity and clinical course.
- Blood pH will need to be reevaluated frequently during treatment with sodium bicarbonate, then rechecked 12–24 hours later to ensure stability.

Possible Complications

- Liver failure/necrosis, renal failure/necrosis, methemoglobinemia, metabolic acidosis, esophageal strictures, GI perforation with septic peritonitis, and aspiration pneumonia.
- Pine needle or pinecone foreign body.

Expected Course and Prognosis

- Prognosis for cats exposed to phenol/phenolic derivatives is poor; that for pine oil is guarded. Small ingestions can quickly result in rapidly progressive signs and require aggressive medical intervention. Even with excellent medical management, death from liver or renal necrosis can occur.
- Most dogs recover uneventfully.

Synonyms

Pine oil: alpha-terpineol, arizole, oleum abietis, terpentinoel, unipine, yarmor

Phenol: benzenol, carbolic acid, carbolic oil, fenosmolin, fenosmoline, hydroxybenzene, monohydroxybenzene, monophenol, oxybenzene, phenic acid, phenol alcohol, phenyl alcohol, phenyl hydrate, phenyl hydroxide, phenylic acid , phenylic alcohol

Phenolic derivatives: cade oil, chlorinated phenols, creosote, creosol, coal tar, cresolic acid, hexachlorophene, hydroquinone, juniper tar (*Juniperus oxycedrus*), paraphenol, phenylphenol, phlorglucinol, pyrocatechol, pyrogallol, resorcin, resorcinol, sulfurated phenols, xylenol

See Also

Acids
Alkalis
Essential Oils/Liquid Potpourri
Tea Tree Oil/Melaleuca Oil

Abbreviations

See Appendix 1 for a complete list.

PEG = percutaneous endoscopic gastrostomy
SAMe = S-adenosyl-L-methionine

Suggested Reading

Chan TY, Sung JJ, Crichley JA. Chemical gastro-oesophagitis, upper gastrointestinal haemorrhage and gastroscopic findings following Dettol poisoning. Hum Exp Toxicol 1995; 14:18–19.

Gieger TL, Correa SS, Taboada J, et al. Phenol poisoning in three dogs. J Am Anim Hosp Assoc 2000; 36(4):317–321.

Gwaltney-Brant SM. Miscellaneous indoor toxicants. In: Peterson ME, Talcott PA, eds. Small Animal Toxicology, 3rd edn. St Louis, MO: Elsevier, 2013; p. 297.

Monteiro-Riviere NA, Inman AO, Jackson H, Dunn B, Dimond S. Efficacy of topical phenol decontamination strategies on severity of acute phenol chemical burns and dermal absorption: in vitro and in vivo studies in pig skin. Toxicol Ind Health 2001; 17(4):95–104.

Rousseax CG, Smith RA. Acute pinesol toxicity in a domestic cat. Vet Hum Toxicol 1986; 28:316–317.

Welker JA, Zaloga GP. Pine oil ingestion: a common cause of poisoning. Chest 1999; 116:1822–1826.

Acknowledgment: The authors and editors acknowledge the prior contributions of Catherine Angle, DVM, MPH, and Ahna G. Brutlag, DVM, MS, DABT, DABVT, who co-authored this topic in the previous edition.

Author: Dominic Tauer, DVM
Consulting Editor: Ahna G. Brutlag, DVM, MS, DABT, DABVT

Soaps, Detergents, Fabric Softeners, Enzymatic Cleaners, and Deodorizers

chapter 88

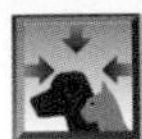

DEFINITION/OVERVIEW

- Soaps, detergents, fabric softeners, and enzymatic cleaners are composed mainly of anionic, cationic, nonionic, or amphoteric surfactants. Some also contain builders such as complex phosphates, sodium carbonate, and sodium silicate or enzymes such as proteases, amylases, or lipases. Deodorizers and soaps contain perfume oils, and some products contain alcohol(s) (e.g., ethanol or isopropanol).
- Most of these products can cause a variety of clinical signs but generally produce a low level of toxicity in veterinary species. The exceptions are the cationic detergents, automatic dishwashing detergents (ADWD), and single-use laundry detergent pods (LDPs).
- Clinical signs of intoxication from these products include, but are not limited to, nausea, vomiting, diarrhea, drooling. More serious but uncommon complications include CNS depression, renal insufficiency, oral or esophageal burns, GI bleeds, convulsions, and coma.

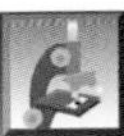

ETIOLOGY/PATHOPHYSIOLOGY

Mechanism of Action

- With polar and nonpolar ends, surfactants reduce water surface tension, thus allowing surfaces to be wet more efficiently.
- Builders reduce water hardness, emulsify grease and oil, and maintain alkalinity. High concentrations of certain builders (e.g., trisodium phosphate) bind calcium and cause hypocalcemia.
- With catalytic action, enzymes in enzymatic cleaners break down organic stains to enhance cleaning efficacy. Enzymes cause release of bradykinin and histamine, resulting in dermal irritation and possible respiratory sensitization/bronchospasm if inhaled.
- ADWD cause toxicosis through a direct effect on tissue and may lead to necrosis. Muscle weakness and paralysis can result from the ganglion-blocking and curare-like activity of quaternary ammonium compounds.

Blackwell's Five-Minute Veterinary Consult Clinical Companion: Small Animal Toxicology, Second Edition.
Lynn R. Hovda, Ahna G. Brutlag, Robert H. Poppenga, and Katherine L. Peterson.

Companion website: www.fiveminutevet.com/toxicology

- Increased severity of LDP exposures compared with traditional detergents is due to the fact that LDPs are both highly concentrated and packaged under pressure. Oral exposures often consist of biting and rupturing the pods, leading to rapid expulsion and aspiration and/or swallowing of the product.

Pharmacokinetics – Absorption, Distribution, Metabolism, Excretion

- These products are generally well absorbed, with peak levels 1 hour post ingestion. Products containing ethanol or isopropanol have significantly enhanced GI absorption. Dermal irritant effects can occur almost immediately.
- Topical absorption is limited with ≤1% absorption in some cases. While healthy skin is a good barrier, absorption can also occur through defects in skin surface.
- Surfactants are metabolized in the liver and resulting metabolites are excreted mainly in the urine and minimally in feces.

Toxicity

- Cationic surfactants are the most toxic, followed by anionic surfactants, and then nonionic and amphoteric surfactants. See table 88.1 for a list of common surfactants.
    - Animals licking or grooming skin surfaces exposed to cationic detergents may develop poisoning. This is an especially common method of exposure in cats, which may show significant tissue injury at concentrations ≤2%.
    - Products containing >7.5% cationic surfactants may be corrosive and cause serious complications. Fatalities have been reported from >20% dermal exposure to cationic products.
    - There is risk of corrosive damage at pH <2 or pH >12, but pH should not be the only determining factor, especially with the cationic detergents where the pH may be neutral or only slightly alkaline.
    - LD_{50} mouse (oral): 1400–4600 mg/kg (anionic and nonionic detergents).
    - LD_{50} rat (oral): 420 mg/kg (cationic detergents).
- Personal care soap, hand dishwashing soaps, regular liquid laundry detergents, deodorizers, and enzymatic cleaners may be irritants causing nausea, vomiting, and diarrhea.
- Median emetic dose in dogs (oral): 6–25 mg/kg (laundry products).
- Builders are irritants at low concentrations but corrosive at high concentrations.
- Perfume oils and alcohols cause irritant effects and drying/defatting of skin.
- Fatal automatic dishwashing detergent dose in dogs is 500–2500 mg/kg.

Systems Affected

- Gastrointestinal – nausea, vomiting, diarrhea, and gastritis are common. There is potential for corrosive injury leading to drooling, dysphagia, epigastric pain, and bleeding from cationic surfactants and highly concentrated products.
- Skin – dryness, dermatitis, and irritation. Hair loss, chemical burns, and necrosis are uncommon except with high concentration cationic surfactants and ADWD.

TABLE 88.1. Common surfactants.

Anionic
• Alkyl sodium sulfate • Alkyl sodium sulfonate • Dioctyl sodium sulfosuccinate • Linear alkyl benzene sulfonate • Sodium lauryl sulfate • Tetrapropylene benzene sulfonate
Nonionic
• Alkyl ethoxylate • Alkyl phenoxy polyethoxy ethanols • Polyethylene glycol stearate
Cationic

• Quaternary ammonium compounds
  ◦ Benzalkonium chloride
  ◦ Benzethonium chloride
• Pyridinium compounds
  ◦ Cetylpyridinium chloride
• Quinolinium compounds
  ◦ Dequalinium chloride

Amphoteric
• Imidazolines • Betaines

- Respiratory – coughing, stridor, dyspnea, and respiratory muscle paralysis (with severe exposures to cationic surfactants).
- Ophthalmic – conjunctive erythema, irritation, pain, stinging, tearing, and potentially corneal damage.
- Cardiovascular – hypotension and shock (only in severe exposures with cationic surfactants).
- Nervous – lethargy, CNS depression, coma (severe poisoning), and seizures (cationic surfactants).
- Endocrine/metabolic – metabolic acidosis (severe poisoning).
- Hemic/immune – hypersensitivity reactions and intravascular hemolysis (rare).

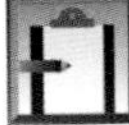

SIGNALMENT/HISTORY

- Any age or breed of animal can be affected.

Risk Factors

- Preexisting liver disease may slow metabolism of surfactants.
- Preexisting chronic skin conditions (e.g., allergic dermatitis) may be exacerbated.
- Preexisting respiratory illnesses (e.g., asthma) may be exacerbated.

Historical Findings

- Exposures to these products is frequently but not always witnessed. Discovery of spilled detergent, soap, or enzymatic cleaners, or chewed-up bars of soap or fabric softeners is common.

CLINICAL FEATURES

- Ingestion: initial clinical signs of nausea, vomiting, or diarrhea and drooling are immediate and common. As intoxication with cationic or other corrosive products progresses, lethargy, vocalization, stridor, or dysphagia may occur. Oral and/or esophageal burns, with bleeding, are possible. Lack of oral ulceration does not rule out the possibility of damage to the esophagus. Serious but uncommon systemic symptoms include restlessness, CNS depression, renal insufficiency, convulsions, and coma.
- Inhalation/aspiration of powdered products or mist deodorizers: initially, coughing, shortness of breath, drooling, stridor, and retractions. As intoxication progresses, respiratory depression or airway compromise may occur but are unlikely with acute exposure.
- Ocular exposure: initially, irritation, redness, and tearing. With delays in treatment and highly concentrated products, there is an increased risk of corneal damage from cationic surfactants and more corrosive products.
- Dermal exposure: initial signs of irritation, pruritus, and erythema, but more serious dermal necrosis with some more concentrated cationic detergents.
- Fatalities are usually associated with respiratory failure, aspiration, asphyxia, and corrosive gastrointestinal injuries resulting from ingestion.

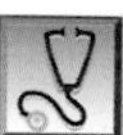

DIFFERENTIAL DIAGNOSIS

- Toxicities.
    - Pesticides.
    - Bleaches (notably, highly concentrated or “ultra” bleaches) and ammonia-based cleaning solutions.
    - Corrosives.
- Primary hypersensitivity to topical products.
- Primary respiratory disease.

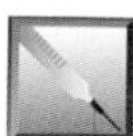

DIAGNOSTICS

- Diagnosis should be made based on patient history, physical examination, symptoms, and clinical suspicion. No specific laboratory testing is useful in confirming the diagnosis.
- Endoscopy should be performed within 12–24 hours of cationic surfactant ingestion if signs of tissue injury are present (drooling, stridor, anorexia, etc.).
- Animals with respiratory symptoms should be evaluated with a thoracic radiograph.

Pathological Findings

- Gross examination at necropsy may reveal mucosal ulceration in fatal cases of corrosive product ingestion.
- There are no specific histopathological findings associated with soap, detergent, fabric softener, enzymatic cleaner, or deodorizer toxicity.

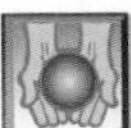

THERAPEUTICS

- Treatment and care following exposures to most soaps, hand dishwashing soaps, detergents, laundry detergents, and deodorizers can be handled at home.
- Goals of treatment include removal from exposure site, prevention of further absorption, and providing necessary supportive and symptomatic care.
- Emesis is not generally indicated or necessary (see Detoxification).
- Exposure to cationic surfactants, LDPs, and ADWD should be carefully evaluated and assessed for potential corrosive and systemic intoxication.
    - Minimal ingestions of low concentrations of cationic detergents (<7.5%) can be handled similarly to hand dishwashing soaps and laundry detergents.
    - Sizeable ingestions of cationic detergents, especially with concentrations >7.5%, should be handled as corrosive exposures.

Detoxification

- Emesis, gastric lavage, and administration of activated charcoal are not generally indicated, especially with cationic detergents, due to risk of further corrosive exposure.
- Evacuation of stomach contents should be considered only when product ingredients, history, and assessment indicate a high potential for serious systemic toxicity.
- Emesis may be induced if the animal has not spontaneously vomited within 30 minutes after ingestion of large quantities of a *non*corrosive product.
- Ocular – flush the eyes with normal saline (preferred) or room temperature water for ≥20 minutes or until the pH of the conjunctival sac is 8 or less (for alkaline exposures). If ocular irritation progresses for >2 hours, if the product's pH is >12, if cationic concentration is >2% or if an ADWD is involved, the animal should be referred to an ophthalmic specialist.
- Dermal – irrigate the exposed topical area(s) for ≥10 minutes with room temperature water (initially use soap in cases of deodorizer or cationic product exposure).

Appropriate Health Care

- Maintain vital functions – secure and protect airway, supply oxygen, and provide respiratory supportive care as needed.
- Aggressively monitor and replace fluids and electrolytes when necessary.
- Ingestion.
    - Oral dilution with water.
    - Monitor for GI bleeding.

  - If excessive vomiting and/or diarrhea occur, consider an antiemetic or antidiarrheal as needed.
  - In cases with a significant potential for gastritis, corrosive injury, or GI bleeding, NSAIDs should be avoided.
- Inhalation of powder or deodorizer mist.
  - No treatment usually necessary other than monitoring for symptom development.
  - Oral or IV corticosteroids (e.g., prednisone 0.5–1 mg/kg PO q 24 hours or equivalent doses of dexamethasone, dogs) and inhaled beta$_2$ agonists (e.g., albuterol 0.05 mg/kg PO q 8 hours, dogs) may help control bronchospasm.
  - Analgesic administration as needed following exposure (e.g., buprenorphine 0.005–0.03 mg/kg IV, IM, SQ q 6–12 hours).

Drugs of Choice and Antidotes

- There are no known effective antidotes.

Precautions/Interactions

- Do NOT try to neutralize the exposure with additional chemicals as this can create an exothermic reaction and cause thermal burns.
- Do not orally dilute with large volumes of water post ingestion as this may increase the risk of vomiting, "sudsing," and aspiration.
- Avoid topical oil-based creams, lotions, or ointments if exposed to potentially corrosive products as this may "trap" the product against the skin.
- Do not induce emesis or administer activated charcoal if you suspect ingestion of a corrosive product (cationic concentration >7.5% or ADWD) or if vomiting has already occurred.
- Be alert to interactions with strong oxidizers, strong reducing agents, strong acids, and metals.
- In cases with a significant potential for gastritis, corrosive injury, or GI bleeding, NSAIDs should be avoided.

Alternative Drugs

- Ingestion of sizeable quantities of phosphate-containing products may require treatment with sevelamer or another oral phosphate-binding medication. Monitor blood levels of calcium, magnesium, and phosphorus until symptoms have abated.
- Calcium gluconate 10% solution (0.5–1.5 mL/kg IV, slowly over 15–30 min) or calcium chloride 10% (0.15–0.50 mL/kg IV, slowly) is indicated as needed for hypocalcemia following ingestion of builder-containing detergents.
- Animal studies have shown corticosteroid (prednisone 0.25–0.5 mg/kg PO q 24 hours × 3–5 days, then q 48 hours × 2 weeks) and prophylactic antibiotic treatment within 48 hours of exposure or ingestion to be helpful in cases of severe burns or esophageal injury.

- Topical hydrocortisone cream, aloe vera gel, lotion, and cold packs are additional options for dermal relief.
- Seizures should be controlled with anticonvulsants (e.g., diazepam 0.5–1 mg/kg IV to effect).

Diet

- If the animal is vomiting or unconscious, keep NPO until signs resolve.

Activity

- Base on signs and severity of exposure.

Surgical Considerations

- Surgical resection of damaged tissue in cases of severe corrosive damage.
- Severely injured patients may need PEG tube placement for nutritional support.

COMMENTS

Client Education

- Readmit patient if pain or signs return/worsen despite appropriate treatment or if the animal is not eating and drinking.

Patient Monitoring

- Monitor electrolytes, fluids, and acid–base status post ingestion.
- Monitor 6–8 hours post vomiting for signs of aspiration, coughing, gagging, or stridor.
- Monitor for intravascular hemolysis. If this occurs, monitor renal function and PCV/TS.
- Monitor serum calcium levels following significant ingestion of detergents containing builders.
- Monitor respiratory signs for up to 12 hours post inhalation.

Prevention/Avoidance

- Prevent access to products in the home, particularly while cleaning or doing laundry.

Possible Complications

- Aspiration post vomiting.
- Irreversible ocular damage, changes in vision.
- Development of esophageal or intestinal strictures.
- Intravascular hemolysis, though uncommon, may occur, especially in animals with liver disease.

Expected Course and Prognosis

- Prognosis depends mainly on the specific ingredients, product pH, concentration, quantity, viscosity, and route of exposure (see Toxicology).
- For animals with exposure to personal care soap, hand dishwashing detergent, laundry detergent, deodorizers, enzymatic cleaners, and other noncorrosive products, the prognosis is generally excellent and the course uneventful.
- For animals with clinical signs such as hypotension, CNS depression, coma, seizures, necrosis, GI bleeds, metabolic acidosis, or dysphagia, the prognosis is guarded. The animal should be monitored for stricture development.

Synonyms

- Air fresheners, surfactants, builders

See Also

Acids
Alkalis
Essential Oils/Liquid Potpourri

Abbreviations

See Appendix 1 for a complete list.

ADWD = automatic dishwashing detergent
LD_{50} = median lethal dose
LDP = laundry detergent pod
NPO = *nil per os* (nothing by mouth)
PEG = percutaneous endoscopic gastrostomy

Suggested Reading

DiCarlo MA. Scientific reviews. Household products: a review. Vet Hum Toxicol 2003; 45(2):256–261.
Gfeller RW, Messonnier SP. Handbook of Small Animal Toxicology and Poisonings, 2nd edn. St Louis, MO: Mosby/Elsevier, 2004; pp. 125–126, 151–156, 299–300.
Gwaltney-Brant SM. Miscellaneous indoor toxicants. In: Peterson ME, Talcott PA, eds. Small Animal Toxicology, 3rd edn. St Louis, MO: Elsevier, 2013; p. 291.
Sioris LJ, Schuller HK. Soaps, detergents, and bleaches. In: Shannon MW, Borron SW, Burns MJ, eds. Haddad and Winchester's Clinical Management of Poisoning and Drug Overdose, 4th edn. Philadelphia, PA: Saunders/Elsevier, 2007; p. 1443.

Acknowledgment: The authors and editors acknowledge the prior contributions of Lauren E. Haak, PharmD, DABVT, who co-authored this topic in the previous edition.
Authors: Leo J. Sioris, PharmD; Christina Fourre, DVM Candidate, Class of 2017
Consulting Editor: Ahna G. Brutlag, DVM, MS, DABT, DABVT

Insecticides and Molluscicides

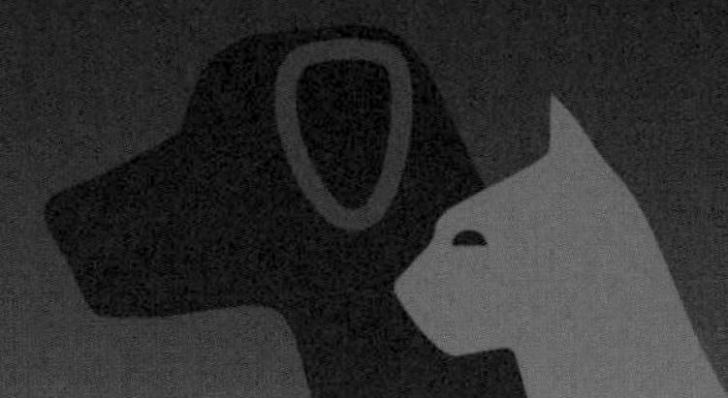

chapter 89

Amitraz

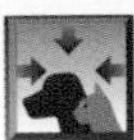

DEFINITION/OVERVIEW

- Amitraz is a formamidine derivative insecticide which is used as an acaracide and miticide in veterinary medicine.
- Amitraz is available in various formulations and concentrations. Formulations include powders, collars, sprays, dips, and topicals for companion animal, livestock, and industrial use.
- Some common trade names include Certifect®, Francodex®, Mitaban®, Mitac®, Mitacur®, Ovasyn®, Preventic®, Taktic®, Triatix®, and Triatox®.
- Amitraz collars contain 9% amitraz (90 mg/g); each 27.5 g collar contains 2500 mg of amitraz.
- Animal exposures resulting in toxicosis are often due to ingestion of amitraz-containing collars or from amitraz product misuse.
- Clinical signs depend on the route of exposure. Topical overdose usually results in transient sedation lasting from 48 to 72 hours. The signs associated with oral exposure are more severe and include depression, head pressing, ataxia, seizures, coma, ileus, diarrhea, vomiting, hypersalivation, polyuria, hypothermia, bradycardia, hyper- or hypotension, and mydriasis.

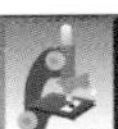

ETIOLOGY/PATHOPHYSIOLOGY

Mechanism of Action

- Amitraz is a diamide topical parasiticide with a poorly understood mechanism of action.
- It primarily acts as a CNS $alpha_2$-adrenergic agonist and as a weak monoamine oxidase inhibitor (MAOI).
- Other suspected actions include mild serotonin and antiplatelet effects.

Pharmacokinetics – Absorption, Distribution, Metabolism, Excretion

- Rapidly absorbed orally; peak plasma levels occur approximately 1.5–6 hours following ingestion, and the elimination half-life in dogs is approximately 12 hours.

Blackwell's Five-Minute Veterinary Consult Clinical Companion: Small Animal Toxicology, Second Edition.
Lynn R. Hovda, Ahna G. Brutlag, Robert H. Poppenga, and Katherine L. Peterson.

Companion website: www.fiveminutevet.com/toxicology

- Dermal absorption is minimal.
- Tissues found to contain the highest concentrations of amitraz are bile, the liver, eye, and intestines.
- Metabolized in the liver to active and inactive metabolites. The main metabolite in dogs is 4-amino-3-methylbenzoic acid, which is inactive.
- Metabolites are excreted primarily in urine; some fecal excretion occurs.

Toxicity

- Some dogs exposed to topical amitraz have developed toxicosis in spite of poor dermal absorption.
- Oral LD_{50} in dogs is 100 mg/kg.
- 4 mg/kg/day PO for 90 days in beagles resulted in CNS depression, ataxia, hypothermia, hyperglycemia, and increased pulse rates. No dogs died during the study.
- Toxicosis associated with ingestion of amitraz-containing collars is significant in all species studied.
    - Ingestion of a 2-inch portion of an amitraz collar (estimated dose 10 mg/kg) resulted in moderate lethargy, mydriasis, bradycardia and hypotension in a dog.
    - Ingestion of a 3.5-inch portion of an amitraz collar (estimated dose 23 mg/kg) resulted in profound depression, recumbency, mydriasis, profound bradycardia, and distended abdomen in a dog.
- Cats are very sensitive to toxicosis and develop signs at much lower doses than dogs.

Systems Affected

- Nervous – depression, ataxia, seizure, and/or coma due to $alpha_2$-adrenergic stimulation.
- Gastrointestinal – hypersalivation, vomiting, diarrhea, bloat or ileus secondary to anticholinergic effects.
- Cardiovascular – hypertension or hypotension, bradycardia secondary to $alpha_2$-adrenergic receptor activity.
- Endocrine/metabolic – hyperglycemia via adrenergic inhibition of insulin release. Hypothermia due to peripheral vasodilation. Hyperthermia due to increased muscle activity from tremors or seizures.
- Respiratory – respiratory depression due to depression of the respiratory center of the brain.
- Ophthalmic – mydriasis due to $alpha_2$-adrenergic receptor activity.
- Renal/urological – polyuria may result at higher overdoses due to suppression of ADH.
- Hemic/lymphatic/immune – DIC can occur secondary to severe hyperthermia.

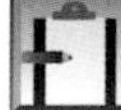

SIGNALMENT/HISTORY

- All ages, sexes, and breeds of dogs are affected. Toy breeds are reported to be more susceptible to the CNS effects.

Risk Factors

- Amitraz is contraindicated for canine patients ≤4 months of age.
- Geriatric and debilitated animals are at greater risk of toxicosis even at normal doses.
- Animals with severe skin inflammation may be at higher risk for dermal absorption, leading to systemic toxicosis.
- Amitraz is not suitable for patients with seizure disorders as it may potentially lower the seizure threshold.

Historical Findings

- History of exposure, which may be witnessed. Pet owners may find chewed amitraz collars in the household, along with symptomatic pets if enough time has elapsed.
- Owners may cause toxicosis in their pets when canine or livestock products are inadvertently or inappropriately applied to pets.

Location and Circumstances of Poisoning

- Exposures generally occur in the home due to unsecured products or via direct application.
- The potential does exist for exposures in the farm environment due to the use of amitraz in livestock and agricultural products.

Interactions with Drugs, Nutrients, or Environment

- Corticosteroids and other immune-suppressing drugs (e.g., azathioprine, cyclophosphamide).
- MAOIs (e.g., selegiline) and those with MAOI-like activity.
- Tricyclic antidepressants (e.g., amitriptyline and clomipramine).
- SSRIs (e.g., fluoxetine and fluvoxamine).
- Atypical antipsychotic agents.
- Anesthetic drugs with known adrenergic activity (e.g., xylazine or medetomidine).

CLINICAL FEATURES

- Onset of signs generally occurs within 30 minutes to 2 hours after ingestion although they may be delayed for up to 10–12 hours.
- Patients may present with CNS depression, tremors, ataxia, mydriasis, hypotension or hypertension, bradycardia and GI signs (including vomiting, hypersalivation, GI stasis). Hypothermia or hyperthermia may be present. Dehydration, tachypnea, and dyspnea are less commonly reported.
- Some patients may present seizing or with an owner history of having seized. Other patients may present minimally responsive or comatose.
- The duration of clinical signs is generally quite long (3–7 days) if reversal agents are not used.

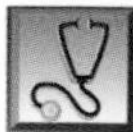

DIFFERENTIAL DIAGNOSIS

- Intoxications.
  - Alpha$_2$-adrenergic agents (e.g., xylazine, dexmedetomidine, tizanidine, imidazoline decongestants)
  - Anticholinesterase insecticides
  - Antidepressants (e.g., SSRIs, TCAs)
  - Benzodiazepines
  - Ethanol, methanol, isopropanol
  - Ethylene glycol
  - Macrocyclic lactone parasiticides (e.g., ivermectin, milbemycin)
  - Marijuana
  - Nicotine
  - Tremorgenic mycotoxins
- Primary or secondary neurological disease.
- Primary metabolic disease (e.g., hepatic encephalopathy, uremic encephalopathy, diabetes mellitus).

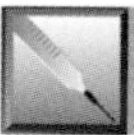

DIAGNOSTICS

- ECG and blood pressure monitoring for bradycardia and hypotension.
- Baseline chemistry and CBC.
- Monitor blood glucose levels frequently, especially for those patients that are known diabetics.
- Gas chromatography-mass spectrometry of gastric contents, plasma, and hair can be used to detect exposure, but long turn-around times make this of little value in emergent cases.

Pathological Findings

- No specific gross or microscopic pathological lesions are expected.

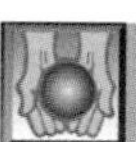

THERAPEUTICS

- The goals of treatment are to manage serious or life-threatening clinical signs, remove the source of the intoxication, monitor for development of complications, and provide supportive care until signs have resolved.

Detoxification

- If the patient is asymptomatic following amitraz collar ingestion, induction of emesis may be attempted. Do not use xylazine or medetomidine as emetic agents.
  - 3% hydrogen peroxide 2 mL/kg PO up to maximum of 45 mL; feeding small, moist meals may improve efficacy.

- Apomorphine (dogs): 0.02–0.04 mg/kg IV, SC, IM; can cause CNS depression, so use with care.

- Induction of emesis is not recommended in animals with clinical signs.
- If incomplete retrieval of collar in asymptomatic or mildly symptomatic patient, consider activated charcoal and cathartics.
    - Activated charcoal 1–3 g/kg PO q 12 hours until collar is retrieved or eliminated in the stools.
    - Nonoily laxative (e.g., sorbitol); when using osmotic diuretics, monitor closely for signs of hypernatremia.
    - Enema to evacuate colon may aid in decreasing intestinal transit time.
    - Bulky diet may aid in decreasing intestinal transit time.
- If the patient is stable and if exposure was topical, bathe with warm water and liquid dish detergent to remove the product.
- Ingested collars or collar pieces may need to be removed via endoscopy or surgery.

Appropriate Health Care

- Patients displaying mild sedation may require no specific treatment beyond monitoring for worsening signs.
- Provide thermoregulation as needed.
- Crystalloid IV fluids to help maintain hydration and treat hypotension. Diuresis does not speed amitraz elimination, but fluids do help to support the cardiovascular system.
- If the patient remains hypotensive, additional therapy may be necessary, including colloid and/or vasopressor therapy.

Antidotes

- $Alpha_2$-adrenergic antagonists can be helpful in reversing the CNS depression, hyperglycemia, and cardiovascular effects of amitraz.
    - Atipamezole 50 μg/kg IM; may need to repeat if collar remnants remain in GI tract and signs persist.
    - Yohimbine 0.1–0.2 mg/kg IV; start with lower end of dose; may need to repeat due to short half-life and/or if collar remnants remain in GI tract and signs persist.

Drugs of Choice

- Tremors/seizures may be treated with diazepam or barbiturates, but the lowest effective dose should be used due to severe sedation.
    - Diazepam 0.1–0.25 mg/kg, IV to effect PRN.
    - Phenobarbital 2–4 mg/kg, IV to effect PRN.
- If vomiting is protracted, consider antiemetic therapy.
    - Dolasetron 0.5–1.0 mg/kg IV q 24 hours.
    - Maropitant 1 mg/kg SQ q 24 hours.
    - Ondansetron 0.1–0.2 mg/kg SQ, IV q 8–12 hours.

Precautions/Interactions

- Atropine should not be used for treatment of bradycardia as it may exacerbate/precipitate hypertension and/or GI stasis.
- Insulin administration should not be used to treat hyperglycemia; administration of alpha$_2$-adrenergic antagonist will restore euglycemia.
- Do not use xylazine or medetomidine as emetic agents.

Nursing Care

- Frequent monitoring of vital signs is essential in symptomatic patients: heart rate, blood pressure, body temperature, respiratory rate (if comatose).
- Monitor urine production.
- Monitor blood glucose.
- Monitor for and manage ileus as needed.
- Observation may be required for 24–72 hours, or up to 5–7 days in severe cases.

Diet

- Return to normal diet at discharge in uncomplicated cases.
- Patients experiencing ileus or GI irritation may require dietary alterations until these signs have resolved.

Activity

- Patients should be kept quiet and secure while symptomatic but can return to normal activity with successful resolution of the case.

Surgical Considerations

- Endoscopic or surgical removal of amitraz-containing collars may be necessary.

COMMENTS

Prevention/avoidance

- Secure all pesticides/medications where they cannot be accessed by pets or children.
- Always use pesticide products per label directions based on dog age and/or weight.
- Never apply/administer a product labeled for dogs only to other species.
- Manufacturer warnings state that amitraz may alter an animal's ability to maintain homeostasis following topical treatment, and treated animals should not be subjected to stress for at least 24 hours following amitraz treatment.

Possible Complications

- Patients with prolonged periods of tremoring, seizure, or hypothermia may develop myoglobinuric renal failure or DIC.
- Gastrotomy to remove collar may increase risk of gastric dilation secondary to gastrointestinal hypomotility.

Expected Course and Prognosis

- Most patients receiving prompt, appropriate treatment will recover within 24–72 hours.
- Patients experiencing severe CNS dysfunction, ileus, or complications from tremors/seizures have a more guarded prognosis.

Abbreviations

See Appendix 1 for a complete list.

MAOI = monoamine oxidase inhibitor

Suggested Reading

Andrade SF, Sakate M. The comparative efficacy of yohimbine and atipamezole to treat amitraz intoxication in dogs. Vet Hum Toxicol 2003; 45(3):124–127.

Richardson JA. Amitraz. In: Peterson ME, Talcott PA, eds. Small Animal Toxicology, 3rd edn. St Louis, MO: Elsevier, 2013; pp. 431–435.

Valtolina C, Adamantos S. Amitraz toxicity. Stand Care 2009; 11(5):8–12.

Acknowledgment: The authors and editors acknowledge the prior contributions of Nancy M. Gruber, DVM, who authored this topic in the previous edition.
Author: Sharon Gwaltney-Brant, DVM, PhD, DABVT, DABT
Consulting Editor: Robert H. Poppenga, DVM, PhD, DABVT

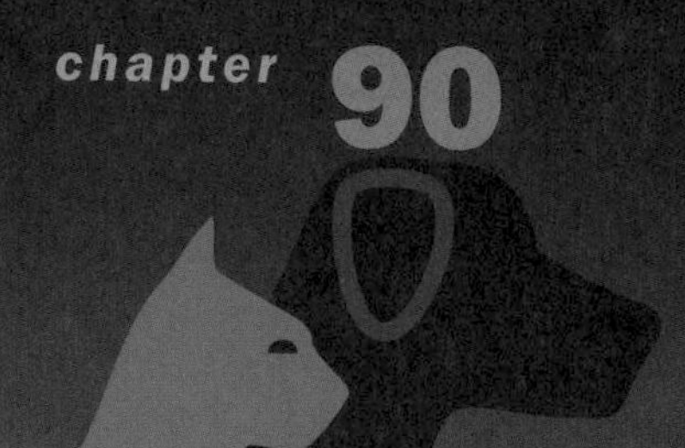

chapter 90

Metaldehyde

 DEFINITION/OVERVIEW

- Metaldehyde is a polycyclic polymer of acetaldehyde.
- Primarily affects the CNS.
- Ingredient of slug and snail baits; also used as solid fuel for some camp stoves and is marketed as a color flame tablet for party goods.
- Snail and slug baits.
    - Purchased as liquids, granules, wettable powders, or pelleted baits.
    - May also contain other toxicants such as arsenate or insecticides.
    - Newer products containing iron phosphate (or iron EDTA) are now available and are considered to be less toxic (see Chapter 95 for a discussion of iron).

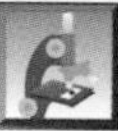 ETIOLOGY/PATHOPHYSIOLOGY

Mechanism of Action

- The exact mechanism is unknown.
    - It has been proposed that metaldehyde is converted to acetaldehyde after ingestion and that acetaldehyde is the primary toxic agent.
    - However, acetaldehyde was not found in the serum of rats during a dosing study and the authors recommended that this theory be reevaluated.
- Recent evidence suggests that metaldehyde may increase excitatory neurotransmitters or decrease inhibitory neurotransmitters; seizure threshold may be decreased.
    - Decreased levels of GABA, NE, and 5-HT are found in experimental mice.
    - MAO concentrations increased in treated mice.
- Metabolic acidosis and hyperthermia may be additional factors in clinical effects.

Pharmacokinetics – Absorption, Distribution, Metabolism, Excretion

- Low water solubility.
- Hydrolyzed, in part, in acid environment of the stomach.

Blackwell's Five-Minute Veterinary Consult Clinical Companion: Small Animal Toxicology, Second Edition.
Lynn R. Hovda, Ahna G. Brutlag, Robert H. Poppenga, and Katherine L. Peterson.

Companion website: www.fiveminutevet.com/toxicology

- Likely metabolized and detoxified by cytochrome P450.
- Acetaldehyde is metabolized to carbon dioxide and eliminated by the lungs.
- Urinary excretion as metaldehyde is less than 1% of dose.

Toxicity

- LD_{50} values.
  - Canine LD_{50}: 210–600 mg/kg BW.
  - Feline LD_{50}: 207 mg/kg BW.
  - Rabbit LD_{50}: 290–1250 mg/kg BW.
  - Guinea pig LD_{50}: 175–700 mg/kg BW.
- Bait concentration ranges from 2.75% to 3.25%.
- At 210 mg/kg (lowest canine LD_{50}) and 3.25% bait, dosage for LD_{50} is 6.5 grams bait/kg BW.

Systems Affected

- Neuromuscular – seizures and muscle tremors.
- Hepatobiliary – delayed hepatotoxicosis has been reported but is not common.
- Multiple organ failure is possible secondary to convulsions and hyperthermia.

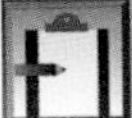

SIGNALMENT/HISTORY

Risk Factors

- Increased poisoning during predominant gardening and growing season.
- Increased risk when baits are overused or placed without protection from pets, or containers are left available or open.
- Dogs are much more likely to be poisoned than cats.
- Breed, age, or sex predilections are not known.

Historical Findings

- Recent history of pets with access to treated garden areas.
- Recent purchase of slug baits.
- Baits not protected from access by pets.
- Occasionally, access to camp stove fuels or other metaldehyde sources.

Location and Circumstances of Poisoning

- Prevalence is highest where slugs are a pest problem.
- Most common usage of baits is in coastal and low-lying areas with high prevalence of snails.
- Most consistent problems are also in warmer temperate to subtropical areas of United States.

Interactions with Drugs, Nutrients, or Environment

- None reported.
- Conditions that inhibit cytochrome P450 might enhance toxicity.

CLINICAL FEATURES

- May occur immediately after ingestion or may be delayed for up to 3 hours.
- Anxiety and panting are early signs.
- Muscle tremors.
- Seizures – may be intermittent early but progress to continuous; not necessarily evoked by external stimuli.
- Hyperthermia – temperature up to 108°F (42.2°C) common; probably caused by excessive muscle activity from convulsions; may lead to DIC or multiple organ failure if uncontrolled.
- Tachycardia and hyperpnea between convulsions – may note muscle tremors and anxiety; may be hyperesthetic to sounds, light, and/or touch.
- Nystagmus or mydriasis possible.
- Hypersalivation, vomiting, or diarrhea possible.
- Ataxia prior to or between seizures.

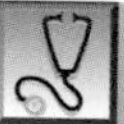

DIFFERENTIAL DIAGNOSIS

- Strychnine toxicosis – causes intermittent seizures that can be evoked by external stimuli.
- Penitrem A or roquefortine toxicosis – mycotoxins usually found in moldy English walnuts or cream cheese; have been reported in other foodstuffs; cause a tremorgenic syndrome.
- Lead toxicosis – may cause seizures, behavior changes, blindness, vomiting, diarrhea.
- Zinc phosphide toxicosis – may cause seizures and hyperesthesia.
- Bromethalin toxicosis – may cause seizures.
- Organochlorine insecticide toxicosis – causes seizures in most mammals.
- Anticholinesterase insecticide (organophosphorus and carbamate insecticides) – may cause seizures; often accompanied by excessive salivation, miosis, lacrimation, dyspnea, urination, and defecation.
- Seizures – may be the result of a host of nontoxic conditions (e.g., neoplasia, trauma, infection, metabolic disorder, and congenital disorder).

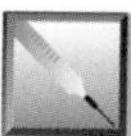

DIAGNOSTICS

- No specific or diagnostic features on CBC, chemistry, or UA.
- Increased serum muscle enzyme activities.

- Metabolic acidosis is typical.
- Changes in renal or hepatic values are possible but most likely secondary to uncontrolled hyperthermia.
- Radiographs may be indicated to evaluate for the presence of gastric material or severity of ingestion. Some metaldehyde bait pellets are radiopaque and may show up on radiographs.
- Metaldehyde testing can be performed on vomitus, stomach contents, serum, urine, or liver.
    - Keep samples frozen after collection.
    - Urine may yield low or negative values (see Pharmacokinetics).
    - Testing capabilities vary widely among laboratories, so check first to see what samples are recommended.

Pathological Findings

- Lesions are not consistent or pathognomonic.
- Odor of acetaldehyde or formaldehyde in stomach contents.
- Hepatic, renal, or pulmonary congestion.
- Pulmonary edema and/or hemorrhage.
- Nonspecific agonal hemorrhages on heart and mucosal surfaces.
- Traumatic bruising or hemorrhage secondary to seizures.

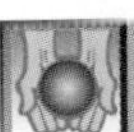

THERAPEUTICS

Detoxification

- Recommend emesis at home if ingestion is reported less than 2 hours previous and animal is asymptomatic.
- Use hydrogen peroxide PO at 1–3 mL/kg BW; if no response, send patient to veterinary hospital.
- In hospital, use apomorphine 0.03 mg/kg IV (preferred) or 0.04 mg/kg IM in dog or cat.
    - Note: some authorities recommend not using apomorphine in cats.
    - Do *not* administer emetic to patients with seizures or that are comatose or hyperesthetic.
- In cats, xylazine at 0.44 mg/kg IM can be used as an emetic.
- Alternative to emetic is gastric lavage with water at 3–5 mL/kg, repeated until lavage fluid is clear.
- Follow gastric clearing with activated charcoal (1–3 g/kg BW) and sorbitol cathartic (4 g/kg BW PO).
- Symptomatic patients should have their symptoms controlled (e.g., muscle relaxant, anticonvulsant, thermoregulation, cooling measures, etc.) and once stabilized, they should be gastric lavaged under sedation or general anesthesia. The airway should be protected with an inflated ETT, and the stomach lavaged to remove any remaining product.

Appropriate Health Care

- Emergency inpatient intensive care management until convulsions cease and hyperthermia is controlled.
- Acute care for metabolic acidosis may be essential to successful treatment.
    - Treat according to laboratory blood gas results.
    - If venous blood gas analysis reveals a severe metabolic acidosis (pH <7.0, BE ≤15, HCO_3 <11), sodium bicarbonate should be considered (0.5–1 mEq/kg slowly over 1–3 hours, IV).
- Control hyperthermia with cool water baths, ice packs, IV fluids, etc., until temperature reaches 103.5°F; cooling measures should be discontinued at this temperature and regulated frequently.
- Monitor to prevent aspiration of vomitus. Consider the use of antiemetics or prokinetics if necessary.
- Aggressive IV fluid therapy is often necessary to aid in cooling measures, to treat the underlying metabolic acidosis, to correct dehydration, to correct electrolyte imbalances, and to aid in perfusion.

Antidote

- No antidote is available.

Drugs of Choice

- Convulsions are controlled with diazepam, barbiturates, or general anesthesia and methocarbamol can be used to control muscle tremors. Seizures are frequently resistant to anticonvulsants and require general inhalant anesthesia for control.
    - Diazepam: 0.5–1 mg/kg IV bolus; repeat 5 minutes later if seizure has not subsided. Supplement with other control methods if seizures continue.
    - Barbiturates: phenobarbital 4–16 mg/kg IV; if control not adequate, consider pentobarbital 3–15 mg/kg IV to effect.
    - Methocarbamol: 50–150 mg/kg IV to effect; do not exceed 330 mg/kg/day.

Precautions/Interactions

- Never induce vomiting in a convulsing patient.

Activity

- Restrict activity so that patient is not injured during convulsions.

COMMENTS

Patient Monitoring

- Periodically allow anticonvulsants to wear off to reevaluate seizure condition.
- Monitor for possible liver or renal damage during convalescence.

Prevention/Avoidance

- Instruct owners/guardians on risks of metaldehyde.
- Advise clients on proper use, placement, and protection of metaldehyde from access by pets.
- Some manufacturers dye the product green or blue to assist with identification, which can result in confusion with other products (e.g., rodenticides).
- Some states require manufacturers to adjust the formulation to decrease palatability to pets.

Possible Complications

- Liver or renal dysfunction is possible several days after recovery from the initial signs and is probably a sequela to the convulsions and hyperthermia.
- Aspiration pneumonia is a concern with any convulsing patient.
- Hyperthermia may lead to DIC or multiple organ failure.
- Temporary blindness or memory loss may occur.
- Concurrent toxicoses from additional ingredients (arsenate or insecticides) if they are present in the molluscicide.

Expected Course and Prognosis

- Prognosis principally depends on the amount ingested, time to treatment, and quality of care.
- Delayed or nonaggressive treatment may result in death within hours of exposure.

Abbreviations

See Appendix 1 for a complete list.

Suggested Reading

Brutlag AG, Puschner B. Metaldehyde. In: PetersonME, TalcottPA, eds. Small Animal Toxicology, 3rd edn. St Louis, MO: Elsevier, 2013; pp. 635–642.

Buhl KJ, Berman FW, Stone DL. Reports of metaldehyde and iron phosphate exposures in animals and characterization of suspected iron toxicosis in dogs. J Am Vet Med Assoc 2013; 242:1244–1248.

Yas-Natan E, Segev G, Aroch I. Clinical, neurological and clinicopathological signs, treatment and outcome of metaldehyde intoxication in 18 dogs. J Small Anim Pract 2007; 48(8):438–443.

Author: Konnie H. Plumlee, DVM, MS, DABVT, DACVIM
Consulting Editor: Robert H. Poppenga, DVM, PhD, DABVT

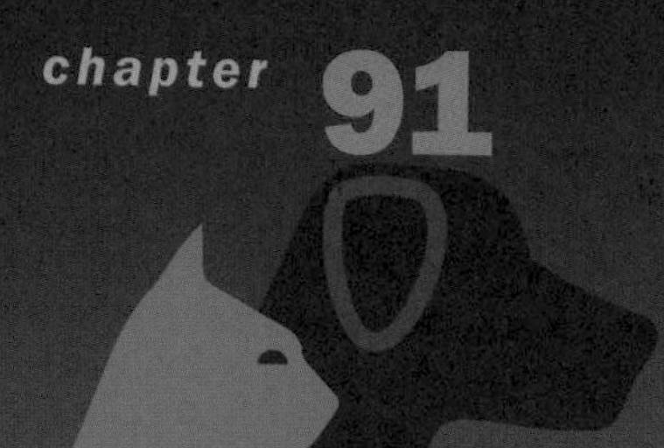

chapter 91

Imidacloprid and Other Neonicotinoids

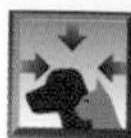

DEFINITION/OVERVIEW

- Neonicotinoids are a relatively new class of insecticides found in a variety of commercial preparations as well as topical spot-on veterinary products.
- Imidacloprid is one of the most widely used of these compounds and was the first commercially successful neonicotinoid insecticide. However, the neonicotinoid class also includes acetamiprid, clothianidin, dinotefuran, nitenpyram, thiacloprid, and thiamethoxam.
- Imidacloprid is used in topical flea products for dogs and cats and has a wide margin of safety given its high specificity for nicotinic receptors in insects. Neonicotinoids generally pose little risk of toxicity to pets.
- Neonicotinoids have been implicated in colony collapse disorder of bees, but this has not been proven.

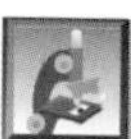

ETIOLOGY/PATHOPHYSIOLOGY

Mechanism of Action

- Neonicotinoids act on several types of postsynaptic nicotinic acetylcholine receptors in the CNS of insects, and these compounds likely have both agonistic and antagonistic effects.
- Binding to nicotinic acetylcholine receptors results in initial spontaneous discharge of nerve impulses with subsequent failure of nerve impulse transmission.
- While mammalian tissues contain multiple subtypes of nicotinic receptors, imidacloprid and other neonicotinoids are highly specific to insect nicotinic receptors and do not cross the blood–brain barrier in vertebrates, thus reducing potential toxicity to mammals.

Pharmacokinetics – Absorption, Distribution, Metabolism, Excretion

- Absorption.
    - Topical imidacloprid spreads quickly over the skin via translocation. The drug is sequestered in hair follicles and glands but exhibits minimal to no systemic absorption.

Blackwell's Five-Minute Veterinary Consult Clinical Companion: Small Animal Toxicology, Second Edition.
Lynn R. Hovda, Ahna G. Brutlag, Robert H. Poppenga, and Katherine L. Peterson.

Companion website: www.fiveminutevet.com/toxicology

  - Ingested imidacloprid is rapidly and almost completely absorbed from the gastrointestinal tract. The same has been shown for multiple neonicotinoids.
- Distribution.
  - Distribution following oral administration occurs quickly, with peak levels generally noted within an hour to several hours, depending on the specific neonicotinoid.
  - With oral administration, imidacloprid and other neonicotinoids distribute widely to tissues but are not distributed to the CNS, fatty tissues, or bone.
  - Imidacloprid, nitenpyram, and other neonicotinoids do not accumulate in tissues.
  - With topical application, imidacloprid is distributed in the fatty layer of the skin.
- Metabolism.
  - Metabolism occurs primarily in the liver.
  - Imidacloprid is oxidatively cleaved to the active metabolite 6-chloronicotinic acid. This metabolite is either conjugated with glycine and eliminated or is reduced to guanidine.
- Excretion.
  - In rats, 90% of imidacloprid is eliminated within 24 hours and 96% eliminated within 48 hours.
  - Routes of elimination for imidacloprid metabolites include urine (70–80%) and feces (20–30%).
  - The other neonicotinoids and their derivatives are also primarily eliminated via the urine.

Toxicity

- Imidacloprid.
  - Topical imidacloprid at 50 mg/kg resulted in no adverse effects in dogs and cats.
  - A 1-year feeding study of imidacloprid in dogs showed a NOEL (no observed effect level) of 41 mg/kg. Higher doses did result in elevated cholesterol levels and increased concentrations of liver cytochrome P450.
  - Dermal LD_{50} of imidacloprid is over 5000 mg/kg in rats.
  - Acute oral LD_{50} of technical-grade imidacloprid has been estimated to be 450 mg/kg in rats and 130–170 mg/kg in mice. Clinical signs and transient mild liver damage have been observed in rats at doses of 300 mg/kg.
  - Imidacloprid is not considered to be carcinogenic, mutagenic, or teratogenic, which is similar across all neonicotinoids. Topical imidacloprid products have been labeled for use in pregnant animals, as well as puppies and kittens as young as 7 weeks. However, reproductive toxicity and fetotoxicity have been noted in experimental studies with other neonicotinoids.
- Nitenpyram.
  - Adult dogs and cats administered up to 10 times the therapeutic dose daily of nitenpyram for a month showed no adverse effects.
  - The NOEL of nitenpyram in a 1-year study in dogs was shown to be 60 mg/kg/day.
  - Cats given 125 times the therapeutic dose of nitenpyram (125 mg/kg) exhibited hypersalivation, lethargy, vomiting, and tachypnea.

  - The acute oral LD_{50} of nitenpyram in rats is 1575–1680 mg/kg, and the acute dermal LD_{50} is >2000 mg/kg.
- Other neonicotinoids.
  - The acute oral LD_{50} of thiacloprid in rats is 396–836 mg/kg. It was not acutely toxic by a dermal route in rabbits.
  - Two studies have shown acetamiprid's acute oral LD_{50} to be 314–417 mg/kg and 146–217 mg/kg in rats. It was not acutely toxic by a dermal route.
  - Thiamethoxam showed an LD_{50} of 1563 mg/kg in rats and 871 mg/kg in mice. It was not acutely toxic by a dermal route in rats.
  - Clothianidin and dinotefuran were not acutely toxic via dermal, oral, or inhalational routes in the rat.

Systems Affected

- Nervous – neonicotinoids block nicotinergic pathways, thus causing a build-up of acetylcholine at the neuromuscular junction. This results in insect hyperactivity, convulsions, paralysis, and eventually death. Signs in dogs and cats may include tremors, muscle weakness, and ataxia.
- Gastrointestinal – oral contact can cause excessive salivation. Nicotinic signs include salivation, vomiting, and diarrhea.
- Skin – signs of hypersensitivity reactions may include erythema, pruritus, and alopecia.
- Hepatobiliary – mild biochemical changes, perturbations of liver function, and liver enlargement with chronic overdose.

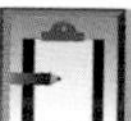

SIGNALMENT/HISTORY

- Dogs and cats with exposure to normal topical application of products containing imidacloprid are not at risk for toxicosis. Exposure to extremely high doses may put pets at risk, especially if ingested.
- Diagnosis is generally based on history and clinical signs.

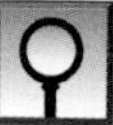

CLINICAL FEATURES

- There is little published data regarding adverse effects in dogs and cats, but clinical signs are generally expected to be mild.
- Signs have been shown to occur within 15 minutes to 2 hours and typically resolve within 24 hours.
- Imidacloprid is bitter, so acute oral contact may cause excessive salivation or vomiting.
- Nicotinic signs in dogs and cats may include lethargy, salivation, vomiting, diarrhea, tremors, muscle weakness, and ataxia.
- Hypersensitivity reactions can occur with any topical product and have been reported. Signs may include erythema, pruritus, and alopecia.

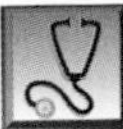

DIFFERENTIAL DIAGNOSIS

- Other oral toxins causing hypersalivation, e.g., corrosive products, insoluble calcium oxalate-containing plants.
- Any other nontoxicant cause of hypersalivation or nausea, e.g., dental disease, oral ulceration or inflammation, other GI disease, kidney disease, liver disease, pancreatitis, etc.

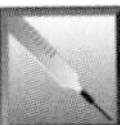

DIAGNOSTICS

- Hair and skin samples – somewhat helpful in establishing diagnosis.
  - Some laboratories can test for imidacloprid in these samples. However, as toxic tissue levels have not been established, this can only confirm exposure.
  - Techniques utilized to detect imidacloprid and 6-chloronicotinic acid residues include high-performance liquid chromatography with UV detection and enzyme-linked immunosorbent assay.
- Chemistry and urinalysis – not helpful in establishing diagnosis.

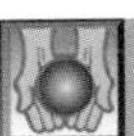

THERAPEUTICS

- The goal of therapy is to reduce absorption and provide symptomatic and supportive care.
- There is no specific antidote for treatment of overdoses.

Detoxification

- If exposure is dermal, bathing with a mild dishwashing detergent or follicle-flushing shampoo is recommended for removal.
- Emetics, adsorbents, or cathartics could be used depending on clinical signs observed, but absorption and elimination are so rapid that this approach is rarely indicated.

Appropriate Health Care

- If exposure is via ingestion, recommended treatment includes dilution with water or milk. Oral therapy is not recommended if there is vomiting.
- Antihistamines or steroids may be utilized for treatment of acute hypersensitivity reactions.

COMMENTS

Expected Course and Prognosis

- Prognosis is generally considered good. The neonicotinoids have a wide margin of safety in mammals and thus seldom pose a problem to companion animals.

- Published reports of intoxication in dogs and cats are rare, but most are expected to recover with appropriate veterinary care in 24–72 hours.

Abbreviations

See Appendix 1 for a complete list.

NOEL = no observed effect level

Suggested Reading

Ensley SM. Neonicotinoids. In: Gupta RC, ed. Veterinary Toxicology: Basic and Clinical Principles, 2nd edn. Boston, MA: Academic Press/Elsevier, 2012; pp. 596–598.

Gwaltney-Brant SM. Atypical topical spot-on products. In: Peterson M, Talcott P, eds. Small Animal Toxicology, 3rd edn. St Louis, MO: Elsevier, 2013; pp. 744–745.

Rose PH. Nicotine and the neonicotinoids. In: Marrs TC, ed. Mammalian Toxicology of Insecticides. Cambridge: Royal Society of Chemistry, 2012; pp. 184–220.

Sheets LP. Imidacloprid: a neonicotinoid insecticide. In: KriegerR, ed. Handbook of Pesticide Toxicology, Vol. 2. San Diego, CA: Academic, 2001; pp. 1123–1130.

Wismer T. Novel insecticides. In: PlumleeKH, ed. Clinical Veterinary Toxicology. St. Louis, MO: Mosby, 2004; pp. 184–185.

Authors: Kate S. Farrell, DVM; Karl E. Jandrey, DVM, MAS, DACVECC
Consulting Editor: Robert H. Poppenga, DVM, PhD, DABVT

chapter 92

Miscellaneous Insecticides

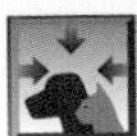

DEFINITION/OVERVIEW

- Fipronil, afoxolaner, and spinosad are three insecticide compounds in current clinical use with small animals. While they have various structural differences, there are important similarities in their mechanisms of action.
- All three compounds have a wide margin of safety due to their relative selectivity for receptors in the insect nervous system. At therapeutic doses and mild-to-moderate overdoses, adverse effects in mammals are generally limited to gastrointestinal upset, lethargy, and dermal irritation.
- One exception to the general safety of these insecticides for mammals is that fipronil is very toxic to rabbits and is absolutely contraindicated in this species.

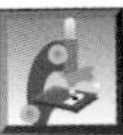

ETIOLOGY/PATHOPHYSIOLOGY

Mechanism of Action

- Fipronil is an antiparasitic agent of the phenylpyrazole class. Mechanistically, it interferes with the function of insect GABA-mediated chloride channels, preventing chloride uptake and leading to excessive neuronal stimulation.
- Afoxolaner is an isoxazoline compound with mechanistic similarities to fipronil. Like fipronil, it works by blocking insect GABA-mediated chloride channels, with the same inhibitory effect on chloride uptake, leading to neuronal hyperstimulation.
- Spinosad is a combination of two macrocyclic lactones, spinosyn A and D. It is a nicotinic acetylcholine receptor agonist with specific activity on the D-alpha receptors in the insect nervous system. Spinosad binding causes hyperexcitation of insect motor neurons, resulting in paralysis and death. Interference with GABA-mediated chloride channels appears to be a secondary mechanism of action.

Blackwell's Five-Minute Veterinary Consult Clinical Companion: Small Animal Toxicology, Second Edition.
Lynn R. Hovda, Ahna G. Brutlag, Robert H. Poppenga, and Katherine L. Peterson.

Companion website: www.fiveminutevet.com/toxicology

Pharmacokinetics – Absorption, Distribution, Metabolism, Excretion

- Fipronil products are labeled for topical use in dogs and cats. Dermally applied fipronil is quite lipophilic, concentrating in skin oils and hair follicles. It spreads across the body surface, via the skin oils, within 24 hours of dermal application. When applied topically, <5% of the drug is absorbed systemically. It may be ingested if an animal licks the product off itself or a housemate. Oral bioavailability is typically 50–85% of the total ingested dose.
- Afoxolaner is labeled for oral use in dogs only. It is rapidly absorbed from the GI tract and is highly protein bound. Half-life in dogs after oral administration ranges from 7.7 to 17.8 days. It is concentrated in the bile and excreted primarily in the feces.
- Spinosad is labeled for oral use in dogs only. It is rapidly absorbed from the GI tract, with a bioavailability of approximately 70%. It is concentrated particularly in adipose tissues, and is eliminated over days to weeks, primarily in the feces.

Toxicity (End Use Products)

- Fipronil: oral LD_{50} (rat): 5000 mg/kg.
- Afoxolaner: oral LD_{50} (rat): >1000 mg/kg.
- Spinosad: oral LD_{50} (rat): >3600 mg/kg.

Systems Affected

- Fipronil.
  - Skin/exocrine – erythema, dermatitis, pruritus, alopecia.
  - Gastrointestinal – transient hyporexia/anorexia. Hypersalivation, vomiting with oral exposures.
  - Nervous – hiding, lethargy. Rabbits may experience ataxia, tremors, and seizures.
- Afoxolaner.
  - Gastrointestinal – vomiting, diarrhea, hyporexia/anorexia.
  - Nervous – lethargy/depression.
  - Skin/exocrine – dry skin, pruritus.
- Spinosad.
  - Gastrointestinal – vomiting, hyporexia/anorexia, diarrhea, hypersalivation.
  - Nervous – depression/lethargy, ataxia, tremoring, seizures.
  - Skin/exocrine – pruritus.

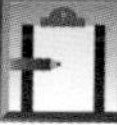

SIGNALMENT/HISTORY

Risk Factors

- Smaller animals are more likely to be accidentally or improperly overdosed with medications labeled for larger animals. This often occurs when a pet owner attempts to split a dose of a large dog product among several smaller pets.

- Afoxolaner and spinosad should both be used with caution in patients with a history of seizures, due to the theoretical potential that they may lower the seizure threshold in these animals.
- Rabbits are at extreme risk from any exposure to fipronil.

Location and Circumstances of Poisoning

- Fipronil is intended for topical application. Overdoses may occur from inadvertent or intentional overapplication of the product, or from using a product labeled for a larger weight class of animal. Topical products are sometimes accidentally given by mouth, or may be licked off the fur/skin of a housemate. Canine and feline labeled products are sometimes unknowingly applied to rabbits.
- Afoxolaner and spinosad are given orally. Overdoses may occur by accidentally repeating a dose or by using a product labeled for a larger weight class of animal on a smaller animal.
- Toxic exposures are more common during warmer months when risk for ectoparasitism is highest and need for these products is the greatest. In warm climates where these products are used year round, incidence of toxicosis shows less seasonal variation.

Interactions with Drugs, Nutrients, or Environment

- Spinosad should not be used concurrently with high-dose ivermectin (e.g., for conditions such as demodectic mange) as it may increase the risk for ivermectin toxicosis. This interaction is not observed when spinosad is used with low-dose ivermectin (e.g., for monthly heartworm prevention).

CLINICAL FEATURES

- Dermatological signs in dogs and cats may be seen within minutes to several days of topical application of fipronil.
- Gastrointestinal signs in dogs and cats may be seen within minutes to 2–3 days after ingestion of fipronil, afoxolaner, and spinosad.
- Rabbits will typically develop signs within a week of exposure to fipronil. Initial signs may be mild and nonspecific, and often include hyporexia/anorexia and lethargy/depression. These may be followed as much as 2–3 weeks later by ataxia, tremors, and seizures.
- Because initial signs in rabbits may be mild and nonspecific, these animals are sometimes not presented for care until more dramatic neurological signs have developed. The owner may be unaware of a link between the fipronil exposure and clinical signs, so a thorough history is essential in order to correctly identify the cause.

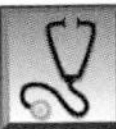

DIFFERENTIAL DIAGNOSIS

- Animals with GI signs – primary gastrointestinal disease of any origin.
- Animals with dermal signs – primary dermatological disease of any origin. Hypersensitivity reaction to other drugs, vaccines, insect or arachnid envenomation.

- Animals experiencing ataxia, seizures, or tremors.
  - Other intoxications, including bromethalin, metaldehyde, baclofen, tremorgenic mycotoxins, ethanol, ethylene glycol, marijuana, ivermectin, benzodiazepines, etc.
  - Epilepsy, either idiopathic or secondary to metabolic disease, intracranial neoplasia, or cerebrovascular disease.
  - Hypoglycemia, particularly in young and/or very small patients.

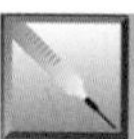

DIAGNOSTICS

- History of use.
- Routine laboratory work-up is typically unrewarding in diagnosing toxicosis caused by these compounds, but may be helpful in ruling out alternative differentials.
- Plasma or serum can be tested for the presence of fipronil, though this service is offered by only a handful of laboratories and would confirm exposure but not necessarily intoxication.

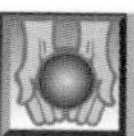

THERAPEUTICS

Detoxification

- Topical fipronil products can be removed from skin and coat by bathing the patient using a liquid dish detergent and rinsing thoroughly. These detergents contain degreasing agents, which remove the lipophilic products from skin and coat more effectively than shampoos labeled for humans or pets. Bathing is most effective if performed within 24–48 hours of product application. In some cases, 1–2 repeat baths may be necessary for full removal.
- Patients that are hypersalivating after grooming a topical product off the coat may benefit from gentle oral irrigation with clean water or isotonic saline solution. Encouraging the animal to drink water or eat food may also help remove the adverse taste from the mouth.
- In case of ophthalmic exposure to a topical product, the eyes should be gently irrigated with room temperature water or an eyewash solution for 10–15 minutes.
- For ingested products, emesis induction may be considered. Chewable tablets are rapidly absorbed, so emesis longer than 60 minutes post ingestion is generally of minimal benefit. Emesis induction is not indicated in rabbits due to their inability to vomit. Emesis should not be induced in any patient showing signs of toxicity, with decreased level of consciousness, or impaired ability to protect the airway.
- A dose of activated charcoal with a cathartic may be considered in patients with large ingestions. The same contraindications apply as with emesis induction.

Appropriate Health Care

- Patients experiencing mild dermatological or gastrointestinal signs can usually be managed on an outpatient basis.

- Patients experiencing neurological signs, including rabbits exposed to fipronil, should be hospitalized.
- Patients that have received spinosad and ivermectin, and are exhibiting signs of ivermectin overdose, should be managed as with other cases of ivermectin toxicity.

Antidotes

- No specific antidotes exist to fipronil, afoxolaner, or spinosad. Treatment of affected patients is symptomatic and supportive.

Drugs of Choice

- Note: Dosages that follow are for dogs, unless otherwise specified. Appropriate drugs and dosages should be confirmed for other species.
- For dermal irritation or pruritus.
  - Steroids – prednisone 0.5–1.1 mg/kg PO divided q 12 hours, tapering dose as needed.
  - Antihistamines – diphenhydramine 2.2 mg/kg PO q 8–12 hours, not to exceed 50 mg per dose.
- For evidence of secondary bacterial infection with open or ulcerated skin – cefpodoxime 5–10 mg/kg PO q 24 hours.
- For severe or persistent vomiting secondary to ingestion of products – maropitant 1 mg/kg SQ q 24 hours.
- For rabbits experiencing seizures after fipronil exposure.
  - Diazepam 0.5–1 mg/kg IV or per rectum.
  - Midazolam 1–2 mg/kg IM or IV.

Precautions/Interactions

- High-dose ivermectin therapy should not be used concurrently in an animal receiving spinosad.

COMMENTS

Prevention/Avoidance

- Rabbit owners should be informed that fipronil is toxic and should never be used in this species.
- In homes shared between rabbits and dogs or cats, safest option is to keep rabbits separated from treated animals for 48 hours after a fipronil product is applied.
- All small animal owners should be cautioned that antiparasitic products should never be used in a manner that deviates from the product label, unless such use is at the specific direction of a veterinarian.

Expected Course and Prognosis

- Prognosis is generally excellent for dogs and cats experiencing gastrointestinal or dermal effects following exposure to fipronil, afoxolaner, or spinosad.
- Any rabbit with exposure to fipronil has a guarded prognosis and requires careful monitoring for 3–4 weeks post exposure.
- Prognosis for rabbits exhibiting neurological signs after exposure to fipronil is poor.

See Also

Ivermectin/Milbemycin/Moxidectin

Abbreviations

See Appendix 1 for a complete list.

Suggested Reading

Anadon A, Gupta RC. Fipronil. In: Gupta RC, ed. Veterinary Toxicology: Basic and Clinical Principles, 2nd edn. New York: Elsevier, 2012; pp. 604–608.

Cooper PE, Penaliggon J. Use of Frontline spray on rabbits. Vet Rec 1997; 140(20):535–536.

Drag M, Saik J, Harriman J, Larsen D. Safety evaluation of orally administered afoxolaner in 8-week-old dogs. Vet Parasitol 2014; 201(3-4):198–203.

Dunn ST, Hedges L, Sampson KE, et al. Pharmacokinetic interaction of the antiparasitic aqents ivermectin and spinosad in dogs. Drug Metab Dispos 2011; 39(5):789–795.

Plumb DC. Spinosad. In: Plumb DC, ed. Plumb's Veterinary Drug Handbook, 8th edn. Ames, IA: Wiley-Blackwell, 2015; pp. 972–973.

Author: James N. Eucher, DVM, DHSc, MS, MPH
Consulting Editor: Robert H. Poppenga, DVM, PhD, DABVT

chapter 93

Organophosphorus and Carbamate Insecticides

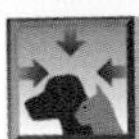 DEFINITION/OVERVIEW

- Organophosphate (OP) and carbamate cholinesterase-inhibiting insecticides are still common causes of toxicosis in dogs and cats, although the incidence has been steadily decreasing nationwide. This is likely due to the removal of several products from the home market and the introduction and increasing popularity of several other less toxic insecticides.
- Chlorpyrifos, once found in flea collars and other pesticide products, was withdrawn in 2000, and diazinon followed in 2004. Older products are still found (and used) in homes, garages, and attics and remain a source of poisoning.
- Products currently licensed for use on animals, in the house, on the lawn and garden, or for farm or agricultural use are all potential sources of poisoning.
- Carbamate *fungicides* that do not inhibit cholinesterase activity are in a different category and not discussed in this chapter.

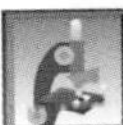 ETIOLOGY/PATHOPHYSIOLOGY

- In addition to systemic exposure, dogs and cats can be poisoned through ophthalmic, respiratory, and dermal routes. Onset and duration of clinical signs and toxicity vary depending on the particular OP or carbamate, as well as the route of exposure.

Mechanism of Action

- Competitive inhibitors of cholinesterase enzymes. Enzyme inhibition allows acetylcholine, a neurotransmitter, to accumulate at nerve junctions in the parasympathetic/sympathetic nervous systems, the peripheral nervous system, and the central nervous system (CNS). This results in initial and excessive stimulation of muscarinic, nicotinic, and CNS cholinergic receptors.
- Two main enzymes with cholinesterase activity.
  - Acetylcholinesterase ("true" cholinesterase) – present in the RBC membrane.
  - Pseudocholinesterase (plasma cholinesterase) – found in the plasma, liver, pancreas, and CNS.

Blackwell's Five-Minute Veterinary Consult Clinical Companion: Small Animal Toxicology, Second Edition.
Lynn R. Hovda, Ahna G. Brutlag, Robert H. Poppenga, and Katherine L. Peterson.

Companion website: www.fiveminutevet.com/toxicology

Pharmacokinetics – Absorption, Distribution, Metabolism, Excretion

- Precise pharmacokinetics vary with each compound.
- Well absorbed across intact skin, lungs, cornea, and GIT.
- Widely distributed and many accumulate in fat.
- Metabolized in liver.
- Excreted in urine as metabolites.
- Organophosphates.
  - Liver microsomal enzymes convert some OPs to a more toxic "oxon" compound. OPs irreversibly bind to cholinesterase enzymes, increasing the toxicity and duration of action.
  - Different OPs bind to cholinesterase with different affinity. Some "age" or become more strongly bound with the passage of time.
- Carbamates.
  - Inhibition of cholinesterase enzymes is due to carbamylation of the enzyme esters. Binding is labile, reversible, and not as long lasting as seen with OPs.

Toxicity

- Varies widely depending on the compound.
- Organophosphorus compounds.
  - Very highly toxic compounds include disulfoton, fensulfothion, parathion, terbufos, TEPP (tetraethyl pyrophosphate), and others.
  - Compounds with intermediate toxicity include coumaphos, famphur, trichlorfon, and others.
  - Intermediate to low toxicity compounds include chlorpyrifos, diazinon, dichlorvos, fenthion, malathion, and others.
  - Oral LD_{50} of chlorpyrifos in cats is very low (10–40 mg/kg).
- Carbamate compounds.
  - Extremely toxic compounds include aldicarb, carbofuran, methomyl, carbofuran, and others.
  - Aminocarb, bendiocarb, and propuxur are among the highly toxic compounds.
  - Moderately toxic compounds include carbaryl and others.

Systems Affected

- Virtually all systems in the body are affected to some extent by OPs or carbamates, with effects dependent on the specific neuroeffector junction involved.
- Accumulation of acetylcholine at autonomic junctions results in stimulation of end organs, with excessive secretions and smooth muscle contractions the expected outcome.
- Variable effects are observed at skeletal muscle junctions where both stimulatory and, to a lesser extent, inhibitory effects occur.
- Gastrointestinal – stimulation of muscarinic synapses results in the acute onset of salivation (S), lacrimation (L), urination (U), defecation (D), and gastroenteritis (GE) (this is where the mnemonic SLUDGE comes from).

- Nervous – stimulation results in variable and diverse signs.
- Neuromuscular – tremors and muscle weakness as part of nicotinic stimulation; paresis or frank paralysis following the acute cholinergic crisis (intermediate syndrome).
- Cardiovascular – inhibitory effect on SA node results in bradycardia.
- Ophthalmic – miosis or mydriasis from either muscarinic or nicotinic stimulation.
- Respiratory – vapors produce irritation to mucous membranes and bronchospasm. Dyspnea can result from bronchoconstriction and fluid accumulations.

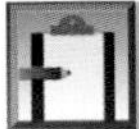

SIGNALMENT/HISTORY

Risk Factors

- Cats are more sensitive than dogs, especially to chlorpyrifos; however, poisonings are more frequently reported in dogs.
- Younger animals may be at greater risk.
- Thin animals or those with a naturally occurring lean body mass may be more susceptible to intoxication from lipophilic OPs.

Historical Findings

- Chewed-up containers or disturbed earth around recently treated rose bushes and shrubs.
- Rapid onset of SLUDGE syndrome (the author has recently begun using the mnemonic DUMBSLED to describe diarrhea, urination, miosis/mydriasis, bradycardia, salivation, lacrimation, emesis and dyspnea).
- Products are often used to intentionally poison pets.

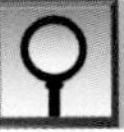

CLINICAL FEATURES

- Local effects from direct contact with the product. Signs may be seen in just a few moments or delayed for days with dermal exposure or following ingestion of delayed-release products (e.g., impregnated ear tags).
- Ophthalmic – irritation, lacrimation, photophobia, and miosis or mydriasis. Pupil size generally returns to normal in 12–36 hours.
- Respiratory – respiratory irritation with bronchospasm; absorption across mucous membranes.
- Dermal – irritation; absorption can occur across intact skin with systemic toxicity if concentration and duration of exposure is high enough.
- Systemic effects may occur as early as 5–60 minutes, usually occur by 6 hours, and rarely after 12 hours unless exposure was dermal or compound was in a delayed-release form.
- CNS – agitation or depression, aggression, seizures, respiratory depression and failure (centrally mediated), death.
- Muscarinic signs – most commonly observed and generally associated with the SLUDGE syndrome. Other signs include bradycardia, dyspnea, and miosis.

- Nicotinic signs – facial twitching (especially in cats), weakness, ataxia, muscle tremors, tachycardia, paralysis, and mydriasis.
- Intermediate syndrome: signs generally occur 24–72 hours after the onset of acute signs and may last from several days to weeks.
  - Occurs most commonly with lipophilic OPs.
  - Acute or chronic; can be seen following prolonged dermal exposure.
  - Due to downregulation of the cholinergic receptors, particularly muscarinic, and eventual fatigue of the nicotinic receptors.
  - Neuromuscular weakness predominantly affects the thoracic limb, neck, and respiratory muscles. Cervical ventroflexion is common.
- Other signs include cranial nerve deficits, anorexia, diarrhea, muscle tremors, abnormal postures or behaviors, miosis or mydriasis, depression, and seizures.
- Death from hypoventilation and respiratory depression.

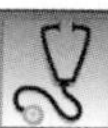

DIFFERENTIAL DIAGNOSIS

- Amphetamine, methylphenidate, methamphetamine, cocaine, and other human CNS stimulant compounds.
- Concentrated pyrethrin/permethrin topical products.
- Metaldehyde.
- Strychnine.
- Toxic mushrooms.
- Chlorinated hydrocarbon pesticides.
- Tremorgenic mycotoxins found in moldy food and compost (penitrem A, roquefortine).
- Zinc phosphide-containing rodenticides.
- Convulsant form of bromethalin intoxication.
- Severe gastroenteritis or pancreatitis from infectious, environmental, or other causes.

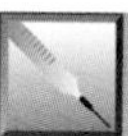

DIAGNOSTICS

- Analysis of stomach contents or vomitus for the parent compound.
- Modern analytical methods can detect OP and carbamate residues and metabolites in body organs such as liver, kidney, and fat.
- Positive response to a test dose of atropine (0.02 mg/kg IV).
- Blood cholinesterase activity antemortem and brain cholinesterase activity postmortem. Levels less than 50% of normal are considered suspicious and less than 25% of normal are diagnostic.
- Cholinesterase testing: cautious interpretation of measured activity, considering onset of signs and when sample was taken. Reversal of cholinesterase inhibition can occur over time, particularly with carbamate exposures. Anemia can lead to low cholinesterase values.
- Plasma cholinesterase – may be more appropriate for cats and avian species; can be used for other species.

- Whole blood cholinesterase – measures cholinesterase in plasma and RBC membranes; can be used for all species, including cats.
- Brain cholinesterase –some inhibitors do not cross the blood–brain barrier well; it has been difficult for laboratories to establish reference ranges for many species, depending on which part of the brain is collected and tested.

Pathological Findings

- Non-specific lesions; endocardial and epicardial petechial hemorrhages; pulmonary edema; pancreatitis in dogs can occur.

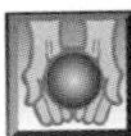

THERAPEUTICS

Detoxification

- Oral exposure.
  - Early induction of emesis depending on the carrier. Many liquid products have petroleum-based carriers, and emesis is NOT indicated for these.
  - If significant emesis occurs spontaneously, induction is unnecessary.
  - Gastric lavage followed by one or two doses of activated charcoal (4 hours apart) with or without a cathartic (depends if diarrhea is already present).
  - Flea collars that are ingested will need to be removed by emesis, whole-bowel irrigation, endoscopy, or surgery.
- Dermal exposure.
  - Clip hair if possible.
  - Bathe thoroughly in warm water and soap. Rinse and repeat several times.
  - Personal protection important when bathing.
- Ophthalmic exposure.
  - Lavage with tepid water for 10–15 minutes.
  - Ophthalmic ointment for irritation.
- Respiratory exposure.
  - Move to fresh air.
  - Humidified oxygen as needed for severe dyspnea.

Appropriate Health Care

- Close monitoring of heart rate. Bradycardia is most common; tachycardia can occur.
- Blood pressure support as needed.
- Oxygen as needed for dyspnea or hypoxemia.
- Severe respiratory depression or secondary aspiration pneumonia can occur; be prepared to provide ventilatory support as needed.
- Venous blood gas monitoring to detect metabolic acidosis; bicarbonate only if severe.
- Monitor closely for pancreatitis (dogs) and hemorrhagic gastroenteritis (dogs and cats).

Antidotes

- Atropine – effective *only* for SLUDGE or DUMBSLED signs. Primarily used to control bronchial secretions and bradycardia. Dosage range for this is very wide.
  - Mild-to-moderate toxicity.
    - Dosage range of 0.1–0.5 mg/kg BW.
    - Give ¼ of dose IV and remainder IM or SQ.
    - Repeat every 1–2 hours as needed until the animal is stable and secretions are controlled.
  - Serious and life-threatening toxicity.
    - Use the high end of the dosage range (1–2 mg/kg BW).
    - Give ¼ of the dose IV, wait 15 minutes and give the remainder SQ or IM.
    - Repeat every 1–2 hours until animal is stable and secretions are controlled.
- Secretions and then heart rate should be the guide to redosing.
- Pay particular attention to respiratory secretions as animals can die from hypoxia if not enough atropine is administered.
- Pralidoxime chloride (2PAM) – used for OP toxicosis to reverse the initial binding of OP with acetylcholinesterase. Questionable efficacy in carbamate toxicoses.
  - 20 mg/kg BW IM or IV q 8–12 hours *slowly* over 15–30 minutes; stop if signs get worse.
  - Rapid IV administration of 2PAM is associated with tachycardia, laryngospasm, neuromuscular blockade, muscle rigidity, and death.
  - Greatest efficacy when given within the first 24 hours after exposure.
  - Generally see effects after 1–2 doses; if no response after 3–4 doses, discontinue use.
  - Has been suggested to be beneficial in treatment of intermediate syndrome, even when signs occur later than 24 hours post exposure. It appears to work well on the most commonly affected muscles, such as the diaphragm and cervical muscles.

Drugs of Choice

- Fluid therapy: IV fluids to maintain hydration. Use PCV/TPP to monitor, but generally run fluids at 2–3× maintenance or greater as significant amounts of fluid are lost with secretions and decontamination procedures.
- Seizures.
  - Diazepam: 0.25–0.5 mg/kg IV, to effect.
  - Phenobarbital: 10–20 mg/kg IV, to effect.
- Antiemetics if vomiting is severe or persistent.
  - Maropitant: 1 mg/kg SQ q 24 hours.
  - Ondansetron: 0.1–0.2 mg/kg IV q 6–12 hours (dogs and cats).
- GI protectants, as needed.
  - H_2 blockers.
    - Famotidine 0.1–0.2 mg/kg PO, SQ, IM, IV q 12 hours for dogs; 0.2 mg/kg q 12–24 hours IM, SQ, PO, IV (slowly) for cats.

- □ Ranitidine 2 mg/kg q 8 hours IV, PO for dogs; 2.5 mg/kg q 12 hours IV or 3.5 mg/kg q 12 hours PO for cats.
- □ Cimetidine 10 mg/kg PO, IM, IV q 6–8 hours.
- Omeprazole: 1–2 mg/kg daily PO for dogs; 1 mg/kg daily PO for cats.
- Sucralfate: 0.5–1 g q 8–12 hours PO for dogs; 0.25 g q 8–12 hours PO for cats.

Precautions/Interactions

- Do NOT use 2 PAM in combination with phenothiazines, morphine, or succinylcholine.
- Use atropine judiciously. Use enough to keep the animal from drowning in secretions. Initial tachycardia should not preclude the use of atropine, but close monitoring is necessary.

Surgical Considerations

- Endoscopic or surgical removal may be necessary if the animal has swallowed a flea collar or pesticide-impregnated cattle ear tag.

Environmental Issues

- Properly dispose of these pesticides to avoid environmental/groundwater contamination.

COMMENTS

Patient Monitoring

- Pay close attention to secretions. Use an appropriate amount of atropine to control secretions. Replace IV fluids to correct fluid losses from secretions and decontamination procedures.
- Monitor heart rate – bradycardia occurs most commonly, tachycardia less so.

Prevention/Avoidance

- Keep pesticides away from pets, follow label directions, and properly dispose of old or unused products.
- Fence or otherwise keep pets out of rose gardens and shrubs and any other areas when pesticides are applied.

Expected Course and Prognosis

- Good with early and aggressive care. Animals developing the intermediate syndrome may need care for several days to weeks. Pancreatitis and hemorrhagic gastroenteritis complicate the recovery.

Abbreviations

See Appendix 1 for a complete list.

DUMBSLED = diarrhea, urination, miosis/mydriasis, bradycardia, salivation,lacrimation, emesis, dyspnea
SLUDGE = salivation, lacrimation, urination, diarrhea, gastroenteritis
TEPP = tetraethyl pyrophosphate

Suggested Reading

Bahri L. Pralidoxime. Compend Contin Educ Vet 2002; 24(11):884–886.

Fikes J. Organophosphorus and carbamate insecticides. Toxicology of selected pesticides, drugs and chemicals. Vet Clin North Am Small Anim Pract 1990; 20(2):353–367.

Frick TW, Dalo S, O'Leary JF, et al. Effects of the insecticide diazinon on pancreas of dog, cat, and guinea pig. J Environ Pathol Toxicol 1987; 7(4):1–11.

Hopper K, Aldrich J, Haskins C. The recognition and treatment of the intermediate syndrome of organophosphate poisoning in a dog. J Vet Emerg Crit Care 2002; 12(2): 99–102.

Means C. Organophosphate and carbamate insecticides. In: Peterson ME, Talcott PA, eds. Small Animal Toxicology, 3rd edn. St Louis, MO: Elsevier, 2013; pp. 715–724.

Tecles F, Panizo C, Subiela SM, et al. Effects of different variables on whole blood cholinesterase analysis in dogs. J Vet Diagn Invest 2002; 14:132–139.

Author: Patricia A. Talcott, DVM, PhD, DABVT
Consulting Editor: Robert H. Poppenga, DVM, PhD, DABVT

Pyrethrins and Pyrethroids

chapter 94

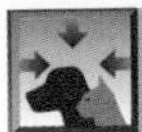

DEFINITION/OVERVIEW

- Pyrethrins are derived from flowers of the genus *Chrysanthemum*, while pyrethroids are synthetic derivatives of pyrethrins. They are commonly used as topical and environmental insecticides and come in a variety of formulations including sprays, shampoos, dips, collars, ear tags, dusts, spot-on/pour-on liquids, and granules.
- Signs associated with toxicosis include hypersalivation, hyper- or hypothermia, dyspnea, paresthesia, vomiting, hyperexcitability, tremors, ataxia, weakness, seizures, and death.

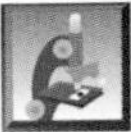

ETIOLOGY/PATHOPHYSIOLOGY

- Pyrethroids and pyrethrins have three general classifications based on chemical structure.
  - **Pyrethrins**: pyrethrin I and II, cinerin I and II, and jasmolin I and II.
  - **Type I pyrethroids** contain no cyano (CN) group: allethrin, bifenthrin, permethrin, phenothrin, resmethrin, sumithrin, tefluthrin, tetramethrin.
  - **Type II pyrethroids** contain a cyano group: cyfluthrin, cyhalothrin, cypermethrin, cyphenothrin, deltamethrin, fenvalerate, flumethrin, fluvalinate, and tralomethrin.
  - Etofenprox contains no cyano group but is classified as a nonester pyrethroid or pyrethroid derivative rather than a Type I pyrethroid. Because of this classification, some manufacturers claim/market etofenprox as a nonpyrethroid; however, its mechanism of action and toxic effects are typical of pyrethroids.
- Synthetic manipulation of pyrethrins to form pyrethroids results in products that are more environmentally stable, therefore having longer-lasting efficacy.
- Pyrethrins and pyrethroids are frequently formulated with other ingredients to enhance the insecticidal activity of the formulation.
  - Methoprene and pyriproxyfen: insect growth regulators that prevent immature insect stages from maturing by interfering with insect-specific growth hormones.
  - Piperonyl butoxide: synergist that inhibits insect metabolism of some insecticides, including pyrethroids.

Blackwell's Five-Minute Veterinary Consult Clinical Companion: Small Animal Toxicology, Second Edition.
Lynn R. Hovda, Ahna G. Brutlag, Robert H. Poppenga, and Katherine L. Peterson.

Companion website: www.fiveminutevet.com/toxicology

Mechanism of Action

- Pyrethrins and pyrethroids cause hyperexcitability of cells by slowing the closing of sodium channels. The duration of action is much longer for Type II versus Type I pyrethroids. Type II pyrethroids may also exhibit activity on GABA-gated chloride channels.
- Sodium channels are found in large numbers in peripheral muscle, salivary glands, and the CNS, which explains the manifestation of signs seen with overdoses.
- The effect on sodium influx is temperature dependent, with increased activity at cooler temperatures.
- Paresthesia effects (tingling, burning, numbing, itching) following topical application of some pyrethroids (e.g., permethrin) are caused by direct action on cutaneous sensory nerves.

Pharmacokinetics – Absorption, Distribution, Metabolism, Excretion

- Rapidly absorbed following ingestion; oral bioavailability in dogs is ~50%.
- Transdermal absorption varies with species, pyrethroid, and formulation, but in general is quite low.
- Pyrethrins and pyrethroids are highly lipophilic and readily distribute to tissues with high lipid concentrations such as the CNS, adipose tissue, liver, kidneys, and milk.
- Pyrethrins and pyrethroids do not cross the placenta or accumulate in the fetus.
- Metabolism occurs in small intestine, liver and blood.
  - Primary routes are hydrolysis of ester bonds and oxidation of acid and alcohol moieties.
  - Metabolites of hydrolysis and oxidation have little to no toxicological action.
  - Sensitivity of cats to pyrethroids is therefore unlikely to be related to a deficiency in glucuronidation ability.
  - Some metabolites are further conjugated with amino acids, glucuronide, or sulfate.
- Metabolites are eliminated primarily through the urine, although some pyrethroids (e.g., permethrin) have significant biliary excretion.

Toxicity

- In mammals, pyrethroids are 50× less toxic than organochlorine, 136× less toxic than organophosphorus and 280× less toxic than carbamate insecticides.
- Toxicity varies with animal species as well as the specific pyrethrin/pyrethroid product, concentration, and formulation.
- Generally, products containing <1% pyrethrin/pyrethroid are well tolerated by mammals, including cats.
- Cats are particularly sensitive to many concentrated (>5%) pyrethroids. Some cats can tolerate concentrated forms of phenothrin, but enough adverse reactions were reported that feline phenothrin spot-on products were removed from the market. Cats do tolerate concentrated (40–60%) etofenprox products when applied at the labeled rate.

- Onset of signs of toxicosis may occur within minutes to several hours following exposure depending on species involved, route of exposure, pyrethrin/pyrethroid, formulation, and dosage.
- Toxicosis is classified as Type I or Type II based on signs seen in rats.
    - This classification is *not* related to the Type I and Type II pyrethroid chemical classification.
    - Type I toxicosis is characterized by progressive body tremors, exaggerated startle response, hyperexcitability, and prostration.
    - Type II toxicosis is characterized by hypersalivation, weakness, ataxia, coarse tremor, and tonic seizures.
    - Some pyrethroids cause syndromes that have characteristics of both Type I and Type II toxicoses.
- Dermal paresthesia at the site of concentrated pyrethroid application can result in signs of agitation, scratching, panting, hyperactivity, or depression and reluctance to move.
- Oral exposure may result in hypersalivation and/or vomiting without neurological involvement.

Systems Affected

- Gastrointestinal – hypersalivation, vomiting, diarrhea, gastritis.
- Skin/exocrine – paresthesia, localized dermal hypersensitivity reaction.
- Nervous – hyperesthesia, hyperexcitability, ataxia, paw/facial twitching, muscle fasciculation, tremor, seizure.
- Endocrine/metabolic – hyperthermia due to prolonged muscle activity; stimulation of the adrenal gland resulting in potential hyperglycemia.
- Ophthalmic – mydriasis, transient blindness, significant contact irritation due primarily to carrier agents in the product.
- Respiratory – respiratory distress secondary to unmanaged neurological symptoms. True anaphylactic or allergic responses generally only occur with natural pyrethrins.
- Renal/urological – myoglobinuria secondary to uncontrolled/prolonged tremors or seizures; potential for ARF.

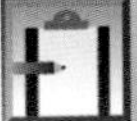

SIGNALMENT/HISTORY

Risk Factors

- Felines are especially sensitive to some concentrated pyrethroids (e.g., 45% permethrin), but tolerate concentrated forms of others (e.g., 40% etofenprox).
- Very young, very old, anemic, sick, debilitated, or stressed animals may be at increased risk of toxicosis.
- Heavy flea, tick, or other parasite infestations may increase risk of toxicosis.

Historical Findings

- Patients may present with a history of product application or misuse within the previous 12–24 hours.
- Some cats present after a canine pyrethroid spot-on product was applied to another pet in the house with which they had physical contact.
- Patients (commonly dogs) may present after having ingested large quantities of pyrethroid-based granular yard insecticides, pyrethroid flea collars, or contents of tubes of topical spot-on products.

Location and Circumstances of Poisoning

- Intentional or accidental exposures generally occur in or around the home.
- Exposure to livestock or agricultural products may occur in farming environments.

Interactions with Drugs, Nutrients, or Environment

- Pyrethroids have no anticholinesterase activity, so potentiation of organophosphorus or carbamate insecticides is not expected if used together.
- Use of more than one pyrethroid product may result in additive effects and increase risk of toxicosis; this is primarily a concern with concentrated (>5%) pyrethroids.

CLINICAL FEATURES

- Onset of clinical signs varies based on formulation of product and route of exposure, ranging from several minutes to several hours.
- Signs include hypersalivation, hyper- or hypothermia, paresthesia, "paw flicking," vomiting, hyperexcitability, tremors, ataxia, weakness, dyspnea, seizures, and death.
- Paresthesia effects may result in reluctance to move, hiding, hyperactivity, agitation, panting, and attempts to scratch the site of application.

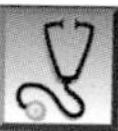

DIFFERENTIAL DIAGNOSIS

- Intoxications: organophosphate or carbamate insecticides, organochlorine insecticides, strychnine, metaldehyde, 4-aminopyridine, methylxanthines, tremorgenic mycotoxins, CNS stimulant drugs (amphetamine, cocaine, etc.), nicotine, xylitol.
- Hepatic encephalopathy, uremic encephalopathy, hypoglycemia, hypocalcemia.
- CNS trauma, CNS neoplasia, CNS inflammation/infection.

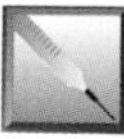

DIAGNOSTICS

- Baseline PCV/TS and blood glucose.
- CBC, serum chemistry, UA, particularly in geriatric patients or those with metabolic disease.

- In cases with severe tremors or seizures, a CK and coagulation panel may be helpful in determining other underlying etiologies or secondary complications (e.g., DIC).
- Gas chromatographic analysis of hair samples or tissues (fat, brain, liver) can confirm exposure to pyrethroids, but potentially long turn-around times make this impractical for diagnosing emergent cases. Tissue pyrethroid concentrations do not correlate with degree of clinical illness.
- No specific gross or microscopic pathological findings are expected.

THERAPEUTICS

- The goals of treatment are to manage clinical signs, provide supportive care, remove the source of the intoxication when feasible, and monitor for development of complications due to prolonged tremors or seizures.
- Minor signs such as hypersalivation, facial/ear twitching, paw flicking, single episodes of vomiting or diarrhea may occur as adverse effects following the appropriate use of pyrethroid products in dogs and cats. These signs are generally transient and do not usually require specific treatment.

Detoxification

- Manage severe clinical signs (tremors, seizures) first before attempting decontamination.
- Oral exposures.
  - Cats, especially, may hypersalivate due to the unpleasant taste of a topically applied product as they attempt to groom themselves. These "taste reactions" can often be managed by offering milk or liquid from canned, water-packed tuna to help dilute the taste of the product.
  - Patients whose exposure is thought to be due to grooming product off themselves or other animals are not likely to have significant product in the GI tract to warrant induction of emesis or administration of activated charcoal.
  - Do not induce emesis in symptomatic patients due to risk of aspiration pneumonia. Do not administer activated charcoal to patients showing more than mild signs due to risk of aspiration pneumonia.
  - Patients that have ingested large quantities of pyrethroid solids (e.g., collars, granules) and are not showing signs may have emesis induced.
  - 3% hydrogen peroxide 2 mL/kg PO up to maximum of 45 mL; feeding a small, moist meal may improve efficacy.
  - Dogs: apomorphine 0.02–0.04 mg/kg IV, SC, IM; can cause CNS depression, so use with care.
  - Cats: alpha$_2$-adrenergic agents (sedative effects can be reversed with atipamezole or yohimbine).
    - Dexmedetomidine 0.001–0.002 mg/kg IV or 0.04 mg/kg IM.
    - Xylazine 0.44 mg/kg IM, SC.

    - Activated charcoal (1–3 g/kg) with cathartic may also be used in asymptomatic patients following ingestion of large amounts of solid pyrethroids.
- Dermal exposures.
    - Medically manage any severe signs first; attempting to bathe tremoring patients may worsen tremors or precipitate seizures.
    - Bathe patients in liquid dish detergent using warm water; several applications of detergent may be necessary. Keep patient warm following bathing.

Appropriate Health Care

- Manage severe tremors and/or seizures. Antitremor therapy will not always eliminate every ear or facial twitch, and care should be taken not to overmedicate in order to eliminate minor tremors or twitching. The goal is to manage tremors to the point that the patient can maintain a normal body temperature, ambulate normally, and eat/drink without problems.
- IV fluids may aid in providing cardiovascular support, maintaining hydration, and cooling hyperthermic patients; fluids will not enhance elimination of pyrethroids, so diuresis is not warranted.
- Thermoregulation is vital. Tremoring/seizing patients frequently present hyperthermic due to muscle activity. Managing tremors/seizures followed by bathing often results in resolution of hyperthermia without need for aggressive cooling measures. Patients not kept warm following bathing risk hypothermia, which can exacerbate muscle tremors as pyrethroids are more potent at lower body temperatures.
- Patients experiencing local paresthesia reactions may respond to one or more of the following.
    - Vitamin E oil applied directly to area of product application often eliminates the uncomfortable sensation. Snip open an oral vitamin E capsule and squeeze contents onto skin.
    - Cool packs applied to the area may provide additional relief.
    - Diphenhydramine may help in cases with persistent signs; more likely due to sedative effect rather than antihistaminic effect.

Antidote

- There is no specific antidote.

Drugs of Choice

- Tremors/seizures can be treated with methocarbamol or other CNS depressants.
    - Methocarbamol 50–220 mg/kg IV; administer ½ of dose at ~2 mL/min, wait for patient to relax, then administer remainder slowly to effect. Some have advocated following bolus with methocarbamol CRI of 8.8–12.2 mg/kg/hour; dosages exceeding 330 mg/kg/day may be required in severe cases but patients receiving these higher dosages should be carefully monitored for methocarbamol-induced respiratory depression.

- Midazolam 0.05–0.31 mg/kg/hour IV CRI +/- propofol; monitor respiration and body temperature closely in anesthetized patients.
- Propofol 1.5–19 mg/kg/hour IV CRI; monitor respiration and body temperature closely in anesthetized patients.
- Phenobarbital 2–8 mg/kg IV to effect; monitor respiration and body temperature closely in anesthetized patients.
- Pentobarbital 4–16 mg/kg IV to effect; monitor respiration and body temperature closely in anesthetized patients.
- Diazepam 0.13–1.5 mg/kg IV, 0.47–1.7 mg/kg per rectum; rarely effective as sole agent for tremors or seizures, but can reduce hyperesthesia when used in combination with methocarbamol.

■ Intravenous lipid emulsions (ILE) have been used successfully in cats with permethrin toxicosis. Until more data is available on appropriate dosages, side effects, etc., such use should be considered investigational and restricted to patients unresponsive to other treatment or where euthanasia is being considered due to cost/duration of treatment.
- ILE, 20% solution, 1.5 mL/kg bolus followed by 0.5 mL/kg/min for 30–60 min; repeat in 4–6 hours if signs still present and serum is not lipemic; discontinue if no effect after two doses. Reported adverse events with ILE therapy include hemolysis and pancreatitis.

Precautions/ Interactions

■ Atropine is not indicated in treating pyrethroid toxicosis.

COMMENTS

Patient Monitoring

■ Monitor for return of tremors in patients that initially responded to treatment. Reassess thermoregulation measures and decontamination effectiveness if tremors continue to recur.

■ Monitor for development of complications from tremors/seizures (e.g., rhabdomyolysis, DIC, renal injury, etc.).

Prevention/Avoidance

■ Secure all pesticides where they cannot be accessed by pets or children.

■ Always use pesticide products per label directions based on animal age and/or weight.

■ Never apply a product labeled only for dogs to other species.

■ Fish and aquatic invertebrates are exquisitely sensitive to pyrethrins and pyrethroids and may die from minimal exposures. Dogs that had topical pyrethroid products applied should not be allowed to enter water containing desirable fish or invertebrates until the product has completely dried.

Possible Complications

- Rhabdomyolysis +/- myoglobinuric ARF due to prolonged muscular exertion from tremors or seizures.
- Prolonged hyperthermia may result in development of DIC.

Expected Course and Prognosis

- Most cases that are treated promptly and aggressively have good outcomes.
- Failure to obtain prompt treatment can result in development of complications (e.g., rhabdomyolysis, DIC) that can worsen prognosis.

Abbreviations

See Appendix 1 for a complete list.

Suggested Reading

Boland LA, Angles JM. Feline permethrin toxicity: retrospective study of 42 cases. J Feline Med Surg 2010; 12(2):61–71.

Draper WE, Boldfer L, Cottam E, McMichael M, Schubert T. Methocarbamol CRI for symptomatic treatment of pyrethroid intoxication: a report of three cases. J Am Anim Hosp Assoc 2013; 49(5):325–328.

Hansen SR. Pyrethrins and pyrethroids. In: Peterson ME, Talcott PA, eds. Small Animal Toxicology, 3rd edn. St Louis, MO: Elsevier, 2013; pp. 769–775.

Kuo K, Odunayo A. Adjunctive therapy with intravenous lipid emulsion and methocarbamol for permethrin toxicity in 2 cats. J Vet Emerg Crit Care 2013; 23(4):436–441.

Acknowledgment: The authors and editors acknowledge the prior contributions of Nancy M. Gruber, DVM, who authored this topic in the previous edition.

Author: Sharon Gwaltney-Brant, DVM, PhD, DABVT, DABT

Consulting Editor: Robert H. Poppenga, DVM, PhD, DABVT

Metals and Metalloids

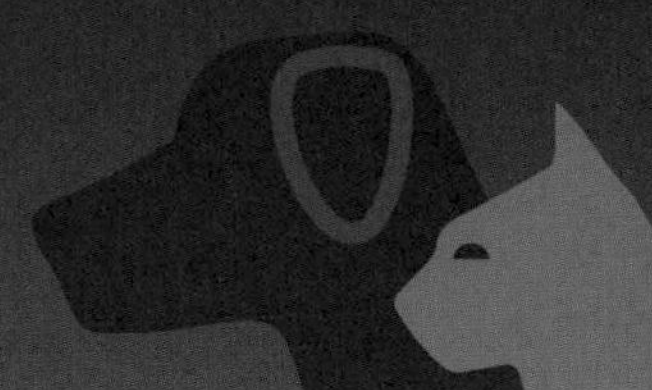

Iron

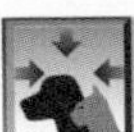

DEFINITION/OVERVIEW

- Iron is an essential element for living organisms in that it is essential for the transport and binding of oxygen, as well as its requirement for many oxidation-reduction reactions.
- In companion animals, oral toxicosis is predominant, but iron can be toxic by injectable routes as well.
- Iron may be lethal when ingested in large quantities due to its oxidation-reduction properties.
- Sources of large concentrations of readily ionizable iron include multivitamins, dietary mineral supplements, human gestational supplements, fertilizers, molluscicides, and some types of hand warmers.
- Large doses of ionizable iron can result in loss of the normal mucosal limitations of iron absorption, likely due to the corrosive effect to the GI mucosa.
- Circulating iron in excess of the total iron-binding capacity (TIBC), also referred to as free iron, is very reactive. It can cause oxidative damage to any cell type, as well as subcellular organelles.
- Damage to mitochondria results in loss of oxidative metabolism.
- Primary systems affected are GI, hepatic, cardiovascular, and CNS.

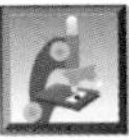

ETIOLOGY/PATHOPHYSIOLOGY

- Iron toxicosis is generally associated with ingestion of iron-fortified pills (e.g., vitamin/minerals or gestational supplements), but other sources include iron-fortified fertilizers, newer molluscicide products, and some types of hand warmers.
- In order for iron to be absorbed and be toxic, it must be in a readily ionizable form.
- Metallic iron, iron-containing alloys, and iron oxide (rust) are not readily ionizable. Thus, they are not associated with iron toxicoses.
- Take care when calculating iron ingestion; iron salts in supplements and medications vary in elemental iron content (between 12% and 63%; see table 95.1).

Blackwell's Five-Minute Veterinary Consult Clinical Companion: Small Animal Toxicology, Second Edition.
Lynn R. Hovda, Ahna G. Brutlag, Robert H. Poppenga, and Katherine L. Peterson.

Companion website: www.fiveminutevet.com/toxicology

TABLE 95.1. **Percentage of elemental iron in common soluble iron salts.**

Salt	Percentage of elemental iron
Iron (as ferric salt)	100
Iron (as ferrous salt)	100
Ferric ammonium citrate	15
Ferric chloride	34
Ferric hydroxide	63
Ferric phosphate	37
Ferric pyrophosphate	30
Ferrocholinate	12
Ferroglycine sulfate	16
Ferrous fumarate	33
Ferrous carbonate	48
Ferrous gluconate	12
Ferrous lactate	24
Ferrous sulfate (anhydrous)	37
Ferrous sulfate (hydrate)	20
Peptonized iron	16

Mechanism of Action

- Large oral doses of ionizable iron can result in loss of the normal mucosal limitations of iron absorption, likely due to the corrosive effect to the GI mucosa.
- Circulating iron in excess of the TIBC (i.e., free iron) is very reactive. It can cause oxidative damage to any cell type, as well as subcellular organelles.
- Reduction-oxidation cycling of iron from ferric to ferrous states and back can result in free radicals that are highly reactive.
- Free circulating iron causes oxidative damage to membranes, resulting in highly reactive hydroxyl ions and hydroxyl radicals. These reactive byproducts cause further membrane damage.
- Predominant damage is focused on tissues of highest exposure to the free iron: GIT, cardiovascular, and hepatic.
- Vasodilatation and vascular damage result in systemic shock, leading to a metabolic acidosis.
- Vascular damage can result in hemorrhage.
- Damage to mitochondria results in loss of oxidative metabolism and further contributes to systemic metabolic acidosis.

Pharmacokinetics – Absorption, Distribution, Metabolism, Excretion

- Iron absorption is typically limited at the site of the GI mucosa.
- Iron must be ionized in order to be absorbed.
- Ferrous iron is more bioavailable than ferric, but ferric can be absorbed to a lesser degree if it is ionized.
- Once absorbed, iron is distributed to tissues bound to iron-binding proteins.
- Saturation of these iron-binding proteins results in "free iron" being circulated in the serum to tissues.
- Unused iron is sequestered in tissues as ferritin molecules.
- Unlike most metals, animals have an inability to excrete excess iron. Even in overdose situations, excess iron is incorporated into ferritin in cells as a means of sequestering it.
- Minimal amounts of iron are lost from the body, primarily via exfoliation of GIT cells or via blood loss.

Toxicity

- Oral toxic dose (dogs).
  - <20 mg/kg of ionizable iron is nontoxic.
  - 20–60 mg/kg of ionizable iron can result in clinical signs.
  - >60 mg/kg of ionizable iron can result in serious clinical disease.
- Injectable iron is more toxic due to much greater bioavailability.

Systems Affected

- Cardiovascular.
  - Free circulating iron reacts with the lipids in cell membranes with which it comes in contact.
  - Oxidative damage occurs to the vascular endothelial cells.
  - Cellular damage results in vasodilatation, vascular leakage, and hemorrhage.
- Metabolic.
  - Hypovolemia and hypotension result in a lactic acidosis, contributing to acid–base imbalances (e.g., metabolic acidosis).
  - Mitochondrial damage by free iron inhibits oxidative metabolism.
- Gastrointestinal.
  - Direct oxidative damage to the mucosal cells results in GI erosions, ulcerations, and hemorrhage.
  - Pills may adhere to mucosal surfaces, resulting in significant localized erosions even when systemic toxic doses have not been ingested.
  - Corrosive damage allows iron to move more freely into systemic circulation.
  - Potential long-term effects are stricture formation in the esophagus or GIT.
- Hepatobiliary.
  - Hepatocytes are exposed to free iron absorbed from the GIT via portal blood flow.
  - Hepatocytes and Kupffer cells extract free iron from the circulation.

    - Free iron damages hepatocellular membranes and subcellular organelles.
    - Cellular damage can result in coagulation deficits.
- Nervous.
    - CNS effects typically secondary to effects on other systems.
    - Vascular damage can result in CNS edema.
    - Hepatic damage can result in hepatic encephalopathy.

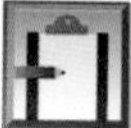

SIGNALMENT/HISTORY

- All species are potentially susceptible, with no age-associated difference in susceptibility.
- Dogs are likely to ingest large amounts of the described iron-containing materials, owing to relatively indiscriminate eating behavior.

Historical Findings

- Owners frequently report ingestion of large numbers of vitamin/mineral pills.

Location and Circumstances of Poisoning

- Most frequent ingestion occurs inside households when dogs gain access to bottles of vitamin/mineral pills.
- Much rarer exposures that result in toxic effects include ingestions of iron-fortified fertilizers or some types of iron-containing hand warmers.
- Exposure of dogs to iron-containing molluscicides has increased due to wider availability of products designed to replace metaldehyde formulations.

CLINICAL FEATURES

- Toxicosis is unlikely to develop in animals that remain asymptomatic for 6–8 hours.
- Iron toxicosis occurs in four phases outlined below.
- Severity and timing of the phases are dependent on the dose and differing amounts of damage among tissues.
- Clinical stages initially present in the GIT, due to first presentation for oral exposures.
    - Stage I (0–6 hours).
        - □ Vomiting
        - □ Diarrhea
        - □ Lethargy
        - □ GI hemorrhage
        - □ Abdominal pain
    - Stage II (6–24 hours).
        - □ Apparent recovery
    - Stage III (12–96 hours).
        - □ Vomiting

- Diarrhea
- Lethargy
- GI hemorrhage
- Shock
- Tremors
- Abdominal pain
- Metabolic acidosis

- **Stage IV (2–6 weeks).**
  - GI obstruction from stricture formation is a secondary effect of the massive mucosal damage that occurs early in the syndrome.

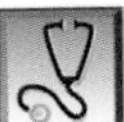

DIFFERENTIAL DIAGNOSIS

- Primary gastrointestinal disease – mesenteric torsion, GDV, foreign body obstruction, pancreatitis, septic peritonitis, hemorrhagic gastroenteritis, viral enteritis, bacterial enteritis, gastroenteritis, infectious, parasitic.
- Secondary gastrointestinal disease – hypoadrenocorticism, endotoxin ingestion from garbage, caustic/corrosive ingestion, heat stroke, "shock gut."
- Primary metabolic disease – renal, hepatic, etc.

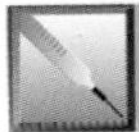

DIAGNOSTICS

- CBC, chemistry, UA, venous blood gas analysis – evidence of leukocytosis, hyperglycemia, metabolic acidosis, normal to high AST, ALT, ALP, and serum bilirubin.
- Serum analysis for total iron and TIBC.
  - Often available through local human hospitals.
  - Normal serum iron binding capacity is 3–4 times the serum iron concentration.
  - Serum iron in excess of TIBC indicates poisoning such that treatment is required.
  - If chewable tablets or a liquid solution are involved, serum iron levels should be checked 2–3 hours post ingestion.
    - Normal level in dogs: 94–122 µg/dL.
    - Level at which chelation is necessary: >350–500 µg/dL.
  - Monitor at 2–3 hours and at 5–6 hours post ingestion in asymptomatic patients (absorption rates vary and serum iron concentrations may change rapidly).
  - Monitor every 6–8 hours in patients on chelation therapy.
- Radiography may be beneficial, as intact iron-containing pills can be radiodense. One may be able to visualize pill bezoars or pills adhered to the esophageal/gastric mucosa.

Pathological Findings

- Primary gross lesions are of damage to the GIT, liver, and vascular systems.
- Damage to the GIT can range from erythema to complete denudation of epithelial cells.

- Hemorrhage in the GIT and liver is often observed, but hemorrhage can be seen in any organ system. Hepatomegaly may also be evident.
- Pathological lesions of edema and hemorrhage in any organ system can occur due to damage to vasculature.
- Cellular damage to vascular endothelium, hepatocytes, and myocardial cells may be seen histologically.

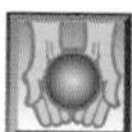

THERAPEUTICS

- General therapy is aimed at minimizing further iron absorption, correcting hypovolemic shock, correcting metabolic acidosis, treating GI signs, and eliminating free iron.

Detoxification

- Activated charcoal does not bind to iron and should not be used.
- Prevent further GI and systemic damage by removal of unabsorbed iron from the stomach. This will lessen the duration and severity of clinical signs.
- Induce emesis in asymptomatic patient, early post ingestion. Caution is advised if evidence of gastric damage is already present.
- Gastric lavage should be performed when emesis is contraindicated or when pill bezoars are identified (e.g., radiographically).
- Emergency gastrotomy may be indicated if lavage fails to remove adherent pills or bezoars, and a toxic amount of iron has been ingested.

Appropriate Health Care

- Treat shock and metabolic acidosis appropriately. (See chapter 2, Emergency Management of the Poisoned Patient, for more information.)
- IV fluids as needed for dehydration and hypovolemia for 24–72 hours or as needed until clinical signs abate; this will also enhance urinary elimination of chelated iron.
- Treat GI damage with gastric antiulcer medication, demulcents, or sucralfate. Maintain gastric demulcents/protectants to decrease GI damage and decrease the potential for stricture formation. This care should continue beyond the use of chelation to remove free iron.

Antidotes

- Chelate the systemic free iron to prevent further oxidative damage to tissues.
    - Deferoxamine mesylate is an effective iron chelator and is given at 15 mg/kg/hour, slow IV infusion or 40 mg/kg IM q 4–6 hours or 40 mg/kg, slow IV q 4–6 hours.
    - For chelation when indicated by serum iron exceeding TIBC, or when serum iron levels are >350–500 µg/dL.
    - Duration of chelation therapy is until TIBC is greater than serum iron.
    - Monitor serum iron and TIBC every 6–8 hours while on chelation therapy.

Drugs of Choice

- Antiemetics.
  - Maropitant 1 mg/kg, SQ q 24 hours.
  - Ondansetron 0.1–0.2 mg/kg, SQ, IV q 8–12 hours.
  - Metoclopramide 0.2–0.5 mg/kg, PO, IM, SQ q 8 hours or 1–2 mg/kg/day, CRI IV.
- H_2 antagonists.
  - Famotidine 0.5–1.0 mg/kg, PO, SQ, IM, or IV q 12–24 hours.
- Proton pump inhibitors.
  - Omeprazole 0.5–1.0 mg/kg, PO q 24 hours in dogs; 0.7 mg/kg, PO q 24 hours in cats.
  - Pantoprazole 1 mg/kg, IV q 24 hours in dogs.
- Sucralfate 0.5–1 g, PO q 8 hours.
- Oral milk of magnesia or aluminum hydroxide will precipitate iron in the GIT as insoluble iron hydroxide.

Precautions/Interactions

- Gastric lavage is contraindicated when hematemesis is present due to increased risk of perforation.
- Intravenous deferoxamine must be given slowly or it may precipitate cardiac arrhythmias.
- Deferoxamine is teratogenic. Use in pregnant patients only if the benefits outweigh the risks.
- Deferoxamine-iron chelates are eliminated in the urine. Caution is advised for patients with poor renal function.

Alternative Drugs

- New iron chelation agents are in development for treating chronic iron overload in humans, but they currently have not been investigated for use in acute iron overload in companion animals.

Diet

- Oral intake should be limited during the first 24 hours in severely affected animals. After thorough evaluation of GI damage, one can determine whether the patient can return to a normal diet or should be placed on a bland, easily digestible, soft food diet for a period of time to allow mucosal repair.

Activity

- Once clinical signs have abated, activity does not need to be limited.

Surgical Considerations

- In cases where a toxic dose has been ingested and (1) pill bezoars are adherent to mucosa, (2) pills are visualized by radiography, or (3) lavage fails to remove materials, emergency gastrotomy is indicated.

COMMENTS

- Care must be taken with induction of emesis or gastric lavage, as cellular damage can predispose to perforating injuries during these procedures.
- It is critical that remaining iron material or pills be removed to prevent further absorption or GI damage.

Patient Monitoring

- Monitor hydration status, serum hepatic enzymes, acid–base status, and GIT effects.
- After chelation therapy is discontinued, appropriate supportive care should be provided for an additional 24 hours in order to monitor the serum iron and TIBC at least once 24 hours post chelation therapy.
- In severely affected animals, owners should be informed to monitor their pet for normal dietary intake and fecal production for up to 6–8 weeks in order to evaluate for the development of strictures.

Prevention/Avoidance

- Prevention is only achieved by limiting the potential animal exposure.

Possible Complications

- As previously outlined, stricture formation is a possible sequel to GI mucosal damage.

Expected Course and Prognosis

- In patients that do not develop clinical signs by 8 hours, the prognosis is very good. These animals are unlikely to develop clinical signs.
- In patients that are adequately decontaminated prior to development of clinical signs, the prognosis is fair to guarded until there is a lack of signs for 8 hours or until the serum iron is less than the TIBC at 6–8 hours post ingestion.
- In symptomatic patients, the prognosis is guarded until chelation therapy results in serum iron levels less than the TIBC. The prognosis is based on the severity of clinical signs and the amount of damage already done.

Abbreviations

See Appendix 1 for a complete list.

Suggested Reading

Albretsen JC. Iron. In: Plumlee H, ed. Clinical Veterinary Toxicology. St Louis, MO: Mosby, 2004; pp. 202–204.

Brutlag AG, Flint CTC, Puschner B. Iron intoxication in a dog consequent to the ingestion of oxygen absorber sachets in pet treat packaging. J Med Toxicol 2012; 8:76–79.

Hall JO. Iron. In: Peterson ME, Talcott PA, eds. Small Animal Toxicology, 3rd edn. St Louis,MO: Elsevier, 2013; pp. 595–600.
Hooser. Iron. In: Gupta RC, ed. Veterinary Toxicology Basic and Clinical Principles, 2nd edn. San Diego: Elsevier, 2012; pp. 517–521.

Author: Jeffery O. Hall, DVM, PhD, DABVT
Consulting Editor: Robert H. Poppenga, DVM, PhD, DABVT

Lead

DEFINITION/OVERVIEW

- Multisystemic intoxication (blood lead >0.4 ppm) following acute or chronic exposure to some form of lead.
- Both acute and chronic intoxications are possible depending on exposure amounts and duration.
- Primarily gastrointestinal and neurological signs. Gastrointestinal signs often precede CNS signs and are more likely with chronic, low-level lead exposure. CNS signs are more common with acute exposures and in younger animals.
- Sources for lead exposure include lead paint and paint residues or dust from sanding; car batteries; linoleum; solder; plumbing materials and supplies; lubricating compounds; putty; tar paper; lead foil; golf balls; lead object (e.g., ammunition, fishing sinkers, drapery weights), leaded glass; use of improperly glazed ceramic food or water bowl. The most common sources of exposure for dogs and cats are lead paint or lead-contaminated dust or soil.

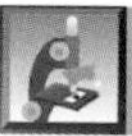

ETIOLOGY/PATHOPHYSIOLOGY

Mechanism of Action

- Cell damage is due to the ability of lead to substitute for other polyvalent cations (especially divalent cations such as Ca and Zn) important for cell homeostasis.
- Diverse biological processes are affected, including metal transport, energy metabolism, apoptosis, ion conduction, cell adhesion, inter- and intracellular signaling, enzymatic processes, protein maturation, and genetic regulation.

Pharmacokinetics – Absorption, Distribution, Metabolism, Excretion

- Bioavailability of lead is dependent on its form (inorganic or organic; if inorganic, salt or pure metal).
- Lead has higher bioavailability in young, growing animals due to absorption via calcium-binding proteins.
- More than 90% of absorbed lead is bound to red blood cells.

Blackwell's Five-Minute Veterinary Consult Clinical Companion: Small Animal Toxicology, Second Edition.
Lynn R. Hovda, Ahna G. Brutlag, Robert H. Poppenga, and Katherine L. Peterson.

Companion website: www.fiveminutevet.com/toxicology

- Unbound lead is widely distributed in tissues.
- Bone serves as a long-term storage site for lead.
- A significant percentage of ingested lead is eliminated via the feces without being absorbed; absorbed lead is eliminated via the urine and bile.
- The half-life of lead is multiphasic; in dogs, lead elimination is triphasic with half-lives of 12 days (blood), 184 days (soft tissues) and >4500 days (bone).

Toxicity

- Not well defined in cats; toxicity noted in cats at 1000 ppm in diet or oral ingestion of 3 mg/kg.
- An acutely toxic oral dose for dogs is approximately 190–1000 mg/kg (dependent on lead form) whereas a chronic cumulative toxic dose is 1.8–2.6 mg/kg/day.

Systems Affected

- Gastrointestinal – unknown mechanism, likely damage to peripheral nerves.
- Nervous – capillary damage; alteration of membrane ionic channels and signaling molecules.
- Renal/urological – damage to proximal tubule cells due to enzyme disruption and oxidative damage.
- Hemic/lymph/immune – interference with hemoglobin synthesis, increased fragility and decreased survival of RBCs, release of reticulocytes and nucleated RBCs from bone marrow, inhibition of 5'-pyrimidine nucleotidase causing retention of RNA degradation products, aggregation of ribosomes resulting in basophilic stippling.

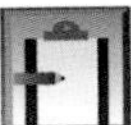

SIGNALMENT/HISTORY

Risk Factors

- Housing in older, nonrenovated buildings where lead-based paint was used.
- Housing in older buildings undergoing renovation where environmental lead contamination is more likely to occur.
- Low socioeconomic status of pet owner.
- Younger animals (<1 year) have higher risk due to greater lead bioavailability.
- Dogs more commonly affected than cats.
- No breed or sex predilections.

Historical Findings

- History of renovation of older house or building or ingestion of lead objects.

Location and Circumstances of Poisoning

- Dogs are more likely to ingest lead-containing paint or lead objects; cats are exposed to lead-containing dusts as a result of grooming.

Interaction with Drugs, Nutrients or Environment

- Lead bioavailablity is enhanced in animals deficient in calcium, zinc, iron, or vitamin D, or fasting animals.
- High dietary zinc and calcium decrease lead bioavailability.

CLINICAL FEATURES

- Primarily gastrointestinal and neurological signs.
- Signs are often insidious in onset and vague and include vomiting, diarrhea, anorexia, weight loss, abdominal pain, colic, regurgitation (secondary to megaesophagus), lethargy, hysteria, seizures, blindness, anemia, PU/PD.
- Cats – central vestibular abnormalities such as vertical nystagmus and ataxia reported.

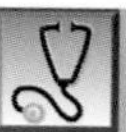

DIFFERENTIAL DIAGNOSIS

Dogs

- Canine distemper
- Infectious encephalitides
- Epilepsy
- Bromethalin, methylxanthine or tremorgenic mycotoxin toxicosis
- NSAID toxicosis
- Heat stroke
- Intestinal parasitism
- Intussusception
- Foreign body
- Pancreatitis
- Infectious canine hepatitis

Cats

- Degenerative or storage diseases
- Hepatic encephalopathy
- Infectious encephalitides
- Organophosphate/carbamate insecticide, bromethalin, or methylxanthine toxicosis

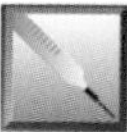

DIAGNOSTICS

CBC/Biochemistry/Urinalysis

- Between 5 and 40 nucleated RBCs/100 WBCs without anemia; absence of nucleated RBC changes does not rule out the diagnosis.

- Anisocytosis, polychromasia, poikilocytosis, target cells, hypochromasia.
- Basophilic stippling of RBCs; often difficult to detect.
- Neutrophilic leukocytosis.
- Cats – elevated AST and ALP reported.
- Urinalysis – mild nonspecific renal damage; glucosuria; hemoglobinuria.

Imaging

- Presence of radiopaque material in the GI tract (presence or absence is not diagnostic).
- Lead lines (precipitation of lead salts) within the epiphyseal plate of long bones is uncommon.

Lead detection

- Toxic – antemortem whole blood: >0.4 ppm (40 μg/dL); postmortem liver and/or kidney: >5 ppm (wet weight).
- Lower values – must be interpreted in conjunction with history and clinical signs.
- No normal "background" blood lead concentrations; typically less than 0.05 ppm.
- Blood concentrations – do not correlate with occurrence or severity of clinical signs.
- $CaNa_2EDTA$ mobilization test – collect one 24-hour urine sample; administer $CaNa_2EDTA$ (75 mg/kg IM); collect a second 24-hour urine sample; with toxicosis, urine lead increases 10–60-fold post EDTA (succimer could conceivably be substituted for $CaNa_2EDTA$).
- While not documented in small animals, in people, a lead mobilization test following administration of succimer has been used to measure the presence of a mobilizable and potentially toxic lead pool.

Pathological Findings

- Gross – might note paint chips or lead objects in gastrointestinal tract.
- Intranuclear inclusion bodies – might note in hepatocytes or renal tubular epithelial cells; intracellular storage form of lead; considered pathognomonic.
- Cerebrocortical lesions – spongiosis, vascular hypertrophy, gliosis, neuronal necrosis, demyelination.

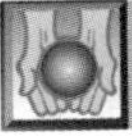

THERAPEUTICS

Detoxification

- Evacuation of gastrointestinal tract – saline cathartics; sodium or magnesium sulfate (dogs, 2–25 g; cats 2–5 g PO as 20% solution or less).
- Sulfate-containing cathartics potentially precipitate lead in the GI tract to the less bioavailable lead sulfate form.
- Endoscopic or surgical removal of lead objects in the GI tract might be warranted in some cases.

Appropriate Health Care

- Inpatient – first course of chelation, depending on severity of clinical signs.
- Outpatient – orally administered chelators.

Antidotes

- Reduction of lead body burden – chelation therapy with $CaNa_2EDTA$ (dogs and cats, 25 mg/kg SC, IM, IV q 6 hours for 2–5 days); dilute to a 1% solution with D5W before administration. May need multiple treatment courses if blood lead concentration is high; allow 5-day rest period between treatment courses. SC administration is preferred.
- Succimer – alternative to $CaNa_2$ EDTA; orally administered chelating agent; 10 mg/kg PO q 8 hours for 5 days followed by 10 mg PO q 12 hours for 2 weeks; allow 2-week rest period between treatments. May administer per rectum if clinical signs such as emesis preclude oral administration. Cats successfully treated with 10 mg/kg PO q 8 hours for 17 days. Advantages over other chelators: can be given PO, allowing for outpatient treatment; does not increase lead absorption from the gastrointestinal tract; not reported to be nephrotoxic; chelation of essential elements such as zinc and copper is not clinically significant.
- $CaNa_2EDTA$ more effective at removing lead from bone; succimer more effective at removing lead from soft tissues.
- Identify sources for lead exposure and eliminate or restrict access.

Drugs of Choice

- Control of seizures – diazepam (given to effect; dogs and cats, 0.5 mg/kg IV) or phenobarbital sodium (administer in increments of 10–20 mg/kg IV to effect).
- Alleviation of cerebral edema – mannitol (0.25–2 g/kg of 15–25% IV, slow infusion over 30–60 minutes) and dexamethasone (2.2–4.4 mg/kg IV).
- Some evidence that antioxidants or thiol-containing drugs might be useful – vitamins C and E, alpha-lipoic acid, N-acetylcysteine; optimal doses not determined.
- B-vitamins, especially thiamine, may also be useful; optimal doses not determined.

Precautions/Interactions

- $CaNa_2EDTA$ – do not administer to patients with renal impairment or anuria; establish urine flow before administration; do not administer orally.
- $CaNa_2EDTA$ – safety in pregnancy not established; teratogenic at therapeutic doses, although in human medicine is recommended over succimer for use in pregnant patients.
- Succimer – safety in pregnancy not established; fetotoxic at doses much higher (100–1000 mg/kg) than recommended therapeutic dose.
- $CaNa_2EDTA$ – depletion of zinc, iron, and manganese with long-term therapy; although succimer also chelates zinc and copper, the degree of chelation is not clinically significant.

Nursing Care

- Balanced electrolyte fluids – Ringer's solution; replacement of hydration deficit.

Diet

- Provide good-quality, nutritionally complete diet.

Surgical Considerations

- Removal of lead objects from the gastrointestinal tract might be warranted in some cases.

COMMENTS

Patient Monitoring

- Assess blood lead values before additional courses of chelation therapy or 10–14 days after cessation of chelation therapy.

Prevention/Avoidance

- Client awareness of potential sources for exposure and avoidance of contact with those sources.
- Test paint, dust, soil prior to animal access if likelihood of lead contamination.

Possible Complications

- Uncontrolled seizures can result in permanent neurological deficits.
- Blindness.

Expected Course and Prognosis

- Signs should dramatically improve within 24–48 hours after initiating chelation therapy.
- Prognosis – favorable with treatment.
- Uncontrolled seizures – guarded prognosis.

Public Health

- Environmental lead contamination and exposure is a significant public health problem.
- Families of affected pets should consult their physicians and have lead determinations made.
- Depending on the circumstances of exposure, environmental clean-up might be warranted.

Synonyms

Plumbism

Abbreviations

See Appendix 1 for a complete list.

$CaNa_2EDTA$ = calcium disodium ethylene diamine tetraacetate

Suggested Reading

Knight TE, Kumar MSA. Lead toxicosis in cats – a review. J Feline Med Surg 2003; 5:249–255.

Knight TE, Kent M, Junk JE. Succimer for treatment of lead toxicosis in two cats. J Am Vet Med Assoc 2001; 218:1946–1948.

Morgan RV. Lead poisoning in small companion animals: an update (1987–1992). Vet Hum Toxicol 1994; 36:18–22.

Ramsey DT, Casteel SW, Fagella AM, et al. Use of orally administered succimer (meso-2,3-dimercaptosuccinic acid) for treatment of lead poisoning in dogs. J Am Vet Med Assoc 1996; 208:371–375.

VanAlstine WG, Wickliffe LW, Everson RJ, et al. Acute lead toxicosis in a household of cats. J Vet Diagn Invest 1993; 5:496–498.

Author: Robert H. Poppenga, DVM, PhD, DABVT
Consulting Editor: Robert H. Poppenga, DVM, PhD, DABVT

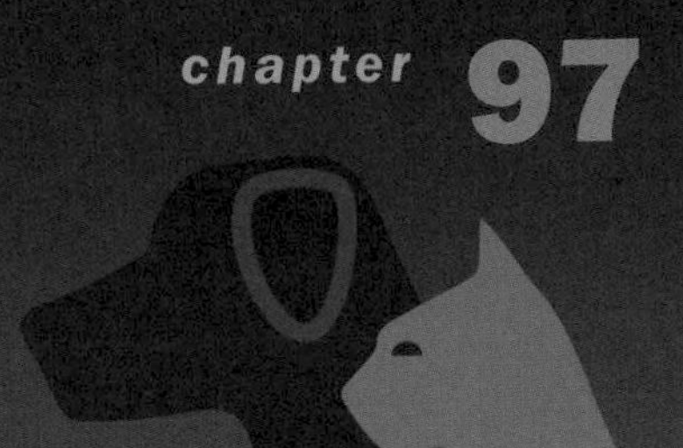

Zinc

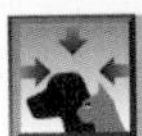

DEFINITION/OVERVIEW

- Zinc (Zn) toxicosis results from the ingestion of zinc-containing objects such as pennies (see later in this chapter), metallic nuts, bolts, staples, galvanized metal (e.g., nails), pieces from board games, zippers, toys, and jewelry or from products containing zinc salts such as zinc oxide.
- Zinc-containing products include the following.
    - Zinc carbonate and gluconate (dietary supplements), Zn acetate (throat lozenges).
    - Zinc chloride (deodorants), Zn pyrithione (shampoo), Zn oxide (sunblock, diaper creams, calamine lotion).
    - Zn sulfide (paint).
    - Metallic zinc (coins, nut, bolts), brass (alloy of zinc and copper).
- The most common cause of Zn toxicosis is penny ingestion.
    - US pennies minted after 1982 contain 97.5% Zn.
    - Canadian pennies minted from 1997 through 2001 contain 96% Zn.
- Toxicosis initially presents as gastrointestinal upset with vomiting and anorexia but can progress to intravascular hemolytic anemia. Secondary multiorgan failure (renal, hepatic, pancreatic, and cardiac), DIC, and cardiopulmonary arrest can occur in severe toxicosis.
- Zinc oxide, a common ingredient in skin protectants such as diaper rash cream and zinc-containing lozenges, can cause gastroenteritis but is not expected to cause Zn toxicosis with acute ingestion.

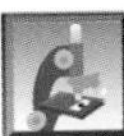

ETIOLOGY/PATHOPHYSIOLOGY

Mechanism of Action

- Unknown: mechanisms have been proposed but none confirmed.
- Intravascular hemolysis is common.
- High concentrations of zinc may be found in serum, red blood cells, liver, kidneys, and pancreas following toxicosis.

Blackwell's Five-Minute Veterinary Consult Clinical Companion: Small Animal Toxicology, Second Edition.
Lynn R. Hovda, Ahna G. Brutlag, Robert H. Poppenga, and Katherine L. Peterson.

Companion website: www.fiveminutevet.com/toxicology

Pharmacokinetic – Absorption, Distribution, Metabolism, Excretion

- Zinc absorption primarily occurs in the small intestine after oral exposure. The acidic environment of the stomach promotes leaching of zinc from ingested objects, allowing for absorption.
- Metabolism occurs in the liver, with metallothionein playing a significant role.
- Excretion occurs primarily via the feces, with a small amount excreted in the urine. Urinary excretion plays a bigger role in toxicosis and with chelation therapy.

Toxicity

- LD_{50} in dogs: 100 mg/kg acute Zn salt ingestion.
- Ingestion of 1 penny (2.5 g) can cause toxicosis in most dogs.
- Acute ingestion of topical Zn-containing products generally causes gastrointestinal upset; chronic exposure has been documented to cause zinc toxicosis.

Systems Affected

- Hemic – intravascular hemolysis, Heinz body anemia, coagulopathy, DIC, leukocytosis with neutrophilia, left shift, monocytosis, lymphopenia.
- Gastrointestinal – anorexia, vomiting, diarrhea.
- Endocrine – pancreatitis.
- Renal – pigmenturia (hemoglobinuria, bilirubinuria), azotemia, oliguria/anuria.
- Nervous – depression, ataxia, seizures.
- Hepatic – hyperbilirubinemia, elevated liver enzymes, hepatic necrosis.

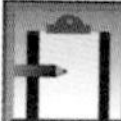

SIGNALMENT/HISTORY

- Toxicosis can occur in any species but is frequently reported in young, small breed dogs (<25 pounds) that are often unable to pass the metallic object out of the stomach.

Risk Factors

- Young animals may ingest more foreign objects due to indiscriminate eating.

Historical Findings

- Ingestion of topical cream or metallic object.
- History of vomiting, lethargy, anorexia, jaundice, abnormal or red-colored urine.

Location and Circumstance of Poisoning

- Most exposures to coins or zinc salts occur in the home.
- Kennels or workplaces may pose added risks for other Zn metal or salt ingestion.

Interaction with Drugs, Nutrients, or Environment

- Zinc may interfere with copper or iron absorption, although this is unlikely to be a concern with acute exposures.
- Zinc absorption may be decreased with high dietary levels of phytates, calcium, or phosphorus and increased with certain amino acids and EDTA.

CLINICAL FEATURES

- The most common signs are anorexia, vomiting, diarrhea, lethargy, depression, pale or icteric mucous membranes, and icteric sclera and skin. Orange-tinged feces and hemoglobinuria may be noted.
- GI signs may begin minutes after ingestion. The onset of hemolysis is dependent upon the rate at which a zinc-containing object breaks down in the stomach, which might take hours to days.
- Animals with hemolytic anemia will often be tachycardic with weak or bounding pulses. A heart murmur may be noted on auscultation.
- Severe depression and seizures can develop at later stages.
- Death is often due to cardiovascular collapse and multiorgan failure.

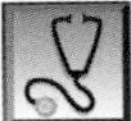

DIFFERENTIAL DIAGNOSIS

- Hemolysis: IMHA, babesiosis, onions, garlic, chives, naphthalene mothballs, acetaminophen, snake and spider envenomation, propylene glycol, and caval syndrome.
- Gastrointestinal signs: primary gastrointestinal infectious and inflammatory diseases, foreign body ingestion, dietary indiscretion, and secondary to metabolic disease.

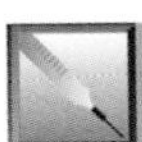

DIAGNOSTICS

- Abdominal radiographs to evaluate for metallic object in GI tract. Repeat after object removal to ensure all metal is removed.
- CBC.
  - Hemolytic anemia, Heinz body formation, regenerative anemia. Spherocytosis and target cells are inconsistently noted.
  - Leukocytosis with neutrophilia, left shift, monocytosis, lymphopenia.
  - Thrombocytopenia in animals with DIC.
- Serum chemistry.
  - Hyperbilirubinemia, elevated AST, ALP, and less commonly GGT and ALT.
  - Azotemia.
  - Elevated amylase and lipase.
- Urinalysis: bilirubinuria, hemoglobinuria, isosthenuria, proteinuria, tubular casts.

- Coagulation panel: prolonged PT/PTT, hypofibrinogenemia, thrombocytopenia, high FDPs suggestive of DIC.
- Serum Zn levels often exceed 5 ppm (normal range 0.7–2 ppm for dogs and cats). Contact reference lab for instruction prior to submission as specific tubes are required.

Pathological Findings

- Gross lesions include icterus, splenomegaly, hepatomegaly, pigmenturia.
- Histological lesions include evidence of pigmentary nephropathy, hepatic necrosis, pancreatic acinar cell necrosis. Macrophages may contain hemosiderin.
- Tissue Zn levels can be measured in liver, kidney, and pancreas samples collected postmortem.

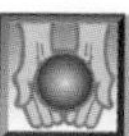

THERAPEUTICS

- Main goal of treatment is stabilization and rapid removal of zinc objects if present.

Detoxification

- Induce emesis in asymptomatic animals with evidence of a metallic foreign object in the stomach. Not always efficacious.
- Removal of the metallic object via endoscopy or laparotomy/gastrotomy after initial stabilization. Zinc levels decrease rapidly after removal of the object.
- Activated charcoal does not bind to zinc and is not indicated.

Appropriate Health Care

- IV fluids to maintain hydration and perfusion.
- Red blood cell transfusion(s) may be needed for patients with clinical signs associated with anemia; plasma transfusion(s) may be needed for coagulopathy.

Drugs of Choice

- H_2 receptor antagonists such as famotidine 0.5–1 mg/kg IV, SQ, IM, PO q 12–24 hours, can be given to help reduce stomach acidity and decrease the rate of Zn release from ingested metal.
- Antiemetics such as maropitant 1 mg/kg SQ q 24 hours can be given for protracted vomiting.

Alternative Drugs

- For stomach acid reduction.
  - Proton pump inhibitors such as omeprazole 0.5–1 mg/kg PO q 24 hours or pantoprazole 0.7–1 mg/kg IV q 24 hours.

- Oral antacid such as calcium carbonate 25–50 mg/kg PO q 2–4 hours can be used in nonvomiting animals.

Precautions/Interactions

- Chelation using $CaNa_2EDTA$ is controversial and should not be necessary once the object or source has been removed. Zinc concentrations will rapidly decrease once the source is removed. Chelation therapy may increase absorption of Zn if initiated before the metal is removed and $CaNa_2EDTA$ can also exacerbate GI signs and cause nephrotoxicity.
- Avoid other nephrotoxic drugs such as NSAIDs and aminoglycosides because of the risk of renal failure.
- The use of blood products from a universal donor in dogs (DEA 1.1 negative) may decrease transfusion reactions if blood type or cross-match cannot be performed prior to blood product administration.

Nursing Care

- Minimize patient stress prior to stabilization.
- Recumbent animals will need soft bedding and positional rotation every 4 hours.

COMMENTS

Patient Monitoring

- Hospitalization and monitoring for 24–72 hours following object removal.
- PCV should be monitored every 6–12 hours. Serum chemistry should be monitored every 12–24 hours. Recheck blood work 1–2 weeks post discharge to assess response to therapy.
- Urinary catheterization can be done to monitor urine output if concerned about acute renal failure.
- Blood and urine Zn levels should decrease rapidly following Zn object removal. If not noted, reassess patient for additional Zn exposure.

Expected Course and Prognosis

- Animals may show improvement within 48–72 hours after object removal.
- Complete recovery is possible.
- Prognosis is guarded to good depending on degree of morbidity prior to object removal.
- Development of multiorgan failure (especially kidney and liver), DIC, seizures, or cardiopulmonary arrest may imply a worse prognosis.

Possible Complications

- Multiple organ failure (especially liver and kidney), DIC, pancreatic disease, cardiopulmonary arrest, and seizures can occur even with aggressive therapy.

Prevention/Avoidance

- Inform clients of the hazard of ingesting zinc-containing objects and products and ensure that pets do not have access to areas where exposure may occur.
- Advise owners to avoid use of topical zinc-containing preparations without veterinary supervision.

See Also

Batteries
Foreign Objects
Lead
Matches and Fireworks
Metallic Toxicants (Appendix 3)

Abbreviations

See Appendix 1 for a complete list.

Suggested Reading

Cummings JE, Kovacic JP. The ubiquitous role of zinc in health and disease. JVECC 2009; 19:215–240.
Gurnee CM, Drobatz KJ. Zinc intoxication in dogs: 19 cases (1991–2003). JAVMA 2007; 230:1174–1179.
Talcott PA. Zinc poisoning. In: Peterson ME, Talcott PA, eds. Small Animal Toxicology, 3rd edn. St Louis, MO: Elsevier, 2013; pp. 847–851.
Van der Merwe D, Tawde S. Antacids in the initial management of metallic zinc ingestion in dogs. J Vet Pharmacol Ther 2008; 32:2003–2006.

Acknowledgment: The authors and editors acknowledge the prior contributions of Dr. Kathryn M. Meurs, DVM, PhD, and Patricia A. Talcott, DVM, PhD, DABVT, who authored this topic in the previous edition.
Author: Katherine L. Peterson, DVM, DACVECC
Consulting Editor: Robert H. Poppenga, DVM, PhD, DABVT

Nondrug Consumer Products

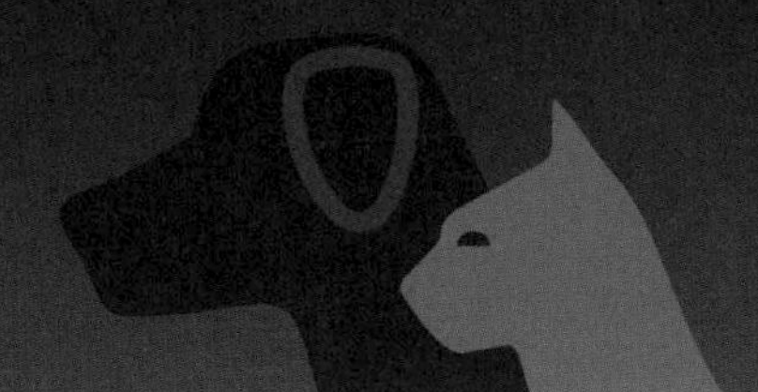

chapter 98

Glow Jewelry (Dibutyl Phthalate)

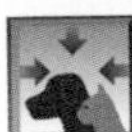

DEFINITION/OVERVIEW

- Most glow jewelry or glow-in-the-dark jewelry contains an oily, chemiluminescent substance known as dibutyl phthalate.
- Common types of glow jewelry include plastic wands, sticks, rings, necklaces, bracelets, and earrings (Fig. 98.1).
- Dibutyl phthalate is also widely used in the manufacturing of products including plastics, glues, dyes, printing ink, solvents for perfume, safety glass, and as insect repellants for use in clothing.
- A few glow stick type products contain hydrogen peroxide in phthalic ester and phenyl oxalate ester or contain batteries; these products are not covered in this chapter.

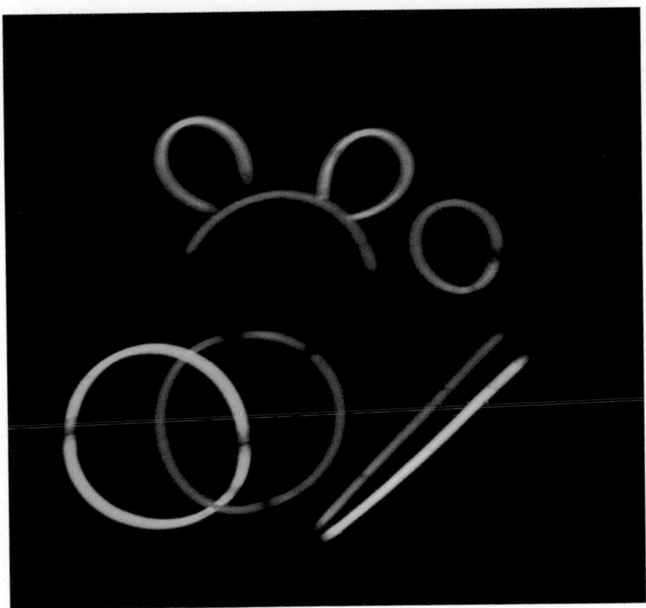

■ **Fig. 98.1.** Glow jewelry. Photo courtesy of Tyne K. Hovda.

Blackwell's Five-Minute Veterinary Consult Clinical Companion: Small Animal Toxicology, Second Edition.
Lynn R. Hovda, Ahna G. Brutlag, Robert H. Poppenga, and Katherine L. Peterson.

Companion website: www.fiveminutevet.com/toxicology

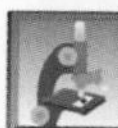

ETIOLOGY/PATHOPHYSIOLOGY

Mechanism of Action

- Dibutyl phthalate is an irritant to the eyes, skin, and mucous membranes.
- It has an unpleasant, bitter taste that tends to limit oral exposure.

Toxicity

- Dibutyl phthalate has a low order of acute toxicity with a wide margin.
- Oral LD_{50} (rats) >8 g/kg; lethal exposure for other species is unknown.
- Rats receiving an oral dose of 1 mg/kg twice a week for 1.5 years had no adverse effects; rats and other laboratory animals tolerated 2 g/kg orally once daily for 10 days.
- Glow jewelry contains small amounts of dibutyl phthalate, with most pieces containing less than 5 mL of liquid. The exterior packaging (fig 98.2.) often states the amount but approximate values are:
  - earrings and bracelets 0.3–0.5 mL
  - necklaces 1–2 mL
  - large wands 3–5 mL.

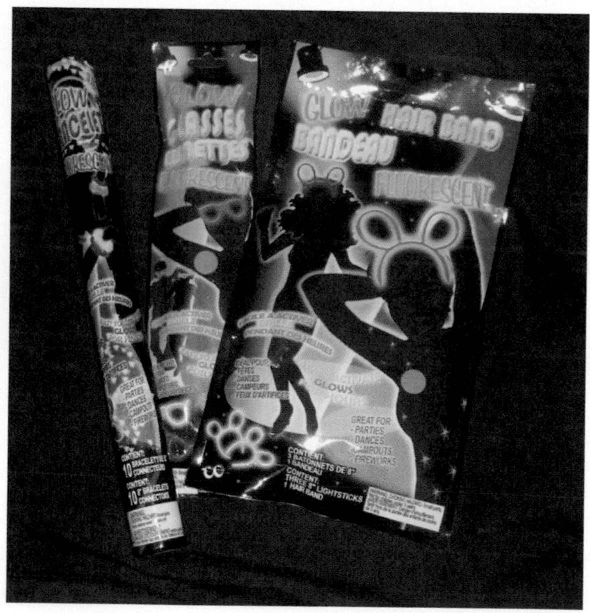

Fig. 98.2. Outside packaging of glow jewelry. Photo courtesy of Tyne K. Hovda.

Systems Affected

- Gastrointestinal – oral irritation, profuse hypersalivation, agitation secondary to oropharyngeal discomfort, vomiting.

- Skin/exocrine – irritation, burning, redness, contact dermatitis.
- Ophthalmic – stinging and burning sensation, profuse lacrimation, photophobia, conjunctival edema, conjunctivitis.
- Respiratory – labored breathing and respiratory paralysis have been noted in experimentally fatally poisoned animals (rare and not reported with glow jewelry).

SIGNALMENT/HISTORY

- Any age or breed of dog or cat may be affected.
- History of biting or chewing product.
- Self-grooming in cats increases potential for oral and ocular exposure.

Location and Circumstances of Poisoning

- The presence of children in the household may increase exposure.

CLINICAL FEATURES

- Pets biting into the sticks or ingesting the liquid should be evaluated in a dark room for evidence of product on their haircoat. If present, it should be removed with a mild soap.
- Clinical signs are typically due to the unpleasant and bitter chemical taste of the product, resulting in an acute onset of profuse hypersalivation or emesis.
- Other clinical signs include agitation, aggressiveness, or abnormal behaviors such as hiding or running away.
- Contact with thin haircoat or hairless areas results in a mild burning and stinging sensation.
- Cats may develop pruritus and can self-traumatize with scratching.
- Ocular exposure may result in conjunctivitis or corneal abrasion. The presence of corneal ulceration should be ruled out with fluorescein staining.

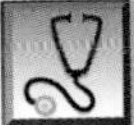

DIFFERENTIAL DIAGNOSIS

- Other irritant products such as perfumes and alcohols.
- Oxalate-containing plants.
- Oral ingestion of topical flea and tick products.

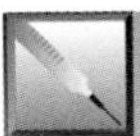

DIAGNOSTICS

- In general, diagnostics are not necessary.
- Consider blood work in significantly symptomatic, pediatric, and geriatric patients, or patients with underlying disorders.

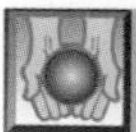

THERAPEUTICS

- Goals of treatment include decontamination, oropharyngeal lavage, antiemetics, fluids, and bathing.

Detoxification

- Emesis and gastric lavage are not indicated.
- Activated charcoal is unnecessary.
- Wipe out the mouth, rinse with cool water or offer a small amount of palatable liquid (e.g., chicken broth, milk, canned tuna water, or canned cat food) to dilute the product and help remove the taste.
- The signs are generally self-limiting and related to the taste of dibutyl phthalate; signs quickly resolve with decontamination.
- Bathe with a mild, noninsecticidal pet shampoo or dish soap and rinse well with tepid water. Examine pet in a darkened room to ensure that all of the glow product has been completely removed from the haircoat.

Appropriate Health Care

- A thorough ocular exam may be necessary if ophthalmic signs are present.
- If ocular exposure to dibutyl phthalate has occurred, the eyes should be lavaged thoroughly with eye wash for 10–15 minutes.
- Slit lamp or fluorescein testing may be necessary to evaluate for corneal ulceration. Ulceration should be treated with ophthalmic medication as deemed medically appropriate.
- Fluids (SQ or IV) may be needed in symptomatic patients.

Antidotes and Drugs of Choice

- No antidote exists.
- Antiemetic – Maropitant 1 mg/kg SQ q 24 hours.

COMMENTS

Prevention/Avoidance

- Pet owners should be informed about the exposure to glow jewelry, particularly during holidays or events.

Expected Course and Prognosis

- Most reactions are self-limiting and can be treated at home without veterinary intervention.
- For symptomatic animals, little treatment is required.

- Many of the signs are associated with the bitter taste of the product and resolve quickly once the product is gone.
- Animals with an ocular exposure often have to evaluated by a veterinarian.
- Prognosis for complete recovery is excellent.

Abbreviations

See Appendix 1 for a complete list.

Suggested Reading

Hoffman RJ, Nelson LS, Hoffman RS. Pediatric and young adult exposure to chemiluminescent glow sticks. Arch Ped Adol Med 2002; 156(9):901–904.

Kamrin MA. Phthalate risks, phthalate regulation, and public health: a review. J Toxicol Environ Health B Crit Rev 2009; 12(2):157–174.

Rosendale ME. Glow jewelry (dibutyl phthalate) ingestion in cats. Vet Med 1999; 94(8):703.

Acknowledgment: The authors and editors acknowledge the prior contributions of Justine A. Lee, DVM, DACVECC, who co-authored this topic in the previous edition.
Author: Tyne K. Hovda, DVM
Consulting Editor: Katherine L. Peterson, DVM, DACVECC

chapter 99

Fluoride

DEFINITION/OVERVIEW

- Fluoride toxicosis can develop from corrosive products (hydrofluoric acid) and noncorrosive products (e.g., sodium fluoride).
- This chapter will focus on noncorrosive fluoride ingestion. See chapter 11, Hydrofluoric Acid, for more information on this toxicant.
- Noncorrosive fluoride products are typically over-the-counter products used for prophylactic dental care, multivitamins, osteoporosis treatment, and insecticides.
- Most common signs of fluoride ingestion include vomiting and diarrhea, which typically require minimal supportive care.
- Concentrated fluoride salts can be caustic to the GIT and in severe toxicosis lead to metabolic disturbances that result in arrhythmias and respiratory muscle paralysis.
- Long-term chronic overdoses without calcium supplementation can cause skeletal fluorosis, leading to fractures and malformations.

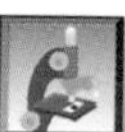

ETIOLOGY/PATHOPHYSIOLOGY

Mechanism of Action

- When fluoride salts are ingested, they react with the acidic environment of the stomach to create hydrofluoric acid, which is highly corrosive.
- Once absorbed, hydrofluoric acid interferes with calcium metabolism and may cause hypocalcemia. It also interferes with Na/K ATPase and causes efflux of K from the cell, resulting in hyperkalemia.
- In severe toxicosis, hypocalcemia and hyperkalemia can be severe enough to cause ECG changes and secondary cardiac arrhythmias may result.
- Respiratory muscle paralysis from hypocalcemia and cardiac arrest from hyperkalemia are the most common causes of death.

Blackwell's Five-Minute Veterinary Consult Clinical Companion: Small Animal Toxicology, Second Edition.
Lynn R. Hovda, Ahna G. Brutlag, Robert H. Poppenga, and Katherine L. Peterson.

Companion website: www.fiveminutevet.com/toxicology

Pharmacokinetics – Absorption, Distribution, Metabolism, Excretion

- Sodium fluoride and other soluble fluorides are rapidly absorbed from the GIT and reach peak plasma levels 30 minutes after ingestion.
- Fluoride is not protein bound and circulates as a free ion until it binds to the bone over several hours after ingestion.
- Fluoride is 50% excreted by the kidneys with the remainder excreted in feces, sweat, and milk or retained by the bone.
- Elimination half-life is 2–9 hours in people with normal kidney function but can be prolonged with kidney disease, unknown half-life in small animals.

Toxicity

- Very little information exists in the veterinary literature regarding acute fluoride toxicosis in small animals.
- Anecdotally, elemental fluoride <5 mg/kg results in mild symptoms; higher doses may require more aggressive care.
- Sodium fluoride is 45% elemental fluoride by weight (1 mg sodium fluoride = 0.45 mg elemental fluoride).
- Fluoride toothpaste typically contains up to 1.1 mg of fluoride per gram of toothpaste. Mouthwashes or rinses typically contain 0.2% sodium fluoride and have approximately 9.1 mg of fluoride/mL of rinse. Verify amounts for each brand.

Systems Affected

- Cardiovascular – cardiac arrhythmias secondary to profound hyperkalemia and hypocalcemia (severe toxicosis).
- Gastrointestinal – GI irritation, nausea, vomiting, anorexia, abdominal pain, HGE, oral irritation, tooth enamel changes can occur in young animals.
- Hemic/lymphatic/immune – hypocalcemia, hyperkalemia.
- Hepatobiliary – increased liver enzymes.
- Respiratory – coughing, respiratory irritation, respiratory muscle paralysis (severe toxicosis).
- Musculoskeletal – painful muscle spasms/tremors, weakness, skeletal fluorosis (chronic).
- Nervous – hyperactive reflexes.
- Skin/exocrine – dermal irritation.

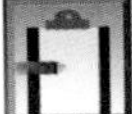

SIGNALMENT/HISTORY

Risk Factors

- Any age, sex, and breed of pet can be affected.
- Animals drinking water from a source with high fluoride content.
- Young animals may be predisposed to tooth damage with chronic exposure.

Historical Findings

- Witnessed ingestion or discovery of chewed-up packaging.
- Owners may report drooling, vomiting, and anorexia.
- Chronic lameness, frequent fractures and bony injury with minimal trauma may be indicative of chronic fluoride toxicosis.

Location and Circumstances of Poisoning

- Exposure typically occurs within the home, specifically in the bathroom, where the pet has access to toothpaste, mouthwash or vitamins containing fluoride.

Interactions with Drugs, Nutrients, or Environment

- Absorption of fluoride may be inhibited with aluminum or magnesium hydroxide products.

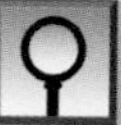

CLINICAL FEATURES

- Clinical signs may be present within a few hours after exposure.
- Mucous membrane erythema, oral irritation, vomiting, hypersalivation, nausea, abdominal pain, or dysphagia may be present.
- Cardiac arrhythmias, muscle tremors, or muscle weakness may be noted with severe toxicosis.

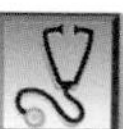

DIFFERENTIAL DIAGNOSIS

- GI symptoms – GI irritants or other corrosives, plants such as azalea or rhododendron, calcium oxalate-containing plants.
- Hypocalcemia – nursing, hypoparathyroidism.
- Hyperkalemia – iatrogenic supplementation, acute kidney failure, urinary obstruction, uroabdomen, hypoadrenocorticism.
- Cardiac arrhythmias – primary cardiac disease, electrolyte derangements.

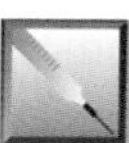

DIAGNOSTICS

- Serum chemistry – hyperkalemia, hypocalcemia, hypomagnesemia, elevated liver enzymes.
- ECG –QT prolongation, arrhythmias secondary to potassium, magnesium and calcium abnormalities.

Pathological Findings

- Primarily limited to irritant or corrosive damage in the GIT.
- Chronic fluorosis causes exostosis of long bones as well as mottled, pitted, or excessively worn teeth/enamel.

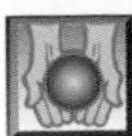

THERAPEUTICS

- Treatment for most fluoride ingestion is supportive care for GI signs.
- Larger exposures may require decontamination, neutralization of the fluoride with calcium, fluid therapy, correction of electrolyte abnormalities, and GI supportive care.

Detoxification

- Before decontamination is initiated, determine which type of fluoride was ingested (e.g., corrosive vs noncorrosive), if possible.
- Noncorrosive.
  - Emesis should be induced if ingestion was within 2 hours for a tablet-based product or 1 hour for a gel or powder.
  - With large recent exposures, if emesis return is low yield, consider gastric lavage with a large-bore stomach tube and an inflated endotracheal tube to protect the airway.
- Corrosive.
  - Emesis is contraindicated.
  - With large exposures, calcium gluconate solution can be administered orally or via stomach tube to bind fluoride ions.

Appropriate Health Care

- Maintain hydration and perfusion with IV fluid therapy until clinical symptoms resolve.
- Correct electrolyte abnormalities.
  - Calcium supplementation: calcium gluconate 10% 50–150 mg/kg IV over 20–30 minutes to effect; monitor heart rate and an ECG during administration. Regular insulin administration and dextrose supplementation can be considered for severe hyperkalemia.
- If indicated, monitor cardiac function with a continuous ECG to evaluate for the presence of arrhythmias.

Drugs and Antidotes of Choice

- No antidote available.
- GI supportive therapy.
  - Cerenia 1 mg/kg SQ q 24 hours for an antiemetic.
  - Famotidine 0.5–1 mg/kg IV, SQ, PO q 12–24 hours.
  - Sucralfate 0.25–1 g/kg PO q 8 hours.
- Aluminum hydroxide 30–100 mg/kg PO per day, divided into 2–4 doses.
- Magnesium hydroxide 5–15 mL q 24 hours.

Precautions/Interactions

- Electrolyte supplementation needs to be performed with cardiac monitoring and regular rechecks of serum levels to determine if further supplementation is necessary.

- Aluminum hydroxide can alter the absorption of other drugs and should be administered 1 hour apart from other oral medications.

Diet

- The additional use of dairy products (e.g., milk, yogurt, etc.) to neutralize the fluoride may be beneficial, provided the patient is not vomiting.
- Calcium supplementation may be needed initially, but no long-term diet changes are recommended.
- Bland diet can be considered in patients with GI signs.

Surgical Considerations

- Ulcerations of the GIT could potentially cause perforation, necessitating surgical intervention (rare).

COMMENTS

Patient Monitoring

- Serum electrolytes should be monitored every 2–4 hours during initial management of severely symptomatic cases to guide supplementation.

Prevention/Avoidance

- Store fluoride-containing products away from pets.

Possible Complications

- In severe cases, if electrolyte abnormalities cannot be corrected, death from cardiac arrest or respiratory muscle paralysis is possible. Mechanical ventilation may be necessary until respiratory muscle paralysis resolves.

Expected Course and Prognosis

- Most OTC noncorrosive fluoride exposures result in mild clinical signs and should resolve with supportive care within 24 hours.
- Prognosis is good with small ingestions or with early intervention and appropriate management. Large ingestions with late intervention have a guarded prognosis.

Synonyms

Skeletal fluorosis, sodium fluoride toxicosis, fluoride silicate toxicosis, fluoridosis

See Also

Hydrofluoric Acid

Abbreviations

See Appendix 1 for a complete list.

Suggested Reading

Augenstein WL, Spoerke DG, Kulig KW. Fluoride ingestion in children: a review of 87 cases. Pediatrics 1991; 88:907–912.

Boink AB, Wemer J, Meulenbelt J, et al. The mechanism of fluoride-induced hypocalcaemia. Hum Exp Toxicol 1994; 13:149–155.

Author: Catherine Angle, DVM, MPH
Consulting Editor: Katherine L. Peterson, DVM, DACVECC

Plants and Biotoxins

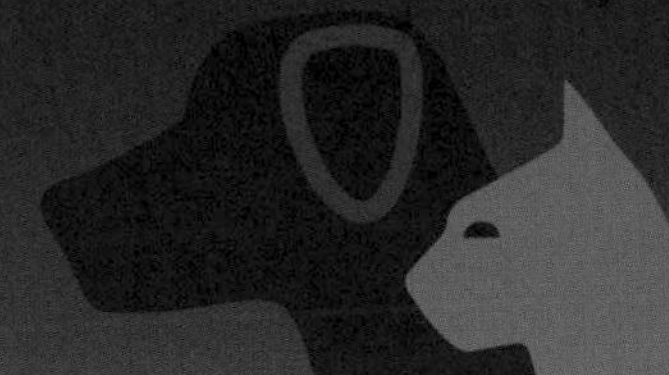

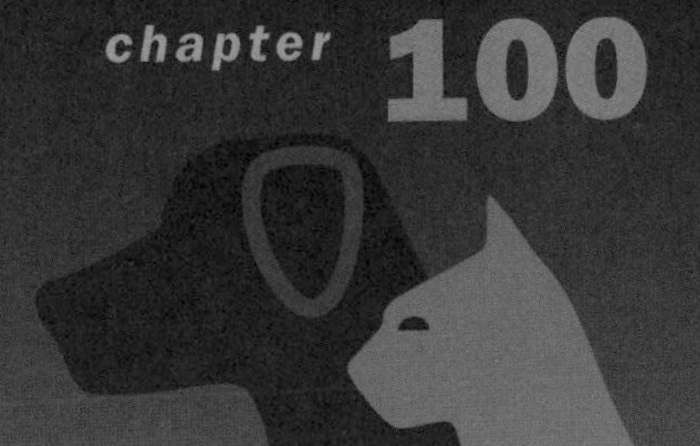

chapter **100**

Azaleas and Rhododendrons

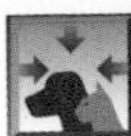

DEFINITION/OVERVIEW

- There are over 1000 species of azaleas/rhododendrons in the Ericaceae family. Typically, the deciduous forms are referred to as azaleas (Fig. 100.1), and the larger evergreen forms are called rhododendrons (Figs 100.2 and 100.3), but there may be some exceptions. Both forms have showy flowers.
- Azaleas/rhododendrons are found on all continents. They occur naturally in nature, cultivated as shrubs or small trees, and as indoor ornamentals.
- Diterpenoid grayanotoxins (previously known as andromedotoxins or rhodotoxins) are found to some extent in all plants in the Ericaceae family.
- All parts of the plant are toxic, but concentrations of toxin may vary between plants.
- Clinical signs usually occur quickly (within a few hours of ingestion), but may be delayed up to 12 hours.

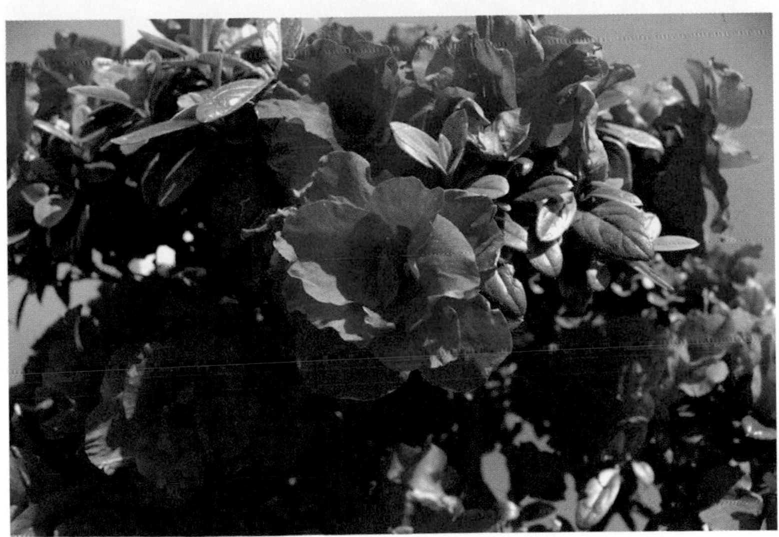

Fig. 100.1. Azalea in full bloom. Photo courtesy of Tyne K. Hovda.

Blackwell's Five-Minute Veterinary Consult Clinical Companion: Small Animal Toxicology, Second Edition.
Lynn R. Hovda, Ahna G. Brutlag, Robert H. Poppenga, and Katherine L. Peterson.

Companion website: www.fiveminutevet.com/toxicology

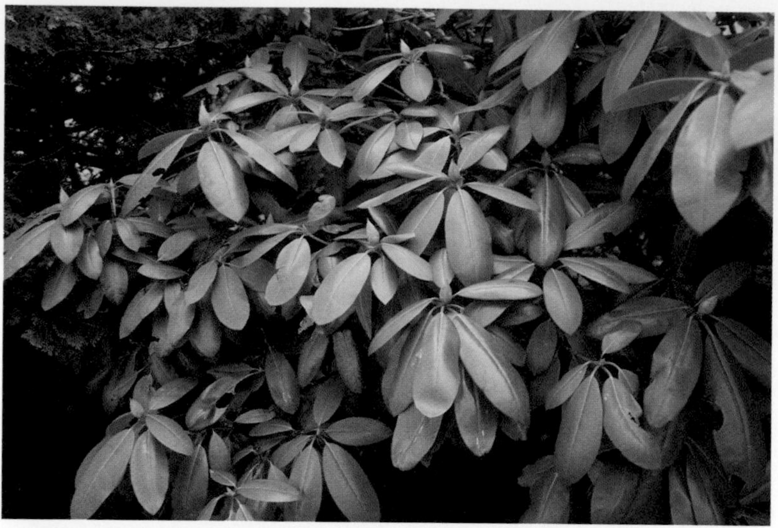

■ **Fig. 100.2.** Rhododendron shrub. Photo courtesy of Tyne K. Hovda.

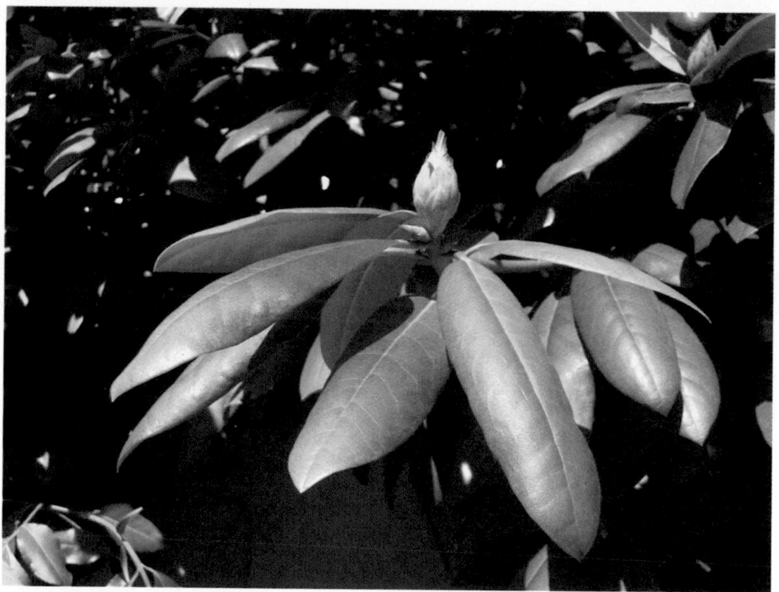

■ **Fig. 100.3.** Close-up of rhododendron leaf and bud. Photo courtesy of Tyne K. Hovda.

ETIOLOGY/PATHOPHYSIOLOGY

Mechanism of Action

- Grayanotoxins bind to group II receptor sites in voltage-gated sodium channels within cells in the heart, nerve, and skeletal muscle, thus increasing permeability of sodium ions, and resulting in prolonged depolarization/excitability of the affected cell membranes.

Pharmacokinetics – Absorption, Distribution, Metabolism, Excretion

- Absorption is thought to be rapid because clinical signs usually occur within a few hours.
- Metabolism and excretion are also thought to be rapid.

Toxicity

- Grayanotoxins I and III are currently considered the principal toxic isomers; I is most common. Concentrations of various grayanotoxins (I through XXV) vary among plants.
- All parts of the plant, including nectar and flowers, and especially leaves, are toxic.
- Secondary products such as Labrador tea, alternative medicine concoctions, and honey ("mad honey disease") may also be toxic.
- Ingestion of 0.2% of animal's body weight (documented in cattle) may cause clinical signs.

Systems Affected

- Gastrointestinal – early onset of hypersalivation and gastroenteritis (with repeated swallowing, anorexia, persistent vomiting, abdominal pain, bloat, diarrhea).
- Cardiovascular – changes in heart rate and rhythm (bradycardia, tachycardia, AV block, hypotension, arrhythmias)
- CNS – ranges from depression or weakness (lasting 2–3 days in some cases) to coma.

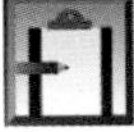

SIGNALMENT/HISTORY

- There is no breed or species predilection.
- Animals with underlying cardiac disease are at increased risk.

CLINICAL FEATURES

- Onset of clinical signs is usually rapid, occurring within the first couple of hours, but signs may be delayed for up to 12 hours.
- Gastrointestinal signs typically predominate (hypersalivation, retching, vomiting, diarrhea [rare], abdominal pain, anorexia, possible hemorrhagic enteritis, bloat).
- Cardiovascular signs include bradycardia or tachycardia (possibly a reflex secondary to hypotension), arrhythmias, hypotension, CV block, cardiopulmonary arrest.
- Neurological signs include depression, weakness, and reluctance to stand (may be related to CV events), tremors, seizures, paralysis, coma.
- Other clinical signs may include transient blindness, dyspnea, vocalization.

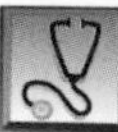

DIFFERENTIAL DIAGNOSIS

- Infectious or metabolic disease (viral, bacterial, HE).
- Other toxicants.
    - *Taxus* spp. and cardiac glycoside-containing plants (foxglove, oleander, etc.).
    - Prescription medications used in veterinary or human medicine for cardiac disease (particularly digitalis).
    - Prescription medications used in veterinary or human medicine that have cardiac effects without being specifically prescribed for cardiac disease.
    - Organophosphate- and carbamate-containing pesticides.
- Underlying cardiac disease.

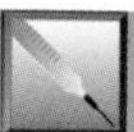

DIAGNOSTICS

- Clinical laboratory tests (serum chemistry and CBC) typically do not show primary abnormalities, but there may be secondary metabolic acidosis (as a consequence of seizures) or dehydration and electrolyte imbalance secondary to prolonged vomiting.
- Diagnosis is typically made through history of ingestion and identification of plant material.
- Liquid chromatography-mass spectrometry is available to determine presence of grayanotoxins in stomach contents, serum, urine.
- Pathological findings are usually nonspecific (plant material in the GIT, mild hemorrhagic enteritis, renal tubular damage, possible aspiration pneumonia).

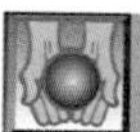

THERAPEUTICS

Detoxification

- Bathe animal if topical contamination.
- Early emesis if CNS signs have not yet developed.
- Gastric lavage to remove large amounts of plant material (retain for toxin identification).
- AC/C × 1 if no risk of aspiration and if GIT motility is normal (measure serum sodium PRN).

Appropriate Health Care

- Pay close attention to hydration (vomiting may be severe).
- Monitor vitals including blood pressure frequently.
- Consider continuous ECG for first 12–18 hours.
- Hospitalize in darkened area without excess stimulation (seizures may occur, and neurological signs may persist for a few days).

Antidote

- There is no specific antidote.

Drugs of Choice

- Early, cautious use of IV fluids to maintain blood pressure and hydration, with care to avoid overloading.
- For bradycardia.
  - Atropine 0.02–0.04 mg/kg IV, IM, or SQ.
  - Glycopyrrolate.
    - Dog: 0.011 mg/kg IV or IM.
    - Cat: 0.005–0.01 mg/kg IV or IM, 0.01–0.02 mg/kg SQ.
  - Temporary pacemaker for severe cases of unresponsive bradycardia.
- Antiarrhythmics may be necessary if persistent tachycardia or if nonresponsive to IV fluids, if severe ventricular dysrhythmias, or if evidence of poor perfusion (hypotension, pulse deficits, tachycardia, pale mucous membranes, prolonged CRT).
  - Lidocaine.
    - Dogs: 2–4 mg/kg IV while monitoring ECG. If effective, follow with CRI of 25–100 µg/kg/min.
    - Cats: 0.25–0.5 mg/kg slow IV while monitoring ECG. If effective, follow with CRI of 10–20 µg/kg/min. Use with caution in cats.
  - Procainamide.
    - Dogs: 2–4 mg/kg IV over 3–5 minutes (up to 20 mg/kg IV bolus), followed by 25–50 µg/kg/min CRI.
- Benzodiazepine or other anticonvulsant medications for seizures.
  - Diazepam 0.25–0.5 mg/kg IV PRN.
  - Phenobarbital 2–5 mg/kg IV PRN for seizures if diazepam unsuccessful.
  - Midazolam 0.1–0.5 mg/kg IV.
- Antiemetics if vomiting is persistent or severe.
  - Maropitant 1 mg/kg SQ q 24 hours.
  - Ondansetron 0.1–0.2 mg/kg IV q 6–12 hours.
- GI protectants as needed.
  - H_2 blockers.
    - Famotidine 0.5–1 mg/kg PO, SQ, IM, IV q 12–24 hours.
    - Ranitidine 1–2 mg/kg PO, SQ, IM, IV q 8–12 hours.
  - Proton pump inhibitor.
    - Omeprazole 0.5–1 mg/kg PO q 24 hours.
    - Pantoprazole 0.7–1 mg/kg IV once daily.
  - Sucralfate 0.25–1 g PO q 8 hours × 5–7 days if evidence of active ulcer disease.

COMMENTS

- Azaleas, rhododendrons, and clippings should be kept out of pet's environment.
- Flowering plants are tempting to cats and should be kept out of reach.

Expected Course and Prognosis

- Prognosis is good with early and appropriate therapy.
- Development of cardiac compromise complicates therapy and decreases prognosis.
- Neurological signs may persist for days.

See Also

Beta Receptor Antagonists (Beta-Blockers)
Calcium Channel Blockers
Cardiac Glycosides
Organophosphorus and Carbamate Insecticides
Yew

Abbreviations

See Appendix 1 for a complete list.

Suggested Reading

Burrows GE, Tyri RJ. Toxic Plants of North America. Ames, IA: ISU Press, 2006; pp. 444–449.

Knight AP. A Guide to Poisonous House and Garden Plants. Jackson, WY: Teton NewMedia, 2006; pp. 235–237.

Jansen SA, Kleerekooper I, Hofmam Z, et al. Grayanotoxin poisoning: 'Mad honey disease'and beyond. Cardiovasc Toxicol 2012; 12(3):208–215.

Milewski LM, Khan SA. An overview of potentially life threatening poisonous plants in dogs and cats. J Vet Emerg Crit Care 2006; 16(1):25–33.

Acknowledgment: The authors and editors acknowledge the prior contributions of Erica Cargill, CVT, and Lynn R. Hovda, RPh, DVM, MS, DACVIM, who co-authored this topic in the previous edition.

Author: Catherine M. Adams, DVM
Consulting Editor: Lynn R. Hovda, RPh, DVM, MS, DACVIM

chapter 101

Blue-green Algae (Cyanobacteria)

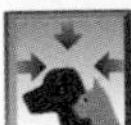

DEFINITION/OVERVIEW

- Blue-green algal (cyanobacterial) proliferations occur in freshwater and brackish ecosystems under certain environmental conditions, potentially resulting in toxin production and leading to harmful algal blooms (Fig. 101.1).
- Supplements containing blue-green algae are potential sources for exposure as well as toxin-contaminated water sources.
- Most blue-green algal blooms do not produce toxins. However, determining toxin production and severity is not possible with the naked eye. All blooms are potentially toxic.
- Blue-green algae exposure can lead to an acute intoxication affecting the liver, skin, or CNS. Hepatotoxic blue-green algae poisonings are more frequently reported than dermal and neurotoxic algal intoxications.

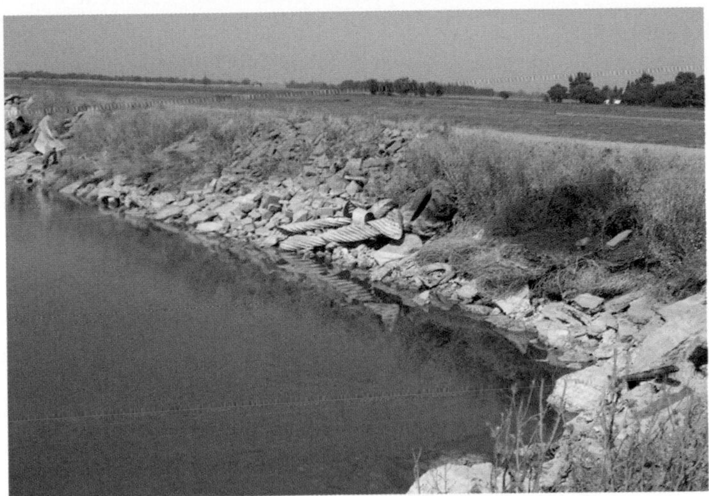

■ **Fig. 101.1.** *Microcystis* sp. algal bloom; pond in Northern California, August 2008. Bloom resulted in illness and death of cattle. Outbreak occurred during a period of high ambient temperature (above 100°F for days) after strong winds had concentrated the algal material at one side of the pond, which was the only water access these cattle had. Photo courtesy of Birgit Puschner.

Blackwell's Five-Minute Veterinary Consult Clinical Companion: Small Animal Toxicology, Second Edition.
Lynn R. Hovda, Ahna G. Brutlag, Robert H. Poppenga, and Katherine L. Peterson.

Companion website: www.fiveminutevet.com/toxicology

- Toxigenic blue-green algae include *Microcystis*, *Anabena*, *Aphanizomenon*, *Oscillatoria*, *Lyngbya*, and *Planktothrix*.
- Microcystins are hepatotoxic blue-green algae toxins that have been found worldwide and are produced by *Microcystis*, *Anabaena*, *Planktothrix*, and other genera.
- Anatoxins, which include anatoxin-a and anatoxin-$a_{s,}$ are neurotoxic blue-green algae toxins produced by *Anabaena*, *Planktothrix*, *Oscillatoria*, *Microcystis*, and other genera.
- Dermatotoxins include lyngbya-, aplysia- and debromoaplysiatoxin produced by *Lyngbya*, *Schizothrix*, and *Planktothrix*.
- Cyanotoxin poisoning has occurred in animals and humans.
- Overall prognosis is poor, with death occurring minutes to hours (neurotoxin) or hours to days (hepatotoxin) after exposure.

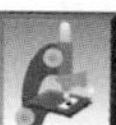

ETIOLOGY/PATHOPHYSIOLOGY

Mechanism of Action

- Microcystins target the liver by inhibiting protein phosphatases 1 and 2A. The resulting disruption of cytoskeletal components and associated rearrangement of filamentous actin within hepatocytes cause severe liver damage. Free radical formation and mitochondrial alterations may also contribute to the pathological changes, most notably acute centrilobular necrosis.
- Anatoxin-a is a potent cholinergic agonist at nicotinic acetylcholine receptors that results in continuous electrical stimulation at the neuromuscular junctions.
- Anatoxin-a_s is a naturally occurring irreversible acetylcholinesterase inhibitor that leads to increased acetylcholine concentrations in the synapse. Anatoxin-a_s is incapable of crossing the blood–brain barrier; therefore, effects and clinical signs are peripheral.
- Lyngbya-, aplysia-, and debromoaplysiatoxins are all activators of protein kinase C, an enzyme important in controlling the function of other proteins.

Pharmacokinetics – Absorption, Distribution, Metabolism, Excretion

- There are very limited data on the kinetics of microcystins. Some data suggest conjugation with glutathione and cystine as major detoxification pathways.
- Data on the toxicokinetics of anatoxin-a and anatoxin-a_s do not exist.
- Lyngbyatoxin A is slightly lipophilic and has been found to penetrate the skin within hours. Other data on the toxicokinetics of lyngbya-, aplysia-, and debromoaplysiatoxins are lacking.

Toxicity

- The LD_{50} for microcystins varies between 50 and 11,000 μg/kg, depending on the exact microcystin structure, the species affected, and the route of administration. In mice, the oral LD_{50} value for microcystin-LR is 10.9 mg/kg, while the IP LD_{50} is 50 μg/kg. Most algal

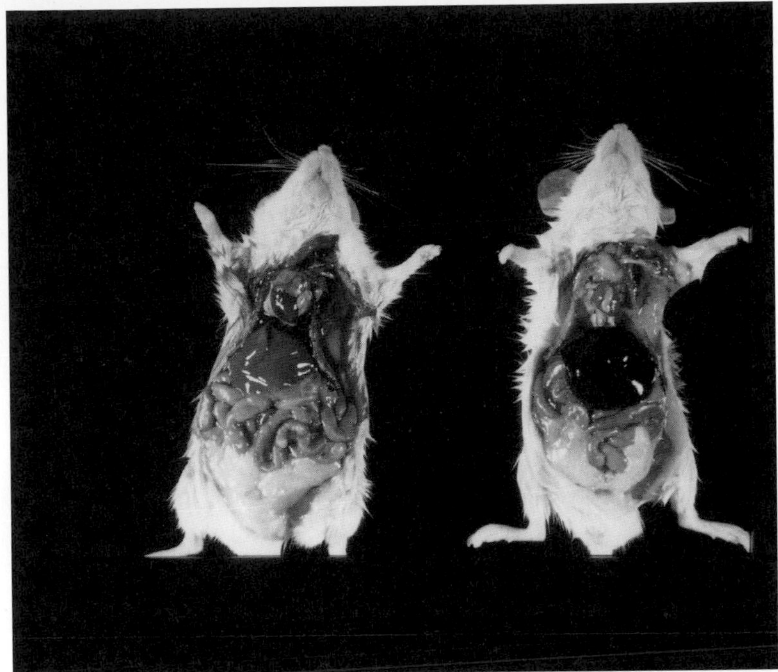

Fig. 101.2. Mouse bioassay: massive hepatic enlargement with dark discoloration subsequent to intraperitoneal injection with 0.5 mL of algal extract (R mouse). Control mouse (L) was given 0.5 mL of deionized water IP. Algal boom had resulted in illness and death of cattle in Northern California and was identified morphologically as a *Microcystis* sp. Photo courtesy of Birgit Puschner.

blooms contain a number of structural variants of microcystins, and thus it is difficult to estimate the potential toxicity of a bloom (Fig. 101.2).

- The reported IP LD_{50} of anatoxin-a in mice is 200 µg/kg while the IV LD_{50} is estimated at less than 100 µg/kg. The oral toxicity of anatoxin-a is much higher, with an oral LD_{50} in mice reported as greater than 5,000 µg/kg.
- Anatoxin-a_s is much more toxic than anatoxin-a. The reported IP LD_{50} in mice is 20 µg/kg.
- Reported IP LD_{50} of lyngbyatoxin A in mice is 0.25 mg/kg.
- Chronic and subchronic toxicity data does exist for domestic animals.

Systems Affected

- Microcystins.
  - Hepatobiliary – diarrhea, weakness, pale mucous membranes, icterus, shock.
- Anatoxin-a and anatoxin-$a_{s.}$
  - Nervous – muscle tremors, muscle rigidity, paralysis, cyanosis, salivation with anatoxin $a_{s.}$
- Lyngbya-, aplysia-, and debromoaplysiatoxins.
  - Dermal – pruritus, erythema, blister formation, dermatitis.

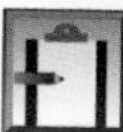

SIGNALMENT/HISTORY

- Dogs are the most common species affected by microcystins and anatoxin-a, although many species may develop toxicosis if a sufficient dose is ingested.
- Backyard ponds that are poorly maintained and allow for cyanobacterial proliferation may pose a risk to dogs.

Risk Factors

- Dogs that enjoy swimming are more likely to consume toxic amounts of an algal bloom than dogs that refrain from water.
- Algal bloom prevalence is higher during increased water temperature and elevated nutrient concentrations in the water.
- Use of a dietary supplement containing naturally harvested blue-green algae.

Historical Findings

- Witnessed exposure to water with or without visible algal bloom. Toxins may persist in the water post bloom.
- Algal material on coat or present in vomit.
- Owners frequently report rapid onset of clinical presentation, usually within 30 minutes of access to water.
- Other animals (especially livestock) may be found dead near the water source.

Location and Circumstances of Poisoning

- Lakes, streams, ponds, removed algal material (bucket).
- Most microcystin-producing algal blooms are found in freshwater, but they have also occurred in saline environments.
- Algal bloom prevalence is highest during increased water temperature and elevated nutrient concentrations in the water.
- Steady winds that propel toxic blooms to shore allow for ingestion by thirsty animals.
- Different algal species reside in the benthic zone (i.e., on the sediment) or in the pelagic zone (water column). Blooms of pelagic species are usually easily detected at the water surface of ponds, rivers, or lakes. Blooms of benthic species are difficult to detect since algae reside on the surface of sediment and stones in rivers or lakes.

CLINICAL FEATURES

- Microcystins – acute hepatotoxicosis with clinical signs of diarrhea, weakness, pale mucous membranes, and shock. Progression of disease is rapid and death generally occurs within several hours of exposure.

- Anatoxin-a – clinical signs include rapid onset of rigidity and muscle tremors, followed by paralysis, cyanosis, and death as a result of potent cholinergic stimulation. Progression is very rapid and death usually occurs within minutes to a few hours of exposure.
- Anatoxin-a$_s$ – rapid onset of excessive salivation (the "s" stands for salivation), lacrimation, diarrhea, and urination associated with muscarinic overstimulation. Clinical signs of nicotinic overstimulation include tremors, incoordination, and convulsions. Respiratory arrest and recumbency may be seen prior to death. Progression is very rapid and animals may die within 30 minutes of exposure.
- Lyngbya-, aplysia-, and debromoaplysiatoxins – acute onset of pruritus and erythema followed by dermatitis with or without blister formation. Prognosis is good.

DIFFERENTIAL DIAGNOSIS

- Microcystin toxicosis – other causes of acute liver failure such as amanitins, aflatoxins, cocklebur, xylitol, cycad palms, acetaminophen.
- Anatoxin-a – strychnine, metaldehyde, avitrol, penitrem A/roquefortine mycotoxins, methylxanthines, pyrethrin/pyrethroid insecticides, organochlorine insecticides, poisonous plants (cyanide, oleander, poison hemlock), illicit substances (amphetamine derivatives), ephedra-containing compounds.
- Anatoxin-a$_s$ – organophosphorus and carbamate insecticides, slaframine.
- Lyngbya-, aplysia-, and debromoaplysiatoxins – other causes of dermatitis such as insect bites, bacterial infections, parasites, and allergic reactions.

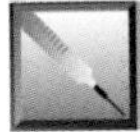

DIAGNOSTICS

- Save gastric contents and water source samples for diagnostic testing.
- Clinical pathology.
    - Microcystins – increase in serum ALP, AST, ALT, and in bilirubin, hyperkalemia, hypoglycemia.
    - Anatoxin-a and anatoxin-a$_s$ – no significant findings.
- Toxicology testing.
    - Toxicity is strain specific and identification of a potential toxin-producing strain should be followed up by toxicant detection to predict toxicity level.
    - Anatoxin-a$_s$ – depressed blood cholinesterase activity.
    - Identification of the algae in the suspect water source or stomach contents; however, positive identification does not confirm intoxication because the toxicity of the cyanobacteria is strain specific, and morphological observations alone cannot predict the hazard level.
    - Detection of microcystins in gastric contents and suspect source material.

- Detection of anatoxin-a in gastric contents, urine, bile, and suspect source material.
- Mouse bioassay (IP injection of algal bloom extract) was used in the past to determine the toxicity of crude algal biomass in suspicious blue-green algae poisonings (see Fig. 101.2).

Pathological Findings

- Microcystins – detection of algal bloom material in GI tract and/or on legs. Grossly evident liver enlargement; histological lesions include progressive centrilobular hepatocyte rounding, dissociation, necrosis; breakdown of the sinusoidal endothelium; and intrahepatic hemorrhage.
- Anatoxin-a and anatoxin-a_s – detection of algal bloom material in GI tract and/or on legs. No lesions are usually present.

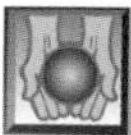

THERAPEUTICS

- The treatment goals are to prevent further exposure and absorption, control CNS signs, and provide supportive care.
- Treatment is often unsuccessful due to the rapid onset of clinical signs and death.
- Microcystin toxicosis – provide supportive therapy to treat hypovolemia and electrolyte imbalances.
- Anatoxin-a toxicosis – general supportive care and specific measures to control seizures should be performed.
- Anatoxin-a_s toxicosis – atropine should be given at a test dose to determine its efficacy in animals with life-threatening clinical signs. After the test dose, atropine can be given repeatedly until cessation of salivation.
- Lyngbya-, aplysia-, and debromoaplysiatoxins – provide supportive therapy to treat pruritus, dermatitis, and potentially secondary bacterial infections.

Detoxification

- Emesis may be induced in asymptomatic animals with recent exposures.
- Activated charcoal can be attempted, but efficacy is questionable.
- Bathe all animals with dermal exposure very thoroughly. Protective clothing must be worn by staff members during bathing (risk of dermatitis).

Appropriate Health Care

- All intoxicated animals will need aggressive and intensive care.
- Ventilation should be closely monitored in patients with severe neurological impairment using venous or arterial (preferred) pCO_2 or end-tidal capnography. Mechanical ventilation is indicated for patients with hypoventilation.

Antidote

- No antidote available.

Drugs of Choice

- Manage acute signs of hepatic hemorrhagic shock with IV crystalloids, colloids, and blood products as needed. Initial shock boluses of 20 mL/kg of crystalloids can be given over 10–20 minutes during initial stabilization.
- The use of blood products (pRBC, WB, FFP, or FP) may be necessary to increase oxygen-carrying capacity and to replace coagulation factors. Patients should be blood typed prior to transfusion.
    - Blood products (whole blood, pRBC, etc.) 10–20 mL/kg IV to effect.
    - FFP or FP 10–20 mL/kg IV over 1–4 hours.
- Seizures.
    - Diazepam 2–5 mg/kg IV. These doses are much higher than normally used for seizure control. In general, if a 2 mg/kg IV dose does not control seizures, switch to phenobarbital.
    - Phenobarbital 2–20 mg/kg IV q 6–12 hours (may have to use very high doses).
- Tremors.
    - Methocarbamol 55–220 mg/kg IV.
- Atropine 0.02–0.04 mg/kg IV to effect in anatoxin-a_s intoxication.
- Vitamin K_1 (phytonadione) 1–5 mg/kg q 24 hours PO, SQ to address clotting issues.
- Hepatoprotectants.
    - SAMe 18–20 mg/kg PO q 24 hours.
    - Silymarin 20–50 mg/kg PO q 24 hours.

Precautions/Interactions

- Wear protective clothing while handling/bathing affected animals. Significant contact dermatitis may occur.

Nursing Care

- Intensive care and monitoring may be needed.
- Anatoxin-a and anatoxin-a_s – thermoregulation and minimize sensory stimulation.

Prevention/Avoidance

- Dogs should be denied access to water with visible algal blooms.
- Reduce fertilizer runoff and applications in fields surrounding ponds used for drinking water.
- Remove algal blooms from ponds immediately and discard material safely.

Public Health

- Toxin-producing algal blooms also pose a significant human health risk. Cases of human contact dermatitis, upper respiratory irritation, and death have occurred.
- Suspect blooms should be reported to local environmental regulatory authorities.
- A guideline value of no more than 1 μg/L of total microcystin-LR in drinking water has been set by the World Health Organization.

COMMENTS

Client Education

- Though most algae blooms do not produce toxins, determining toxicity is not possible with the naked eye. Therefore, warn clients to avoid all visible algal blooms.
- Toxin-producing algal blooms also pose a risk to humans. Do not allow children to play in or near suspect blooms.

Patient Monitoring

- Microcystin toxicosis – monitor liver function, coagulation status.
- Anatoxin-a and anatoxin-a_s – monitor biochemical profile, blood gases, and respiratory function.

Possible Complications

- DIC, rhabdomyolysis, and myoglobinuria with subsequent renal failure are possible if prolonged, untreated tremors/seizures or hyperthermia present.

Expected Course and Prognosis

- Animals poisoned with blue-green algae toxins are often found dead.
- Blue-green algae intoxications progress so rapidly that treatment is often too late.
- Prognosis is poor.

Abbreviations

See Appendix 1 for a complete list.

Suggested Reading

Puschner B, Roegner A. Cyanobacterial (blue-green algae) toxins. In: Gupta RC, ed. Veterinary Toxicology: Basic and Clinical Principles, 2nd edn New York: Elsevier, 2012; pp. 953–965.

Puschner B, Brent H, Tor ER. Diagnosis of anatoxin-a poisoning in dogs from North America. J Vet Diagn Invest 2008; 20:89–92.

Acknowledgment: The authors and editors acknowledge the prior contributions of *Amber Roegner, BS,* who co-authored this topic in the previous edition.
Authors: Adrienne Bautista, DVM, PhD, DABVT; Birgit Puschner, DVM, PhD, DABVT
Consulting Editor: Lynn R. Hovda, RPh, DVM, MS, DACVIM

Cardiac Glycosides

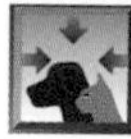

DEFINITION/OVERVIEW

- A significant number of plants (and smaller number of animals) contain naturally occurring cardiotoxic cardenolides or bufadienolides that cause GI disturbances as well as severe cardiac arrhythmias. Approximately 400 cardiac cardenolides have been described. Digoxin and digitoxin, the most widely known of these toxins, were first used to treat congestive heart failure in human beings, and are still occasionally used in human and veterinary medicine. Ingestion of pharmaceutical products containing these compounds is generally associated with more severe toxicity than ingestion of plants.
  - Common plants containing cardiac glycoside toxins include the following.
  - Desert rose (*Adenium obesum;* Fig. 102.1)
  - Dogbane (*Apocynum* spp.)
  - Purple or common foxglove (*Digitalis purpurea*; Figs 102.2 and 102.3)
  - Giant milkweed (*Calatropis* spp.)
  - Kalanchoe (*Kalanchoe* spp.; Fig. 102.4)
  - Lily of the valley (*Convallaria majalis*; Fig. 102.5)
  - Milkweed (*Asclepias* spp.)
  - Oleander (*Nerium oleander*; Figs 102.6 and 102.7)
  - Star of Bethlehem (*Ornithogalum umbellatum*)
  - Wooly foxglove (*Digitalis lantana*)
  - Yellow oleander (*Thevetia peruviana*)
- Common names are often used interchangeably to describe any of several different plants. Confirming the scientific name is essential for accurate identification.
- Different plants may have varying levels of toxicity, and concentrations of these glycosides may differ in separate parts of the plant (i.e., stem, leaves, seeds, or fruit).
- Plants can be cultivated for indoor and outdoor uses, and may also be found growing in the wild.

Blackwell's Five-Minute Veterinary Consult Clinical Companion: Small Animal Toxicology, Second Edition.
Lynn R. Hovda, Ahna G. Brutlag, Robert H. Poppenga, and Katherine L. Peterson.

Companion website: www.fiveminutevet.com/toxicology

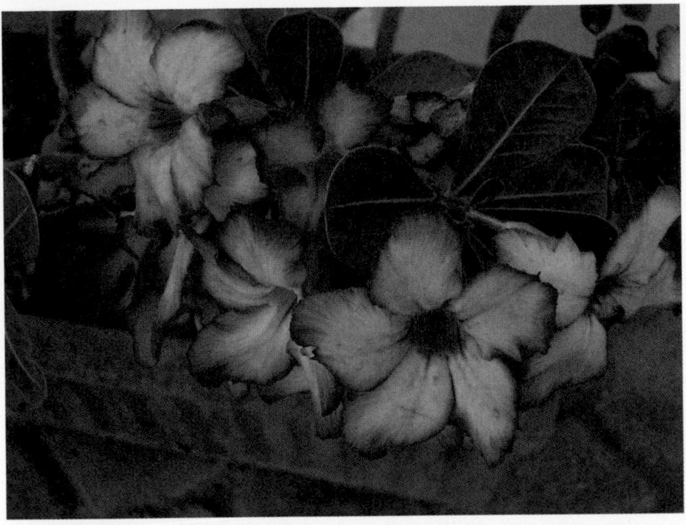

■ **Fig. 102.1.** Desert rose (*Adenium obesum*). Photo courtesy of Lynn R. Hovda.

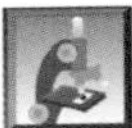

ETIOLOGY/PATHOPHYSIOLOGY

Mechanism of Action

- Cardiac glycosides have an inhibitory effect on sodium/potassium ATPase, resulting in an increase in intracellular sodium and decrease in intracellular potassium. This effect is particularly pronounced in cardiac muscle and vascular smooth muscle.

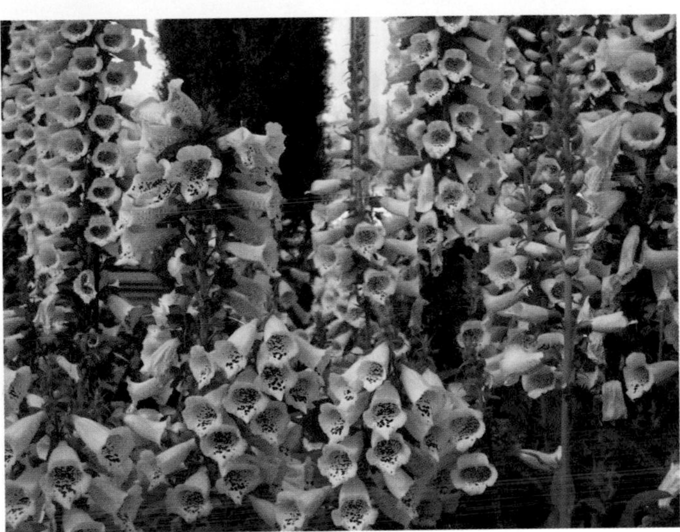

■ **Fig. 102.2.** Common foxglove (*Digitalis purpurea*). Photo courtesy of Tyne K. Hovda.

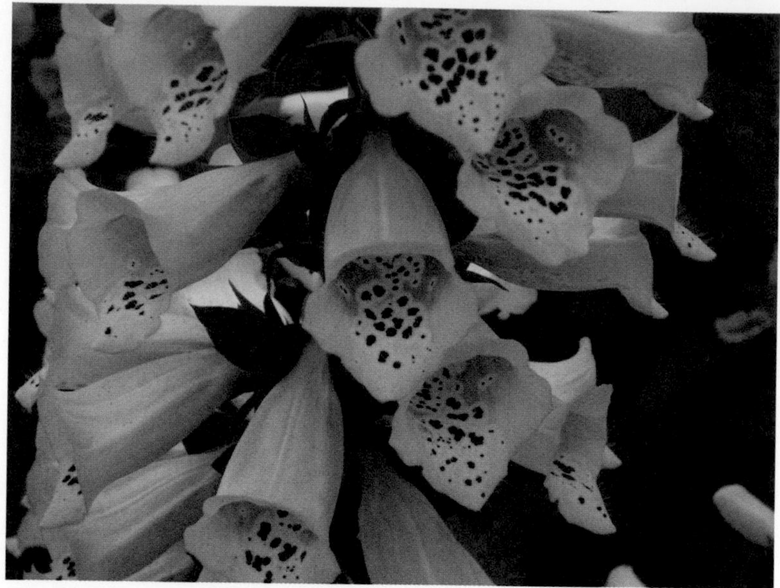

■ **Fig. 102.3.** Close-up of common foxglove (*Digitalis purpurea*). Photo courtesy of Lynn R. Hovda.

- The cell's resting membrane potential shifts in a positive direction (i.e., the cell becomes relatively less polarized) and eventually a complete loss of normal myocardial electrical function occurs.
- Extracellular potassium rises, leading to a marked hyperkalemia and loss of cardiac excitability.

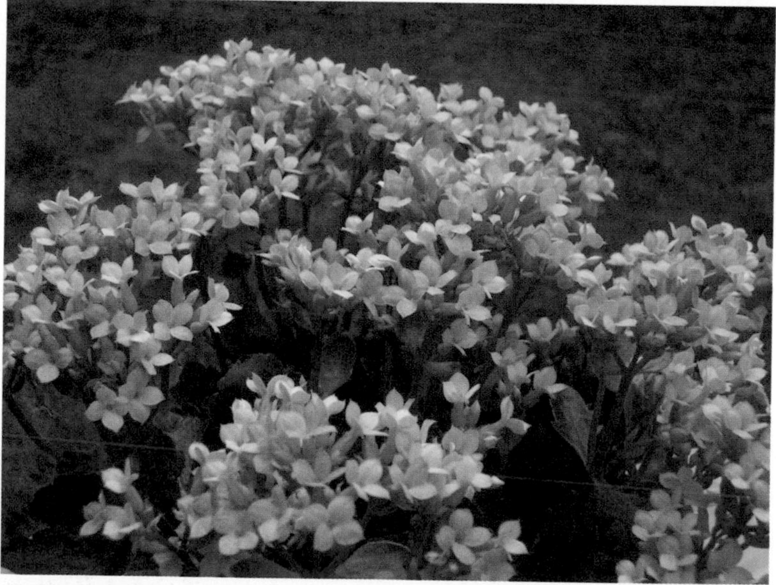

■ **Fig. 102.4.** Kalanchoe (*Kalanchoe* spp.). Photo courtesy of Tyne K. Hovda.

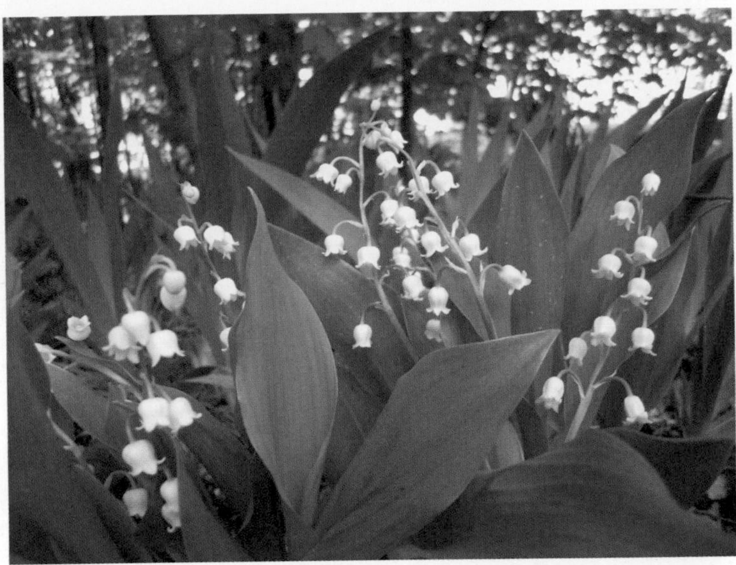

■ **Fig. 102.5.** Lily of the valley (*Convallaria majalis*). Photo courtesy of Tyne K. Hovda.

Pharmacokinetics – Absorption, Distribution, Metabolism, Excretion

- Absorption is rapid, with signs developing from 30 minutes to a few hours post ingestion.
- Food delays absorption in all species. In cats, the presence of food in the stomach may decrease the total amount absorbed by as much as 50%.

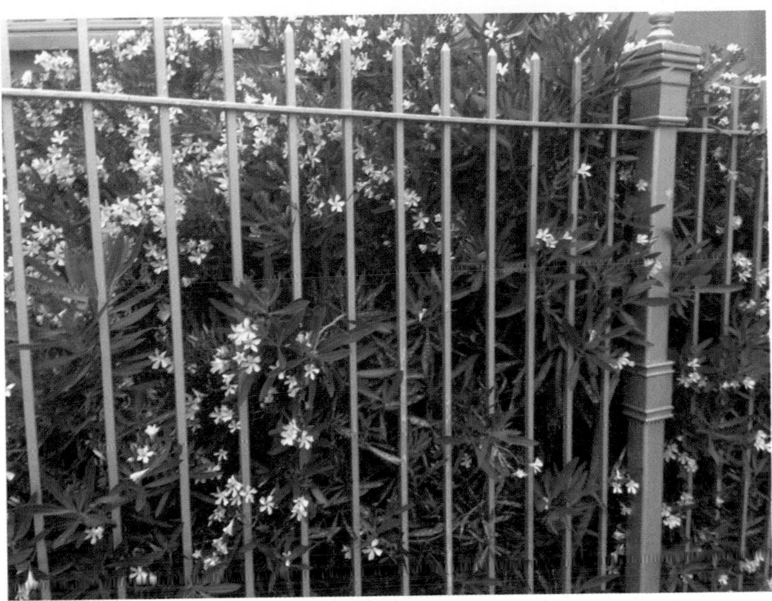

■ **Fig. 102.6.** Oleander plant (*Nerium oleander*). The plant was found growing along the street in New Orleans, LA. Photo courtesy of Lynn R. Hovda.

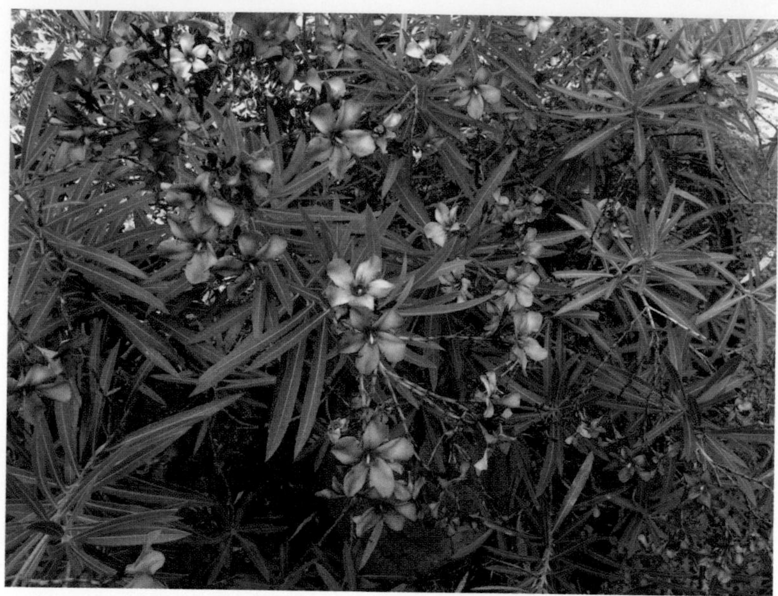

■ **Fig. 102.7.** Oleander flower (*Nerium oleander*). Photo courtesy of Tyne K. Hovda.

- Widely distributed in body tissues, particularly heart, kidney, liver, stomach, muscle.
- 20–30% protein bound. Elimination is primarily renal.
- Some hepatic metabolism and enterohepatic recirculation occurs, but the extent to which this is clinically relevant remains somewhat controversial.
- Renal dysfunction may greatly slow the rate of elimination.

Toxicity

- Digitalis is a steroidal glycoside. The various plant toxins are structurally similar and present the same toxic profile.
- Several hundred different plant toxins have been identified, most specific to a particular plant species.
  - The degree of toxicity varies depending on the particular plant, plant part, and amount consumed.
  - Most of the cardiac glycoside plants can cause toxicosis if either fresh or dried plant matter is consumed.
  - All plant parts are considered toxic. Even water from vases containing bouquets of these plants is potentially hazardous. Ingestion of just a few seeds or one to two leaves may be enough to cause serious clinical signs.

Systems Affected

- Gastrointestinal – signs occur most frequently and include hypersalivation, vomiting, and diarrhea with or without blood.

- Cardiovascular – abnormalities include bradycardia, all degrees of AV block, and a variety of arrhythmias. Rarely, tachycardia may occur. Death occurs from asystole.
- Neuromuscular – signs are vague and may be secondary to decreased cardiac output and hypotension.
- Ophthalmic – mydriasis can occur.

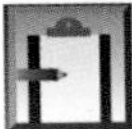

SIGNALMENT/HISTORY

- No breed or species predilection for exposure.
- Cats may be more sensitive than dogs; male cats are more sensitive than females.
- Dogs with ABCB1 (formerly referred to as MDR-1) gene mutation (e.g., Collies, Australian Shepherds, etc.) are more sensitive to the CNS effects of glycoside toxicity.

Risk Factors

- Animals with a prior history of renal disease or cardiac disease, especially those currently receiving digoxin or other cardiac drugs.
- Obese animals may experience toxicity at lower doses than lean animals.

Historical Findings

- Owner often reports that the animal gained access to medications such as digoxin, chewed or dug up relevant plants, or knocked over a vase in which plants were located and drank the water.

Location and Circumstances of Poisoning

- Can occur anywhere. Some species of the plants are widely distributed throughout the United States.
- Oleander tends to occur with greater frequency in the warmer portions of the country.
- Most of the plants are fairly unpalatable but may be ingested by bored or confined animals.

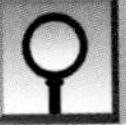

CLINICAL FEATURES

- Vomiting with or without blood, diarrhea with or without blood, and hypersalivation are the most commonly reported signs, often occurring within 30–45 minutes of ingestion. Weakness and depression often precede the onset of cardiac abnormalities. Varying degrees of bradycardia or tachycardia, weak and irregular pulses, hypotension, AV block, and arrhythmias can occur. Other signs include mydriasis, tremors, and coma.
- Animals may be found dead.

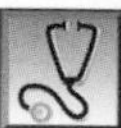

DIFFERENTIAL DIAGNOSIS

- Primary cardiac disease of any origin.
- Calcium channel blocker or beta-blocker ingestion.
- Ingestion of *Taxus* spp. or plants in *Ericaceae* family (azaleas, rhododendrons).
- Ingestion of other pharmaceuticals with known cardiac effects.
- Severe GI disease associated with viral, bacterial, or parasitic infection.

DIAGNOSTICS

- Presence of pills or plants in stomach or GIT.
- Serum chemistry with early and marked hyperkalemia. May change to hypokalemia as time passes.
- Serum digoxin levels may be available from human hospitals. If a plant ingestion is suspected, be sure the laboratory is running an assay that includes the toxin associated with the specific plant in question.
- Detection of cardiac glycosides in tissue or urine is rarely performed but can be done by chromatography if the specific glycoside is known.

Pathological Findings

- Gross findings depend on the time of death, but plant pieces may be found in the stomach and small intestine. The epicardium may have a mottled appearance with clotted blood in the ventricles.
- Histopathological findings include venous and capillary congestion throughout the body with severe, diffuse hepatic congestion and marked caudal vena cava distension.

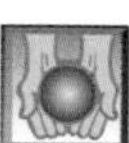

THERAPEUTICS

Detoxification

- Induction of emesis if recent exposure and the animal is not already vomiting.
- In massive ingestions, consider sedation, endotracheal intubation (with a cuffed, inflated tube), and gastric lavage.
- Activated charcoal with a cathartic × 1 dose followed by activated charcoal every 4–6 hours for up to 24 hours, if no risk for aspiration and sodium level can be monitored.

Appropriate Health Care

- Hospitalize animals with known ingestions for at least 12 hours. Clinical signs are often evident at 30–45 minutes post ingestion but may be delayed for several hours, depending on the particular material ingested.

- ECG monitoring for a minimum of 24 hours in animals with clinical signs. Treat arrhythmias as they develop.
- Baseline serum chemistry with special attention to potassium and renal indices. Venous blood gases to monitor for metabolic acidosis. Correct electrolyte and acid–base abnormalities as needed.
- Judicious use of IV fluids with close monitoring of patient response – goal is to support, but not overload, the cardiovascular system.

Antidote

- Digoxin-specific Fab fragments (Digibind) have been used in dogs to reverse the cardiac effects of digoxin and oleander, and may be effective for other cardiac glycoside toxins as well. High cost often precludes their use. A wide variety of doses have been suggested. If used, best option is to monitor serum digoxin levels and adjust dose accordingly.

Drugs of Choice

- Early yet cautious use of IV fluids to maintain blood pressure and perfusion.
- Bradycardia.
  - Atropine 0.02–0.04 mg/kg IV, IM, or SQ.
  - Glycopyrrolate 0.01–0.02 mg/kg SQ, IM, or IV.
  - In severe cases of bradycardia unresponsive to medical management, the use of a temporary pacemaker may be indicated.
- The use of antiarrhythmics (lidocaine, procainamide) may be necessary if the patient is persistently tachycardic and nonresponsive to IV fluids, has severe ventricular dysrhythmias, or has evidence of poor perfusion (hypotension, pulse deficits, tachycardia, pale mucous membranes, prolonged CRT).
  - Lidocaine.
    - Dogs: 2–4 mg/kg IV over 1–2 minutes to effect. If effective follow with CRI at 25–100 mcg/kg/min. ECG must be monitored carefully during use.
    - Cats: 0.25–0.5 mg/kg slow IV while monitoring ECG. If effective use CRI of 10–20 mcg/kg/min cautiously in cats.
  - Procainamide.
    - Dogs: 2–4 mg/kg IV over 3–5 minutes (up to 20 mg/kg IV bolus), followed by 20–50 mcg/kg/min CRI.
- Antiemetics if vomiting is severe or persistent.
  - Maropitant 1 mg/kg SQ q 24 hours.
  - Ondansetron 0.1–0.2 mg/kg IV q 8–12 hours.
- GI protectants as needed.
  - H_2 blockers.
    - Famotidine 0.5–1 mg/kg PO, SQ, IM, IV q 12 hours.

 - □ Ranitidine 1–2 mg/kg PO, SQ, IM, IV q 8–12 hours.
 - □ Cimetidine 5–10 mg/kg PO, SQ, IM, IV q 6 hours.
- Omeprazole 0.5–1 mg/kg PO q 24 hours.
- Sucralfate 0.25–1 g PO q 8 hours for 5–7 days if evidence of active ulcer disease.

Alternative Drugs

- Fructose-1, 6-diphosphate has been used experimentally to decrease the severity of cardiac effects in dogs. The mechanism of action is not understood.

Precautions/Interactions

- Hawthorn, an herbal supplement, should not be used as it exacerbates the toxicity of cardiac glycosides.
- Calcium channel blockers and beta-blockers can have additive effects on AV conduction and should be avoided as they may result in complete heart block.

Nursing Care

- Palpation of extremities for coldness; may indicate decreased perfusion secondary to hypotension.
- Severely affected patients may require 3–6 days of hospitalization.

COMMENTS

Client Education

Avoid the use of herbal or alternative supplements such as hawthorn until the animal has recovered completely.

Patient Monitoring

- Continuous ECG for first 24 hours and then as needed to monitor effect of cardiac drugs.
- Serial blood pressure monitoring, especially early in toxicity. Hypotension may become severe.
- Baseline and repeat serum electrolytes. Hyperkalemia may be early and marked; hypokalemia has been reported but generally occurs later.

Prevention/Avoidance

- Owners should know the common plants in their home, yard, and geographical location.
- Oleander commonly grows wild in the south west, especially in California, Arizona, New Mexico, and Texas. Off-leash dogs in these areas should be watched carefully for any signs of exposure.

Expected Course and Prognosis

- Prognosis is guarded to good with appropriate care and timely intervention.
- Cardiac arrhythmias may complicate recovery but are not insurmountable if treated early.

See Also

Beta Receptor Antagonists (Beta-Blockers)
Calcium Channel Blockers
Azaleas and Rhododendrons
Yew

Abbreviations

See Appendix 1 for a complete list.

Suggested Reading

Atkinson KJ, Fine DM, Evans TJ, et al. Suspected lily-of-the-valley (*Convallaria majalis*) toxicosis in a dog. J Vet Emerg Crit Care 2008; 18(4):399–403.

Bandara V, Weinstein SA, White J, et al. A review of the natural history, toxinology, diagnosis and clinical management of *Nerium oleander* (common oleander) and *Thevetia peruviana* (yellow oleander) poisoning. Toxicon 2010; 56(3):273–281.

Milweski LM, Safda AK. An overview of potentially life-threatening poisonous plants in dogs and cats. J Vet Emerg Crit Care 2006; 16(1):25–33

Smith G. Kalanchoe species poisoning in pets. Vet Med 2004; 99(11):913–936.

Tiwary AK, Poppenga RH, Puschner B. In vitro study of the effectiveness of three commercial adsorbents for binding oleander toxins. Clin Toxicol 2009; 47(3):213–218.

Acknowledgment: The authors and editors acknowledge the prior contributions of Erica Cargill, CVT, and Krishona L. Martinson, PhD, who co-authored this topic in the previous edition.

Author: James N. Eucher, DVM, DHSc, MS, MPH
Consulting Editor: Lynn R. Hovda, RPh, DVM, MS, DACVIM

chapter 103

Lilies

DEFINITION/OVERVIEW

- Toxicosis is associated with ingestion of many plants in the genera *Lilium* and *Hemerocallis*.
- Cats are the target species.
- Kidneys are the target organs.
- Ingestion of plant parts can result in vomiting, anorexia, lethargy, oliguria or anuria, acute kidney injury, and, rarely, pancreatitis.
- Lilies are frequently cultivated as garden and house plants, found growing in nature, and used in many floral bouquets and baskets.

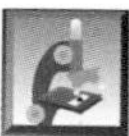

ETIOLOGY/PATHOPHYSIOLOGY

- Ingestion of plant material (leaves, stems, and flowers).
- Ingestion of pollen and water contaminated with pollen or plant material.
- Aqueous floral extract contains the highest amounts of toxic compound.
- Includes Asiatic hybrid lilies such as the stargazer (*Lilium* spp.), Asiatic lily (*Lilium asiatic;* Fig. 103.1), Easter lily (*L. longiflorum*; Fig. 103.2), Japanese show lily (*L. speciosum;* Fig. 103.3), Oriental lily (*L. orientalis*; Fig. 103.4), red lily (*L. umbellatum*), tiger lily (*L. tigrinum or L. lancifolium*), Western lily (*L. occidentale*), wood lily (*L. philadelphicum*), and daylily (*Hemerocallis* spp.; Figs 103.5 and 103.6).

Mechanism of Action

Renal tubular necrosis with intact basement membrane.

Toxicity

- The toxin has not been identified but is known to be water soluble.
- Doses of 568 mg/kg of aqueous leaf extract and 291 mg/kg of aqueous flower extract of Easter lily have elicited toxicosis in cats.
- Deaths have occurred after ingestion of only one or two plant pieces.

Blackwell's Five-Minute Veterinary Consult Clinical Companion: Small Animal Toxicology, Second Edition.
Lynn R. Hovda, Ahna G. Brutlag, Robert H. Poppenga, and Katherine L. Peterson.

Companion website: www.fiveminutevet.com/toxicology

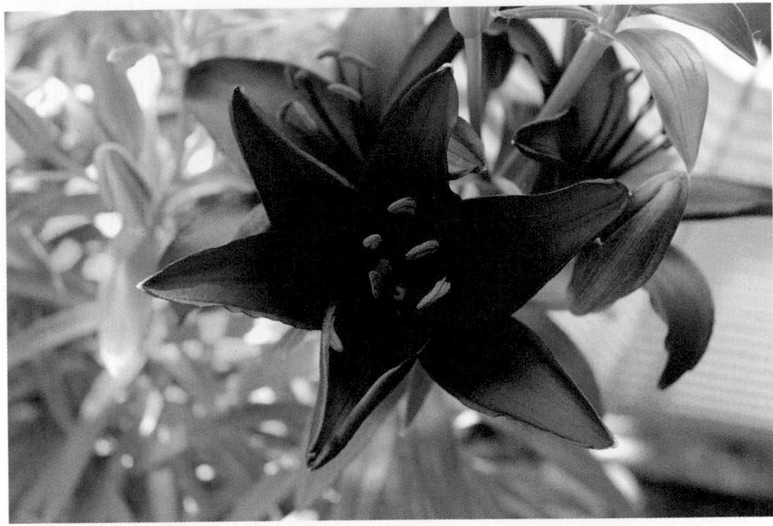

■ **Fig. 103.1.** Asiatic lily (*Lilium asiatic*). Photo courtesy of Lynn R. Hovda.

Systems Affected

- Renal – acute kidney injury.
- Gastrointestinal – vomiting, diarrhea, anorexia, hypersalivation.
- Neurological – depression, ataxia, tremors, seizures.

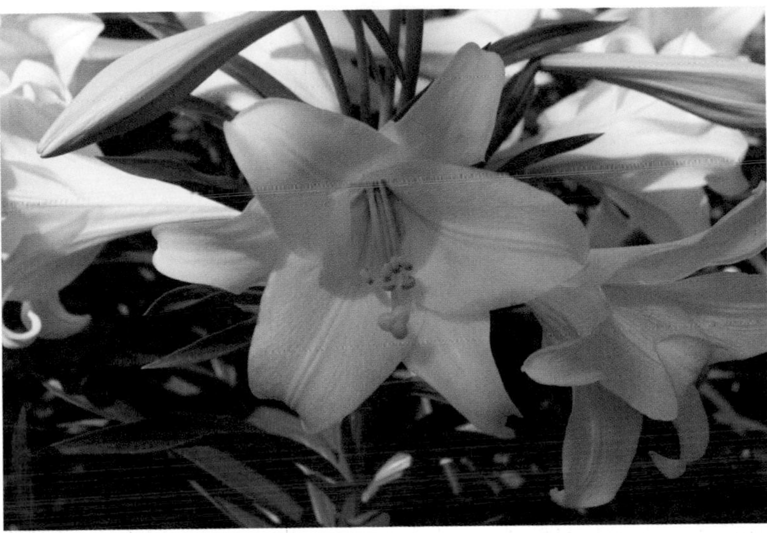

■ **Fig. 103.2.** Easter lily (*Lilium longiflorum*). Photo courtesy of Tyne K. Hovda.

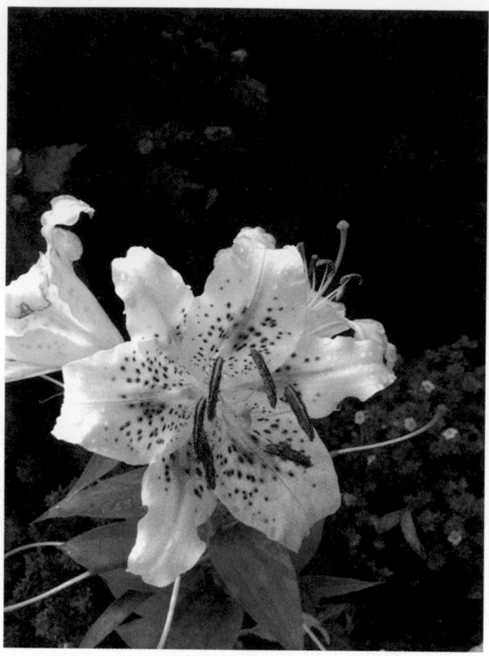

■ **Fig. 103.3.** Japanese show lily (*Lilium speciosum*). Photo courtesy of Lynn R. Hovda.

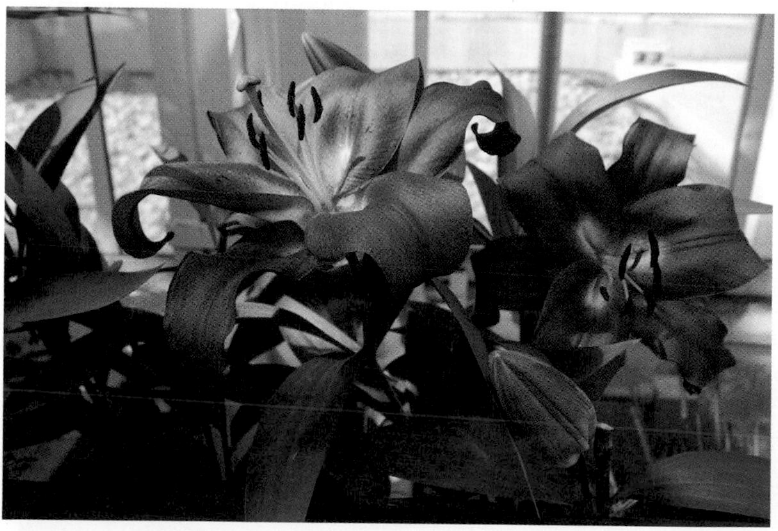

■ **Fig. 103.4.** Oriental lily (*Lilium orientalis*). Photo courtesy of Lynn R. Hovda.

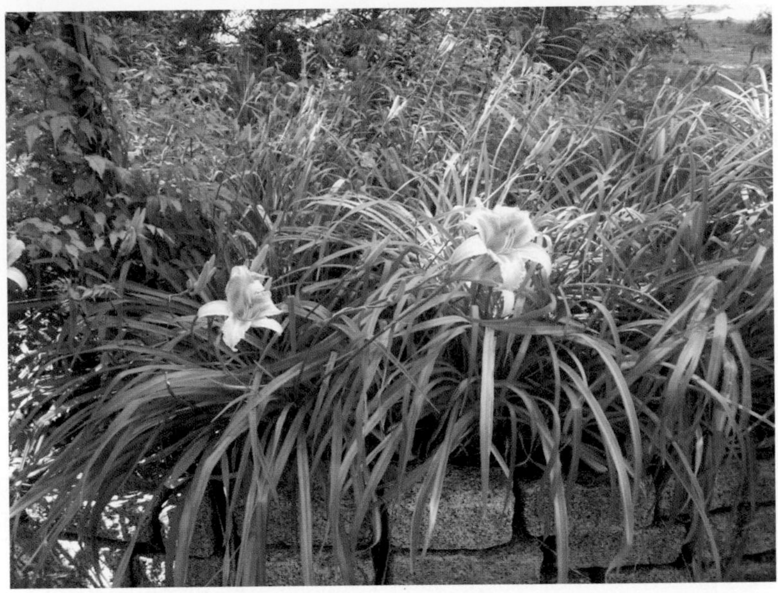

■ **Fig. 103.5.** Daylily plant (*Hemerocallis* spp.). Note the many leaves arranged in a grass-like cluster. Photo courtesy of Tyne K. Hovda.

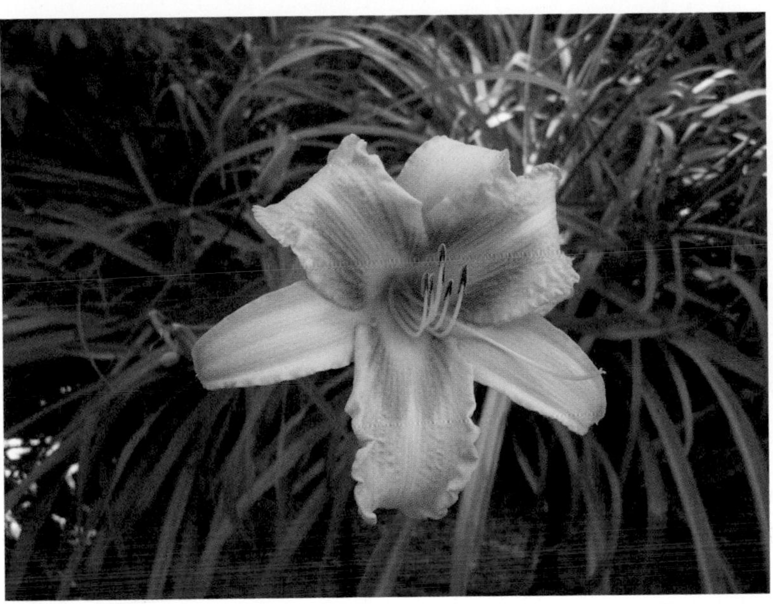

■ **Fig. 103.6.** Close-up of daylily flower (*Hemerocallis* spp.) Photo courtesy of Tyne K. Hovda.

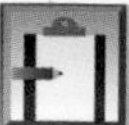

SIGNALMENT/HISTORY

- Most cases are reported in cats.
- Dogs are thought to be affected, but attempts to reproduce the disease in dogs (and rabbits) have been unsuccessful.
- Most exposures occur around holidays or other festive occasions where lilies are used as house plants or found in floral arrangements.

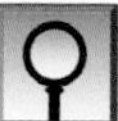

CLINICAL FEATURES

- All parts of the lily are considered toxic; however, the leaves are most commonly ingested.
- Signs usually develop within 6–12 hours of exposure.
- Early signs include vomiting, anorexia, and lethargy followed by acute kidney injury.
- Clinical signs of acute kidney injury include polyuria, oliguria, or anuria, dehydration, vomiting, diarrhea, and depression.
- Some cats also present with CNS signs such as ataxia, head pressing, disorientation, tremors, and seizures.
- Severe pancreatitis has also been reported, but is considered rare.

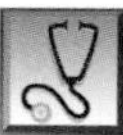

DIFFERENTIAL DIAGNOSIS

- Toxins.
  - Ethylene glycol
  - Grapes or raisins
  - Nonsteroidal antiinflammatory drugs and nephrotoxic drugs
  - Soluble oxalate plants
- Infectious diseases.
- Physical abnormalities (ureteral obstruction, nephrolith).

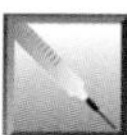

DIAGNOSTICS

- Serum chemistry findings include increases in blood urea nitrogen (BUN), creatinine, phosphorus, and potassium. BUN and creatinine generally increase within 18–24 hours of exposure. Creatinine may be disproportionately elevated.
- Urinalysis typically shows glucosuria, proteinuria, and isosthenuria. Epithelial casts usually can be seen in urine 12 hours after exposure.
- Renal ultrasound reveals changes consistent with acute tubular necrosis.

Pathological Findings

- Gross examination shows swollen, edematous kidneys and systemic congestion. Pancreatic necrosis may be present.

- Histopathological examination of the kidneys shows acute proximal convoluted renal tubular necrosis with or without mineralization. The collecting ducts may contain granular or hyaline casts, and the basement membrane, while intact, may contain mitotic figures.

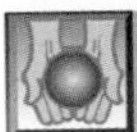

THERAPEUTICS

- Treatment of lily toxicosis consists primarily of early and aggressive supportive care including early decontamination, prevention of renal damage, and maintenance of fluid, electrolyte, and acid–base balance.
- Baseline BUN, creatinine, and electrolytes should be obtained on admission and repeated daily until they have returned to normal.

Detoxification

- Bathe cats contaminated with pollen.
- Emesis within 1–2 hours of ingestion. Hydrogen peroxide is not recommended in cats. Dexmedetomidine (7 mcg/kg IM or 3.5 mcg/kg IV) is an effective emetic in cats. Xylazine (0.44–1.1 mg/kg IM or SQ) is less effective.
- Activated charcoal with a cathartic × 1 dose.

Appropriate Health Care

- Early and aggressive use of IV fluids to prevent renal damage.
- Baseline serum chemistries to include BUN and creatinine. Monitor daily.
- Monitor urine output and add diuretics as needed.

Antidote

- No antidote available.

Drugs of Choice

- IV fluid therapy at 2–3 times maintenance for 48 hours, then decrease depending on BUN and creatinine levels.
  - Choice of fluid therapy depends on electrolyte and glucose levels.
  - IV fluids should be started within 18 hours of exposure; SQ fluids are not effective.
- Diuresis in oliguric cats once they are well hydrated.
  - Furosemide CRI at 1–2 mg/kg/hour IV.
  - Mannitol bolus at 1–2 g/kg IV, followed by CRI if needed.
- GI protectants as needed.
  - H_2 blockers.
    - Famotidine 0.5–1 mg/kg PO, SQ, IM, IV q 12 hours.

    - □ Ranitidine 1–2 mg/kg PO, SQ, IM, IV q 8–12 hours.
    - □ Cimetidine 5–10 mg/kg PO, SQ, IM, IV q 6 hours.
  - Omeprazole 0.5–1 PO mg/kg daily.
  - Sucralfate 0.25–1 g PO q 8 hours × 5–7 days if evidence of active ulcer disease.
- Peritoneal or renal dialysis may be useful in anuric cats.

COMMENTS

Client Education

- Any exposure to lilies in cats, regardless of the amount, should be considered harmful, and immediate veterinary intervention sought.

Prevention/Avoidance

- Keep Easter lilies and floral arrangements with lilies out of households with cats.
- Do not plant or maintain lilies in a garden if an outside cat can gain access to them.

Expected Course and Prognosis

- Delaying treatment 18 hours or longer after exposure usually results in acute kidney injury.
- The prognosis for cats aggressively treated prior to 18 hours post exposure is good. Once oliguria or anuria develops, the prognosis becomes fair to grave. Chronic renal impairment may occur in these cats even after treatment.
- Mortality rate from Easter lily toxicosis is reported to be as high as 100% if treatment is delayed and renal failure occurs.

See Also

Ethylene Glycol and Diethylene Glycol

Grapes and Raisins

Abbreviations

See Appendix 1 for a complete list.

Suggested Reading

Berg RI, Francey T, Segev G. Resolution of acute kidney injury in a cat after lily (*Lilium lancifolium*) intoxication. J Vet Intern Med 2007; 21(4):857–859.

Bennett AJ, Reineke EL. Outcome following gastrointestinal tract decontamination and intravenous fluid diuresis in cats with known lily ingestion: 25 cases (2001–2010). J Am Vet Med Assoc 2013; 242:1110–1116.

Hadley RM, Richardson JA, Gwaltney-Brant SM. A retrospective study of daylily toxicosis in cats. Vet Hum Toxicol 2003; 45(1):38–39.
Milweski LM, Safdar AK. An overview of potentially life-threatening poisonous plants in dogs and cats. J Vet Emerg Crit Care 2006; 16(1):25–33.
Rumbeiha WK, Jayaraj AF, Fitzgerald SD, et al. A comprehensive study of Easter lily poisoning in cats. J Vet Diagn Invest 2004; 16(6):527–541.

Acknowledgment: The authors and editors acknowledge the prior contributions of Krishona L. Martinson, PhD, and Lynn R. Hovda, RPh, DVM, MS, DACVIM, who co-authored this topic in the previous edition.
Author: Amanda L. Poldoski, DVM
Consulting Editor: Lynn R. Hovda, RPh, DVM, MS, DACVIM

chapter 104

Mushrooms

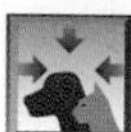

DEFINITION/OVERVIEW

- Several thousand species of mushrooms are found in North America, but fewer than 100 are toxic.
- There is no simple test that distinguishes poisonous from nonpoisonous mushrooms.
- The most toxic mushrooms contain amanitin toxins.
- The number of reported mushroom poisonings in animals is low, although this is likely to be a result of the lack of diagnostic work-up and methods to confirm exposure.
- Amanitins.
    - The majority of confirmed mushroom poisonings in animals are caused by hepatotoxic mushrooms that contain amanitins.
    - Poisoned animals develop gastrointestinal signs between 6 and 24 hours after ingestion. After a period of "false recovery," fulminant liver failure develops generally 36–48 hours after exposure. During the final stage, renal failure can also develop.
    - While a number of mushroom genera (*Amanita*, *Galerina*, and *Lepiota*) contain the hepatotoxic cyclopeptides, *Amanita phalloides* (Fig. 104.1), also known as death cap or death angel, and *A. ocreata* (Fig. 104.2), also known as the destroying angel, are the species most frequently reported in poisonings.
    - Aggressive therapeutic measures are required to improve prognosis and include decontamination, supportive care, and administration of drugs that may reduce the toxin uptake into hepatocytes.
- Other toxic mushrooms (not further discussed in detail in this chapter).
    - Mushrooms that contain muscarine (e.g., *Inocybe* spp., *Clitocybe* spp.) are relatively common but do not appear to be a major risk for poisoning in animals. Poisoned animals show signs of salivation, lacrimation, vomiting, diarrhea, bradycardia, and miosis. Atropine and decontamination procedures are important treatment strategies.
    - Mushrooms that contain muscimol and ibotenic acid (e.g., *Amanita muscaria*, *Amanita pantherina*) are common in the Pacific Northwest. Ingestion can result in ataxia, sedation, muscle spasms, and seizures, but with aggressive supportive care, full recovery is expected within 1–2 days.

Blackwell's Five-Minute Veterinary Consult Clinical Companion: Small Animal Toxicology, Second Edition.
Lynn R. Hovda, Ahna G. Brutlag, Robert H. Poppenga, and Katherine L. Peterson.

Companion website: www.fiveminutevet.com/toxicology

- False morel (*Gyromitra* spp.) ingestion can lead to vomiting, abdominal pain, and diarrhea followed by convulsions. With supportive care, poisoned animals are likely to recover within several days of exposure.
- Hallucinogenic mushrooms (*Psilocybe*, *Panaeolus*, *Conocybe*, and *Gymnopilus* spp.) contain psilocybin. Poisoned animals can develop ataxia, vocalization, overt aggression, nystagmus, and increased body temperature. The management of hallucinogenic mushroom poisoning is essentially supportive, and in most cases, treatment is not necessary.
- Many mushrooms are capable of causing gastrointestinal irritation (*Agaricus*, *Boletus*, *Chlorophyllum*, *Entoloma*, *Lactarius*, *Omphalotus*, *Rhodophyllus*, *Scleroderma*, and *Tricholoma* spp.). In most exposures, vomiting and diarrhea develop between 1 and 6 hours after ingestion, with complete recovery within 24–48 hours.

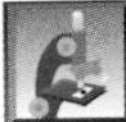

ETIOLOGY/PATHOPHYSIOLOGY

- *A. phalloides* (commonly known as death cap; see Fig. 104.1) is found throughout North America and grows most commonly under oak, birch, pine, and other hardwoods. It can also be found in open pastures.

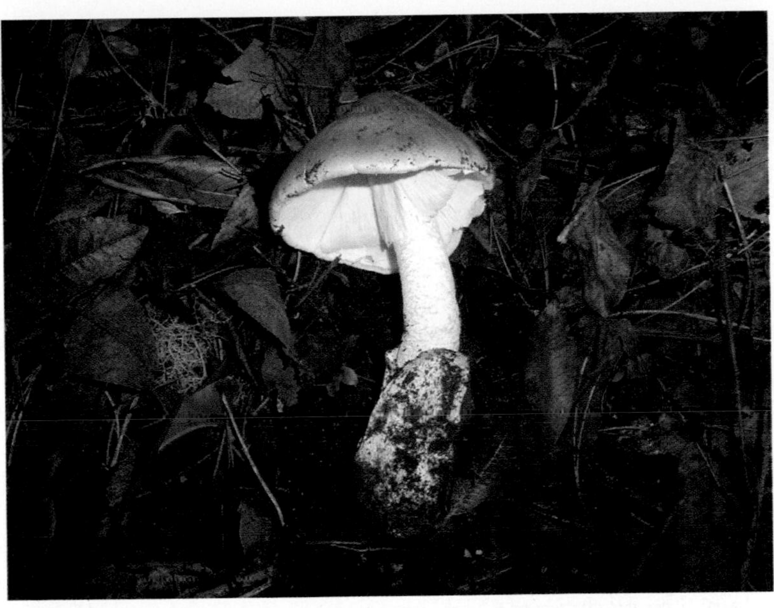

Fig. 104.1. *Amanita phalloides*. Photo courtesy of R. Michael Davis.

- *A. ocreata* (commonly known as Western North American destroying angel; see Fig. 104.2) grows from Baja California, Mexico, along the Pacific Coast to Washington. *A. ocreata* is most commonly found in sandy soils under oak or pine.

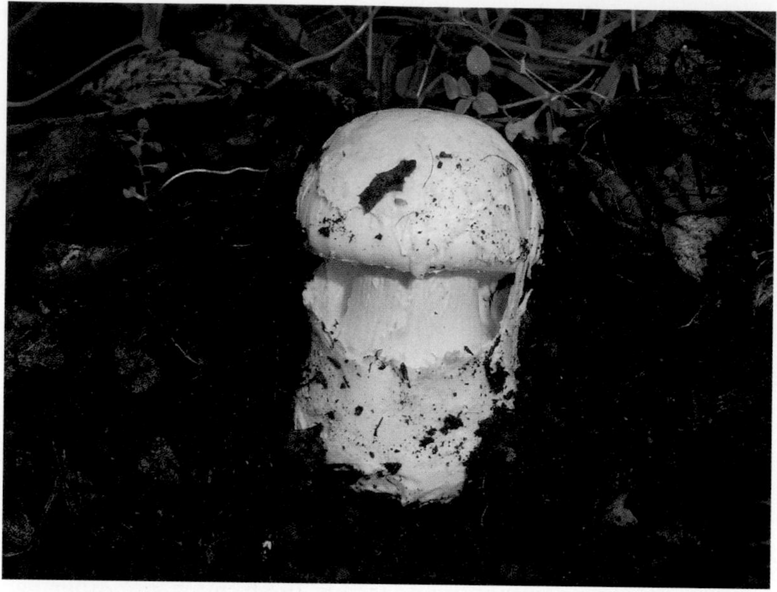

■ **Fig. 104.2.** *Amanita ocreata.* Photo courtesy of R. Michael Davis.

- Amanitins (alpha-, beta-, gamma-, and epsilon-amanitins) are bicyclic octapeptides that are found in approximately 35 mushroom species from three different genera: *Amanita*, *Galerina*, and *Lepiota*. The toxins are not degraded by cooking, freezing, or the acidic environment of the stomach.

Mechanism of Action

- Amanitins inhibit nuclear RNA polymerase II, resulting in decreased protein synthesis and cell death. Hepatocytes, crypt cells, and proximal convoluted tubules are especially susceptible to the effect because of their high metabolic rate.
- Other toxic mechanisms are likely to play an important role in the toxicity of amanitins.

Pharmacokinetics – Absorption, Distribution, Metabolism, Excretion

- After exposure, amanitins exert toxic effects on intestinal cells. Amanitins are rapidly absorbed from the gastrointestinal tract and distributed (not plasma protein bound) to liver and kidney. The plasma half-life of amanitins in dogs is short, ranging from 25 to 50 minutes. Amanitins are largely excreted unchanged in urine and can be detected in urine well before clinical signs occur. Only a small amount of amanitins is excreted in the bile.
- Species-specific data on the bioavailability of amanitins are largely unavailable, but it appears that the absorption rate in dogs is much greater than in mice and rabbits and much less than in people. Rodents appear resistant to the effects of amanitins.

Toxicity

- Amanitins are extremely toxic. The IV LD_{50} of alpha-amanitin in dogs is 0.1 mg/kg BW. An oral LD_{50} for methyl-gamma-amanitin was estimated to be 0.5 mg/kg BW. In humans, the estimated oral LD_{50} of alpha-amanitin is 0.1 mg/kg BW.
- Toxin concentrations in *Amanita* spp. vary depending on growing conditions, moisture, and time of year. Hence, it is very difficult to estimate the minimum amount of mushroom material needed to cause poisoning. Considering the average concentration of amanitins per mushroom of 4 mg/g, the ingestion of two *A. phalloides* has the potential to be lethal to an adult dog, while a smaller amount may kill a puppy.

Systems Affected

- Gastrointestinal – vomiting, diarrhea, and severe abdominal pain begin approximately 8–12 hours after exposure.
- Hepatobiliary – fulminant liver failure develops approximately 36–48 hours after exposure.
- Renal/urological – if the animal survives liver failure, renal and multiorgan failure can develop.
- Hemic – coagulopathy can develop as a result of liver failure.
- Nervous – encephalopathy can develop as a result of liver failure.

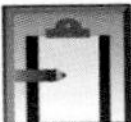

SIGNALMENT/HISTORY

- All breeds and genders are equally susceptible.
- Puppies are at greater risk of being poisoned than adults.
- Cases have been documented in dogs, cats and cattle.
- There are no known genetic predispositions.
- Severe gastrointestinal signs such as vomiting, diarrhea, and abdominal pain occurring hours after an observed mushroom ingestion.
- Severe gastrointestinal signs such as vomiting, diarrhea, and abdominal pain present hours after unobserved roaming in the woods, especially during mushroom season.
- Liver failure occurring after a period of recovery, although gastrointestinal signs were present prior to the recovery phase.

Location and Circumstances of Poisoning:

- Amanitin-containing mushrooms are very common in the San Francisco Bay area, the Santa Cruz Mountains, the Pacific Northwest, and the Northeast.
- Toxic mushrooms are most abundant in warm, wet years and are often found under certain trees (oak, cork, spruce, birch, pine).
- In California, toxic mushrooms are typically found from mid-autumn through late winter.

- In the Northeast, toxic mushrooms are most commonly found from late September through late October.

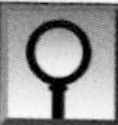

CLINICAL FEATURES

- The chief complaints of amanitin poisoning are vomiting and diarrhea within 24 hours of mushroom exposure and icterus, lethargy, ataxia, seizures, and coma approximately 36–48 hours after exposure.
- The clinical course of amanitin toxicosis can be separated into four phases with characteristic clinical features for each phase. However, not every case presents with the classic four stages.
    - The first phase is a latency period of approximately 8–12 hours after ingestion of amanitin-containing mushrooms without any clinical signs.
    - The second phase begins approximately 6–24 hours after mushroom exposure and is characterized by vomiting, diarrhea, and abdominal pain.
    - The third phase is a period of false recovery during which the animal appears to have recovered. This phase can last from several hours to a few days. During this third phase, close monitoring of liver and kidney function is essential in order to prevent misdiagnosis. In this phase, the breakdown of liver glycogen can lead to severe hypoglycemia.
    - The last phase is characterized by fulminant liver failure and begins between 36 and 84 hours after exposure to amanitins. In this stage, renal and multiorgan failure can also occur and affected animals are icteric, lethargic, and ataxic and have polyuria, polydypsia, anorexia, clotting abnormalities, seizures, or coma. Seizures and coma can also be a direct result of severe hypoglycemia. If large amounts of amanitin-containing mushrooms are ingested, or if a puppy ingested a toxic mushroom, it is possible that the animal may die acutely within 24 hours or just be found dead.

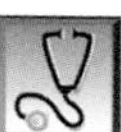

DIFFERENTIAL DIAGNOSIS

- Caustics.
- Viral, bacterial, rickettsial, and parasitic diseases.
- Mushrooms that cause gastrointestinal signs (without liver involvement) – collect mushrooms in area of exposure and have them identified.
- Dietary indiscretion such as ingestion of garbage or spoiled food.
- Other causes of acute liver failure.
- Severe acute pancreatitis.
- Toxicants.
    - Acetaminophen overdose
    - Aflatoxins

- Cocklebur (*Xanthium* spp.)
- Cycad palms (*Cycas* spp.)
- Heavy metals (e.g., lead, zinc)
- Microcystins (hepatotoxic blue-green algae toxins)
- Organophosphate and carbamate insecticides
- Ricin and abrin

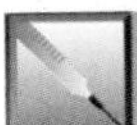

DIAGNOSTICS

- Identification of mushrooms found in the environment or gastric contents. Accurate mushroom identification will require consultation with an experienced mycologist. DNA sequencing of mushroom material is also possible.
- Serum chemistry: beginning with the second or third phase, see increases in AST, ALT, ALP, and bilirubin; hypoglycemia develops.
- Coagulation panel: beginning with the third phase, see prolonged PT and PTT.
- Detection of alpha-amanitin in serum, urine, gastric contents, liver, or kidney. This testing is provided by select veterinary toxicology laboratories.
    - In live animals, urine is considered of superior diagnostic use compared to serum. Amanitins can be detected in urine well before any clinical sign has developed, whereas routine laboratory tests such as serum chemistry profiles are unremarkable until liver or kidney damage has occurred. Amanitins are excreted in urine for several days (up to 72 hours) post exposure. Because of the short half-life of amanitins in plasma, amanitins are usually only detected for approximately 36 hours post exposure. Plasma and urine amanitin concentrations do not seem to correlate with clinical severity or outcome.
    - Postmortem, kidney contains higher amanitin concentrations than liver and is considered the sample of choice, especially if the animal survived for a longer period of time.

Pathological Findings

- The liver may be swollen and distended. No other significant gross abnormalities may be noticed. Histopathologically, the liver has massive hepatocellular necrosis with collapse of hepatic cords. Acute tubular necrosis is seen in dogs that develop renal failure.

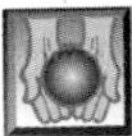

THERAPEUTICS

- No specific therapy has proven to be effective. Even with supportive measures, the mortality rate from amanita poisoning in dogs is high. Amanitin poisoning requires immediate and aggressive treatment to improve prognosis. The key components of therapy are close monitoring, fluid replacement, and supportive care.

Detoxification

- Emesis in animals where exposure occurred less than 2 hours prior to presentation.
- Activated charcoal: multidose activated charcoal at 1–4 g/kg PO q 2–6 hours until 2–3 days post ingestion.

ANTIDOTE

- No specific antidote is available.

Drugs of Choice

- Intravenous fluids – maintain hydration, induce diuresis, correct hypoglycemia.
- 50% dextrose 1 mL/kg IV slow bolus (1–3 min).
- Furosemide 2–4 mg/kg IV q 8–12 hours.
- Vitamin K_1 0.5–1.5 mg/kg SQ or IM q 12 hours; 1–5 mg/kg PO q 24 hours.
- Blood products – dependent on hemostatic test results.
- Silibinin – may be beneficial, but controlled studies are lacking. Experimentally, silibinin was shown to be effective when given twice to dogs at a dose of 50 mg/kg IV, 5 and 24 hours after exposure to *A. phalloides*. An oral form is available that can be given at 2–5 mg/kg PO q 24 hours (silibinin complexed with phosphatidylcholine).
- Penicillin G – reduces the uptake of amanitins into hepatocytes; 1000 mg/kg IV as soon as possible after exposure.

Alternative Drugs

- N-acetylcysteine (NAC) – antioxidant; no data on efficacy in amanitin toxicosis available. This glutathione precursor can be included in the treatment regimen for acute fulminant hepatic failure at 140 mg/kg IV load, followed by 70 mg/kg IV q 6 hours for seven treatments.
- S-adenosylmethionine (SAMe) – antioxidant and hepatoprotectant; no data on efficacy in amanitin toxicosis available. 20 mg/kg PO q 24 hours.
- Ascorbic acid and cimetidine – hepatocyte protectors; no data on efficacy in amanitin toxicosis available. Can be given for supportive therapy.

Precautions/Interactions

- A variety of decontamination procedures are used in humans, including hemodialysis, hemoperfusion, plasmapheresis, forced diuresis, and nasoduodenal suctioning. Controversy remains about the efficacy of these procedures, as specific data do not exist.
- The use of steroids and thioctic acid is no longer recommended in the treatment of amanitin poisoning.

Prevention/Avoidance

- Advise owner to closely scrutinize the environment for mushrooms. Suggest that owner have mushrooms identified by mycology expert and get additional information on the seasonality of amanita mushrooms in their geographic region.

Surgical Considerations

- Biliary drainage through serial gall bladder aspiration or cannula placement has been proposed as a means of removing amatoxins from enterohepatic circulation. Risk for the development of bile peritonitis or other bleeding complications must be considered. A study in pigs found that amatoxins were no longer present in the enterohepatic circulation 24 hours after exposure, suggesting that biliary drainage after such time may be poorly effective as a treatment.

Public Health

- Amanitins are very toxic to humans. Even with supportive measures, the reported mortality rate from amanita poisoning in humans is 20–40%.

COMMENTS

Client Education

- Warn client that temporary improvement can be followed by severe hepatic and renal failure.
- Monitoring in the clinical setting for the first 2–3 days in suspected amanitin exposure.

Patient Monitoring

- Monitor blood glucose, electrolytes, CBC, serum biochemistry, and coagulation parameters at least daily.
- Prevent hypothermia.
- Monitor urine output.

Possible Complications

- DIC
- Hepatic encephalopathy
- Progressive hepatic failure
- Renal failure

Expected Course and Prognosis

- It takes 3–5 days to estimate prognosis.

- Progressive worsening of liver and kidney function and unresponsiveness to supportive treatments are negative indicators.

Synonyms

Amanita toxicosis, death cap intoxication, amatoxin poisoning, hepatotoxic mushroom poisoning, amanitin poisoning

See Also

Acetaminophen
Organophosphorus and Carbamate Insecticides
Sago Palm

Abbreviations

See Appendix 1 for a complete list.

Suggested Reading

Enjalbert F, Rapior S, Nouguier-Soule J, et al. Treatment of amatoxin poisoning: 20-year retrospective analysis. J Toxicol Clin Toxicol 2002; 40:715–757.

Magdalan J, Ostrowska A, Piotrowska A, et al. Failure of benzylpenicillin, N-acetylcysteine and silibinin to reduce alpha-amanitin hepatotoxicity. In Vivo 2009; 23:393–399.

Puschner B. Mushroom toxins. In: Gupta RC, ed. Veterinary Toxicology: Basic and Clinical Principles, 2nd edn. San Diego, CA: Elsevier, 2012; pp. 1140–1151.

Puschner B., Wegenast C. Epidemiology of mushroom poisoning cases in dogs and cats (incidences, respiratory failure, hepatotoxic, nephrotoxic, diagnosis treatment). Vet Clin North Am Small Anim Pract 2012; 42:375–387.

Puschner B, Rose HH, Filigenzi MS. Diagnosis of amanita toxicosis in a dog with acute hepatic necrosis. J Vet Diagn Invest 2007; 19:312–317.

Authors: Adrienne Bautista, DVM, PhD, DABVT; Birgit Puschner, DVM, PhD, DABVT
Consulting Editor: Lynn R. Hovda, RPh, DVM, MS, DACVIM

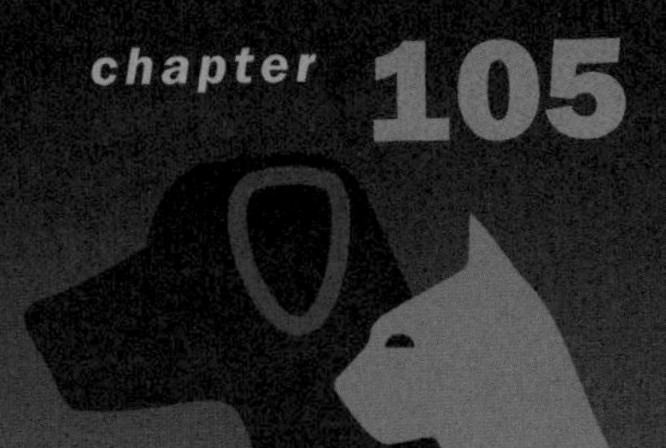

chapter 105

Oxalates – Insoluble

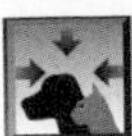

DEFINITION/OVERVIEW

- Insoluble oxalate crystals are found naturally in plants of the Araceae family.
- Roughly 200 species worldwide contain insoluble oxalate crystals.
- *Dieffenbachia* spp. is most commonly associated with problems in animals.
    - Oxalate crystals occur in several layers in leaves and stems.
    - Plants are present in many homes and offices.
- Common names vary tremendously from plant to plant and accurate plant identification must include the scientific name.
- The most commonly reported plants associated with toxicity include the following:
    - Anthurium, flamingo flower (*Anthurium* spp.; Fig. 105.1)
    - Arrowhead vine (*Syngonium* spp.; Fig. 105.2)
    - Calla lily (*Zantedeschia* spp.; Fig. 105.3)
    - Chinese evergreen (*Aglaonema commutatum*; Fig. 105.4)
    - Dumbcane (*Dieffenbachia* spp.; Fig. 105.5)
    - Fruit salad plant (*Monstera deliciosa*; Fig. 105.6)
    - Peace lily (*Spathiphyllum* spp.; Fig. 105.7)
    - Philodendron, sweetheart vine (*Philodendron* spp.; Fig. 105.8)
    - Pothos, hunter's robe, devil's ivy (*Epipremnum* spp.; Fig. 105.9)
    - Umbrella plant (*Schefflera actinophylla*; Fig. 105.10)
    - Upright elephant's ear (*Xanthosoma* spp.; Fig. 105.11)

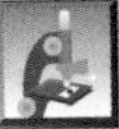

ETIOLOGY/PATHOPHYSIOLOGY

Mechanism of Action

- Insoluble crystals are needle sharp and arranged in bundles called raphides. In many plants, bundles of raphides are organized into specialized cells called idioblasts.

Blackwell's Five-Minute Veterinary Consult Clinical Companion: Small Animal Toxicology, Second Edition.
Lynn R. Hovda, Ahna G. Brutlag, Robert H. Poppenga, and Katherine L. Peterson.

Companion website: www.fiveminutevet.com/toxicology

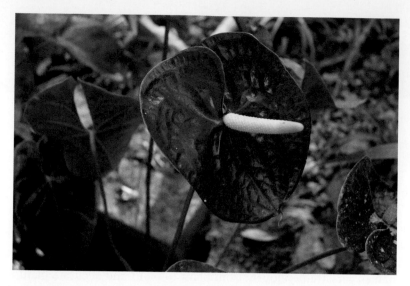

■ **Fig. 105.1.** Anthurium (*Anthurium* spp.). Photo courtesy of Tyne K. Hovda.

- Chewing or biting into plant material rapidly releases the crystals until the idioblast is emptied.
  - The double-edged crystals act much like miniature spears or needles and function primarily as mechanical irritants to the mucous membranes.
  - They also act as chemical irritants, penetrating cells and allowing the entrance of other substances such as prostaglandins, histamine, proteolytic enzymes, or oxalic acid.

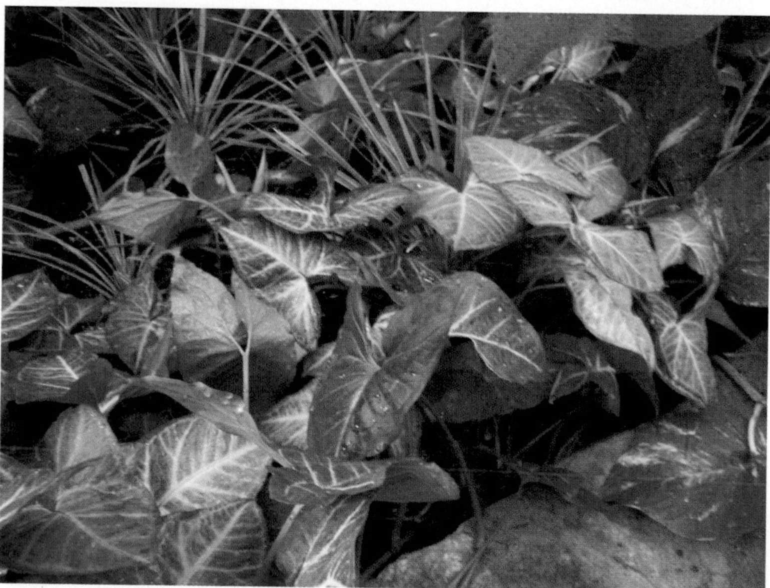

■ **Fig. 105.2.** Arrowhead (*Syngonium* spp.). Photo courtesy of Tyne K. Hovda.

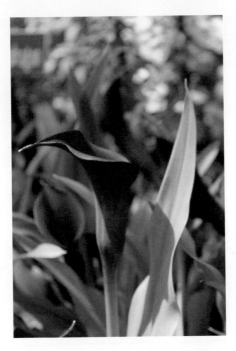

■ **Fig. 105.3.** Calla lily (*Zantedeschia* spp.). Photo courtesy of Tyne K. Hovda.

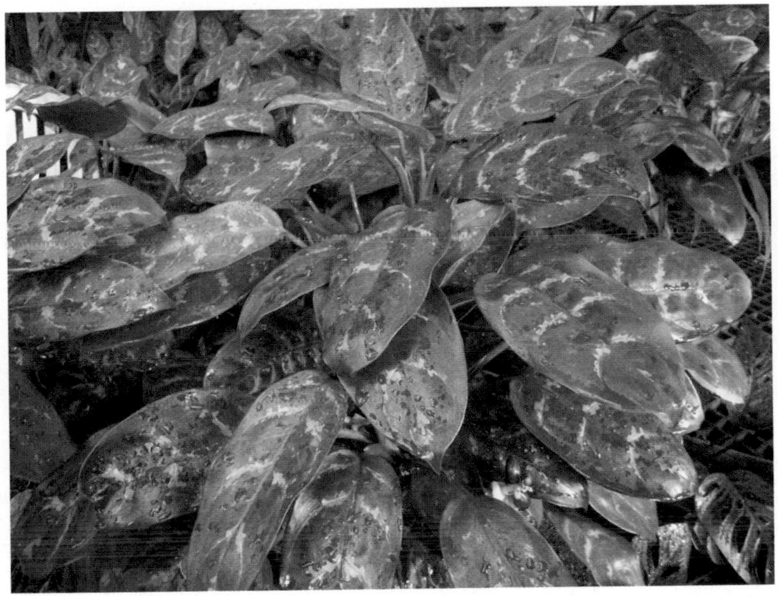

■ **Fig. 105.4.** Chinese evergreen (*Aglaonema commutatum*). Photo courtesy of Tyne K. Hovda.

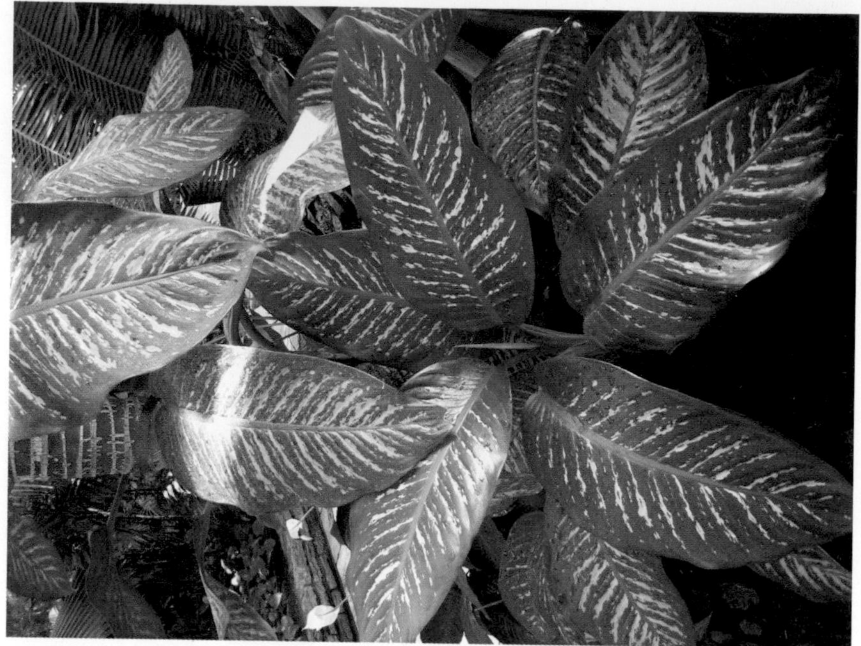

■ **Fig. 105.5.** Dumbcane (*Dieffenbachia* spp.). Photo courtesy of Tyne K. Hovda.

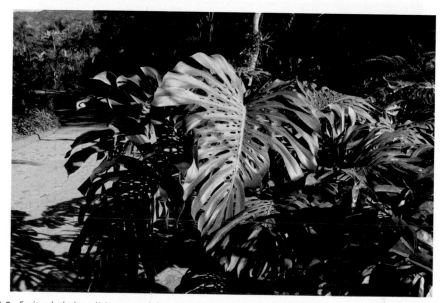

■ **Fig. 105.6.** Fruit salad plant (*Monstera deliciosa*). Photo courtesy Lynn R. Hovda.

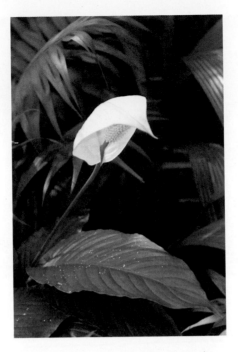

■ **Fig. 105.7.** Peace lily (*Spathiphyllum* spp.). Photo courtesy of Tyne K. Hovda.

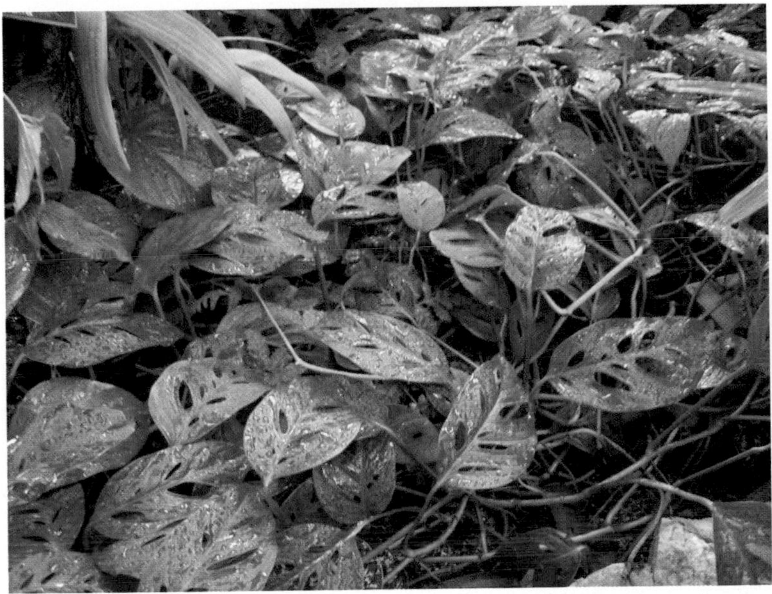

■ **Fig. 105.8.** Philodendron vine (*Philodendron* spp.). Photo courtesy of Tyne K. Hovda.

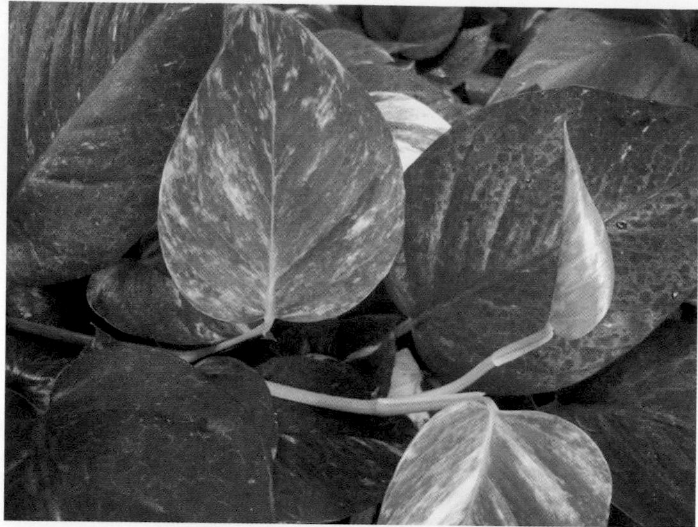

■ **Fig. 105.9.** Golden pothos (*Epipremnum aureum*). Photo courtesy of Tyne K. Hovda.

Pharmacokinetics – Absorption, Distribution, Metabolism, Excretion

- Onset of action is very rapid, occurring within minutes of chewing on the plant.

Toxicity

- Generally are all regarded as mild-to-moderate toxicants.
- Severe cases have occurred and, rarely, death has been reported.

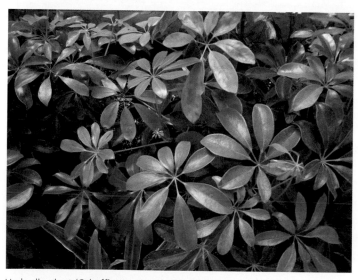

■ **Fig. 105.10.** Umbrella plant (*Schefflera actinophylla*). Photo courtesy of Tyne K. Hovda.

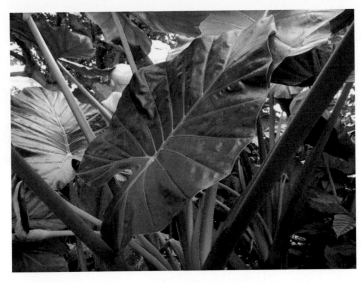

■ **Fig. 105.11.** Upright elephant ear (*Xanthosoma* spp.). Photo courtesy of Tyne K. Hovda.

- *Dieffenbachia* spp. has been associated with more serious outcomes, including death, in dogs and cats.
- Cats ingesting philodendrons may exhibit a wider array of clinical signs.

Systems Affected

- Gastrointestinal – immediate onset of oral pain with vocalization, pawing at the muzzle, and hypersalivation; anorexia and vomiting; and edema of lips, tongue, and/or pharynx.
- Respiratory – rarely dyspnea from inflammation and laryngeal swelling.
- Ophthalmic – plant juices in the eye are associated with severe pain, photophobia, and conjunctival swelling; crystals may be present on the corneal epithelium.

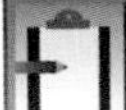

SIGNALMENT/HISTORY

- Indoor dogs and cats are at a higher risk, as most poisonings are associated with houseplants.
  - Dogs tend to chew and destroy the entire plant, often ingesting leaves and stems.
  - Cats are generally fastidious and tend to nibble on the leaves.
- All ages can be affected, although ingestions by younger pets, curious or bored by confinement, tend to occur more often.
- The most common immediate signs are related to the severe pain in the oropharynx and include hypersalivation, head shaking, and pawing at the muzzle area. Signs occurring shortly after exposure include edema of the lips and tongue, vomiting, and anorexia. Airway obstruction and dyspnea are more rare occurrences. Ophthalmic exposure results in severe pain, photophobia, lacrimation, blepharospasm, and swelling of the lids.

Risk Factors

- Presence of plants in animal's environment.
- Boredom, confinement.

CLINICAL FEATURES

- Gastrointestinal – evidence of immediate oral pain (hypersalivation, head shaking, pawing at muzzle) within minutes of exposure; redness or irritation to mucous membranes in oropharynx occurring a short time later; vomiting minutes to hours after exposure.
- Respiratory – dyspnea and airway obstruction if inflammation is severe (rare).
- Ophthalmic – issues only if plant juices have been squirted or rubbed into the eye.

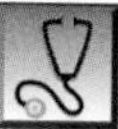

DIFFERENTIAL DIAGNOSIS

- Systemic diseases associated with oral lesions and GI signs.
- Toxicants.
    - Other agents causing oral irritation (capsaicin, topically applied permethrins, detergents).
    - Caustic agents (alkalis, acids in household, and drain cleaners).
    - Plants containing bitter volatile oils.
    - Stinging nettle ingestion.

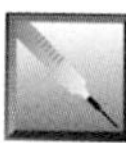

DIAGNOSTICS

- Rarely performed as crystals are insoluble and not absorbed; signs are primarily local in nature and self-limiting.
- Serum electrolytes and chemistry if vomiting persists.

Pathological Findings

- Death rarely occurs, and in the few reported cases, severe and extensive erosive and ulcerative glossitis was present.

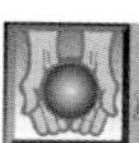

THERAPEUTICS

- Therapy is generally limited and includes appropriate detoxification and supportive care. Many animals respond in 2–4 hours, while some may take 12–24 hours for a complete response.

Detoxification

- Wash the mouth and oral cavity with copious amounts of cool fluids.
- Provide small amounts of milk, yogurt, or other calcium-containing products to bind the oxalate crystals. Give enough to coat the oropharynx but not to cause GI upset and diarrhea.
- If ophthalmic exposure is evident, lavage the eye for 15 minutes and treat as needed.

Appropriate Health Care

- Observe closely for evidence of dyspnea, especially those animals that chewed or ingested large amounts of plants.
- Thorough ophthalmic examination after lavage; fluorescein dye or slit lamp examination.

Antidote

- No specific antidote is available.

Drugs of Choice

- IV fluids if dehydration occurs secondary to hypersalivation and vomiting.
- Antiemetic agents as needed.
  - Dolasetron 0.5–1.0 mg/kg IV q 24 hours.
  - Maropitant 1 mg/kg SQ q 24 hours.
  - Ondansetron 0.1–0.2 mg/kg IV q 8–12 hours.
- GI protectants as needed.
  - H_2 blockers.
    - Famotidine 0.5 mg/kg PO, SQ, IM, IV q 12–24 hours (cautious IV use in cats).
    - Ranitidine 1–2 mg/kg PO, SQ, IM, IV q 8–12 hours.
    - Cimetidine 5–10 mg/kg PO, SQ, IM, IV q 6 hours.
  - Omeprazole 0.5–1 mg/kg daily.
  - Sucralfate 0.25–1 g PO q 8 hours × 5–7 days if evidence of active ulcer disease.
- Nonsteroidal antiinflammatory agents if needed for pain and inflammation.
  - Carprofen.
    - Dogs: 2.2 mg/kg PO q 12–24 hours.
    - Cats: 1–2 mg/kg SQ q 24 hours. Limit dosing to 2 days.
  - Deracoxib 1–2 mg/kg PO q 24 hours (dogs).
  - Robenacoxib 1 mg/kg PO q 24 hours (cats only). Limit to 3 doses.
- Corticosteroid use is controversial, but dexamethasone phosphate 0.125–0.5 mg/kg IV, IM, or SQ may be useful in cases with severe inflammation.

Public Health

- Human beings, especially young children and vulnerable adults, are equally at risk if they chew or ingest plant pieces.

COMMENTS

Expected Course and Prognosis

- Prognosis is excellent as most signs are mild to moderate, have a short duration of action, and require no therapy.

Prevention/Avoidance

- Identify plants presently in the household and place them far out of the animal's reach.
- Learn the scientific names of poisonous plants and keep them out of the household.

Abbreviations

See Appendix 1 for a complete list.

Suggested Reading

Botha CJ, Penrith M. Potential plant poisonings in dogs and cats in southern Africa: review article. J S Afr Vet Assoc 2009; 80(2):63–74.

Burrows GE, Tyrl RJ. Toxic Plants of North America, 2nd edn. Ames, IA: Wiley–Blackwell, 2012; pp. 131–145.

Ellis W, Barfort T, Mastman GJ. Keratoconjunctivitis with corneal crystals caused by Dieffenbachia plant. Am J Ophthalmol 1973; 76:143–146.

Knight AP. A Guide to Poisonous House and Garden Plants. Jackson Hole, WY: Teton NewMedia, 2006; pp. 203–204.

Peterson K, Beymer J, Rudloff E, et al. Airway obstruction in a dog after Dieffenbachia ingestion. J Vet Emerg Crit Care 2009; 19(6):635–639.

Severino L. Toxic plants and companion animals. CAB Rev 2009, 4: 1–6. Available at: www.researchgate.net/publication/248908982_Toxic_plants_and_companion_animals

Acknowledgment: The authors and editors acknowledge the prior contributions of Erica Cargill, CVT, who co-authored this topic in the previous edition.

Author: Lynn R. Hovda, RPh, DVM, MS, ACVIM

Consulting Editor: Lynn R. Hovda, RPh, DVM, MS, AVCIM

chapter 106

Oxalates – Soluble

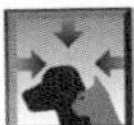

DEFINITION/OVERVIEW

Oxalate toxicity includes both oxalic acid and oxalate salts.

- Oxalic acid is a dicarboxylic acid found naturally in plants of the Araceae, Oxalidaceae, Liliaceae, Polygonaceae, Chenopodiaceae, and Amaranthus families.
- Soluble salts (ammonium, calcium, potassium, sodium) of oxalic acid are also found in a number of plants in these families.

- Most of these plants are weeds growing in pastures and are only associated with problems in livestock grazing on them. A few have been cultivated as houseplants and if ingested in large enough quantities, are a potential source of poisoning to dogs and cats.
- Common household plants with soluble oxalates include the following:
  - Common or garden rhubarb (*Rheum rhabarbarum*; Fig. 106.1)

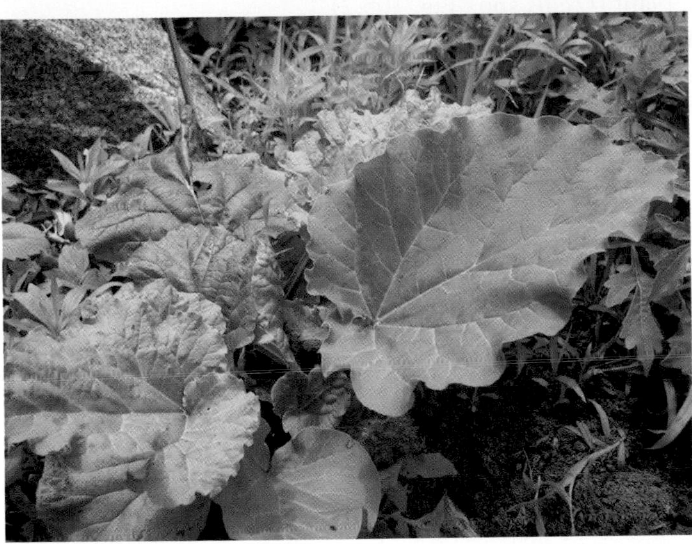

■ **Fig. 106.1.** Rhubarb (*Rheum rhabarbarum*). Photo courtesy of Tyne K. Hovda.

Blackwell's Five-Minute Veterinary Consult Clinical Companion: Small Animal Toxicology, Second Edition.
Lynn R. Hovda, Ahna G. Brutlag, Robert H. Poppenga, and Katherine L. Peterson.

Companion website: www.fiveminutevet.com/toxicology

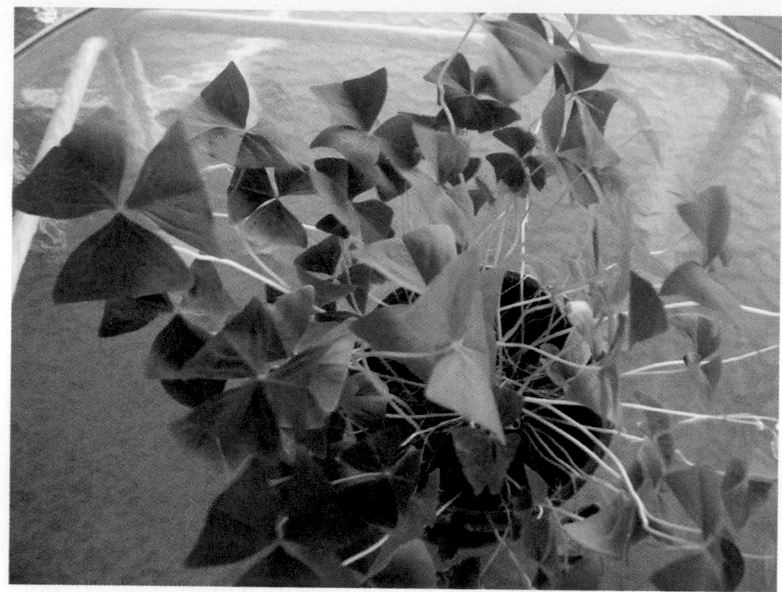

■ **Fig. 106.2.** Shamrock (*Oxalis* spp.). Photo courtesy of Tyne K. Hovda.

- Shamrock plant (*Oxalis* spp.; Fig. 106.2)
- Purple shamrock plant (*Oxalis* spp.; Fig. 106.3)
- Star fruit – esp. sour variety (*Averrhoa carambola*; Figs 106.4 and 106.5)
- Hybrid plants, *Oxalis* spp.

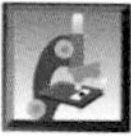

ETIOLOGY/PATHOPHYSIOLOGY

Mechanism of Action

- Soluble oxalates and free oxalic acid are present to varying degrees in all parts of the plant. Total oxalate material in many of the pasture plants is about 16%, with 7–10% of this in the form of an oxalate salt.
- Rhubarb stems are edible, the leaves are not.
- Star fruit presents an interesting dilemma, with soluble oxalates found in much greater concentrations in the sour fruit versus sweet fruit.
  - The sour fruit is generally recognized as inedible, the sweet fruit and juices as edible.
  - Additional mechanisms may contribute to onset of acute renal injury.
- Ingestion of plants results in both free oxalic acid and soluble salts.
- Soluble oxalate salts are absorbed through the GI tract and bind with systemic calcium, resulting in a sudden drop in serum calcium. The accumulation of calcium oxalate crystals causes nephrosis and renal failure.
- Free oxalic acid may be responsible for GI irritation.

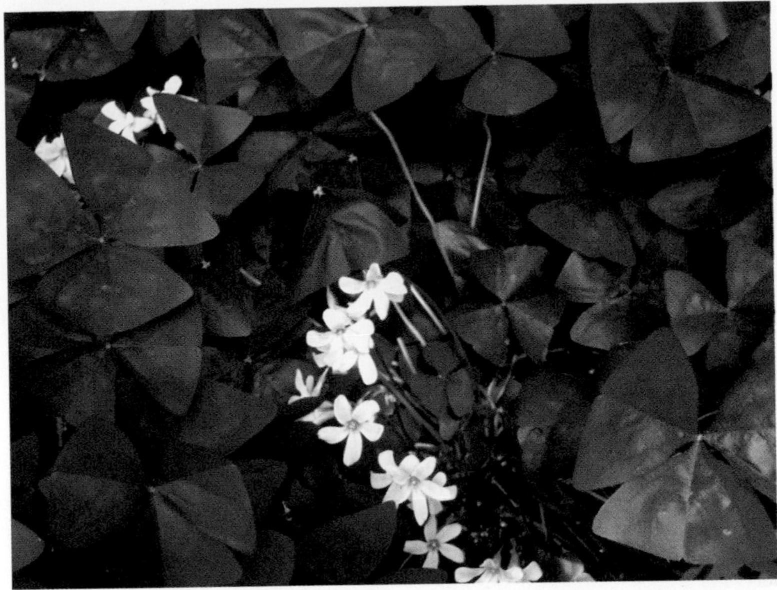

■ **Fig. 106.3.** Purple shamrock (*Oxalis* spp.). Photo courtesy of Lynn R. Hovda.

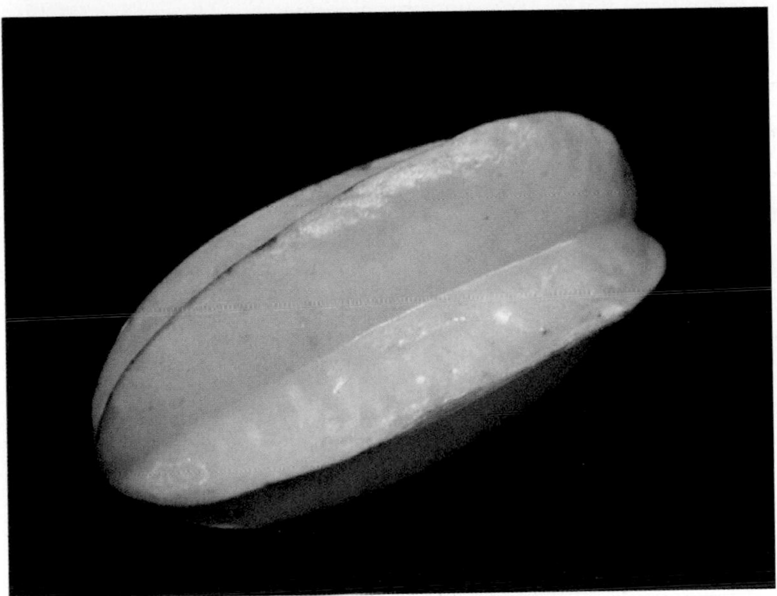

■ **Fig. 106.4.** Star fruit intact (*Averrhoa carambola*). Photo courtesy of Tyne K. Hovda.

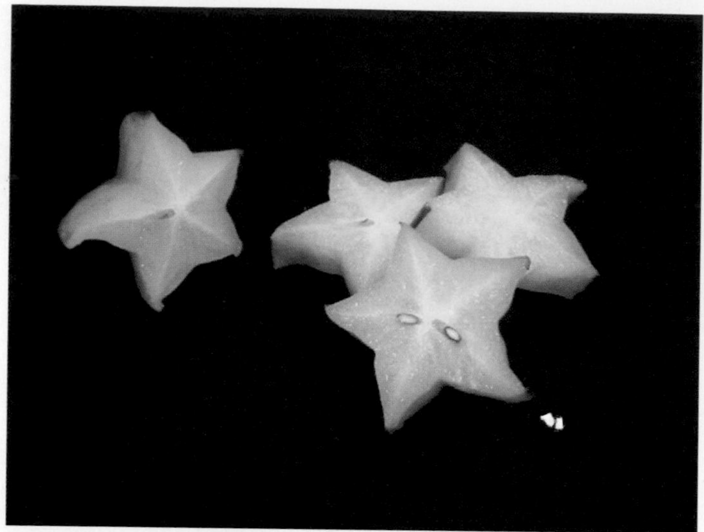

■ **Fig. 106.5.** Star fruit cut sections (*Averrhoa carambola*). Photo courtesy of Tyne K. Hovda.

Pharmacokinetics – Absorption, Distribution, Metabolism, Excretion

- Little is known about the toxicokinetics in animals.

Toxicity

- Unlikely to be an issue unless large amounts are ingested. The sap is very bitter tasting and this may limit absorption in most animals.
- Stems or stalks of rhubarb are edible; leaves are not.
- Star fruit and star fruit juices are usually only a problem when ingested and absorbed in large quantities or in the presence of dehydration or underlying renal disease.

Systems Affected

- Gastrointestinal – GI irritation with vomiting (with or without blood) and diarrhea (with or without blood).
- Renal/urological – renal failure from formation of calcium oxalate crystals.
- Neuromuscular – signs associated with hypocalcemia.
- Musculoskeletal – tetany secondary to hypocalcemia.

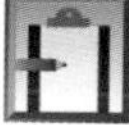

SIGNALMENT/HISTORY

- All small animals, indoors and out, are susceptible to toxicity.

Risk Factors

- Preexisting GI or chronic renal disease.
- Boredom in confined animal.

Historical Findings

- Confirmation of chewed-up plant in animal's environment.
- Leaves from rhubarb plants that have not been adequately disposed of and are ingested.
- Ingestion of a large number of star fruits or large volumes of juices.

CLINICAL FEATURES

- Hypersalivation and anorexia are the earliest signs, followed by vomiting with or without blood and diarrhea with or without blood.
- Depression, weakness, tremors, tetany, and coma follow if the ingestion is large enough to result in systemic hypocalcemia.
- Acute renal failure secondary to calcium oxalate crystal formation results in polydypsia, polyuria, or oliguria with oxaluria, hematuria, and albuminuria. Signs develop at 24–36 hours post ingestion.

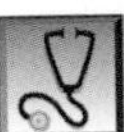

DIFFERENTIAL DIAGNOSIS

- Diabetes mellitus (ketoacidosis or hypoglycemic shock).
- Toxicants.
  - Calcipotriene (Dovonex®).
  - Cholecalciferol rodenticides.
  - Ethylene glycol.
  - Other plant ingestions, including lilies in cats.
- Underlying diseases such as acute renal failure, pancreatitis, or diabetes mellitus.
- Viral or bacterial gastroenteritis (garbage can toxicosis).

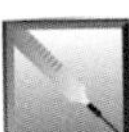

DIAGNOSTICS

- Serum chemistry with early attention to calcium, magnesium, BUN, and creatinine.
- Urinalysis initially may be normal but later will show crystaluria (oxaluria), hematuria, and albuminuria.

Pathological Findings

- Gross pathology yields only renal lesions (swollen and edematous kidneys) and systemic congestion. Histopathological lesions include moderate-to-severe, diffuse acute renal tubular necrosis.

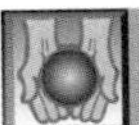

THERAPEUTICS

Detoxification

- Emesis early after ingestion.
- Activated charcoal with cathartic × 1 dose.

Appropriate Health Care

- In severe cases with systemic hypocalcemia and oxaluria, aggressive IV fluid therapy for a minimum of 48 hours to preserve renal function.
- Monitor serum calcium and electrolytes, BUN, and creatinine daily until they have returned to normal limits.

Antidotes

- No true specific antidote, although some may consider the administration of IV calcium an antidote.

Drugs of Choice

- Hypocalcemia.
  - 10% calcium gluconate IV at 5–15 mg/kg (0.5–1.5 mL/kg) over 20–30 minutes.
  - Stop if bradycardia or arrhythmias develop; once CV system is stable, reinstitute at a slower rate.
- Vigorous IV fluid therapy at 2–3X maintenance and adjust as needed for dehydration, electrolyte changes, and urine output. SQ fluids will not be effective in preventing renal damage if oxaluria is present.
- Monitor urine output for development of oliguria (0.5 mL/kg/hour of urine) or anuria (<0.5 mL/kg/hour of urine). If decreased urinary output, consider individually or in combination.
  - Furosemide 2–4 mg/kg IV intermittent boluses in both dogs and cats.
  - Dopamine 2–5 μg/kg/min IV.
  - Mannitol 0.25–1 gram/kg IV over 10–40 minutes.
- Antiemetics if vomiting is severe or persists.
  - Dolasetron 0.5–1 mg/kg IV q 24 hours.
  - Maropitant 1 mg/kg SQ q 24 hours.
  - Ondansetron 0.1–0.2 mg/kg IV q 8–12 hours.
- GI protectants as needed.
  - H_2 blockers.
    - Famotidine 0.5–1 mg/kg PO, SQ, IM, IV q 12 hours (cautious IV use in cats).
    - Ranitidine 1–2 mg/kg PO, SQ, IM, IV q 8–12 hours.
    - Cimetidine 5–10 mg/kg PO, SQ, IM, IV q 6 hours.
  - Omeprazole 0.5–1 mg/kg daily PO.
  - Sucralfate 0.25–1 g PO q 8 hours × 5–7 days if evidence of active ulcer disease.
- Nonsteroidal antiinflammatory agents or other analgesics for pain.
  - Carprofen.
    - Dogs: 2.2 mg/kg PO q 12–24 hours.
    - Cats: 1–2 mg/kg SQ q 24 hours. Limit dosing to 2 days.
  - Deracoxib 1–2 mg/kg PO q 24 hours (dogs).
  - Robenacoxib 1 mg/kg PO q 24 hours (cats). Limit dosing to 3 days.

COMMENTS

Prevention/Avoidance

- Keep these and other toxic plants out of the reach of animals.
- Properly dispose of rhubarb leaves after picking the stems.

Possible Complications

- Chronic renal disease.

Expected Course and Prognosis

- In general, few problems other than GI irritation occur with ingestion of these plants by healthy animals, and the prognosis for recovery is excellent.
- Rarely, systemic hypocalcemia with secondary renal disease develops. If treated early, the prognosis is very good for a full recovery. The prognosis decreases considerably for those animals treated after acute renal disease has occurred.

See Also

Ethylene Glycol and Diethylene Glycol

Abbreviations

See Appendix 1 for a complete list.

Suggested Reading

Burrows GE, Tyrl RJ. Toxic Plants of North America, 2nd edn. Ames, IA: Wiley–Blackwell, 2012; pp. 131–145.

Chen CL, Fang HC, Chou KJ. Acute oxalate nephropathy after ingestion of a star fruit. Am J Kidney Disease 2001; 37:418–422.

Fang HC, Lee PT, Lu PJ, et al. Mechanisms of star fruit-induced acute renal failure. Food Chem Toxicol 2008; 46(5):1744–1752.

Knight AP. A Guide to Poisonous House and Garden Plants. Jackson Hole, WY: Teton NewMedia, 2006; pp. 203–204.

Nakata PA. Plant calcium oxalate crystal formation, function, and its impact on human health. Front Biol 2012; 7(3):254–266.

Acknowledgment: The authors and editors acknowledge the prior contributions of Erica Cargill, CVT, who co-authored this topic in the previous edition.

Authors: Lynn R. Hovda, RPh, DVM, MS, DACVIM

Consulting Editors: Lynn R. Hovda, RPh, DVM, MS, DACVIM

chapter 107

Sago Palm (Cycads)

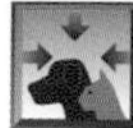

DEFINITION/OVERVIEW

- Toxicosis is caused by ingestion of any part of the sago palm plant (Figs 107.1 and 107.2).
- Cycads is a general term encompassing those plants found in the class Cycadopsia, order Cycadales, families Cycadaceae and Zamiaceae.
    - Cycadaceae has one genus (*Cycas*).
    - Zamiaceae has nine genera with *Zamia* and *Macrozamia* the most well-known.

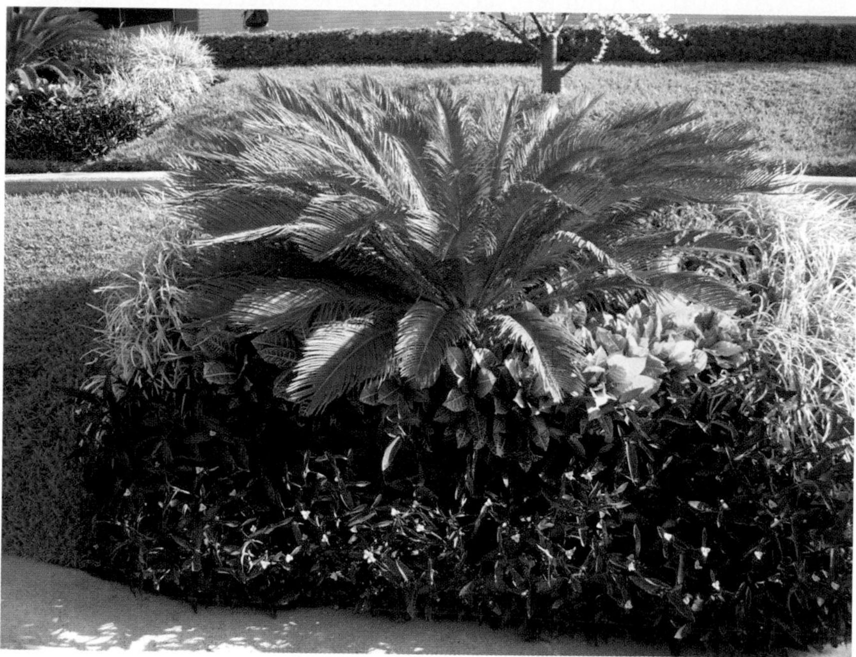

Fig. 107.1. Sago palm (*Cycas* spp.). Photo courtesy of Lynn R. Hovda.

Blackwell's Five-Minute Veterinary Consult Clinical Companion: Small Animal Toxicology, Second Edition.
Lynn R. Hovda, Ahna G. Brutlag, Robert H. Poppenga, and Katherine L. Peterson.

Companion website: www.fiveminutevet.com/toxicology

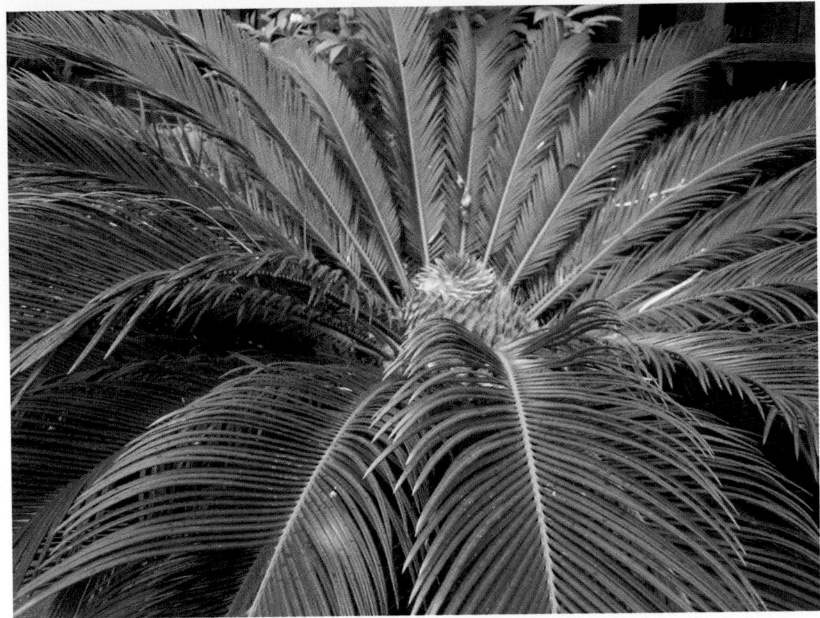

■ **Fig. 107.2.** Cone or flower found at center of sago palm (*Cycas* spp.). Photo courtesy of Lynn R. Hovda.

- *Cycas revulota*, the best known of the many Cycas species, is commonly referred to as the sago palm.
    - Poisoning from members of the Zamiaceae family has been reported in several animal species, including dogs.
- The sago palm is not really a palm. It belongs to a group of plants that date back to the dinosaur era and are often referred to as "living fossils."
- All parts of the plant are toxic; the seeds (nuts) found in the center of the plant are the most toxic part of the plant as they contain the highest amounts of cycasin, the principal toxin (see Fig. 107.2).
- Target species is the dog.
- Target organ is the liver. The most common response to exposure is an early onset of vomiting followed by severe, acute liver failure.
- Hepatic injury is dose dependent and depends not only on what part of the plant but how much has been ingested.

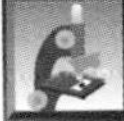

ETIOLOGY/PATHOPHYSIOLOGY

- The incidence of sago palm toxicosis is most common in the southern United States and Hawaii due to the geographic location of the plant.
- Toxicosis is becoming more common in colder climates where sago palms are kept as household "container" plants.
- Other "cycads" including *Zamia* spp. and *Macrozamia spp.* cause similar poisonings.

Mechanism of Action

- Three types of toxins are present.
    - Azoxyglycosides – cycasin, macrozamin, neocycasin.
        - Methylazoxymethanol (MAM is the toxic metabolite).
        - Produce GI signs, hepatotoxicity, and carcinogenicity.
    - β-Methylamino-l-alanine (BMAA). May be responsible for neurological signs.
    - Unidentified high molecular weight compound. May be responsible for neurological signs.

Pharmacokinetics – Absorption, Distribution, Metabolism, Excretion

- Toxins are ingested orally and MAM cleaved from them by β-glucosidase, an enzyme present in the gastrointestinal tract.
- MAM is absorbed by the portal vein, oxidized by cytochrome P450, undergoes glucuronidation, and excreted in the bile.
- Once in feces, MAM is cleaved again and undergoes enterohepatic recirculation, increasing the toxicity.

Toxicity

- All parts of the plant are poisonous, but the seeds contain the highest concentration of toxins. Ingestion of 1–2 seeds has resulted in toxicosis and death.

Systems Affected

- Gastrointestinal – vomiting (+/-blood), hypersalivation, anorexia, and diarrhea (+/- blood) occur early (15 minutes to several hours).
- Hepatobiliary – acute, severe hepatic necrosis develops in 2–3 days.
- Nervous – lethargy, weakness, ataxia, tremors, seizures or coma may occur early or with the onset of hepatic disease.

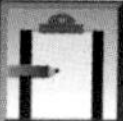

SIGNALMENT/HISTORY

- Dogs are the species known to be affected by this toxicity.
- No breed or sex predilection.
- Ages reported to be affected range from 8 weeks to 11 years, although any age can be affected if the plant is ingested.
- Highest case presentation occurs in southeastern USA from March through August and correlates with outdoor activities and highest seed availability.

Risk Factors

- Environmental exposure to sago palm trees or plants.
- Animals with known or underlying hepatic injury and neurological disease are at the highest risk.

Historical Findings

- History of ingesting sago palm plant or seeds followed by vomiting.

Location and Circumstances of Poisoning

- Most cases occur in the southern United States and Hawaii due to the sandy soil and natural geographic location of the plant.
- Toxicosis is becoming more common in other locales it can now be found as a dwarf or bonsai ornamental houseplant or sold as a seasonal, outdoor plant.

CLINICAL FEATURES

- Clinical signs develop in 15 minutes to 3 days and the duration ranges from 24 hours to 9 days. Gastrointestinal signs occur first, followed by hepatic enzyme changes (2–3 days). In a retrospective study, 95% developed GI signs and 53% developed nervous system signs.
- Vomiting with or without blood is the most common sign followed by lethargy, anorexia, and diarrhea.
- Icterus occurs as the liver enzymes rise.

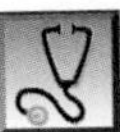

DIFFERENTIAL DIAGNOSIS

- Any toxin or disease process that would cause vomiting and acute hepatic failure.
- Common toxicants.
  - Acetaminophen
  - Amanita mushrooms
  - Blue-green algae
  - Iron
  - Nonsteroidal antiinflammatory drugs
  - Xylitol
- Disease processes.
  - Chronic hepatic necrosis/fibrosis
  - Leptospirosis
  - Septicemia
  - Severe pancreatitis

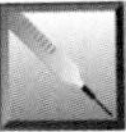

DIAGNOSTICS

- Abdominal/hepatic ultrasound is usually normal shortly after ingestion, but by 24–72 hours may show ascites and evidence of severe liver damage.
- Serum chemistry abnormalities primarily indicate liver damage.
  - Liver enzyme elevations can be very large.

    - Increased ALT; may be well into thousands.
    - Increased AST.
    - Increased ALP.
    - Increased conjugated bilirubin.
    - Increased bile acids.
  - Hypoalbuminemia, hypocholesterolemia.
  - Hypoglycemia or hyperglycemia.
  - Azotemia – increases in BUN and creatinine.
  - Electrolyte abnormalities.
- Complete blood count.
  - Leukocytosis (generally neutrophilia).
  - Neutropenia rarely occurs.
  - Increased hematocrit and decreased total protein.
  - Anemia if blood loss severe.
- Coagulation abnormalities.
  - Thrombocytopenia.
  - Increased PTT.
  - Increased PT.
  - Increased ACT.
- Urinalysis.
  - Bilirubinuria.
  - Hematuria.
  - Glucosuria.

Pathological Findings

- Gross findings include icterus, petechial and ecchymotic hemorrhages, dark, tarry ingesta in the stomach, and evidence of liver damage.
- Histopathological findings include cirrhosis with focal centrilobular and midzonal necrosis and evidence of generalized hemorrhagic disease.

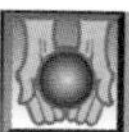

THERAPEUTICS

- The primary objectives of treatment are to prevent further toxin absorption, provide supportive care, and correct clotting abnormalities.

Detoxification

- Induce emesis if within several hours of ingestion. Later emesis may be effective, especially if seeds have been ingested as they may still be in the stomach.
- If emesis is ineffective, consider gastric lavage.
- Activated charcoal with a cathartic once, then administer activated charcoal every 6–8 hours for two additional doses.

Appropriate Health Care

- Monitor closely for signs of liver or renal failure and abnormal bleeding.
- Repeat serum chemistries daily until stabilized.
- Hepatoprotectants may need to be administered for a minimum of 4–6 weeks; some dogs may require them for the remainder of their lives.

Antidote

- There is no antidote.

Drugs of Choice

- Aggressive IV fluid therapy with frequent monitoring of plasma proteins.
  - Nonlactate crystalloids – supply dextrose and B vitamins in addition to maintaining hydration.
  - Colloids if hypoproteinemic.
  - Fresh or frozen plasma if coagulation abnormalities.
- Seizure control.
  - Diazepam 0.25–0.5 mg/kg IV PRN.
  - Phenobarbital 3–5 mg/kg IV PRN.
- Antiemetics to prevent vomiting.
  - Maropitant 1 mg/kg SQ every 24 hours.
  - Ondansetron 0.1–0.2 mg/kg IV q 8–12 hours.
- GI protectants.
  - H_2 blockers.
    - Famotidine 0.5 mg/kg PO, SQ, IM, IV q 12–24 hours.
    - Ranitidine 1–2 mg/kg PO, SQ, IM, IV q 8–12 hours.
  - Omeprazole 0.5–1 mg/kg daily.
  - Sucralfate 0.25–1 g PO q 8–12 hours.
- Vitamin K_1 2–5 mg/kg PO q 24 hours or divided q 12 hours for coagulopathies.
- Blood transfusion for cases of severe hemorrhage.
- Hepatoprotectants.
  - SAMe 20 mg/kg/day PO for 2–4 weeks.
  - Silymarin (milk thistle) 20–50 mg/kg/day PO.
  - Vitamin E 100–400 IU q 12 hours PO.
- Broad-spectrum antibiotics for acute liver failure.
  - Clavulanic acid/amoxicillin 13.75 mg/kg PO q 12 hours.
  - Amoxicillin 22 mg/kg PO, SQ, IM q 12 hours.
  - Ampicillin 15–25 mg/kg PO, IV with metronidazole 7.5 mg/kg PO q 12 hours.

Precautions and Interactions

- Cimetidine should be avoided as it inhibits cytochrome P450 oxidation in the liver.

Alternative Drugs

- N-acetylcysteine (anecdotal use): loading dose of 140 mg/kg IV or PO followed by 70 mg/kg q 6 hours IV or PO for 7–17 doses.

Diet

- Oral intake should be avoided until vomiting is controlled, after which a low-protein diet should be fed.

COMMENTS

Client Education

- Educate the client on the serious consequences associated with ingestion of sago palm plant pieces and seeds.

Patient Monitoring

- Liver enzymes should be monitored at 24, 48, and 72 hours post exposure. If no elevations have occurred by 48–72 hours, the animal is unlikely to develop further problems.
- Symptomatic animals should have liver enzymes monitored until clinical signs have resolved, and then every 1–2 weeks until they normalize.

Prevention/Avoidance

- Remove sago palm plants from the environment or restrict the dog's access to them.

Possible Complications

- Severe chronic active hepatitis
- Permanent hepatic dysfunction
- Hepatic fibrosis

Expected Course and Prognosis

- Varies depending on the use of early and aggressive therapy and the quantity and part of the plant material ingested.
- Prognosis is generally fair with immediate decontamination prior to clinical signs and aggressive therapy.
- Prognosis becomes guarded once clinical signs develop (mortality up to 50%).
- The reported recovery rate after treatment is approximately 33–50%. Most animals will survive with supportive care, but require prolonged hepatic support.
- Long-term survival may be poor. Death may occur in recovered animals 8–12 weeks after initial exposure due to neuronal DNA damage.

Synonyms

Cootie palm, King palm

See Also

Acetaminophen
Mushrooms
Xylitol

Abbreviations

See Appendix 1 for a complete list.

Suggested Reading

Albretsen JC, Khan SA, Richardson JA. Cycad palm toxicosis in dogs: 60 cases (1987–1997). J Am Vet Med Assoc 1998; 213(1):99–101.

Fatourechi L, Del Giudice LA, Sookhoo N. Sago Palm toxicosis in dogs. Compendium 2013; 35(4):E1–E8.

Ferguson D, Crowe M, McLaughlin L, et al. Survival and prognostic indicators for cycad intoxication in dogs. J Vet Intern Med 2011; 25(4)831–837.

McLean MK, Hansen SR. An overview of trends in animal poisoning cases in the United States: 2002–2010. Vet Clin North Am Small Anim Pract 2012; 42(2):219–228.

Mills JN, Lawley MJ, Thomas J. Macrozamia toxicosis in a dog. Aust Vet J 1996; 73(2):69–72.

Youssef H. Cycad toxicity in dogs. Vet Med 2008; 103(5):242–244.

Acknowledgment: The authors and editors acknowledge the prior contributions of Christy A. Klatt, DVM, who authored this topic in the previous edition.
Author: Jean Ihnen, DVM
Consulting Editor: Lynn R. Hovda, RPh, DVM, MS, DACVIM

chapter 108

Spring Bulbs

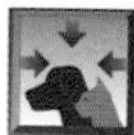

DEFINITION/OVERVIEW

- Poisoning is associated with exposure to many plants belonging to several genera including *Crocus*, *Hippeastrum*, *Hyacinthus*, *Narcissus*, and *Tulipa*.
- Gastrointestinal (GI) signs predominate but cardiovascular (CV), respiratory, and neurological signs may also occur, depending on the amount and genus ingested.
- In much of the US, bulbs are generally planted in the fall with blooms occurring in the spring, although many varieties are shipped and planted in spring with equal success. In growing zones in the southern US, bulbs may be shipped and planted at virtually any time of the year.
- May be found in gardens, as potted houseplants, or in cut flower arrangements (Fig. 108.1).

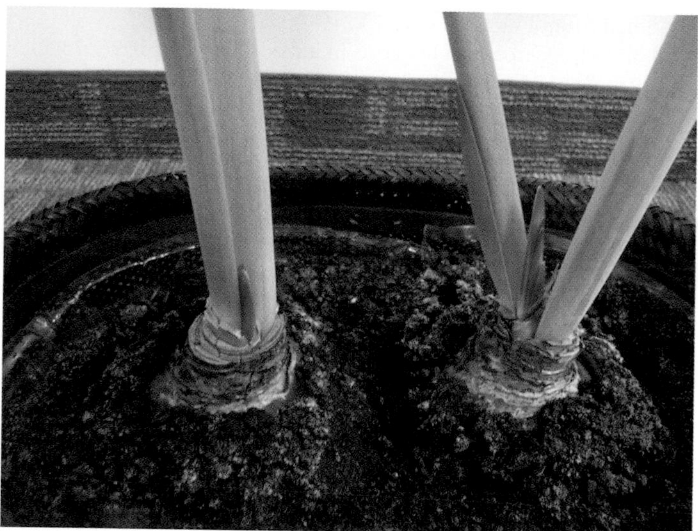

Fig. 108.1. Spring bulb growing as potted indoor plant. Photo courtesy of Lynn R. Hovda.

Blackwell's Five-Minute Veterinary Consult Clinical Companion: Small Animal Toxicology, Second Edition.
Lynn R. Hovda, Ahna G. Brutlag, Robert H. Poppenga, and Katherine L. Peterson.

Companion website: www.fiveminutevet.com/toxicology

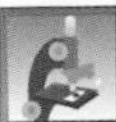

ETIOLOGY/PATHOPHYSIOLOGY

- Ingestion of plant material (leaves, stems, flowers, and bulbs).
- Includes *Crocus* spp. (spring-blooming crocus; Figs 108.2 and 108.3), *Hippeastrum* spp. (amaryllis; Fig. 108.4), *Hyacinthus* spp. (hyacinth; Fig. 108.5), *Narcissus* spp. (daffodil, jonquil, narcissus, paperwhite; Fig. 108.6), and *Tulipa* spp. (tulip; Fig. 108.7).

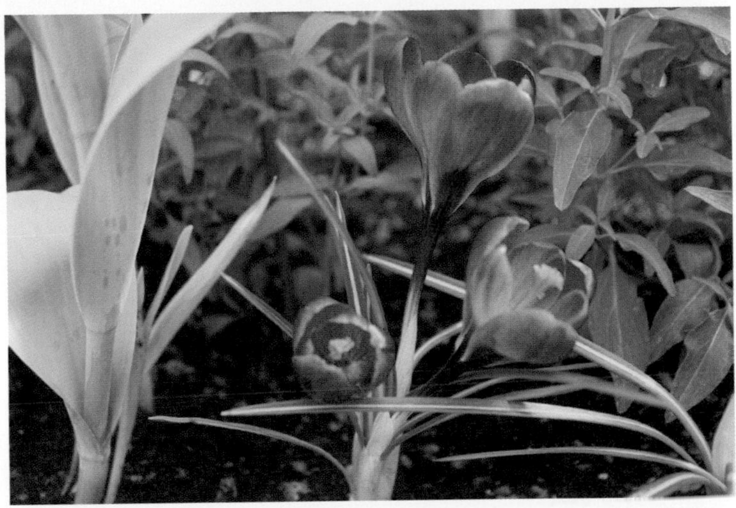

Fig. 108.2. Spring-flowering crocus (*Crocus* spp.). Photo courtesy of Catherine Adams.

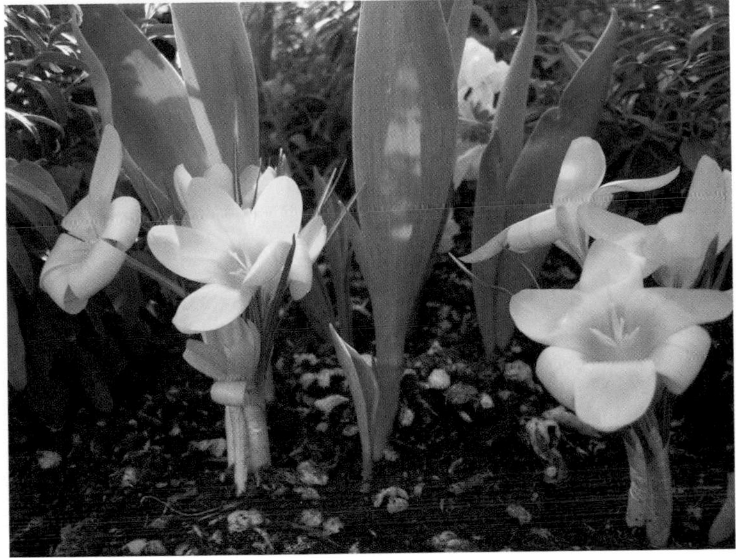

Fig. 108.3. Spring-flowering crocus close-up. Photo courtesy of Ahna Brutlag.

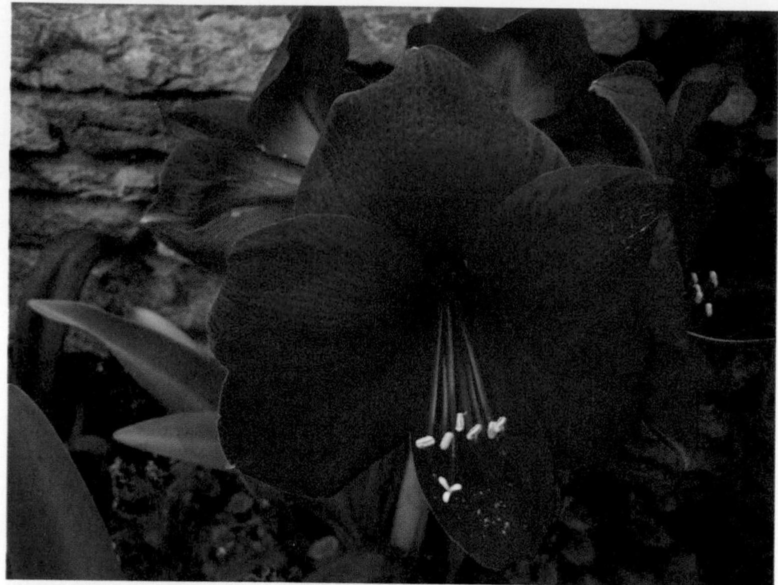

■ **Fig. 108.4.** Amaryllis (*Hippeastrum* spp.). Photo courtesy of Lynn R. Hovda.

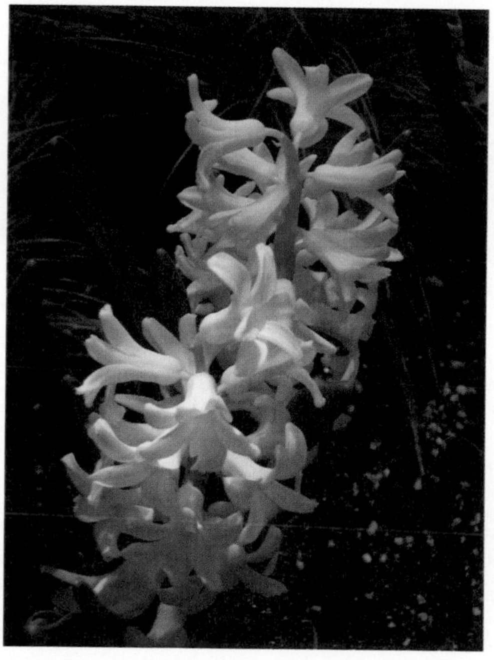

■ **Fig. 108.5** Hyacinth (*Hyacinthus* spp.). Photo courtesy of Tyne K. Hovda.

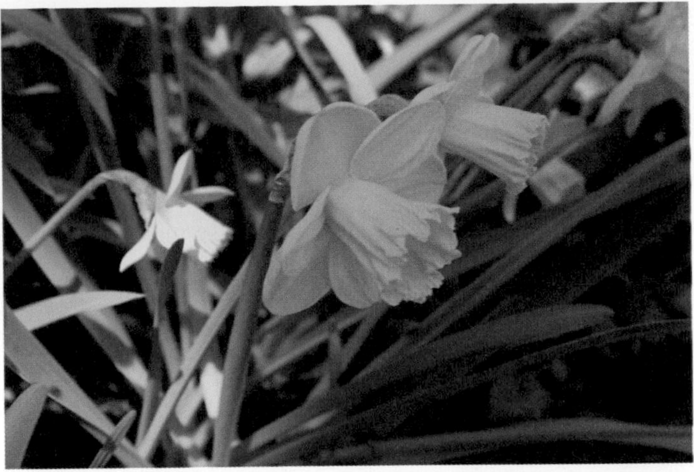

■ **Fig. 108.6.** Daffodils (*Narcissus* spp.). Photo courtesy of Lynn R. Hovda.

Mechanism of Action

- *Crocus* spp. – GI irritation (not to be confused with autumn-blooming crocus or *Colchicum* spp. which contains colchicine).
- *Hippeastrum* spp. and *Narcissus* spp. – Phenanthridine alkaloids (most commonly lycorine) lead to GI signs, hypotension, arrhythmias, and rarely CNS signs; calcium oxalate raphides (needle-like crystals) lead to oral and GI irritation, possible contact dermatitis and dyspnea.
- *Hyacinthus* spp. – GI irritation and possible contact dermatitis due to calcium oxalate raphides and unknown compounds.
- *Tulipa* spp. – Irritant and allergenic lactones tuliposides A and B along with calcium oxalate raphides cause GI signs and possible contact dermatitis, dyspnea, and tachycardia.

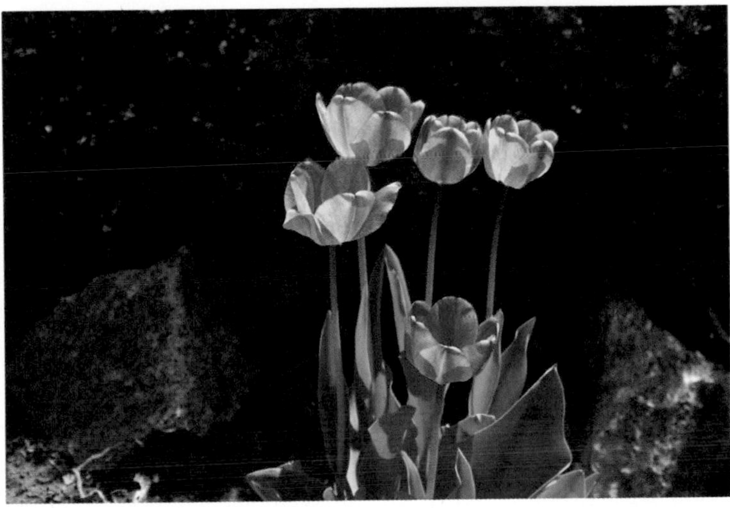

■ **Fig. 108.7.** Tulips (*Tulipa* spp.). Photo courtesy of Lynn R. Hovda.

Pharmacokinetics – Absorption, Distribution, Metabolism, Excretion

- Onset of signs is typically rapid, occurring within minutes of ingestion; rarely delayed up to 24 hours.

Toxicity

- Ingestion of small amounts of plant material tends to cause mild signs; ingestion of large amounts of foliage and/or bulbs may cause moderate-to-severe signs.
- Toxins tend to occur in higher concentrations in the bulbs.
- Exposure to plants in the *Narcissus* spp. has been associated with more serious outcomes. Deaths have been reported but are considered rare.

Systems Affected

- Gastrointestinal – hypersalivation, vomiting, diarrhea, abdominal pain, oral irritation, anorexia.
- Cardiovascular – hypotension, arrhythmias.
- Nervous – ataxia, depression, tremors, seizures (rare).
- Respiratory – dyspnea rarely occurs secondary to oropharyngeal swelling.
- Skin – contact dermatitis and erythema may occur but this is more common in humans.

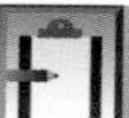

SIGNALMENT/HISTORY

- Dogs and cats are at risk for toxicosis if plant material is ingested.
- Dogs tend to ingest larger amounts of foliage and/or bulbs than cats and are at higher risk for moderate-to-severe clinical signs.

Risk Factors

- Presence of plants in the animal's environment (either indoor or outdoor).
- Boredom, curiosity.

Historical Findings

- Observations and signs often reported by the owner.
  - Ingestion may or may not be witnessed by the owner but damage to plants, missing, or dug-up bulbs may be noted.
  - Initial reported signs tend to be GI in nature with possible progression to weakness, dyspnea, and CNS signs in severe cases.

Location and Circumstances of Poisoning

- Indoors – ingestion of leaves and flowers from potted plants, bouquets, or floral arrangements.
- Outdoors – ingestion of plants present in gardens or bulbs freshly planted or left unattended.

CLINICAL FEATURES

- Signs may be noted within minutes of exposure but rarely may be delayed up to 24 hours.
- Gastrointestinal – evidence of oral irritation or pain (hypersalivation, pawing at the mouth, head shaking) within minutes; redness or irritation to the mucous membranes and oropharynx; vomiting, diarrhea, and abdominal pain within minutes to hours.
- Cardiovascular – lethargy and weakness may be noted in patients experiencing hypotension or arrhythmias following large exposure, especially to *Narcissus* spp.
- Nervous – ataxia, tremors, and seizures are possible following large ingestion of *Narcissus* spp. but rarely occur.
- Respiratory – dyspnea and airway obstruction if severe inflammation of the oropharynx occurs (rare).
- Skin – erythema, pruritus, edema, and pustular rash are rarely reported in animals.

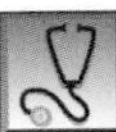

DIFFERENTIAL DIAGNOSIS

- Other toxins.
  - Plants containing irritants including insoluble calcium oxalate crystals.
  - Household products causing oral irritation (dilute cleaning agents, topical insecticides, many fertilizers).
  - Caustic agents (strong acids or alkalis, drain cleaners, batteries, some detergents).
- Foreign body obstruction.
- Systemic diseases associated with GI signs.

DIAGNOSTICS

- Clinical laboratory tests (serum chemistry and CBC) are not specifically diagnostic. Changes related to dehydration and persistent GI signs may be noted.
- Diagnosis is most often made by identification of the plant ingested

Pathological Findings

- Deaths are rare but reddened GI mucosa may be noted; possible cardiac ventricular dilation with exposure to *Narcissus* spp.

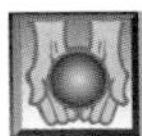

THERAPEUTICS

- Treatment of spring-blooming plant or bulb poisoning consists primarily of symptomatic and supportive care, including management of GI signs, correction of dehydration, and treatment of cardiovascular and CNS signs in severe cases. Small exposures typically only require at-home monitoring and nursing care.

Detoxification

- Extensive decontamination is generally not required in cases involving minimal exposure.
- Rinse the oral cavity with cool water to dilute irritants from the mouth.
- Early emesis should be employed in cases where large amounts of plant material and/or bulbs were ingested, provided the patient is not already vomiting.
- Activated charcoal with a cathartic × 1 dose (following large ingestion only).

Appropriate Health Care

- Minor exposures can often be managed at home with dilution and monitoring.
- SQ or IV fluid therapy as needed depending upon hydration status and severity of GI signs.
- Frequent monitoring of blood pressure and ECG for 12–24 hours in severe cases.
- Close monitoring of CNS status following large ingestion.
- Monitor for dyspnea and airway obstruction in cases involving significant oropharyngeal swelling.

Antidote

- No specific antidote.

Drugs of Choice

- Fluid therapy.
  - SQ fluids in cases with minor signs.
  - IV fluids as needed to correct dehydration, support perfusion, and maintain adequate blood pressure.
- Antiemetic agents as needed.
  - Maropitant 1 mg/kg SQ q 24 hours.
  - Ondansetron 0.1–0.2 mg/kg IV q 8–12 hours (extra-label in both dogs and cats).
- GI protectants.
  - H_2 blockers.
    - Famotidine 0.5 mg/kg PO, SQ, IM, IV q 12–24 hours.
    - Ranitidine 1–2 mg/kg PO, SQ, IM, IV q 8–12 hours.
    - Cimetidine 5–10 mg/kg PO q 6–8 hours.
  - Proton pump inhibitors.
    - Omeprazole 0.5–1 mg/kg PO q 24 hours.
    - Pantoprazole 0.7–1 mg/kg IV over 15 minutes q 24 hours.
  - Sucralfate 0.25–1 g PO q 8 hours × 5–7 days if evidence of active ulcer disease.

- Antiarrhythmics may be necessary if the patient is persistently tachycardic and nonresponsive to IV fluids, has severe ventricular dysrhythmias, or evidence of poor perfusion (hypotension, pulse deficits, tachycardia, pale membranes, prolonged CRT).
  - Lidocaine.
    - Dogs: 2–4 mg/kg IV over 1–2 minutes while monitoring ECG.If effective, switch to CRI at 25–100 μg/kg/min.
    - Cats: 0.25–0.5 mg/kg slow IV while monitoring ECG. If effective switch to CRI of 10–20 μg/kg/min. Use judiciously in cats!
  - Procainamide.
    - Dogs: 2–4 mg/kg IV over 2–5 minutes (may repeat up to 20 mg/kg IV total), followed by 20–50 μg/kg/min CRI.

Diet

- Depending on the severity of GI signs, consider keeping the patient NPO initially then feeding a bland or highly digestible diet.

COMMENTS

Prevention/Avoidance

- Identify plants presently in the household or on the property and limit exposure by placing them out of the animal's reach or restricting access to gardens and flowerbeds.
- Do not leave unplanted bulbs unattended while gardening or in areas that are generally accessible to pets, especially dogs.

Expected Course and Prognosis

- Prognosis is generally excellent to good as most cases develop only mild-to-moderate signs of short duration and require minimal therapy.

See Also

Oxalates – Insoluble

Abbreviations

See Appendix 1 for a complete list.

Suggested Reading

Burrows GE, Tyrl RJ. Toxic Plants of North America, 2nd edn. Ames, IA: John Wiley & Sons, 2013; pp. 720, 770–776, 778–780.

Knight AP. A Guide to Poisonous House and Garden Plants, Jackson: Teton NewMedia, 2006; pp. 123–124, 137–138, 192–194, 290–291.

Lieske CL. Spring-blooming bulbs: a year-round problem. Vet Med 2002; 97:580–588.
Plants – Amaryllidaceae. In: POISINDEX® System. Available at www.micromedexsolutions.com/micromedex2/librarian/ND_T/evidencexpert/ND_PR/evidencexpert/CS/A209F7/ND_AppProduct/evidencexpert/DUPLICATIONSHIELDSYNC/F9AC46/ND_PG/evidencexpert/ND_B/evidencexpert/ND_P/evidencexpert/PFActionId/evidencexpert.IntermediateToDocumentLink?docId=682&contentSetId=51

Authors: Amanda L. Poldoski, DVM; Lynn R. Hovda, RPh, DVM, MS, DACVIM
Consulting Editor: Lynn R. Hovda, RPh, DVM, MS, DACVIM

chapter 109

Yesterday, Today, and Tomorrow Plant

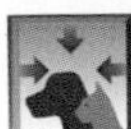

DEFINITION/OVERVIEW

- The genus *Brunfelsia* contains some 30–40 species, several of which are of toxic importance to the small animal veterinarian. Collectively, *Brunfelsia* spp. are considered members of the nightshade group. They are native to subtropical regions in South and Central America as well as the West Indies.
- The plants are valued as ornamentals due to their brightly colored flowers. They can be grown outdoors in warmer climates, as well as indoors in any region. Shortly after the buds open, the flowers rapidly undergo a color change from deep blue/purple to light blue/purple and then to white (Figs 109.1 and 109.2). This process occurs over approximately 3 days, a phenomenon which inspired the common name "yesterday, today, and tomorrow plant."

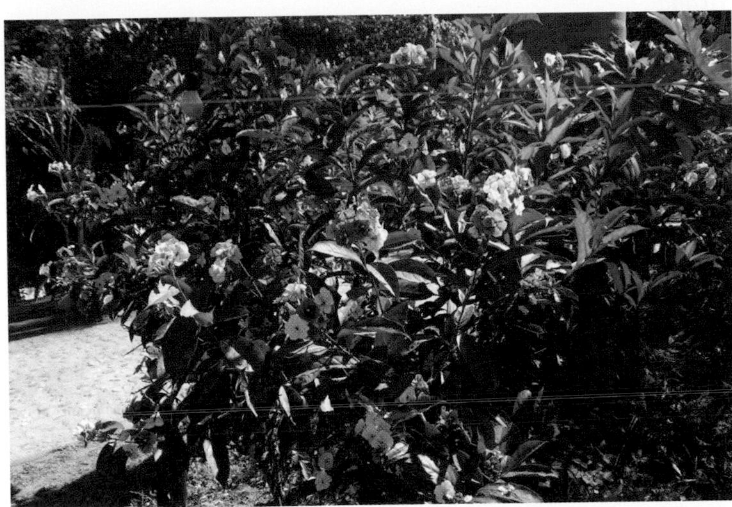

■ **Fig. 109.1.** *Brunfelsia* spp. tree in bloom at the Botanical Gardens, Puerto Vallarta, Mexico. Photo courtesy of Lynn R. Hovda.

Blackwell's Five-Minute Veterinary Consult Clinical Companion: Small Animal Toxicology, Second Edition.
Lynn R. Hovda, Ahna G. Brutlag, Robert H. Poppenga, and Katherine L. Peterson.

Companion website: www.fiveminutevet.com/toxicology

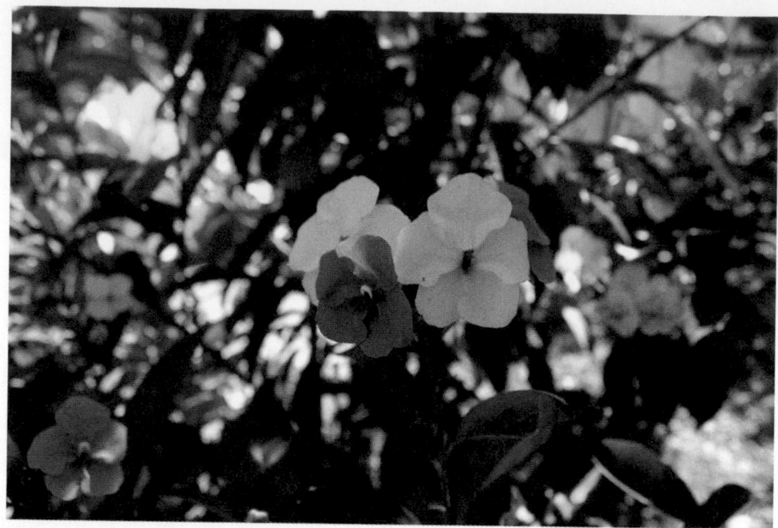

■ **Fig. 109.2.** Close-up of *Brunfelsia* spp. flower. Photo courtesy of Lynn R. Hovda.

- Commonly encountered species of potential toxicity include:
  - *B. australis*
  - *B. americana*
  - *B. calcyina var. floribunda*
  - *B. grandiflora*
  - *B. uniflora* (aka *B. hopeana*).
- Toxicity of *Brunfelsia* spp. is often described as "strychnine-like" and may include vomiting, diarrhea, ataxia, muscle tremors, and seizures.

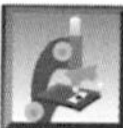

ETIOLOGY/PATHOPHYSIOLOGY

Mechanism of Action

- Three toxins of relevance have been identified in *Brunfelsia* spp. In order of greatest to least contribution to the toxicity caused by the plant, they are the following.
  - Brunfelsamidine causes neuroexcitatory effects, probably by inhibition of glycine receptors. This leads to excess stimulation of motor neurons, manifested by tremors and seizures. Tremor effects may take up to a week to resolve.
  - Hopeanine causes neurodepressant effects, including impaired neurotransmission and paralysis, and is also tremorgenic with ability to lower the seizure threshold.
  - Scopoletin appears to have cardiovascular depressant effects including vascular smooth muscle relaxation, hypotension, decreased cardiac contractility, bradycardia,and diminished cardiac output.
- Affected animals can show signs characteristic for any or all of the three toxins, but brunfelsamidine effects predominate in most clinically affected patients.

- All parts of the plant are potentially toxic if ingested. Berries and seeds are frequently ingested and may contain higher levels of the toxic constituents than other plant structures.

Pharmacokinetics/Toxicity

- Neither specific kinetic data nor LD50 values have been derived for dogs or cats.

Systems Affected

- Gastrointestinal – often the first signs noted may include hypersalivation, anorexia, vomiting, and diarrhea.
- Nervous – lethargy/depression, anxiety, agitation, hyperesthesia, vocalization.
- Musculoskeletal – ataxia, tremors, seizures, opisthotonus.
- Cardiovascular – bradycardia, hypotension, and decreased cardiac output with tissue hypoperfusion.

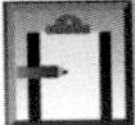

SIGNALMENT/HISTORY

Risk Factors

- Dogs are the most commonly affected small animal species, probably due to their propensity to consider a wide variety of materials as potentially edible. Toxicity has been reported in many other vertebrate species including cats, birds, cattle, and humans.

Historical Findings

- Affected animals may have a past medical history of pica or demonstrated willingness to ingest plant material.
- Owners may note animals displaying interest in the plants, damage consistent with chewing may be found on the plants, or ingestion may be directly observed.
- Berries or other plant material may be found in vomitus or feces.

Location and Circumstances of Poisoning

- *Brunfelsia* spp. are most frequently encountered outdoors in warm portions of the United States, particularly California, the Gulf Coast, and Florida.
- These plants can be grown indoors in any region.

CLINICAL FEATURES

- From 2010 to 2015, 17 cases of dogs ingesting *Brunfelsia* spp. were reported to Pet Poison Helpline. Of these, 16 dogs were symptomatic. Most common signs displayed by symptomatic dogs included depression/lethargy (56% of all symptomatic dogs), ataxia (50%),

seizures (50%), tremors (38%), vocalization (13%), muscle weakness (13%), ptyalism (13%), and anorexia (13%). Of the 17 reported cases, 11 occurred in California, three in Florida, two in Texas, and one in North Carolina.
- Subsequent to ingestion, clinical signs typically develop within 30 minutes to several hours. Fatalities have been reported within 10 hours of ingestion in severe cases.
- Signs persist from hours to several days. Full recovery may require up to a week post ingestion.

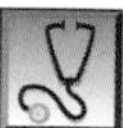

DIFFERENTIAL DIAGNOSIS

- Other intoxications, including ethanol, ethylene glycol, metaldehyde, bromethalin, tremorgenic mycotoxins, baclofen, ivermectin, methylxanthines, marijuana, and strychnine.
- Other than toxic causes of CNS signs, including idiopathic epilepsy, intracranial neoplasia, cerebrovascular accident, hepatic encephalopathy, infectious and parasitic disease.
- Other causes of acute gastroenteritis, including dietary indiscretion, pancreatitis, infectious and parasitic disease.

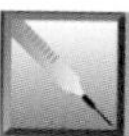

DIAGNOSTICS

- History of known or suspected ingestion.
- Identification of plant material in the vomitus or feces.
- Routine laboratory work-up is typically unrewarding in diagnosing toxicity caused by these compounds, but may be helpful in ruling out alternative differentials.
- Specific diagnostics to rule out other causes of neurological disease may include advanced imaging (CT or MRI), CSF tap, *Toxoplasma* titers, etc.

Pathological Findings

- No specific necropsy findings have been identified.
- Mild pulmonary congestion and hyperemia of the GI mucosa are occasionally reported, but are nonspecific.

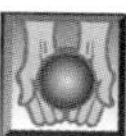

THERAPEUTICS

Detoxification

- Due to the potential for rapid onset of signs, emesis at home is not recommended.
- Survey radiographs may be useful to evaluate for presence, amount, and location of ingesta in the GI tract.
- Emesis induction under direct veterinary supervision should be considered in asymptomatic patients within 2–4 hours of ingestion, so long as the patient can adequately protect the airway.

- Gastric lavage with a cuffed endotracheal tube should be considered in symptomatic patients, those at increased risk of aspiration, or those ingesting very large amounts of plant matter.
- An oral dose of activated charcoal with a cathartic may be considered in asymptomatic patients.
- For patients being decontaminated via gastric lavage, a dose of activated charcoal with cathartic can be given via orogastric tube prior to removing the tube.
- If ingested plant material is present in the lower GI tract, warm water enemas can be used to stimulate colonic peristalsis and speed up transit time.

Appropriate Health Care

- Patients with mild gastrointestinal signs may be monitored at home. Owners should be advised that the patient must be rechecked immediately if any neurological signs develop.
- Patients with severe GI signs, cardiovascular or neurological signs should be hospitalized.
- Treatment is symptomatic and supportive.

Antidote

- No specific antidote exists.

Drugs of Choice

- Balanced IV crystalloids to support hydration, blood pressure, and normothermia. Fluid rate should be increased in animals with prolonged tremors/seizures as they are at increased risk for hyperthermia, rhabdomyolysis, and secondary nephrotoxicity.
- Note: Dosages that follow are for dogs, unless otherwise specified. Appropriate drugs and dosages should be confirmed for other species.
- For control of seizure activity.
    - Diazepam 0.5–1 mg/kg IV or per rectum.
    - Midazolam 0.25–0.5 mg/kg IV or IM.
- For seizures refractory to benzodiazepines.
    - Phenobarbital 5–8 mg/kg IV, repeat doses q 4–6 hours until seizures are controlled.
- For treatment of muscle tremors.
    - Methocarbamol 44–220 mg/kg IV. Recommend not to exceed a maximum total dose of 330 mg/kg/day.
- For severe or persistent vomiting.
    - Maropitant 1 mg/kg SQ q 24 hours.
    - Ondansetron 0.1–0.2 mg/kg IV q 8–12 hours.

Precautions/Interactions

- Atropine may be ineffective in treating bradycardia caused by *Brunfelsia* spp, and should only be considered for use if bradycardia is severe. It is not helpful with treatment of seizures caused by these plants. Atropine should be used sparingly, if at all, because signs of atropine overdose may closely resemble those caused by *Brunfelsia* spp.

Nursing Care

- Temperature should be closely monitored as affected patients can become hyperthermic, particularly with persistent seizures or tremors.
- Patients should be carefully monitored for any evidence of rhabdomyolysis and myoglobinuria.
- Patients may benefit from being kept in a cool, quiet, dark area because overstimulation may precipitate or worsen signs.

COMMENTS

Client Education

- · Owners should be warned of the toxic potential of these plants, particularly in areas where they are commonly grown.

Expected Course and Prognosis

- Patients remaining asymptomatic, or those with mild signs, typically have an excellent prognosis.
- Development of neurological signs, particularly severe tremors and seizures, is associated with a more guarded prognosis.

Synonyms

Franciscan rain tree, kiss me quick, morning, noon, and night.

Abbreviations

See Appendix 1 for a complete list.

Suggested Reading

Burrows GE, Tyrl RJ. Toxic plants of North America, 2nd edn. Ames, IA: Iowa State University Press, 2001; pp. 1107–1108.

Clipsham R. Brunfelsia australis (yesterday, today, and tomorrow tree) and solanum poisoning in a dog. J Am Anim Hosp Assoc 2012; 48(2):139–144.

Delaporte J, Means C. Plants. In: Poppenga RH, Gwaltney-Brant SM, eds. Small Animal Toxicology Essentials. Ames, IA: Wiley-Blackwell, 2011; pp. 157–158.

Singh M, Cowan S, Child G. Brunfelsia spp. 'Yesterday, today, tomorrow" toxicity in four dogs. Austr Vet J 2008; 86(6):214–218.

Spainhour CB, Fiske RA, Flory W, Reagor JC. A toxicological investigation of the garden shrub Brunfelsia calcyina var. floribunda (yesterday-today-and-tomorrow) in three species. J Vet Diagn Invest 1990; 2:3–8.

Author: James N. Eucher, DVM, DHSc, MS, MPH
Consulting Editor: Lynn R. Hovda, RPh, DVM, MS, DACVIM

chapter 110

Yew

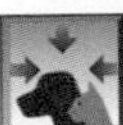

DEFINITION/OVERVIEW

- In the northern hemisphere, the *Taxus* spp. is referred to as the "tree of death." The most common toxic members found in the United States include Japanese yew (*Taxus cuspidata*), English yew (*Taxus baccata*), American yew (*Taxus canadensis*), and Chinese yew (*Taxus chinensis*). The Pacific or western yew (*Taxus brevifolia*) is generally considered to be less toxic than other yews.
- It is commonly used as an ornamental landscape plant in all parts of the country, usually along foundations or walls (Fig. 110.1).

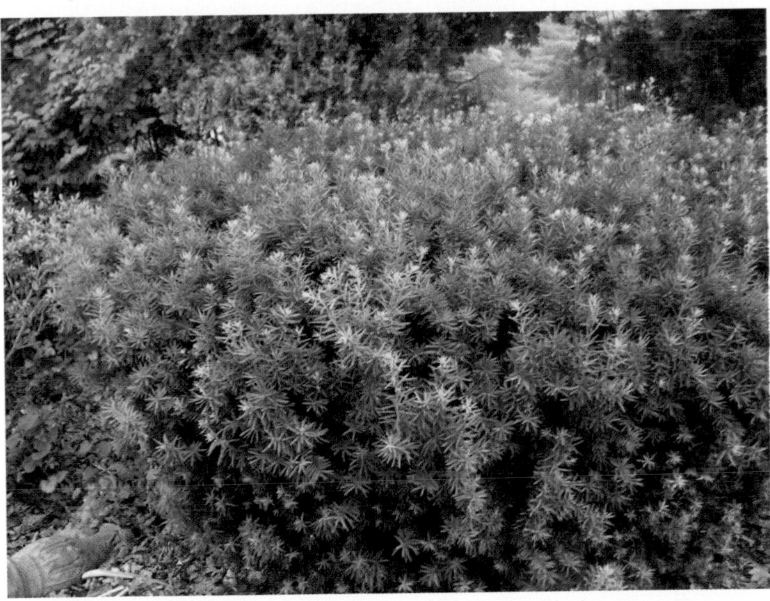

■ **Fig. 110.1.** Japanese yew (*Taxus cuspidata*) shrub. Photo courtesy of Tyne K. Hovda.

Blackwell's Five-Minute Veterinary Consult Clinical Companion: Small Animal Toxicology, Second Edition.
Lynn R. Hovda, Ahna G. Brutlag, Robert H. Poppenga, and Katherine L. Peterson.

Companion website: www.fiveminutevet.com/toxicology

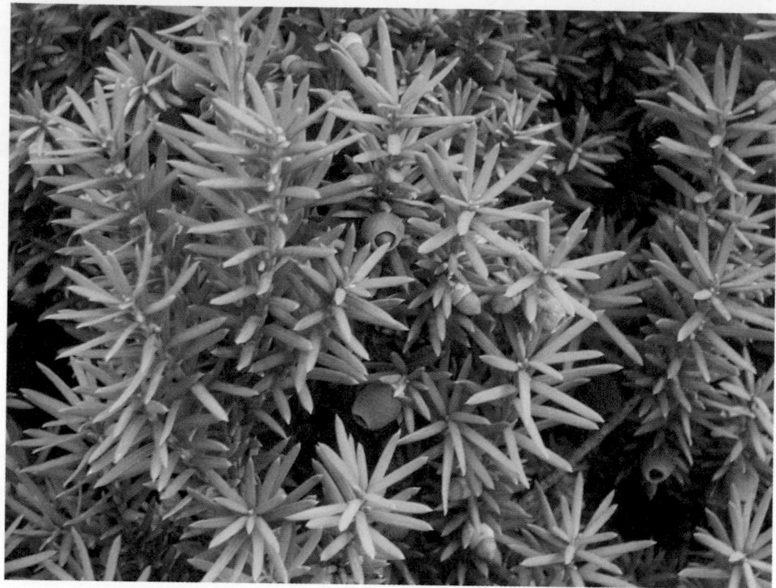

■ **Fig. 110.2.** Fruit of Japanese yew (*Taxus cuspidata*) shrub. Photo courtesy of Tyne K. Hovda.

- Leaves are easily identified. They are simple, alternate, spirally arranged, needle-like, 2–3 cm in length, are dark green on the top and have yellow longitudinal lines underneath.

■ Yews are dioecious plants. The male tree is considered more toxic than the female tree.

- The leaves, bark, and seeds are toxic; the fleshy part of the red fruit is not toxic (Fig. 110.2).
- Toxicosis may be caused by ingestion of either fresh or dried plant material.
- The maximal taxine concentrations occur in the winter.
- $LD_{(min)}$ in dogs is about 2.3 g of leaves/kg (about 11.5 mg/kg of taxine alkaloids).

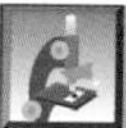

ETIOLOGY/PATHOPHYSIOLOGY

Mechanism of Action

■ Taxines A and B are the primary toxic agents.

- Both are cardiotoxic, but taxine B is more potent and associated with atrioventricular conduction delays, resulting in widening of the QRS complex and depressed p waves on an ECG.
- Taxine B also reduces cardiac contractility and the rate of cardiac depolarization.
- Both taxines A and B are direct calcium channel antagonists at the cardiac cellular level, with lesser effects on other organs.

■ Paclitaxel, a human antineoplastic drug isolated from *T. brevifolia*, has anticancer and antimitotic effects and may be arrhythmogenic in people, but is not the major toxic principle of the plant.

Pharmacokinetics – Absorption, Distribution, Metabolism, Excretion

- Absorption and distribution are rapid.
- Taxines are pseudoalkaloids, metabolized in the liver by P450 enzymes, and excreted as benzoic acid in the urine.

Toxicity

- Taxines A and B are considered the most toxic components, with taxine B being worst.
- $LD_{(min)}$ in dogs is 2.3 g leaves/g BW (11.5 mg/kg BW taxine alkaloids).

Systems Affected

- Cardiovascular – bradycardia, cardiovascular collapse.
- Gastrointestinal – gastroenteritis.
- Central nervous system – behavior changes, ataxia, seizures.

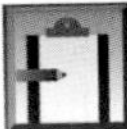

SIGNALMENT/HISTORY

- Yew is toxic to all species. Toxicosis occurs far more frequently in horses and ruminants than in companion animals and humans.
- The bitter, irritant oil in the bark and leaves limits ingestion in companion animals.

Location and Circumstances of Poisoning

- The incidence and degree of intoxication depend on the particular *Taxus* species.
- The Pacific yew (*Taxus brevifolia*) has low levels of taxine alkaloids and thus a much lower potential for toxicity.

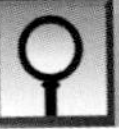

CLINICAL FEATURES

- The overall effect of taxine alkaloids in poisoned animals is peracute cardiovascular collapse and death due to disruption of cardiovascular function with arterial vasodilatation and hypotension.
- Subacute poisoning has been observed and clinical signs include bradycardia, ventricular fibrillation, nonspecific cardiac dysrhythmias, dyspnea, hyperthermia, ataxia, muscle tremors, aggressive behavior, mydriasis, recumbency, seizures, collapse, and death.
- Surviving animals develop gastroenteritis secondary to the volatile oil irritants found in the bark and leaves.

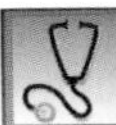

DIFFERENTIAL DIAGNOSIS

- Cardiac disease.
- Other toxicants.

- Arsenic, cyanide, and nitrate either in plant material or as direct toxins.
- Cardiac glycoside-containing plants (foxglove, rhododendron, oleander, others).
- Other pharmaceutical agents not specific to the cardiovascular system, but with known cardiac side effects.

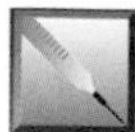

DIAGNOSTICS

History and Environment

- Presence of *Taxus* spp. should be confirmed in the animal's environment and the stomach contents examined for the presence of the plant. Recovered lavage material should be examined for yew and submitted for taxine alkaloid determination.
- Analysis of serum samples by GC/MS or LC/MS has been successful in some yew poisonings.

Bloodwork

- CBC and serum chemistry abnormalities in surviving companion animals may include an increased hematocrit, decreased total protein, hyponatremia, hypochloremia, hypoalbuminemia, and elevated alkaline phosphatase.

Pathological Findings

- Gross and histopathological lesions are generally absent due to the sudden onset of toxicity and death.
- Yew leaves and bark may be found in the stomach, and the mucous membranes of the gastrointestinal tract may be red and inflamed from the volatile irritant oils.
- Other nonspecific findings include pulmonary congestion or edema and hemorrhage secondary to cardiovascular collapse.

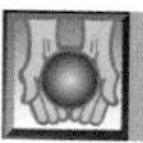

THERAPEUTICS

- Death often occurs almost immediately, leaving little opportunity for therapeutic intervention.
- Additional supportive treatment for surviving animals may be required for several weeks.

Detoxification

- Emesis only if within minutes of witnessed ingestion.
- Gastric lavage followed by activated charcoal with a cathartic × 1 dose.

Appropriate Health Care

- Continuous ECG monitoring for several days, with appropriate use of cardiac-specific medication as needed.
- Monitor and treat hyperthermia PRN, but not below 103.5°F.

Antidote

- No specific antidote is available.

Drugs of choice

- Judicious early IV fluid use, maintaining blood pressure and cardiovascular perfusion, but not overloading the cardiovascular system.
- Antiarrhythmics (lidocaine, procainamide) may be necessary if persistent tachycardia is nonresponsive to IV fluids, if there are ventricular dysrhythmias, or if there is evidence of poor perfusion (hypotension, pulse deficits, tachycardia, etc.).
  - Lidocaine.
    - Dogs: 2–4 mg/kg IV to effect while monitoring ECG. If effective, follow with a CRI of 25–200 µg/kg/min.
    - Cats: 0.25–0.5 mg/kg slow IV while monitoring ECG. If effective follow with CRI of 10–20 µg/kg/min. Use judiciously in cats!
  - Procainamide.
    - Dogs: 2–4 mg/kg IV over 3–5 minutes (up to 20 mg/kg IV bolus), followed by 20–50 µg/kg/min CRI.
- For bradycardia.
  - Atropine 0.02–0.04 mg/kg IV, IM, or SQ.
    - Most effective if administered early in the course, if needed. Humans have shown resistance to atropine administration.
  - Glycopyrrolate.
    - Dog 0.011 mg/kg IV or IM.
    - Cat 0.005–0.01 mg/kg IV or IM, 0.01–0.02 mg/kg SQ.
  - Temporary pacemaker for severe cases of unresponsive bradycardia.
- Seizure or aggressive behavior control as needed.
  - Diazepam 0.25–0.5 mg/kg IV PRN.
  - Phenobarbital 2–5 mg/kg IV PRN for seizures after diazepam use.
  - Midazolam 0.1–0.5 mg/kg IV.
- Antiemetics if vomiting is severe or persistent.
  - Maropitant 1 mg/kg SQ q 24 hours.
  - Ondansetron 0.1–0.2 mg/kg IV q 6–12 hours.
- GI protectants as needed.
  - H_2 blockers.
    - Famotidine 0.5–1 mg/kg PO, SQ, IM, IV q 12–24 hours.
    - Ranitidine 1–2 mg/kg PO, SQ, IM, IV q 8–12 hours.
  - Proton pump inhibitor.
    - Omeprazole 0.5–1 mg/kg q 24 hours.
    - Pantoprazole 0.7–1 mg/kg IV once daily.
  - Sucralfate 0.25–1 g PO q 8 hours × 5–7 days if evidence of active ulcer disease.

Nursing Care

- Avoid unnecessary restraint, exercise, additional stress or excitement for several days.

COMMENTS

Patient Monitoring

- ECG monitoring should occur for several days after initial insult.

Prevention/Avoidance

- *Taxus* spp. should not be planted where pets have access.
- Yew branches should not be used as playthings or chew sticks for pets.
- Yew clippings should be gathered and discarded far from pets.

Expected Course and Prognosis

- Peracute death is likely, although some dogs and cats have survived.

See Also

Beta Receptor Antagonists (Beta-Blockers)
Calcium Channel Blockers
Cardiac Glycosides
Other plant ingestions (rhododendron, azalea, etc.)

Abbreviations

See Appendix 1 for a complete list.

Suggested Reading

Botha CJ, Penrith ML. Potential plant poisonings in dogs and cats in southern Africa: review article. J S Afr Vet Assoc 2009; 80(2):63–74.
Burrows GE, Tyri RJ. Toxic Plants of North America. Ames, IA: ISU Press, 2006; pp. 1177–1185.
Cope RB. The dangers of yew ingestion. Vet Med 2005; 100(9):646–650.
Evans KL, Cook JR. Japanese yew poisoning in a dog. J Am Anim Hosp Assoc 1991; 27:300–302.
Pierog J, Kane B, Kane K, et al. Management of isolated yew berry toxicity with sodium bicarbonate: a case report in treatment efficacy. J Med Toxicol 2009; 5(2):84–89.
Wilson CR, Hooser SB. Toxicity of yew (Taxus spp.) alkaloids. In: GuptaRC, ed. Veterinary Toxicology: Basic and Clinical Principles, 2nd edn. New York: Elsevier, 2012; pp. 1121–1127.

Acknowledgment: The authors and editors acknowledge the prior contributions of Krishona Martinson, PhD, who authored this topic in the previous edition.
Author: Catherine M. Adams, DVM
Consulting Editor: Lynn R. Hovda, RPh, DVM, MS, DACVIM

Rodenticides

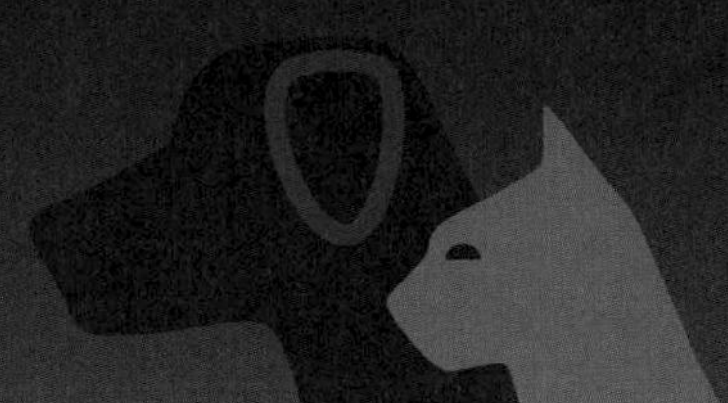

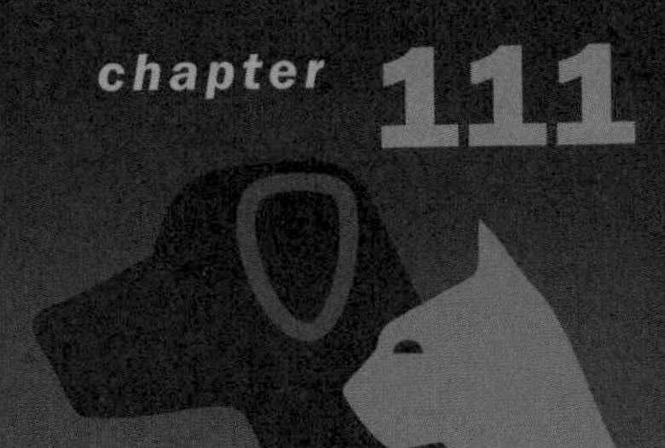

Anticoagulants

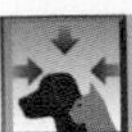

DEFINITION/OVERVIEW

- Anticoagulant rodenticides result in a coagulopathy caused by reduced vitamin K_1-dependent clotting factors in circulation.
- Second-generation anticoagulants (SGAR) were developed in recent decades; they generally are more toxic and some persist longer in the liver, resulting in greater risk (and requirement for a longer duration of treatment) than older first-generation anticoagulants (FGAR).
- Anticoagulant rodenticides are commonly marketed as pellets or paraffin blocks under a variety of trade names (Fig. 111.1).
- Recent restrictions on availability of SGAR through consumer outlets are designed to decrease exposure of nontarget species such as dogs and cats to products containing them.

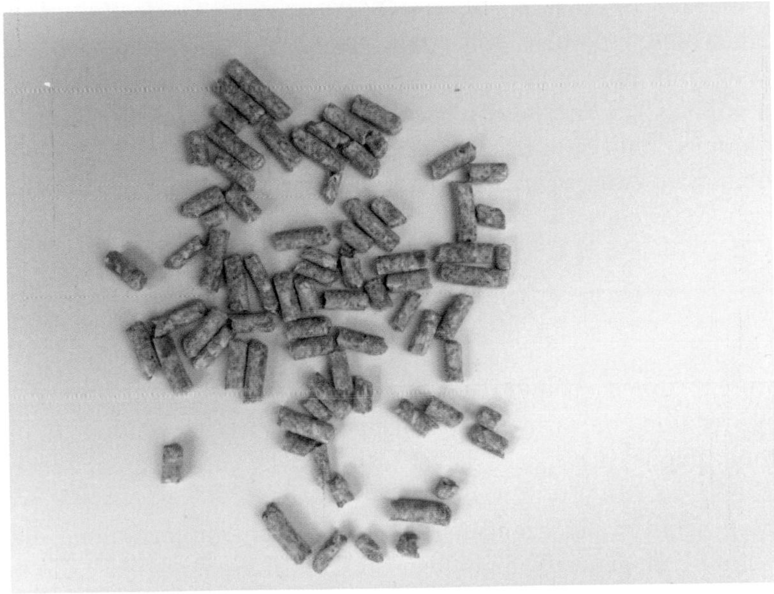

Fig. 111.1. Common form of commercially available anticoagulant rodenticide bait pellets.

Blackwell's Five-Minute Veterinary Consult Clinical Companion: Small Animal Toxicology, Second Edition.
Lynn R. Hovda, Ahna G. Brutlag, Robert H. Poppenga, and Katherine L. Peterson.

Companion website: www.fiveminutevet.com/toxicology

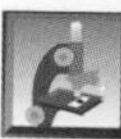

ETIOLOGY/PATHOPHYSIOLOGY

Mechanism of Action

- Reduced vitamin K_1 is required for carboxylation to activated vitamin K-dependent clotting factors: II, VI, IX, and X.
- Carboxylation of clotting factors oxidizes vitamin K_1 to the inactive epoxide form.
- Anticoagulants inhibit vitamin K_1 epoxide reductase, DT diaphorase, and possibly other enzymes involved in the reduction of vitamin K_1-epoxide to vitamin K_1.
- Uncarboxylated clotting factors do not bind calcium sufficiently to participate in clot formation.
- Carboxylated clotting factors decline with time after anticoagulant rodenticide exposure to a point after which coagulation function is inadequate.

Pharmacokinetics – Absorption, Distribution, Metabolism, Excretion

- Readily absorbed (90%) from GIT.
- Peak plasma concentrations occur 1–12 hours post ingestion.
- Bind to plasma proteins, providing an inactive reservoir until released and transported to liver.
- Concentrated in liver; may involve enterohepatic recycling.
- Some are metabolized in the liver to hydroxyl metabolites that are excreted in urine.
- Plasma half-life ranges from hours for some FGAR products like warfarin to days for others such as brodifacoum, chlorphacinone, diphacinone, and other long-lasting compounds.
- Warfarin passes into human milk; evidence of secretion of anticoagulant rodenticides in the milk of animals has also been reported. Clinically, it is best to assume that nursing puppies or kittens could be at risk if the dam has been exposed.
- Limited numbers of cases of transplacental transfer of some anticoagulant rodenticides have also been reported.

Toxicity

- General.
  - Exposure to anticoagulant rodenticide products.
  - First-generation coumarin anticoagulants (i.e., warfarin, pindone, diphacinone and chlorophacinone) have been largely replaced by more potent second-generation anticoagulants.
  - Second-generation anticoagulants (i.e., brodifacoum, bromadiolone, difethialone and difenacoum) are generally more toxic and persist longer before excretion than first-generation agents.
  - Consumption of bait often precedes clinical hemorrhage by 2–3 days.
- Dogs.
  - Difethialone is highly toxic to rats and mice (0.52 mg/kg and 0.47 mg/kg, respectively); toxic to dogs (LD_{50} = 4 mg/kg).
  - Brodifacoum: LD_{50} = 0.25–2.5 mg/kg.

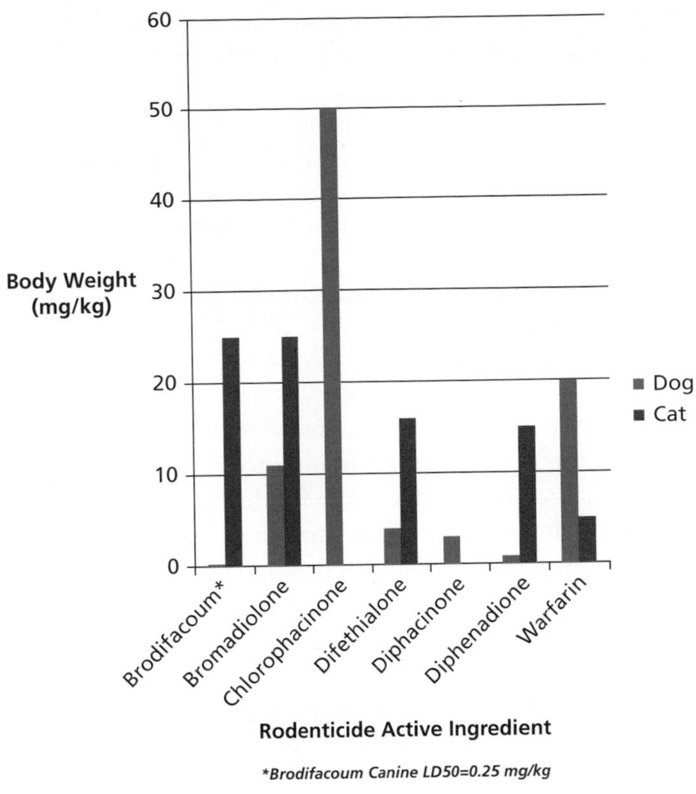

■ **Fig. 111.2.** Comparative LD_{50} values for anticoagulant rodenticides in dogs and cats. Cats are generally more resistant to second-generation (long-acting) anticoagulants than are dogs.

- Bromadiolone: LD_{50} = 11–20 mg/kg.
- Chlorophacinone: LD_{50} = 50–100 mg/kg.
- Warfarin: LD_{50} = 20–50 mg/kg.
- Diphacinone: LD_{50} = 3–7.5 mg/kg.
- See Fig. 111.2 for a graphic comparison of toxicity from common rodenticides.

■ Cats.
- Difethialone (D-Cease): LD_{50} >16 mg/kg.
  - ☐ Concentration in baits lower (0.0025% or 25 ppm) than that of other second-generation rodenticide baits (0.005% or 50 ppm).
  - ☐ Dogs and cats may tolerate higher intake of bait material.

Systems Affected

- Hemic/lymphatic/immune – depletion of activated clotting factors resulting in hemorrhage.
- Gastrointestinal – oral, gastric, intestinal or colonic bleeding.
- Respiratory – massive pulmonary hemorrhage and hemothorax often cause sudden death.

- Neuromuscular – hemorrhage within the CNS compresses neural tissue in the cranium or spinal canal, causing ataxia, tetraparesis, and seizures in rare cases; muscle hemorrhage occurs in response to trauma.
- Musculoskeletal – large intramuscular hematomas following injection, lameness secondary to hemarthrosis.
- Renal hemorrhage – leads to hematuria.
- Reproductive – placental hemorrhage can lead to abortion; vaginal bleeding may also occur.

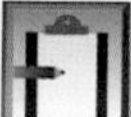

SIGNALMENT/HISTORY

Risk Factors

- Risk of exposure to SGAR is expected to be reduced in urban areas beginning in 2015. The EPA has restricted consumer rodenticide products to those containing FGAR or nonanticoagulant rodenticides. See Suggested Reading for details of the decision.
- Major market share of rodenticides in North America is second-generation anticoagulants.
- Rodenticide products are more commonly used in the spring and fall, so exposure increases during these times.
- Dogs and cats primarily affected, with a much higher prevalence in dogs.
- No breed or gender predilections.
- Younger animals may ingest bait more readily than older animals, due to their curious nature.

Historical Findings

- Baits are often sold as pellets or blocks of various sizes.
- Most baits are colored to distinguish them as a pesticide. However, specific identification of one type of product is difficult based on color alone. Colors: green, blue-green, red, or brown/tan.
- Coughing, dyspnea, tachypnea, or exercise intolerance are often the first clinical signs noted.
- Less commonly, SQ swellings, joint swelling, or bleeding from body orifices are observed.
- Rarely, death is the first evidence of poisoning.

Location and Circumstances of Poisoning

- Often in or around buildings where rodent baits are placed.
- Prevalence increased by careless placement without protective bait stations.
- Exposure may be acute with single large dose or multiple small doses.

Interactions with Drugs, Nutrients, or Environment

- Sulfonamides, phenylbutazone, and other highly protein-bound compounds may displace anticoagulant rodenticides from plasma binding sites, leading to more free toxicant and toxicosis.
- Concurrent use of NSAIDs or other drugs that inhibit platelet function is discouraged due to the risks of exacerbating coagulopathy or bleeding.

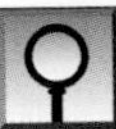

CLINICAL FEATURES

Physical Examination

- Evidence of hemorrhagic shock (i.e., tachycardia, hypovolemic, hypotensive, poor pulse quality, pallor).
- Coughing, dyspnea, tachypnea, pale mucous membranes.
- Hemarthrosis, lameness, presence of SQ hematomas.
- Exercise intolerance, lethargy, depression.
- Hematomas – often ventral and at venipuncture sites.
- Bleeding from body orifices, periorbital bleeding.
- Epistaxis, vaginal or rectal bleeding.
- Muffled heart or lung sounds.

Systemic Signs

- Clotting factor depletion results in generalized ecchymotic hemorrhages and often frank bleeding from many body sites.
- Oral, gastric, intestinal, or colonic bleeding characterized by epistaxis, hemoptysis, hematemesis, melena, or hemorrhagic diarrhea; severe hemorrhage can result in anemia.
- Coughing, dyspnea, abnormal auscultation (i.e., moist rales, increased bronchovesicular sounds, dull ventral lung sounds, etc.), muffled heart sounds, massive pulmonary hemorrhage, hemothorax, exercise intolerance.
- Acute anemia, hypoxemia, respiratory arrest, and sudden death may follow acute pulmonary bleeding.
- Evidence of hemorrhagic shock secondary to blood loss, hypovolemia, or poor cardiac filling may be seen.
- Pericardial effusion (seen as muffled heart sounds, presence of VPCs, pulse deficits, vomiting, collapse, etc.) may be seen with toxicosis, resulting in poor cardiac filling and signs of hypovolemic shock.
- Hemarthrosis results in general or asymmetrical lameness.
- Rarely, hemorrhage compresses neural tissue in cranium or spinal canal, resulting in CNS signs including ataxia, lethargy, blindness, and occasionally seizures. Spinal bleeding can cause paraplegia or quadriplegia.
- Muscle hemorrhage occurs in response to trauma or IM injection.
- Hematuria.
- Placental hemorrhage can lead to abortion; vaginal bleeding possible.

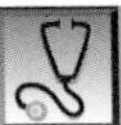

DIFFERENTIAL DIAGNOSIS

- IMT – platelet count <10,000–15,000 × 10^3/µL.
- Coagulation factor deficiency from prolonged liver disease. Assay for related factor deficiencies, for example, factor VII, liver function, bile acids.

- DIC – association with neoplasia, sepsis, pancreatitis, concurrent disease; laboratory evidence of elevated PT, PTT, FDP, d-dimers with thrombocytopenia.
- Hemophilia – congenital clotting factor deficiencies. Assay for related factor deficiencies, for example, factor VIII.
- Fat malabsorption.
- Hemorrhagic shock from trauma, neoplasia, bone marrow suppression, IMHA.

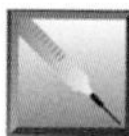

DIAGNOSTICS

Clinical Laboratory Findings

- Anemia – with marked hemorrhage, often acute and nonregenerative.
- Thrombocytopenia from consumptive bleeding (typically 50,000–150,000 × 10^3/μL).
- Prolonged PT and PTT support exposure to rodenticide; PT/PTT prolongation seen at 36–48 hours after ingestion but will normalize with vitamin K_1 therapy. Typically, PT is prolonged more extensively and earlier (6–18 hours earlier) than PTT.
- ACT >150 seconds supports coagulopathy.
- PIVKA assay, although this is rarely used.
- Anticoagulant analysis of blood or liver confirms exposure to a specific product.
- Anticoagulant assay of stomach or intestinal contents is not reliable because of delay between consumption of bait and appearance of clinical signs.

Imaging

- Thoracic radiography may detect pleural effusion (i.e., hemothorax), multilobular, alveolar infiltration (i.e., pulmonary hemorrhage), or an enlarged cardiac silhouette (i.e., pericardial effusion).

Diagnostic Procedures

- Thoracocentesis in dyspneic patients; may confirm hemothorax.
- Preliminary ultrasound of both the pleural and peritoneal cavities may reveal effusion consistent with hemorrhage.

Pathological Findings

- Free blood in the thoracic cavity, lungs, and abdominal cavity is a common finding.
- Hemorrhage into the cranial vault, GIT, and urinary tract is less common; may also see hemorrhage in the subcutaneous space or within muscle bellies.

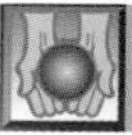

THERAPEUTICS

Detoxification

- If recent ingestion has occurred, immediate emesis induction followed by activated charcoal with a cathartic can be performed.

- If clinical signs have already developed, or if the patient is already coagulopathic (based on diagnostic testing), oral detoxification is often ineffective.
  - However, oral activated charcoal has been proposed to reduce the risk of enterohepatic recirculation of the longer lasting second-generation compounds.

Appropriate Health Care

- Inpatient care necessary for acute crisis.
- Outpatient care can be considered once the coagulopathy is stabilized.
- Correct acute signs of hemorrhagic shock with IV crystalloids, colloids, and blood products as needed. Initial shock boluses of 20 mL/kg of crystalloids can be given over 15–20 minutes during initial stabilization. Repeat 2–3× as needed to effect to increase blood pressure.
- The use of pRBC, WB, FFP, or FP may be necessary to increase oxygen-carrying capacity (increasing RBC count) and to replace coagulation factors. Patients should be blood typed prior to transfusion.
- Correct life-threatening cardiac tamponade or hemothorax. If volume resuscitation (listed above) does not improve clinical signs of hemorrhagic shock, or if dyspnea is severe, pericardiocentesis or thoracocentesis may be indicated. If the patient is stable and responding to therapy, these procedures should be avoided due to the coagulopathic state of the patient. With time, the blood will be reabsorbed and clinical signs should improve. If, however, there is no response to therapy, an autotransfusion of the patient's blood from the pericardial sac or thoracic cavity can be performed via aseptic technique.

Antidote and Drugs of Choice

- Administration of vitamin K_1 – avoid IM injections and give orally (if there are no contraindications such as vomiting) or SQ (with a small needle, in multiple locations if needed). Bioavailability of oral absorption is enhanced by the concurrent feeding of a small amount of a fatty meal, such as canned dog food.
- Vitamin K_1 – 2.5–5.0 mg/kg PO q 24 hours 5 days to 6 weeks (depending on the specific product) or divided PO q 12 hours for first-generation anticoagulant toxicosis.
- Vitamin K_1 administration – continued for 3–4 weeks with suspected second-generation anticoagulant toxicosis.

Precautions/Interactions

- Vitamin K_3 – not efficacious in the treatment of anticoagulant rodenticide toxicosis; contraindicated.
- Intravenous vitamin K_1 – reported anaphylactic reactions; avoid this route of administration.
- Avoid unnecessary surgical procedures and unnecessary parenteral injections until coagulation parameters are within normal limits (e.g., PT, PTT).
- Minimize stress, trauma, and jugular venipuncture or cystocentesis. Catastrophic bleeding may occur as a result.

- Use the smallest possible needle when giving an injection or collecting samples. Phlebotomy sites should be held off adequately to ensure appropriate clot formation.
- Sulfonamides, phenylbutazone, and other highly protein-bound drugs may displace anticoagulant rodenticides from plasma binding sites, leading to more free toxicant and toxicosis.

Diet

- Feed a nutritious high-quality protein diet to support coagulation factor synthesis.

Activity

- Confine patient during the early stages; activity enhances blood loss.

Surgical Considerations

- Thoracocentesis may be important for removing free thoracic blood, which causes dyspnea and respiratory failure, but should only be performed when life-threatening, severe dyspnea or hypoxemia is evident.
- Coagulopathies must be corrected prior to surgery.

COMMENTS

Patient Monitoring

- ACT and PT – assess efficacy of therapy; monitor for 48–72 hours after discontinuation of treatment; if PT is still prolonged, an additional 1–2 weeks of vitamin K_1 therapy should be given.
- There is no need to check PT, ACT, or PTT while patients are on vitamin K_1 therapy, as these coagulation panels should be normal while on therapy. Follow-up blood work should be monitored upon discontinuing vitamin K_1 therapy.
- Do not discontinue vitamin K_1 medication, even if the patient appears completely healthy, without treating for the adequate duration of time.

Prevention/Avoidance

- Do not allow animals to have access to anticoagulant rodenticides; place out of reach of pets and children.
- Bait stations are now required although their effectiveness is unknown.
- Baits transported and hoarded by rodents could be consumed by desirable nontarget species.

Possible Complications

- Warn client that reexposure could be a serious problem; remove all bait from the environment!
- Stress importance of continuing vitamin K_1 for the full prescribed period otherwise serious recurrence of hemorrhage can occur.

- Pregnant animals can abort after acute crisis due to placental hemorrhage and detachment.
- A nursing mother that ingested a toxic amount should be treated; the puppies or kittens will also need to be treated for the full duration of time with vitamin K_1 therapy.

Expected Course and Prognosis

- If the patient survives the first 48 hours of acute coagulopathy, the prognosis improves.
- Prolonged vitamin K_1 therapy is important to continued improvement.

Abbreviations

See Appendix 1 for a complete list.

FGAR = first-generation anticoagulant rodenticide
SGAR = second-generation anticoagulant rodenticide
FFP = fresh frozen plasma

Suggested Reading

EPA decision: www2.epa.gov/rodenticides/restrictions-rodenticide-products

Haines B. Anticoagulant rodenticide ingestion and toxicity: a retrospective study of 252 canine cases. Aust Vet Pract 2008; 38:38–50.

Luiz JA, Heseltine J. Five common toxins ingested by dogs and cats. Comp Cont Ed Pract Vet 2008; 30:578–587.

Murphy MJ. Rodenticides. Vet Clin North Am Small Animal Pract 2002; 32(2):469–484.

Murphy MJ, Talcott PA. Anticoagulant rodenticides. In: Peterson ME, Talcott PA, eds. Small Animal Toxicology, 2nd edn. St Louis,MO: Elsevier, 2006; pp. 563–577.

Author: Michael Murphy, DVM, JD, PhD, DABVT, DABT, RAC
Consulting Editor: Robert H. Poppenga, DVM, PhD, DABVT

chapter 112

Bromethalin

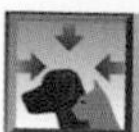

DEFINITION/OVERVIEW

- Bromethalin is a rodenticide that produces marked CNS effects. Rodenticide baits often contain 0.01% or 0.025% bromethalin.
- Toxic doses are approximately 0.3 and 2.5 mg/kg in cats and dogs, respectively.
- Chemical name: N-methyl-2,4-dinitro-N-[2,4,6-tribromophenyl]-6-[trifluoromethyl] benzeneamine.

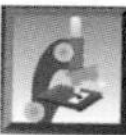

ETIOLOGY/PATHOPHYSIOLOGY

- Poisonings arising from exposure to bromethalin-based rodenticides are increasingly observed in veterinary medicine. Most veterinary cases will involve accidental ingestion but deliberate exposures have also been reported.
- Trade names for rodenticdes that contain bromethalin include Vengeance®, Assault®, Trounce®, No Pest Rat & Mice Killer®, CyKill®, Fastrac®, and others.

Mechanism of Action

- Bromethalin is not an anticoagulant rodenticide and vitamin K_1 is not an antidote.
- Bromethalin uncouples oxidative phosphorylation, resulting in reduced ATP production, impaired sodium and potassium pump function, cerebral edema, and elevated CSF pressure.
- Lipid peroxidation also occurs.

Pharmacokinetics – Absorption, Distribution, Metabolism, Excretion

- Bromethalin is rapidly absorbed from the gastrointestinal tract.
- Peak plasma concentrations occur within 4–6 hours of ingestion.
- Bromethalin is highly lipophilic and is widely distributed to the brain, fat, liver, and kidney.
- Hepatic metabolism to an N-demethylated intermediate is required for toxicity to occur. Species with limited N-demethylase activity (e.g., guinea pigs) are generally resistant to bromethalin poisoning.

Blackwell's Five-Minute Veterinary Consult Clinical Companion: Small Animal Toxicology, Second Edition.
Lynn R. Hovda, Ahna G. Brutlag, Robert H. Poppenga, and Katherine L. Peterson.

Companion website: www.fiveminutevet.com/toxicology

- Bromethalin is excreted in the bile and undergoes enterohepatic recirculation that can delay clearance from the body (half times of elimination >3–6 days).

Toxicity

Dogs

- LD_{50} in dogs is 2.4–3.7 mg bromethalin/kg BW.
- Minimum lethal dose is approximately 1 mg bromethalin/kg BW.

Cats

- LD_{50} in cats is 0.54 mg bromethalin/kg BW.
- Minimum lethal dose is approximately 0.25 mg bromethalin/kg BW.

Systems Affected

- Nervous – CNS depression, ataxia, muscle tremors, seizures, paresis/paralysis, hyperthermia, coma.
- Ophthalmic – abnormal PLR, anisocoria, nystagmus.
- Gastrointestinal—Anorexia, nausea, vomiting (uncommon)
- Respiratory – respiratory depression (may be cause of death).

SIGNALMENT/HISTORY

- Canines are more commonly reported to ingest rodenticides, including bromethalin-based products, than felines.
- Younger animals tend to be more likely to consume rodenticides.
- No breed or age specificity is seen.

Risk Factors

- Cats are much more sensitive to toxicosis than dogs.
- Cats may be at risk of relay toxicity from the ingestion of poisoned rodents.
- Repeated ingestions may produce clinical signs of toxicosis.

Historical Findings

- Owners may report tan, green, or greenish blue material in the feces.
- Owners may observe the exposure or see evidence of exposure (e.g., damaged bait boxes, rodenticide packages).
- The pet owner often notes clinical signs including ataxia, CNS depression, and lethargy.

Location and Circumstances of Poisoning

- Often occurs in the garage and other locations where rodenticides are used or stored.

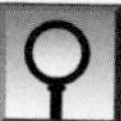

CLINICAL FEATURES

- Ingestion of supra-lethal doses of bromethalin ($\geq LD_{50}$) may result in an acute onset of CNS excitation, muscle tremors, and seizures.
- Ingestion of lower doses of bromethalin ($<LD_{50}$) may result in a delayed syndrome that develops within 2–7 days following ingestion; however, delays of up to 2 weeks may occur.
- Common clinical signs include anorexia, progressive ataxia, paresis and hindlimb paralysis, moderate-to-severe CNS depression, fine muscle tremors, and focal motor or generalized seizures. Abnormal PLR, anisocoria, and nystagmus are often seen.
- Forelimb extensor rigidity and decerebrate postures are often seen.
- With mild poisoning, clinical signs may resolve within 1–2 weeks of onset of clinical signs, although signs can persist for up to 4–6 weeks in some animals.
- Prognosis is very guarded in severely affected animals.

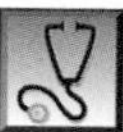

DIFFERENTIAL DIAGNOSIS

- Other toxicants with sedative and/or CNS depressant effects.
- Primary neurological disease (e.g., inflammatory, infectious, infiltrative).
- Primary metabolic disease (e.g., hypoglycemia, hepatic encephalopathy).

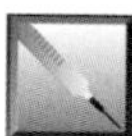

DIAGNOSTICS

Clinical Laboratory Findings

- Diagnosis is dependent upon the presence of an exposure history to a potentially toxic dose of a bromethalin-based rodenticide and the development of consistent clinical signs, the presence of diffuse white matter vacuolization on postmortem examination, and analytical confirmation of bromethalin or its desmethyl metabolite in tissues.
- Alterations in routine serum electrolytes and chemistries are not anticipated unless dehydration is present.
- CSF from bromethalin-poisoned dogs generally reveals normal cytology, protein concentration, specific gravity, and cell count.
- EEG abnormalities may include spike and spike-and-wave activity, marked voltage depression, and abnormal high-voltage, slow-wave activities.

Pathological Findings

- Lesions are generally confined to the CNS.
    - Gross evidence of cerebral edema may occur but is relatively mild.
    - Histopathological changes include spongy degeneration (white matter vacuolization) in the cerebrum, cerebellum, brainstem, spinal cord, and optic nerve white matter due to myelin edema.

- Analytical chemical confirmation of bromethalin or its desmethyl metabolite in fresh frozen fat, liver, kidney, and brain tissue.
- Bromethalin has been detected in formalin-fixed human liver and brain samples by gas chromatography with mass spectrometry detection.
- Neuroimaging (MRI) may reveal generalized brain edema.

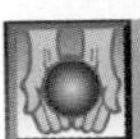

THERAPEUTICS

Detoxification

- Gastrointestinal tract decontamination including early induction of emesis in asymptomatic animals.
- Repeated administration of activated charcoal (0.5–1 mg/kg PO q 4–8 hours for at least 2–3 days). An osmotic cathartic (sodium sulfate, 125 mg/kg PO) is given once with the first dose of activated charcoal.
- The ASPCA Animal Poison Control Center (APCC) has recommended the judicious use of intravenous lipid emulsions (ILE) in cases of severe intoxication with bromethalin. 20% intravenous lipid emulsions: bolus dose of 1.5 mL/kg over 2–3 min or a continuous rate infusion of 0.25 mL/kg/min for 30–60 min. Check serum q 2 hours until it becomes clear; repeat as needed; if no clinical improvement after three doses, discontinue. Adverse effects of ILE may relate to contamination of the lipid product or direct reaction to the emulsion.

Appropriate Health Care

- Hospitalization is often required to manage severe CNS and respiratory depression.
- If respiratory function is compromised, a cuffed endotracheal tube should be placed and ventilation supported mechanically as required.
- Maintaining normal body temperature is important.
- Bromethalin toxicosis can result in severe CNS depression/coma, and appropriate nursing care is imperative. Patients should be kept in a padded cage and should be turned every 6 hours to prevent atelectasis.

Antidote

- There are no known effective antidotes for bromethalin.

Drugs of Choice

- Control of cerebral edema with mannitol (250 mg/kg, q 6 hours IV), dexamethasone (2 mg/kg, q 6 hours IV), and furosemide (1–2 mg/kg, q 6 hours IV) has been recommended but shown to have limited clinical efficacy.
- Diazepam (1–2 mg/kg, as needed, IV) and/or phenobarbital (5–15 mg/kg, as needed, IV) may be given to abolish severe muscle tremors and seizures.

- Methocarbamol (55–220 mg/kg IV, to effect PRN) for control of muscle tremors. Do not exceed 330 mg/kg in 24 hours. Monitor for excessive sedation and respiratory depression with high-dose therapy.

Precautions/Interactions

- Contraindications for the use of mannitol include renal disease, pulmonary edema, dehydration, and intracranial hemorrhage.
- Animals receiving mannitol therapy may become dehydrated during treatment.
- Rehydration of some animals is associated with a worsening of clinical signs, possibly due to rebound cerebral and pulmonary edema. Maintenance of hydration is important and can be more safely accomplished through the administration of oral fluids.

Nursing Care

- Provide respiratory support and mechanical ventilation if needed (very poor prognosis).
- Monitor temperature, heart rate, and respiratory rate.
- Monitor blood pressure and blood glucose frequently and treat appropriately.
- Ophthalmic lubrication may be necessary every 6 hours.
- Keep the patient clean and dry.

Diet

- Moderately to severely affected animals should have food and water withheld to prevent aspiration pneumonia.
- Enteral or parenteral feeding if prolonged neurological complications preclude oral nutrition.

Follow-up

- Follow-up is generally unnecessary, as patients are clinically normal once signs resolve.

Activity

- Patients should be restricted from activity until clinical signs resolve, as ataxia and CNS depression will be apparent. Once clinical signs resolve, no exercise restriction is necessary.

Prevention/Avoidance

- Prevent access of pets to all pesticides, including bromethalin-based rodenticides.

COMMENTS

Client Education

- Prevention is critical. Advise clients that all rodenticides are potentially dangerous for their pets and children.

- Early treatment is also important. Clients should be taught to contact their veterinarian if a pesticide exposure has occurred or an animal is displaying unusual clinical signs.

Patient Monitoring

- Acid–base monitoring is recommended in symptomatic animals.
- Blood glucose concentrations should be monitored frequently.

Expected Course and Prognosis

- Cases involving only mild signs may resolve with close monitoring and supportive care within a 3–7-day period.
- The prognosis is guarded to poor in cases involving severe CNS or respiratory system depression, coma, or paralysis.

Abbreviations

See Appendix 1 for a complete list.

Suggested Reading

Coppock R. Advisory: Bromethalin rodenticide – No known antidote. Can Vet J 2013; 54(6):557–558.

Gwaltney-Brant S, Meadows I. Use of intravenous lipid emulsions for treating certain poisoning cases in small animals. Vet Clin North Am Small Anim Pract 2012; 42:251–262.

Pasquale-Styles MA, Sochaski MA, Dorman DC. Fatal bromethalin poisoning. J Forensic Sci 2006; 51(5):1154–1157.

Peterson ME. Bromethalin. Top Compan Anim Med 2013; 28(1):21–23.

Author: David C. Dorman, DVM, PhD, DABVT, DABT
Consulting Editor: Robert H. Poppenga, DVM, PhD, DABVT

Cholecalciferol

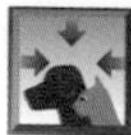

DEFINITION/OVERVIEW

- Cholecalciferol, the chemical name for vitamin D_3, is a necessary part of dietary requirements. Sources are through ingested food, vitamin supplements, and dermal exposure to the sun.
- Rodenticides are another source of cholecalciferol and are the primary cause of vitamin D_3 toxicosis in dogs and cats.
- Human medications containing vitamin D analogs are currently used for treating a variety of human diseases and can be accidentally ingested by pets.
- Intoxication has been documented in dogs fed pet foods containing excessive vitamin D concentrations.
- Vitamin D_3 is expressed either as mg/kg or as IU; 1 μg vitamin D_3 is equivalent to 40 IU.

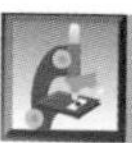

ETIOLOGY/PATHOPHYSIOLOGY

Mechanism of Action

- 1,25-dihydroxycholecalciferol (calcitriol) is the most active metabolite of cholecalciferol.
- Cholecalciferol is converted in the liver by 25-hydroxylase to 25-hydroxycholecalciferol (calcifediol). This is then converted to 1,25-dihydroxycholecalciferol (calcitriol) in the kidneys by 1-alpha-hydroxylase.
- In toxic exposures, calcitriol exerts negative feedback and suppresses renal hydroxylase. There is almost no feedback by calcium, calcitriol, or calcifediol to liver hydroxylase, so calcifediol continues to be produced.
- Calcitriol increases calcium absorption from the GIT, stimulates bone resorption, and increases calcium absorption in the renal distal tubules. This results in increased serum calcium and increased serum phosphorus, causing mineralization of soft tissues.

Pharmacokinetics – Absorption, Distribution, Metabolism, Excretion

- Cholecalciferol undergoes enterohepatic recirculation.
- Cholecalciferol half-life is 19–25 hours. The terminal half-life is weeks to months because it is highly fat soluble.

Blackwell's Five-Minute Veterinary Consult Clinical Companion: Small Animal Toxicology, Second Edition.
Lynn R. Hovda, Ahna G. Brutlag, Robert H. Poppenga, and Katherine L. Peterson.

Companion website: www.fiveminutevet.com/toxicology

- Calcifediol plasma half-life is ≥10 days.
- Calcitriol plasma half-life is 3–5 days.

Toxicity

- The LD_{50} of cholecalciferol in dogs is 85 mg/kg. These calculations are based on a cholecalciferol rodenticide concentration of 0.075%.
- Clinically, normal dogs and cats have developed hypercalcemia at cholecalciferol dosages of 0.5 mg/kg (20,000 IU/kg).
- Signs of toxicosis (i.e., vomiting, anorexia, weakness) have occurred in clinically normal dogs and cats at cholecalciferol dosages of 0.1 mg/kg (4000 IU/kg).
- Vitamin D analogs are potentially lethal at much lower doses than cholecalciferol.

Systems Affected

- Renal – renal tubular necrosis, impaired calcium and phosphorus homeostasis, metastatic calcification.
- Cardiovascular – bradycardia, ventricular arrhythmias, ECG changes (e.g., shortened QT interval and prolonged PR interval), metastatic calcification.
- Gastrointestinal – metastatic calcification of muscularis in stomach and GIT.
- Respiratory – pulmonary metastatic calcification, decreased lung compliance.
- CNS – variable, from depression and lethargy to seizures.
- Musculoskeletal – excessive calcium mobilization from bones, metastatic calcification, periarticular calcification.

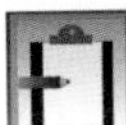

SIGNALMENT/HISTORY

- All breeds and ages of cats and dogs are susceptible to this toxicity.
- Cats and dogs under 6 months of age may be more susceptible.

Risk Factors

- Animals with preexisting diseases such as renal disease or hyperparathyroidism.
- Animals ingesting diets high in calcium and phosphorus.

CLINICAL FEATURES

- The overt clinical signs are vomiting, weakness, lethargy, melena, hemorrhagic diarrhea, depression, PU/PD, and death.
- With examination and diagnostics, hypercalcemia, hyperphosphatemia, renal failure, metabolic acidosis, and bradycardia are found.
- Clinical signs usually begin to occur within 12–36 hours of ingestion.
- Renal failure will occur at 12–36 hours with toxic ingestion.

- Surviving animals may have renal impairment and develop cardiac and GI complications because of calcium deposition and bradycardia.
- Clinical signs may last for weeks because of the slow release of the product from fat stores.

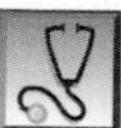

DIFFERENTIAL DIAGNOSIS

- Chronic renal failure
- Ethylene glycol toxicosis
- Grape/raisin toxicosis
- Idiopathic hypercalcemia of cats
- Hypercalcemia of malignancy
- Primary hyperparathyroidism
- Ingestion of prescription skin products containing calcipotriene or tacalcitol
- Ingestion of high-dose oral vitamin D supplements
- Hypoadrenocorticism
- Juvenile hypercalcemia

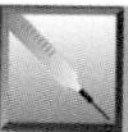

DIAGNOSTICS

- Toxicosis is potentially life threatening when the serum calcium is greater than 12.5 mg/dL, serum phosphorus levels are over 7 mg/dL, and hyposthenuria is documented.
- Phosphorus levels show an increase about 12 hours prior to the calcium level increase and act as a good indicator for treatment with pamidronate or salmon calcitonin.
- Radiographs or ultrasound may show calcification of renal, GI, or vascular tissues.
- Confirmatory tests include serum parathyroid hormone (iPTH), total and ionized calcium, calcifediol (25-monohydroxy D3), and calcitriol (1,25-dihydroxy D3). The combination of tests will differentiate between the various etiologies of hypercalcemia.
  - iPTH is low, total and ionized calcium concentrations are high, calcifediol concentration is high, and calcitriol concentration is normal to low.
- Specific tests for levels of calcipotriene and tacalcitol are not available.

Pathological Findings

- At necropsy, renal tubular degeneration and necrosis; mineralization of the renal tubules, coronary arteries, GIT, and other soft tissues; hemorrhage of gastric mucosa may be evident.
- Concentration of calcifediol levels can be found in renal tissue.

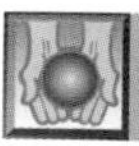

THERAPEUTICS

Detoxification

- Early emesis or gastric lavage.
- Activated charcoal with a cathartic initially, followed by activated charcoal *without* a cathartic q 8 hours for 1–2 days to decrease enterohepatic circulation.

Appropriate Health Care

- Baseline laboratory work (CBC, chemistry panel, venous blood gas, UA, and USG).
- Repeat calcium and phosphorus daily.
- The goal of treatment is to keep the calcium level at less than 12.5 mg/dL and the phosphorus level at less than 7 mg/dL.

Antidote

- No specific antidote is available for vitamin D intoxication.

Drugs of Choice

- Institute 0.9% NaCl diuresis at 2–3 times maintenance until calcium levels decrease.
- If urine output decreases in face of adequate hydration, add the following.
    - Furosemide CRI at 1–2 mg/kg/hour IV.
    - Mannitol bolus at 1–2 g/kg.
- To increase calcium excretion.
    - Furosemide 0.5 mg/kg/hour IV or 2.5–4.5 mg/kg PO TID.
    - Dexamethasone 0.2 mg/kg IV q 12 hours *or* prednisone 2–3 mg/kg PO BID.
- Phosphate binders to keep the calcium × phosphorus product at less than 60 or 70.
    - Aluminum hydroxide 2–10 mL PO q 6 hours if phosphorus levels are high.
- Bisphosphonates to inhibit bone reabsorption and minimize hypercalcemia.
- Currently, pamidronate is the most widely used, although others have been tried.
- Pamidronate disodium (Aredia®).
    - 1.3–2 mg/kg IV diluted in saline and infused over 2 hours for one dose only.
    - Expect serum calcium and phosphorus levels to decrease in 24–48 hours.
    - If levels decrease and then rebound, a second dose may be needed in 5–7 days. Anecdotally, extremely large ingestions have needed redosing in just 3–4 days.
- Antiemetics as needed for persistent vomiting.
    - Maropitant 1 mg/kg SQ q 24 hours.
    - Ondansetron 0.1–0.2 mg/kg IV q 8–12 hours.
- GI protectants.
    - H_2 blockers.
        - □ Famotidine 0.5–1 mg/kg PO, SQ, IM, IV q 12 hours.
        - □ Ranitidine 1–2 mg/kg PO, SQ, IM, IV q 8–12 hours.
        - □ Cimetidine 5–10 mg/kg PO, SQ, IM, IV q 6 hours.
        - □ Omeprazole 0.5–1 mg/kg daily.
        - □ Sucralfate 0.25–1 g PO TID × 5–7 days if evidence of active ulcer disease.

Precautions/Interactions

- Thiazide diuretics are contraindicated as they decrease clearance of calcium.
- Bisphosphonates should rarely be used in combination with calcitonin and then only in the most refractory cases. There is some evidence that the combined use may increase soft tissue mineralization.

- Excessive doses of pamidronate can cause hypocalcemia, and treatment with calcium carbonate may be needed. In severe cases, IV calcium gluconate may be used.

Alternative Drugs

- Salmon calcitonin (Calcimar®, Micalcin®) at 4–7 IU/kg SQ q 8–12 hours.
- Currently used less often than pamidronate due to inconsistencies in treatment and development of resistance after several days of treatment.
- Used instead of pamidronate. All other treatment recommendations remain the same.
- Occasionally both pamidronate and salmon calcitonin must be used to get nonresponsive animals to respond to treatment, but there is some concern for possible soft tissue calcification as a result. Pamidronate is used as the first treatment. If unresponsive, the pet may then receive salmon calcitonin.

Diet

- Low-calcium diet.

COMMENTS

Expected Course and Prognosis

- Outcome depends on the length of and severity of hypercalcemia.
- If calcification has already occurred in the heart, kidneys, lungs or GIT, the prognosis is guarded.
- Hematemesis is associated with a poor prognosis.
- The full course of treatment may take from 1 week to several weeks.

Abbreviations

See Appendix 1 for a complete list.

Calcifediol = 25-monohydroxy D3 = 25-monohydroxycholecalciferol
Calcitriol = 1,25 dihydroxy D3 = 1,25-dihydroxycholecalciferol
iPTH = intact parathyroid hormone
IU = international unit

Suggested Reading

Hare WR, Dobbs C, Slaymen S, et al. Calcipotriene poisoning in dogs. Vet Med 2000; 10:770–778.

Hostutler RA, Chew D, Jaeger J, et al. Uses and effectiveness of pamidronate disodium for treatment of dogs and cats with hypercalcemia. J Vet Int Med 2005; 19:29–33.

Martin TM, De Lorimer LP, Fan TM, et al. Pharmacokinetics and pharmacodynamics of a single dose of zoledronate in healthy dogs. J Vet Pharmacol Ther 2007; 30:492–495.

Pesillo SA, Khan S, Rozanski E, et al. Calcipotriene toxicosis in a dog successfully treated with pamidronate disodium. J Vet Emerg Crit Care 2002; 12(3):177–181.
Rumbeiha WK, Fitzgerald S, Kruger J, et al. Use of pamidronate disodium to reduce cholicalciferol-induced toxicosis in dogs. Am J Vet Res 2000; 61(1):9–13.

Author: Catherine M. Adams, DVM; Robert H. Poppenga, DVM, PhD, DABVT
Consulting Editor: Robert H. Poppenga, DVM, PhD, DABVT

chapter 114

Sodium Monofluoroacetate (Compound 1080)

DEFINITION/OVERVIEW

- Sodium monofluoroacetate (Compound 1080) is a highly water-soluble natural pesticide for mammals that was initially developed in the 1940s.
- It was principally used for the control of gophers, ground squirrels, prairie dogs, rodents, coyotes, and other carnivores in North America. In the USA, 1080 use has been restricted to a livestock protection collar to protect sheep and goats from coyotes.
- It is used for the control of unwanted introduced animals in New Zealand and Australia.
- Sodium monofluoroacetate produces marked CNS and cardiovascular effects.

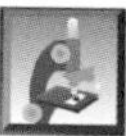

ETIOLOGY/PATHOPHYSIOLOGY

- Poisonings arising from exposure to 1080-based pesticides are rarely observed in veterinary medicine in the USA. Most veterinary cases will involve accidental ingestion although deliberate exposures have also been reported.

Mechanism of Action

- The primary mode of action of 1080 is mediated via its toxic metabolite, fluorocitrate.
- Following absorption, intracellular conversion of 1080 within an animal produces fluorocitrate, which inhibits energy production in the tricarboxylic acid (Krebs) cycle.
- The tricarboxylic acid cycle is a metabolic pathway that breaks down carbohydrates to provide energy for normal cell functions. The inhibition of this metabolic pathway results in accumulation of citrate in the tissues and blood. At high concentrations, citrate binds serum calcium, resulting in hypocalcaemia and ultimately heart failure.
- Death may result from cardiac failure or ventricular fibrillation, progressive CNS depression with either cardiac or respiratory failure as the terminal event, or respiratory arrest following severe convulsions.
- Seizures likely result from altered neurotransmitter concentrations in the CNS.

Blackwell's Five-Minute Veterinary Consult Clinical Companion: Small Animal Toxicology, Second Edition.
Lynn R. Hovda, Ahna G. Brutlag, Robert H. Poppenga, and Katherine L. Peterson.

Companion website: www.fiveminutevet.com/toxicology

Pharmacokinetics – Absorption, Distribution, Metabolism, Excretion

- 1080 is rapidly absorbed from the gastrointestinal tract and lungs. It is not readily absorbed through intact skin.
- Peak plasma concentrations occur within 0.5–3 hours of ingestion.
- 1080 is highly water soluble and is rapidly distributed to most tissues.
- 1080 is excreted in the urine as both the parent (unchanged) chemical and as a range of nontoxic metabolites.
- In most veterinary species the elimination half-life in blood is 1–12 hours.
- The latent period between the time fluoroacetate is ingested and the appearance of clinical signs in mammals is between 0.5 and 3 hours.

Toxicity

Dogs

- LD_{50} in dogs is 0.7 mg/kg BW.

Cats

- Estimated LD_{50} for immature cats is 0.4 mg/kg BW.
- Estimated LD_{50} for cats is 0.2–0.4 mg/kg BW.

Ferrets

- Estimated LD_{50} for ferrets is 1–1.4 mg/kg BW.

Systems Affected

- Nervous – CNS excitation, tremors, seizures.
- Gastrointestinal – nausea, salivation, vomiting.
- Respiratory – cyanosis, respiratory depression (may be cause of death).
- Cardiovascular – cardiac arrhythmias and cardiovascular depression.

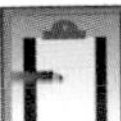

SIGNALMENT/HISTORY

- Canines are more commonly reported to ingest 1080 than felines.
- Younger animals tend to be more likely to consume 1080.
- No breed or age specificity is seen.

Risk Factors

- Dogs are much more sensitive to toxicosis than other species.
- The acute toxicity of 1080 is reduced in New Zealand possums at low ambient temperatures.
- Resistance reportedly can develop after repeated use.

Historical Findings

- The pet owner often notes clinical signs including muscle tremors, severe CNS excitation, and seizures which are not specific for 1080 intoxication.

Location and Circumstances of Poisoning

- Often occurs in locations where the pesticide is used or stored.
- Relay toxicosis from the ingestion of animals poisoned with 1080 has been reported.

CLINICAL FEATURES

- Ingestion may result in an acute onset of CNS excitation, muscle tremors, and seizures.
- Common clinical signs seen include marked CNS disturbances. Poisoned dogs often run uncontrollably, retch and vomit, and appear distressed and agitated with prolonged involuntary muscle contractions exacerbated by seizures prior to death from respiratory failure.
- Prognosis is very guarded in severely affected animals.

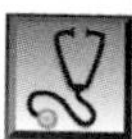

DIFFERENTIAL DIAGNOSIS

- Other toxicants with CNS excitatory effects.
- Primary neurological disease (e.g., inflammatory, infectious, infiltrative, etc.).

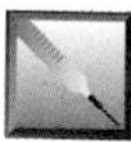

DIAGNOSTICS

Clinical Laboratory Findings

- Diagnosis is dependent upon the presence of an exposure history to a potentially toxic dose of the chemical, the development of appropriate clinical signs, and analytical confirmation of 1080 residues in tissues. Laboratories able to detect 1080 in postmortem samples are limited.
- Alterations in routine serum electrolytes and chemistries are not anticipated unless dehydration is present.
- Variable ECG abnormalities including a prolonged QT interval may also be observed.

Pathological Findings

- Lesions are often absent or nonspecific. Poisoned sheep have developed inflammation, necrosis, and scattered foci of fibrous tissue in the myocardium, pulmonary edema, and inflammation of the lung.
- Analytical chemical confirmation of 1080 residues in fresh frozen muscle, gastric contents, liver, and kidney tissue.

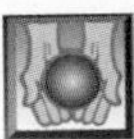

THERAPEUTICS

Detoxification

- Gastrointestinal tract decontamination including early induction of emesis in asymptomatic animals has been reportedly used in Australia; however, neurological signs can rapidly occur and would be a contraindication for emetic use.
- Administration of activated charcoal (0.5–1 mg/kg PO) and an osmotic cathartic (sodium sulfate, 125 mg/kg PO) should be given.

Appropriate Health Care

- Hospitalization is often required to manage severe CNS excitation and respiratory or cardiovascular depression.
- If respiratory function is compromised, a cuffed endotracheal tube should be placed and ventilation supported mechanically as required.
- Maintaining normal body temperature is important.
- Animals should be kept in a padded cage to prevent injury during seizures.

Antidote

- There are no known effective antidotes for 1080.

Drugs of Choice

- A variety of drugs including glycerol monoacetate (at 2–4 g/kg BW, IM), 4-methylpyrazole (20 mg/kg BW, IV), or acetamide partially protect 1080-poisoned animals; however, these treatments are most effective when administered immediately after 1080 ingestion.
- Diazepam (1–2 mg/kg, IV as needed) and/or phenobarbital (5–15 mg/kg, IV as needed) may be given to abolish severe muscle tremors and seizures.
- Methocarbamol 55–220 mg/kg IV, to effect PRN, for control of muscle tremors. Do not exceed 330 mg/kg in 24 hours.
- Judicious calcium administration is also used with confirmed cases of hypocalcemia.

Precautions/Interactions

- Monitor for excessive sedation and respiratory depression with high-dose methocarbamol therapy.

Nursing Care

- Provide respiratory support and mechanical ventilation if needed (very poor prognosis).
- Monitor temperature, heart rate, and respiratory rate.
- Monitor blood pressure and blood glucose frequently and treat appropriately.

Diet

- Moderately to severely affected animals should have food and water withheld to prevent aspiration pneumonia.
- Enteral or parenteral feeding if prolonged neurological complications preclude oral nutrition.

Follow-up

- Follow-up is generally unnecessary, as patients are clinically normal once signs resolve.

Activity

- Patients should be restricted from activity until clinical signs resolve. Once clinical signs resolve, no exercise restriction is necessary.

Prevention/Avoidance

- Prevent access of pets to all pesticides, including 1080-based rodenticides.

COMMENTS

Client Education

- Prevention is critical. Advise clients that all pesticides designed for mammalian pest control are potentially dangerous for their pets and children.
- Early treatment is also important. Clients should be taught to contact their veterinarian if a pesticide exposure has occurred or an animal is displaying unusual clinical signs.

Patient Monitoring

- Acid–base monitoring is recommended in symptomatic animals.
- Blood glucose concentrations should be monitored frequently.

Expected Course and Prognosis

- The survival rate of a poisoned dog is influenced by early recognition by the owner and prompt veterinary management (emesis, lavage, sedation, IV fluids).
- Cases involving only mild signs may resolve with close monitoring and supportive care within a 3–7-day period.
- Veterinary experience in Australia suggests that the survival rate in poisoned dogs is low (approximately 25%).

Abbreviations

See Appendix 1 for a complete list.

Suggested Reading

Eason C, Miller A, Ogilvie S, Fairweather A. An updated review of the toxicology and ecotoxicology of sodium fluoroacetate (1080) in relation to its use as a pest control tool in New Zealand. NZ J Ecol 2011; 35(1):1–20.

Hope A, Smith NA, Temple WA. Treatment of 1080 poisonings in canines – a survey of New Zealand veterinarians. Clin Toxicol 2008; 46(5):382.

Proudfoot AT, Bradberry SM, Vale JA. Sodium fluoroacetate poisoning. Toxicol Rev 2006; 25(4):213–219.

Author: David C. Dorman, DVM, PhD, DABVT, DABT
Consulting Editor: Robert H. Poppenga, DVM, PhD, DABVT

chapter 115

Phosphides

DEFINITION/OVERVIEW

- Zinc phosphide has been used as a rodenticide since the 1930s and is used to control rats, mice, voles, ground squirrels, prairie dogs, nutria, muskrats, feral rabbits, and gophers.
- Aluminum phosphide is also used as a fumigant in grain storage silos and grain transport vehicles.
- OTC products containing 2% zinc phosphide are available in many states; often they are labeled only for below-ground use to control gophers and moles.
- Zinc phosphide is a gray crystalline powder commonly available in 2–10% concentrations as grain- or sugar-based baits in powder, pellet, paste, or tablet formulations.
- Formulations of phosphides commonly have a distinctive odor described as similar to acetylene, rotten fish, or garlic.
- Toxicity is secondary to the production of phosphine gas following ingestion which leads to GI, respiratory, and CNS effects.

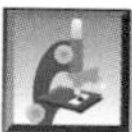

ETIOLOGY/PATHOPHYSIOLOGY

- Zinc (or aluminum and magnesium) phosphide exerts toxic effects due to ingestion, inhalation, or by absorption through broken skin. The most common type of exposure is ingestion with subsequent phosphine gas production.
- Phosphine gas is produced by hydrolysis in a moist or acid environment. The phosphine gas is considered a corrosive and is a direct irritant to the GIT, leading to anorexia, vomiting, and possible hematemesis or melena. The production of phosphine gas within the stomach may lead to gastric or abdominal distension ("bloat") and often pain.
- Profound cardiovascular and respiratory effects can lead to circulatory collapse, cardiac arrhythmias, pulmonary edema, or pleural effusion.
- The smell of rotten fish or acetylene may be noted on the patient's breath or from the vomitus.

Blackwell's Five-Minute Veterinary Consult Clinical Companion: Small Animal Toxicology, Second Edition.
Lynn R. Hovda, Ahna G. Brutlag, Robert H. Poppenga, and Katherine L. Peterson.

Companion website: www.fiveminutevet.com/toxicology

Mechanism of Action

- Zinc phosphine gas is produced by hydrolysis in a moist or acid environment.
- Significant hydrolysis of zinc phosphide occurs at a pH of less than 4, whereas aluminum or magnesium phosphide will undergo hydrolysis at a neutral pH.
- Phosphine gas is considered to have direct corrosive effects on the GIT (esophagus, stomach, and duodenum).
- Phosphine is rapidly absorbed from the GI mucosa and systemically distributed.
- Phosphine may lead to the production of free radicals and oxidative stress, which cause cellular damage and inhibit aerobic respiration.

Pharmacokinetics – Absorption, Distribution, Metabolism, Excretion

- Kinetics of phosphides are not well described.
- Given the rapid onset of clinical signs and the broad range of effects typically seen, there is presumed rapid GI absorption and broad distribution of phosphine gas.
- Oral doses of phosphides result in significant elimination in expired air; available information suggests this may occur within 12 hours after ingestion.

Toxicity

- The approximate toxic dosage of zinc phosphide is believed to be 20–40 mg/kg.
- Several factors affect toxicity, including the amount of food in the stomach, the gastric acid level, and the formulation of zinc phosphide; therefore, the toxic dose varies depending on when the animal last ate.
- Anecdotally, animals that have ingested up to 300 mg/kg on an empty stomach have survived. Consumption of much lower dosages is toxic when consumed with food as a result of increased gastric acid production that promotes hydrolysis.
- Zinc phosphide ingestion can lead to emesis; therefore, the toxicity may be self-limiting in some cases.
- A dose that may produce clinical signs is estimated to be 1/10 of a lethal dose.
- Clinical signs often occur within 15 minutes to 4 hours; death has been reported to occur within 3–48 hours.

Systems Affected

- Gastrointestinal – anorexia, vomiting, hematemesis, melena.
- Cardiovascular – direct myocardial damage, arrhythmias, decreased contractility, hypotension.
- Respiratory – pulmonary edema, pleural effusion.
- Hemic/lymphatic/immune – methemoglobinemia, Heinz body production.
- Nervous – ataxia, weakness, tremors, hyperesthesia, seizures.
- Renal/urological – azotemia, acute renal failure.
- Hepatobiliary – increased ALT, AST, and total bilirubin.

- Endocrine/metabolic – metabolic acidosis; electrolyte imbalances (e.g., potassium and magnesium).
- Musculoskeletal – weakness, ataxia.

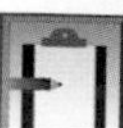

SIGNALMENT/HISTORY

- No known breed or sex predilection.
- Common presenting complaints may include the following.
  - Acute GI signs of vomiting, hematemesis, anorexia, bloating, abdominal pain, and melena.
  - Respiratory distress.
  - Neurological signs of ataxia, tremors, seizures, coma, or sudden death.

Risk Factors

- Ingestion of food will decrease the gastric pH and lead to rapid phosphine gas release.
- Pet owners should be told not to feed their affected pet after exposure (e.g., piece of bread).

Historical Findings

- Determine if there has been potential exposure to rodenticide, and if so, determine the active ingredient of the product used.
- Owners may report acute abdominal distension, pain, emesis, and a malodor noted on the animal's breath.
- In severe cases, respiratory distress, ataxia, seizures, and sudden death have occurred.

Location and Circumstances of Poisoning

- These may be used as household, environmental, or commercially placed baits.

Interactions with Drugs, Nutrients, or Environment

- The toxicity of this product varies depending on the exposure parameters.
- Zinc phosphide will remain stable when placed in a dry environment for 2 weeks, but excessive heat will lead to decreased efficacy of the baits (>122°F).
- Exposure to moisture will cause deterioration of the product.
- Exposure to acid will lead to rapid hydrolysis and phosphine production.
- Some products are formulated to preserve stability in outdoor environments, so occasionally toxicity can persist for extended periods.

CLINICAL FEATURES

- The most common initial clinical signs are vomiting, nausea, and hematemesis.
- The animal may have considerable abdominal distension or pain on palpation.

- A rotten fish odor from the animal's breath or the vomitus is characteristic.
- As phosphine gas is absorbed, there is progression to respiratory distress with labored or raspy breathing and tachypnea.
- Signs may progress to include neurological signs such as ataxia, agitation, aimless wandering or pacing, wild running and barking, tremors, and seizures.
- On PE, the gums may appear cyanotic (hypoxemia) or brown (methemoglobinemia).
- On thoracic auscultation, crackles may be noted.
- Heart rate may be rapid or slow, and arrhythmias may be evident.
- Shock can occur, as demonstrated by rapid heart rate, decreased pulse quality, and cool extremities.
- Neurological assessment will vary depending on the degree of CNS effects.

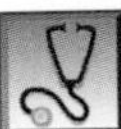

DIFFERENTIAL DIAGNOSIS

- Cholinesterase-inhibiting insecticides (e.g., organophosphorus or carbamates).
- Metaldehyde.
- Serotonin syndrome.
- NSAIDs.
- Tremogenic mycotoxins.
- Primary gastrointestinal disease (e.g., HGE, acute gastroenteritis, parvovirus, etc.).
- Primary cardiac disease (e.g., congestive heart failure).
- Secondary cardiopulmonary disease (e.g., noncardiogenic pulmonary edema from near drowning, seizures, electrocution, ARDS).
- Metabolic disease (renal, hepatic, pancreas).

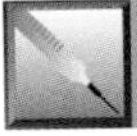

DIAGNOSTICS

- There is no in-house confirmatory test for phosphide rodenticide exposure.
- A suspected exposure, along with consistent clinical signs and an acetylene or rotten fish smell, may support the diagnosis.
- Confirmation using gas chromatography or a Dräger detector tube test can be performed through a diagnostic laboratory. The Dräger test has been validated using canine stomach contents and vomitus. Other postmortem samples for detection of phosphine include the liver and kidney.
- Blood work findings may include the following.
  - Methemoglobinemia or Heinz body formation with evidence of secondary hemolysis.
  - Clinical chemistry panel may reveal azotemia, increased liver enzymes (ALT, AST, and total bilirubin).
  - Electrolyte abnormalities, such as hypokalemia and hypomagnesemia.
  - Other changes may include decreased cholinesterase activity, increased myocardial troponin, metabolic acidosis, and hypoxemia.

Pathological Findings

- Postmortem findings are nonspecific and include venous congestion, capillary breakdown, pulmonary congestion, interlobar lung edema, pleural effusion, hepatic and renal congestion, renal tubular necrosis (in some cases), myocardial necrosis with mononuclear infiltration and fragmentation of fibers, valvular (mitral and aortic) inflammation, and desquamated respiratory epithelium.

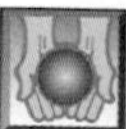

THERAPEUTICS

- Treatment goals are to perform a safe and effective decontamination followed by symptomatic and supportive care.
- Given the risk of phosphine gas exposure to veterinary staff (and owners), clinical judgment and treatment in a well-ventilated area are important considerations. Depending on the patient's clinical presentation, detoxification may include induction of emesis or gastric lavage.
- Administration of an oral liquid antacid may increase gastric pH and thus limit the production of phosphine gas.
- Activated charcoal may decrease toxic effects in zinc phosphide cases.
- Treatment should include gastroprotectants; monitoring for any respiratory, CNS, electrolyte, liver, or kidney effects; and subsequent supportive care.

Detoxification

- Increasing the gastric pH via administration of an oral liquid antacid may decrease or stop the production of phosphine gas.
- Activated charcoal may help decrease the toxicity of zinc phosphide.

Appropriate Health Care

- Symptomatic and supportive care.
- Monitoring for the development of signs in the asymptomatic patient for 12 hours is warranted.
- Hospitalization and care should be continued until life-threatening symptoms resolve.

Antidotes

- There is no antidote available.

Drugs of Choice

- Liquid antacids (such as aluminum hydroxide, magnesium hydroxide, or calcium carbonate) or 5% sodium bicarbonate administered at a dose of 0.5 mL/kg to 1 mL/kg orally may help increase the gastric pH, which may slow or stop the production of phosphine gas. These given prior to emesis induction or at the time of gastric lavage may also protect the veterinary staff due to decreased phosphine gas production.

- Single dose of charcoal at 1–4 g/kg PO.
- Respiratory – if there is evidence of hypoxemia, then oxygen supplementation or mechanical ventilation may be indicated.
- In the presence of shock and for renal protection, IV fluid therapy with either crystalloids or colloids is warranted.
- Gastroprotectants should be used due to the corrosive effects of phosphine gas on the GI mucosa.
  - Famotidine 0.5–1 mg/kg IV q 12 hours.
  - Omeprazole 0.5–1 mg/kg PO q 24 hours.
  - Misoprostol (synthetic prostaglandin analog) may be helpful, 2–5 µg/kg PO q 8 hours.
  - Sucralfate 0.25–1 g PO q 8–12 hours.
- Anticonvulsants to control seizures.
  - Diazepam 0.5 mg/kg IV to effect or CRI at 0.5–1 mg/kg/hour IV.
  - Phenobarbital 4–16 mg/kg IV to effect.
  - Propofol 1–8 mg/kg IV to effect followed by a CRI at 0.1–0.6 mg/kg/hour IV.
- Methocarbamol 50–220 mg/kg IV, to effect; up to 330 mg/kg/day may be effective for tremors.
- Hepatic support.
  - S-adenosyl-methionine 18 mg/kg PO q 24 hours.
  - Silymarin/milk thistle 50–250 mg/day PO q 24 hours.
  - Vitamin K_1 2–3 mg/kg PO q 12–24 hours.
  - Low-protein diet.
- Antioxidants (free radical scavengers and antioxidants may protect tissues from damage).
  - N-acetylcysteine (NAC) may help replace depleted glutathione stores, be directly cytoprotective to the myocardium, and may prevent damage by reactive oxygen species formed due to phosphine gas.
- Methemoglobinemia can be treated with NAC.
  - NAC: loading dose 140 mg/kg IV or PO, followed by intermittent dosing 70 mg/kg IV or PO q 4–6 hours for up to 72 hours.
- Analgesics may be indicated.

Precautions/Interactions

- Examination and emesis should be performed in a well-ventilated area to avoid human exposure to the phosphine gas.
- Do not feed these animals prior to induction of emesis as it may lead to increased phosphine gas production due to the lowering of the gastric pH.

Alternative Drugs

- Magnesium supplementation – there are some reports of hypomagnesemia as a result of zinc phosphine toxicosis and controversy regarding supplementation exists.

- Magnesium plays a key role in the synthesis and activity of glutathione and other antioxidants, which may help counteract some of the damage caused by phosphine gas.
- Pralidoxime (2-PAM).
  - Rat studies have shown that phosphine causes some acetylcholinesterase inhibition.
  - Improved survival is reported with administration of pralidoxime (and atropine) in rats poisoned with aluminum phosphide.
- Melatonin has been shown to decrease tissue damage caused in several organs (brain, heart, liver, kidney, and lungs) by phosphine gas.
- Lipids
  - There are a few clinical reports of the use of coconut oil to decrease phosphine gas production.
  - Studies on the administration of oil (vegetable or paraffin) have been shown in vitro to decrease phosphine gas release.

Nursing Care

- Monitor acid–base status, electrolytes, liver and kidney function, and signs of hypoxemia; intervention should be based on clinical presentation and progression.

Diet

- Due to the GI effects and irritation, a bland diet is indicated for 5–7 days.

Activity

- Case dependent, but should be able to return to normal activity level.

Prevention/Avoidance

- Client education to allow safe use or placement of baits in the animal's environment.

Public Health

- Risk of exposure to phosphine gas by owners (or veterinary staff) if emesis is induced at home, occurs in the car or clinic and not in a well-ventilated area.

COMMENTS

- This can be a very serious or lethal toxicosis.
- Decontamination should take priority, followed by symptomatic and supportive care. The owner should drive with windows down to prevent exposure to phosphine gas should the dog vomit during transport. Veterinary staff should exercise caution and perform any decontamination procedures in a well-ventilated area.

Patient Monitoring

- Close monitoring of the patient in hospital will help guide treatment.
  - Evaluation of respiratory status and hypoxemia should be done frequently on initial presentation.
  - Pulse oximetry monitoring and arterial blood gas analysis may help direct therapy.
  - Presence of hypoxemia and brown-appearing blood should alert the clinician to possible methemoglobinemia.
  - Monitoring of the acid–base status and electrolytes (i.e., ionized calcium, ionized magnesium, sodium, potassium, and chloride) may be indicated.
  - Evaluation of liver and kidney function should be repeated to assess for delayed injury.
- At-home monitoring post treatment for any evidence of GI ulceration or possible perforation.
  - Signs such as weakness, lethargy, anorexia, vomiting, retching, malaise, labored breathing, painful abdomen, etc., should prompt an immediate recheck.
  - Delayed hepatic insults have been reported.
  - Owners should watch for PU/PD, anorexia, vomiting, weight loss, icterus, etc.
  - Acute tubular necrosis is also possible.
  - Animals should be monitored for evidence of renal failure, PU/PD, vomiting, anorexia, and decreased urine production.

Prevention/Avoidance

- Discontinue use and remove baits or discontinue access to bait.

Possible Complications

- Acute renal failure and hepatic damage may follow sublethal exposures.
  - A follow-up clinical chemistry should be evaluated following discharge.

Expected Course and Prognosis

- Asymptomatic patients should be monitored for up to 12 hours.
- Symptomatic patients should be monitored for 48–72 hours or until life-threatening signs resolve and the dog is stable enough for at-home care.

Abbreviations

See Appendix 1 for a complete list.

Suggested Reading

Gray SL, Lee JA, Hovda LR, et al. Potential zinc phosphide rodenticide toxicosis in dogs: 362 cases (2004–2009). J Am Vet Med Assoc 2011; 239(5):646–651.

Schwartz A, Walker R, Sievert J, et al. Occupational phosphine gas poisoning at veterinary hospitals from dogs that ingested zinc phosphide – Michigan, Iowa, and Washington, 2006–2011. *MMWR* 2012; 61(16):286–288.

Fessesswork GG, Stair EL, Johnson BW, et al. Laboratory diagnosis of zinc phosphide poisoning. Vet Hum Toxicol 1994; 36:517–518.

Knight MW. Zinc phosphide. In: Peterson ME, Talcott PA, eds. Small Animal Toxicology, 3rd edn. St Louis, MO: Elsevier, 2013; p. 853.

Proudfoot AT. Aluminum and zinc phosphide poisoning. Clin Toxicol 2009; 47:89–100.

Author: Sarah L. Gray, DVM, DACVECC
Consulting Editor: Robert H. Poppenga, DVM, PhD, DABVT

chapter 116

Strychnine

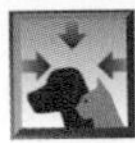 DEFINITION/OVERVIEW

- Strychnine is a very potent alkaloid toxin, derived from the seeds of *Strychnos nux-vomica* and *S. ignatii*. It is used to kill/control ground squirrels, mice, chipmunks, prairie dogs, rats, moles, gophers, birds, and occasionally used on larger predators (e.g., coyotes, wolves, dogs).
- Strychnine is very rapidly absorbed, with onset of clinical signs within 10 minutes to 2 hours.
- Strychnine reversibly blocks the binding of the inhibitory neurotransmitter glycine, resulting in an unchecked reflex stimulation.
- Clinical signs progress from hyperextension of all limbs, extensive muscle rigidity (i.e., with the extensor muscles being more severely affected due to more dominance), seizures, and finally respiratory arrest from paralysis of muscles or respiration.
- Strychnine is eliminated as hepatic metabolites; the parent compound is eliminated in the urine.
- Cause of death is due to apnea, hypoxemia, and respiratory arrest.
- Baits are available in multiple forms and concentrations, and typically range from <0.5% to >0.5%. Lower concentrations are available to the general public in some states, but concentrations >0.5% are limited to use by certified applicators.

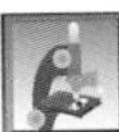 ETIOLOGY/PATHOPHYSIOLOGY

- Malicious poisoning is a relatively common means of exposure.
- Direct exposure to baits is more common in dogs than other domestic species, due to their indiscriminate feeding behavior.
- Relay toxicosis can occur via the ingestion of poisoned rodents and birds.
- Due to more rigid state control and regulation, strychnine toxicosis is less commonly seen.

Mechanism of Action

- Strychnine reversibly blocks the binding of glycine, an inhibitory neurotransmitter in the dorsal horn of the spinal cord and in the CNS.
- The loss of the inhibitory effect in the nervous system results in unchecked spinal reflexes and nerve excitability to the skeletal muscles.

Blackwell's Five-Minute Veterinary Consult Clinical Companion: Small Animal Toxicology, Second Edition.
Lynn R. Hovda, Ahna G. Brutlag, Robert H. Poppenga, and Katherine L. Peterson.

Companion website: www.fiveminutevet.com/toxicology

- Muscle tremors, extensor rigidity, seizures, and respiratory failure develop secondary to toxicosis.

Pharmacokinetics – Absorption, Distribution, Metabolism, Excretion

- Strychnine absorption is very rapid and occurs primarily from the small intestine. A significant amount may also be absorbed from the stomach as well.
- It is widely distributed in the tissues.
- Strychnine is actively metabolized by the liver.
- Parent compound is excreted in the urine.
- Complete elimination should occur by 48–72 hours post ingestion.

Toxicity

- Oral lethal dosage.
  - Dogs: 0.2 mg/kg.
  - Cats: 0.5 mg/kg.
  - Rodents: 1–20 mg/kg.

Systems Affected

- Neuromuscular – uninhibited nerve stimulation leads to continuous muscle stimulation and eventually to tetanic contracture.
- Nervous – uninhibited nerve stimulation leads to seizures.
- Metabolic – continual muscle stimulation leads to metabolic acidosis.
- Musculoskeletal – trauma from the seizure activity can lead to musculoskeletal damage.
- Respiratory –terminal rigidity of respiratory musculature results in apnea and death.

SIGNALMENT/HISTORY

- Occasional history of "rodenticide exposure," but more commonly owners do not know of the exposure.
- Dogs and cats are quite susceptible, as well as all other species.
- All ages of animals are equally susceptible. Unsupervised, outdoor dogs that roam pastures, fields, etc., are at higher risk.
- The most common clinical sign is seizure activity.
- Often, owners do not see the initial signs of muscle tremors.
- Hyperthermia and metabolic acidosis are commonly observed, secondary to the extreme muscle exertion.

Historical Findings

- In the author's experience, the most common history is of malicious poisoning suspicions.
- Occasionally, histories of carcass ingestion are reported.

Location and Circumstances of Poisoning

- Most strychnine poisonings occur in rural areas and agricultural communities. However, it could occur in any area.

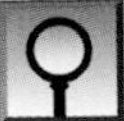

CLINICAL FEATURES

- Clinical signs can develop within 10–120 minutes of ingestion.
- Violent tetanic seizures may be initiated by physical, visible, or auditory stimuli.
- Extensor rigidity.
- Muscle stiffness.
- Opisthotonus.
- Tachycardia.
- Hyperthermia.
- Metabolic acidosis.
- Apnea.
- Vomiting – very rare.
- Death.
- Recovery should be less than 48–72 hours.

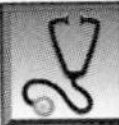

DIFFERENTIAL DIAGNOSIS

- Other toxicants.
  - 1080 (fluoroacetate)
  - 4-aminopyridine
  - Amphetamines
  - Antidepressants
  - Caffeine
  - Chocolate
  - Cocaine
  - Lead
  - LSD
  - Metaldehyde
  - Nicotine
  - Organochlorine insecticides
  - Pyrethrins or pyrethroids
  - Tremorgenic mycotoxins
  - Zinc phosphide
- Systemic diseases: uremia, electrolyte abnormalities (e.g., hypocalcemia) and hepatic encephalopathy, CNS neoplasia, hypoglycemia, encephalitides, heat stroke, trauma, ischemia, tetanus, epilepsy.

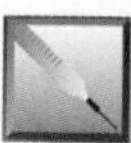

DIAGNOSTICS

- Serum chemistries will identify high CK and lactate dehydrogenase, as well as a systemic metabolic acidosis on venous blood gas analysis.
- Evidence of myoglobinuria may be present on UA.
- Analysis of stomach contents, liver, kidney, blood, or urine for the presence of strychnine.
  - If death is too rapid, kidney and urine may be negative.
- Death from strychnine intoxication is often rapid, with significant bait material still present in the stomach on autopsy.
  - Often, the color-coded grains or pellets (red or green) are obvious in the stomach contents.
  - The sample of choice for testing is generally stomach contents.

Pathological Findings

- Gross and histological pathology is associated with trauma from the seizure activity.
- Red or green pellets or bait stations are often found in the stomach contents.

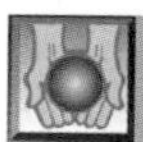

THERAPEUTICS

- Inpatient therapy may require treatment for as long as 48–72 hours.
- Primary goals are preventing dehydration, controlling seizures, maintaining cerebral perfusion, reducing ICP, preventing hypoxemia, and treating muscle rigidity. This often requires care in a 24/7 facility, mechanical ventilation with aggressive sedation, the use of mannitol (to decrease ICP), oxygen therapy, IV fluid therapy, thermoregulation, and nursing care.

Detoxification

- Early decontamination is imperative to minimize duration and severity of clinical signs.
  - Decontamination – activated charcoal (2 g/kg PO); cathartic (sorbitol at 2.1 g/kg PO; magnesium sulfate at 0.5 g/kg PO).
- In asymptomatic patients, immediate emesis induction should be performed, followed by activated charcoal with a cathartic. Because strychnine undergoes enterohepatic recirculation, an additional dose of activated charcoal, this time without a cathartic, should be given orally q 6–8 hours for 24 hours.
- In symptomatic patients, sedation, control of the airway (with an inflated ETT), and gastric lavage are imperative for recent ingestion. Activated charcoal should be administered with a gastric tube once the stomach has been thoroughly lavaged.

Appropriate Health Care

- Patients should be sedated in a quiet, dimly lit room, with cotton earplugs in place to prevent auditory stimulation.

- Patients should be treated with IV fluid therapy q 8 hours for 24 hours to maintain hydration, perfusion, and aid in strychnine elimination and urinary excretion.
- Control tremors and seizures. The use of anticonvulsants is imperative with strychnine toxicosis.
- Supportive care and nursing care.
  - Minimize animal stimulation to avoid inducing a seizure.
  - Control hyperthermia. Monitor temperature q 2–4 hours; implement cooling measures when temperatures exceed 105.5°F. Cooling measures should be stopped when temperatures reach 103.5°F.
  - Change body position and lubricate eyes q 4–6 hours.
  - Avoid nutritional feeding (orally) until clinical signs resolve in order to prevent aspiration pneumonia.

Antidote

- No specific antidote.

Drugs of Choice

- Seizure control.
  - Phenobarbital 4–16 mg/kg IV q 2–6 hours PRN.
  - Potassium bromide 100 mg/kg PO or rectally q 6 hours × 4 doses.
  - Diazepam 0.5–1 mg/kg IV to effect.
- Tremor control.
  - Methocarbamol 55–100 mg/kg IV q 2–6 hours PRN.
  - Glycerol guaiacolate 110 mg/kg IV, repeated as needed.
- Urinary acidification – ammonium chloride (150 mg/kg) is reported to enhance elimination, based on the principle of ion trapping, but this has not been shown to be a practical clinical application and is not commonly done.

Precautions/Interactions

- Do not induce emesis in symptomatic patients due to risks of aspiration pneumonia and seizure stimulation.
- Do not acidify with ammonium chloride if the patient is acidotic, based on venous blood gas analysis.

Activity

- Normal activity should resume upon recovery, unless traumatic injuries limit activity.

COMMENTS

- Although anesthetic intervention does not directly treat the cause of the seizures, it provides the time necessary for the animal to eliminate the offending compound.

- CAUTION: Do not induce a seizure with a stimulus as a means of diagnosing strychnine. This is *not* diagnostic and may be lethal.
- Due to potential exposure to and poisoning of children, the source of the exposure should be investigated and eliminated.
- Strychnine is degraded by soil organisms.
- Strychnine poisoning is *not* treatable at home. If exposure has occurred, have the owner bring the animal to the clinic immediately. If clients wait until clinical signs occur, the animal may be dead before it reaches the clinic.

Patient Monitoring

- Monitor for secondary renal damage from myoglobinuria and possible tubular cast development. Aggressive treatment with IV fluids should be used to prevent this.
- With sedation/anesthesia to control the seizures, the animal can be gradually withdrawn periodically to evaluate the reoccurrence of seizure activity as a means of determining how long the treatment must be continued.
- Early significant decontamination will shorten the duration of required treatment.

Prevention/Avoidance

- Prevention is limited to keeping animals away from baits or poisoned carcasses, and supervising dogs at all times (instead of free roaming).
- Prevent reexposure by removing the source of the toxin.

Possible Complications

- Dependent on the initiation of therapy, hypoxemia that occurred prior to therapy can have permanent neurological effects.
- Renal damage secondary to myoglobinuria will gradually repair.

Expected Course and Prognosis

- Prognosis is poor until seizures are controlled.
- Prognosis is good after seizures are controlled, but prior hypoxemia and secondary renal effects should be discussed with the owner.
- Animals that have normal neurological function at 48–72 hours should have no permanent effect.

See Also

Decontamination and Detoxification of the Poisoned Patient
Emergency Management of the Poisoned Patient

Abbreviations

See Appendix 1 for a complete list.

Suggested Reading

Gupta RC. Non-anticoagulant rodenticides. In: Gupta RC, ed. Veterinary Toxicology Basic and Clinical Principles. San Diego, CA: Elsevier, 2012; pp. 698–711.

Osweiler GD. Strychnine poisoning. In: Kirk RW, ed. Current Veterinary Therapy VIII. Philadelphia, PA: Saunders, 1983; pp. 98–100.

Talcott PA. Strychnine. In: Peterson ME, Talcott PA, eds. Small Animal Toxicology. Ames, IA: Elsevier, 2013; pp. 827–831.

Author: Jeffery O. Hall, DVM, PhD, DABVT
Consulting Editor: Robert H. Poppenga, DVM, PhD, DABVT

Toxic Gases

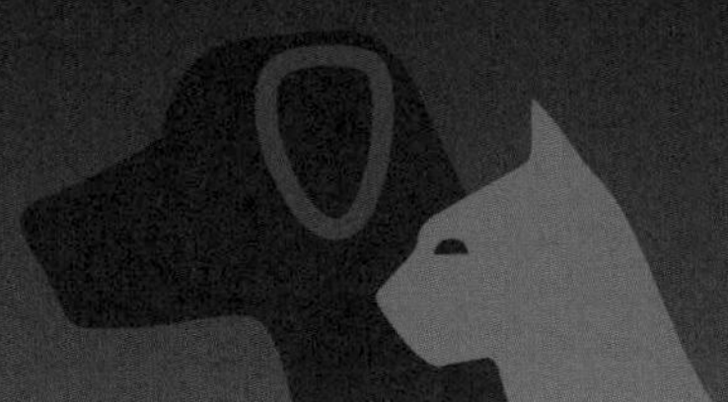

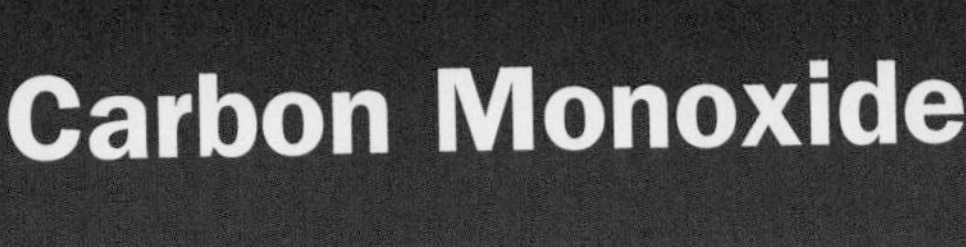

chapter 117

Carbon Monoxide

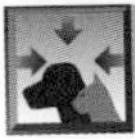

DEFINITION/OVERVIEW

- Carbon monoxide (CO) is a colorless, odorless, toxic gas; common sources of CO include fires, generators, motor vehicle exhaust, and heaters.
- The majority of reported exposures in veterinary medicine are secondary to smoke inhalation from structural fires.
- Clinical effects include respiratory distress, cardiovascular effects, and neurological signs.

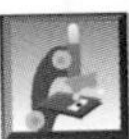

ETIOLOGY/PATHOPHYSIOLOGY

Mechanism of Action

- Tissue and cellular hypoxia are hallmarks of CO toxicity. Hemoglobin binds CO (COHb) with very high affinity, resulting in decreased oxygen (O_2) binding and decreased oxygen content in the blood. Additionally, COHb shifts the oxyhemoglobin saturation curve to the left, impairing release of O_2 at the tissues.
- Organs with high oxygen demand such as the brain and heart are most severely affected by hypoxia.
- Acute and delayed (days to weeks) neurological signs have been reported secondary to CO exposure. The cause is likely multifactorial and may include hypoxic insult to the brain, cerebral hypoperfusion secondary to hypotension, and lipid peroxidation damaging neurons.

Systems Affected

- Cardiovascular – tachycardia, arrhythmias, hypotension, brick red mucous membranes.
- Central nervous system – acute and delayed neurological signs can be observed such as altered mentation, ataxia, blindness, deafness, and seizures.
- Respiratory – tachypnea, increased respiratory effort, increased lung sounds, bronchospasm; may have concurrent smoke inhalation injury (see Chapter 118 – Smoke Inhalation).

Blackwell's Five-Minute Veterinary Consult Clinical Companion: Small Animal Toxicology, Second Edition.
Lynn R. Hovda, Ahna G. Brutlag, Robert H. Poppenga, and Katherine L. Peterson.

Companion website: www.fiveminutevet.com/toxicology

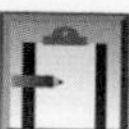

SIGNALMENT/HISTORY

- No species or breed predilection.

Historical Findings

- Dogs and cats presenting with CO toxicosis often have a history of being in a fire or in an enclosed space without adequate ventilation.

CLINICAL FEATURES

- Physical exam findings include hypothermia, increased respiratory effort, abnormal lung sounds, tachycardia, arrhythmias.
- Acute neurological signs can include altered mentation, ataxia, blindness, deafness, and seizures.
- Other clinical signs following exposure to fire/smoke inhalation may include dermal burns, corneal ulcers, and respiratory distress due to thermal damage to upper airways and bronchoconstriction.

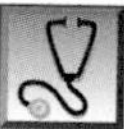

DIFFERENTIAL DIAGNOSIS

- Primary respiratory disease (pneumonia, bronchitis, asthma, pulmonary edema).
- Primary CNS disease (metabolic, infectious, neoplastic, immune mediated).
- Metabolic disease (e.g., hepatic encephalopathy).
- Toxicities – neurotoxins, drug ingestion/overdose.

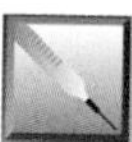

DIAGNOSTICS

- A minimum database, including CBC, serum chemistry, and urinalysis should be performed to evaluate organ function and eliminate other potential causes for neurological signs.
- Blood COHb levels should be obtained at presentation and monitored q 24 hours until normal. This requires CO-oximetry which is available at most human hospitals and some veterinary referral hospitals; COHb levels of $<1\%$ are considered normal in dogs.
- Arterial blood gas should be performed if available.
- Pulse oximetry (SpO_2) is not useful in evaluation of animals with CO toxicity as the value is falsely elevated. The pulse oximeter cannot distinguish between oxyhemoglobin and carboxyhemoglobin. All patients with CO exposure should be assumed to have decreased blood oxygen content.

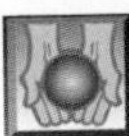

THERAPEUTICS

Detoxification

- Patients should be removed from the environment and provided with fresh air and oxygen supplementation as soon as possible.

Appropriate Health Care

- Supplemental O_2 therapy is the cornerstone of therapy as it expedites elimination of COHb.
  - On room air (FiO_2 21%), the half-life of COHb is 4–6 hours.
  - Half-life is reduced to 40–80 minutes if a patient is intubated and breathing 100% oxygen.
  - Most patients can be managed in an oxygen cage (FiO_2 40–60%) or with nasal O_2 (FiO_2 40–60%) until COHb levels return to normal (typically within 24–48 hours).
- In severe cases or where available, hyperbaric oxygen can be considered.
- IV fluids should be administered to promote normal tissue perfusion and prevent hypotension.

Antidote

- There is no antidote to CO toxicosis.

Nursing Care

- Patients should have recumbent patient care.
- Dogs should have respiratory rate and effort, heart rate/ECG, and blood pressures monitored every 2–6 hours as needed.
- Gloves should be worn at all times in patients with concurrent burns and open wounds.

Activity

- Restrict activity until COHb levels are normal.

COMMENTS

Patient Monitoring

- COHb levels should be monitored q 24 hours until normal.
- Serial neurological evaluation and seizure monitoring while in the hospital.

Prevention/Avoidance

- Patients should not be left in a confined space with a generator or engine running.

Possible Complications

- Neurological signs can develop hours to days after exposure to CO despite initial improvement in clinical signs.

Expected Course and Prognosis

- Prognosis is fair to poor.
- Recent case reports have demonstrated that even animals with very elevated levels of COHb can survive with appropriate oxygen therapy and supportive care.
- Neurological recovery is variable and signs may improve over days to weeks.

See Also

Smoke Inhalation

Abbreviations

See Appendix 1 for a complete list.

COHb = carboxyhemoglobin
HbO_2 = oxyhemoglobin

Suggested Reading

Ashbaugh EA, Mazzaferro EM, McKiernan BC, et al. The association of physical examination abnormalities and carboxyhemoglobin concentrations in 21 dogs trapped in a kennel fire. J Vet Emerg Crit Care 2012; 22(3):361–367.

Ayres, DA. Pulse oximetry and CO-oximetry. In: Burkitt-CreedonJM, ed. Advanced Monitoring and Procedures for Small Animal Emergency and Critical Care. Chichester, West Sussex: Wiley–Blackwell, 2012; pp. 274–285.

Berent AC, Todd J, Sergeeff J. Carbon monoxide toxicity: a case series. J Vet Emerg Crit Care 2005; 15(2):128–135.

Kent M, Creevy KE, deLahunta A. Clinical and neuropathological findings of acute carbon monoxide toxicity in chihuahuas following smoke inhalation. J Am Anim Hosp Assoc 2010; 46:259–264.

Acknowledgment: The authors and editors acknowledge the prior contributions of Lisa L. Powell, DVM, DACVECC, who authored this topic in the previous edition.
Author: Jennifer M. Hall, DVM, DACVECC
Consulting Editor: Katherine L. Peterson, DVM, DACVECC

chapter 118

Smoke Inhalation

DEFINITION/OVERVIEW

- Smoke inhalation represents an uncommon form of pulmonary injury and neurological impairment in veterinary patients, which likely reflects high prehospital admission mortality as opposed to infrequent occurrence.
- Carbon monoxide (CO), cyanide, direct thermal injury, combustion products, and particulate matter that result from burned materials in the fire contribute to the pathophysiology of smoke inhalation.
- Common clinical signs include neurological impairment and respiratory distress, both of which may be delayed in onset.
- Treatment is aimed at alleviating clinical signs and addressing the toxic effects of combusted materials.
- Provision of supplemental oxygen is the highest treatment priority, especially if possible before hospital admission. Additional management strategies include judicious fluid therapy, pain management, and specific treatment of known inhaled toxins.
- The use of empirical antibiotic therapy is not indicated unless a secondary bacterial pneumonia is present. Corticosteroids are not recommended.
- There are limited studies in veterinary patients treated for smoke inhalation; sources indicate a fair to good prognosis when severe skin burns are not present. Significant neurological dysfunction may worsen prognosis.

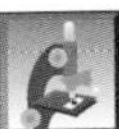

ETIOLOGY/PATHOPHYSIOLOGY

Mechanism of Action

- The severity of smoke inhalation insult is determined by:
  - amount of time spent in the fire
  - type of materials burned
  - amount of heat generated
  - amount of oxygen available
  - animal's health status.

Blackwell's Five-Minute Veterinary Consult Clinical Companion: Small Animal Toxicology, Second Edition.
Lynn R. Hovda, Ahna G. Brutlag, Robert H. Poppenga, and Katherine L. Peterson.

Companion website: www.fiveminutevet.com/toxicology

- The mechanism of action is usually attributed to nonirritant gases (e.g., CO, hydrogen cyanide, CO_2), thermal injury, and smoke toxicosis from released irritant gases and particulate matter.
- Carbon monoxide is believed to be the leading cause of death in animals exposed to fires and smoke. Carbon monoxide's generation, mechanism of action, and toxicity are discussed in chapter 117.
- Common sources of cyanide in household fires include the combustion of fabrics, photographic film, photocopier paper, polyfluorocarbons, polyvinyl acetate, resins, polyurethane foam, and plastic.
- Cyanide toxicosis causes histotoxic hypoxia due to inhibition of oxidative phosphorylation. With impaired oxygen extraction and utilization, there is conversion to anaerobic metabolism in order to facilitate cellular respiration. The end result is accumulation of lactic acid and lactic acidosis.
- Increased inspired CO_2 is not only a nonirritating asphyxiant gas, but it also functions to increase respiratory rate, which further increases inhalation of the other components of smoke.
- The majority of thermal injury secondary to smoke inhalation is restricted to the oral and nasal cavities and larynx due to effective mechanisms for heat dissipation in the upper airway. These effects can be delayed for approximately 24–72 hours.
- Unless steam or superheated particulate matter is inhaled, thermal injury to the lower airways and pulmonary parenchyma is uncommon.
- Chemicals released from burned materials, as well as particulate matter, contribute to the toxicosis of inhaled smoke and the resultant mucosal damage, pulmonary injury, and bronchoconstriction.
- Common inhaled irritants within smoke include ammonia, acrolein, hydrogen chloride, and chlorine gas.

Pharmacokinetics – Absorption, Distribution, Metabolism, Excretion

- For specific information about the pharmacokinetics, absorption, metabolism, and excretion of carbon monoxide, please see chapter 117.
- Cyanide inhalation results in rapid development of clinical signs within seconds to minutes. Most cyanide is converted to thiocyanate, which is formed primarily in the liver and then excreted by the kidneys.
- Carbon dioxide produced in fires is inhaled. Due to its rapid diffusion across the alveoli, it causes increased pCO_2 within the arterial circulation, and subsequent increased respiratory rate secondary to brainstem response. Hyperventilation is effective at decreasing the pCO_2, but it also increases the inhalation of other toxins within the smoke.
- Irritants can be absorbed by inhalation (most common) or by ingestion if there is deposition of the chemical on the pet's haircoat and ingestion during grooming.
- Due to the variety of chemicals released from fire, there is very limited information about the metabolism and excretion of inhaled chemicals in small animals.

Toxicity

- The toxicity of carbon monoxide is discussed in chapter 117.
- There are no documented cases of cyanide toxicosis secondary to smoke inhalation in small animals; however, cyanide toxicosis is thought to have a role in the toxicity of smoke inhalation.
- In small animal patients, there are no standard or known toxic doses for the other toxins released from fires.

Systems Affected

- Respiratory.
    - Oropharyngeal, nasopharyngeal, and laryngeal burns, ulcers, erosions, inflammation, and/or edema.
    - Coughing, tachypnea, dyspnea due to the following.
        - Inhibition of mucociliary escalator function and mucosal sloughing.
        - Deposition of particulate matter along the lower airways and alveoli.
        - Tracheobronchitis.
        - Intraalveolar hemorrhage.
    - Bronchospasm, bronchoconstriction, and obstruction of small airways.
    - Hypoxemia.
    - Hyper- or hypoventilation.
    - Pulmonary edema.
    - ARDS and ALI.
    - Bacterial pneumonia.
- Nervous.
    - Cerebral vasodilation.
    - Cerebral hypoxia.
    - Cerebral edema.
    - Direct effect of toxins on the CNS.
    - Seizures/stupor/coma.
- Cardiovascular.
    - Hyperemic mucous membranes due to CO and cyanide toxicosis and local vasodilation.
    - Myocardial and tissue hypoxia.
    - Carbon monoxide-induced cardiotoxic dysfunction.
    - Mitochondrial cytochrome oxidase dysfunction.
    - Vasodilation (systemic).
    - Methemoglobinemia.
    - Hypovolemia and hypotension.
- Ophthalmic.
    - Direct corneal injury/ulcers from heat, smoke, and particulate matter.
    - Local irritation from chemicals and particulate matter.
- Skin/exocrine.
    - Direct burn and chemical injury, especially to nonhaired skin.

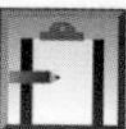

SIGNALMENT/HISTORY

- There are no species, breed, or sex predilections.
- Studies on smoke exposure in dogs and cats showed a median age of approximately 3 years. The young median age is speculated to be due to younger animals' better survival of smoke inhalation and arrival at a veterinary hospital for treatment, in contrast to older pets.

Risk Factors

- Those animals that are commonly kept as pets in the home, or housed in barns and stalls, are at the highest risk.
- May occur more in colder months, from November to March, when more animals are indoors, windows are closed, and heaters are being used with greater frequency.
- Very large animals or animals with underlying disease, such as cardiovascular, respiratory, or musculoskeletal diseases, may be at higher risk of prolonged exposure or death from smoke inhalation if they are physically unable to get out of the burning structure or if they are unable to be moved by their owners or emergency responders.

Historical Findings

- Signs reported at the scene of the fire include the following.
  - Dyspnea.
  - Vocalizing.
  - Coughing, gagging.
  - Open-mouthed breathing (cats).
  - Loss of consciousness.
  - Lethargy (cats).
  - Weakness and ataxia.
  - Foaming from the mouth and/or hypersalivation.
  - Smoke smell on the haircoat.

Location and Circumstances of Poisoning

- Animals have a history of being exposed to a fire or smoke-filled enclosure.

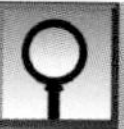

CLINICAL FEATURES

- Respiratory – tachypnea, respiratory distress, open-mouthed breathing (cats; Fig. 118.1), increased bronchovesicular sounds, wheezes, crackles, or moist lung sounds on auscultation, coughing, nasal discharge.
- Nervous – lethargy, depression, ataxia, stupor, coma, excitement/agitation, seizures.
- Cardiovascular – hyperemic mucous membranes, gray/cyanotic mucous membranes, tachycardia, decreased pulse quality, decreased heart sounds on auscultation (cats), gallop rhythm (cats).

- Ophthalmic – blepharospasm, corneal ulceration, third eyelid elevation, conjunctival hyperemia, miotic or mydriatic pupils, epiphora.
- Skin/exocrine – smoke odor to fur, singed hair or burnt skin (especially on the face and footpads) (Fig. 118.2), soot on the skin, skin lacerations.
- Gastrointestinal – hypersalivation (cats).

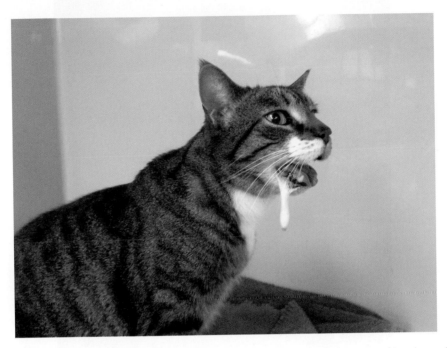

Fig. 118.1. Open mouth breathing and marked hypersalivation in a cat after being trapped in a house fire. Photo courtesy of Dana L. Clarke.

DIFFERENTIAL DIAGNOSIS

- Inhalation of other toxins or substances.
- Pulmonary parenchymal disease such as pneumonia or pulmonary fibrosis.
- Lower airway disease such as asthma, bronchitis, or chronic lower airway disease.
- Upper airway obstruction such as laryngeal paralysis, brachycephalic airway syndrome, or tracheal collapse.
- Pleural space disease such as pneumothorax and pleural effusion.
- Primary cardiac disease with or without congestive heart failure.
- Primary neurological disease such as seizures, toxins, or inflammatory CNS disorders.
- Anaphylaxis.
- Systemic inflammatory response syndrome (SIRS).
- Septic or distributive shock.

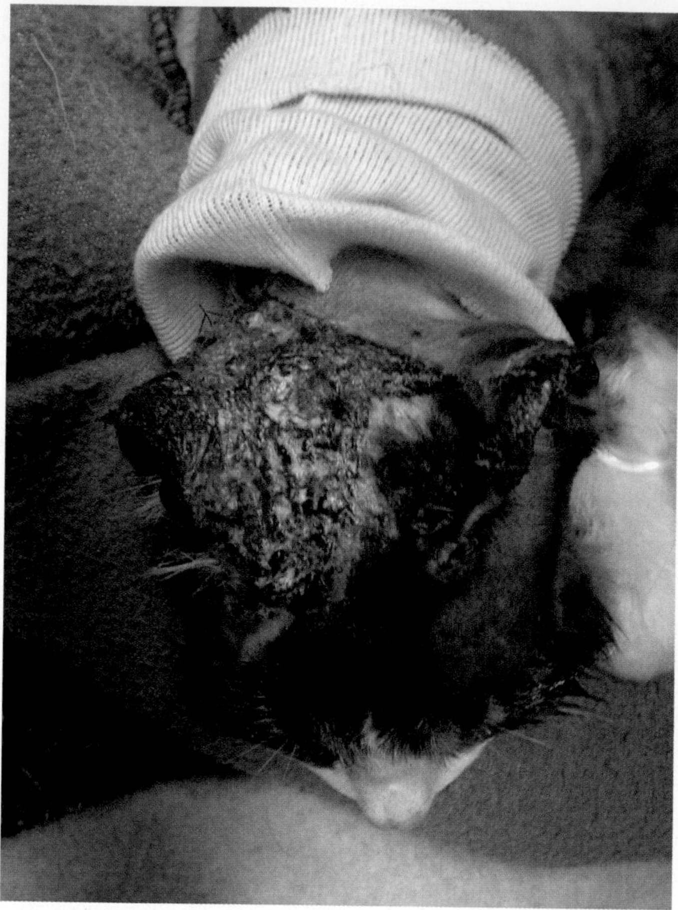

■ **Fig. 118.2.** Significant facial burns and pinna loss in a cat that was maliciously set on fire. Photo courtesy of Dana L. Clarke.

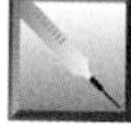

DIAGNOSTICS

- Diagnostics needed to confirm carbon monoxide toxicity are discussed in chapter 117.
- Blood cyanide levels are the gold standard for diagnosing cyanide toxicosis; not widely available. Lethal blood cyanide level in dogs was found to be 438 ± 40 µg/dL in experimental studies.
- Severe lactic acidosis with adequate perfusion suggests cyanide and/or carbon monoxide toxicosis; this can be measured on a handheld lactometer or via blood gas analysis.
- Pulse oximetry is a readily available, noninvasive, rapid diagnostic tool to assess oxygen saturation of hemoglobin. Results must be interpreted with caution since carboxyhemoglobin or MetHb can cause overestimation of the true saturation of hemoglobin with oxygen.
- Minimum database (PCV/TS, blood glucose, and BUN) should be obtained at presentation and reassessed every 4–6 hours, especially in response to IV fluid therapy. Studies have

found that cats and dogs more severely affected by smoke inhalation have a higher PCV and lower BG.

- Blood gas analysis.
    - Arterial blood gas analysis to assess acid–base status, ventilation and oxygenation, even in the presence of carboxyhemoglobin and MetHb.
    - Venous blood gas analysis can also provide similar information but cannot assess oxygenation status.
- Thoracic radiographs – common radiographic changes include diffuse or focal bronchial, interstitial, and alveolar patterns, or any combination of these patterns (Fig. 118.3). Other described changes include pleural effusion and right middle lung lobe consolidation.
- Complete ocular examination is warranted, including measurement of tear production, fluorescein staining, and thorough examination of the conjunctiva, scleral, cornea, and eyelids.
- CBC, serum chemistry, and coagulation profile are warranted in any symptomatic patient.
- Endotracheal or transtracheal wash and/or protected specimen brush sample cytology and aerobic culture are helpful to confirm smoke inhalation (when carbon particulate matter is retrieved) and when there is concern for the presence of pneumonia (e.g., aspiration, complication of severe pulmonary parenchymal injury, ventilator-associated pneumonia).

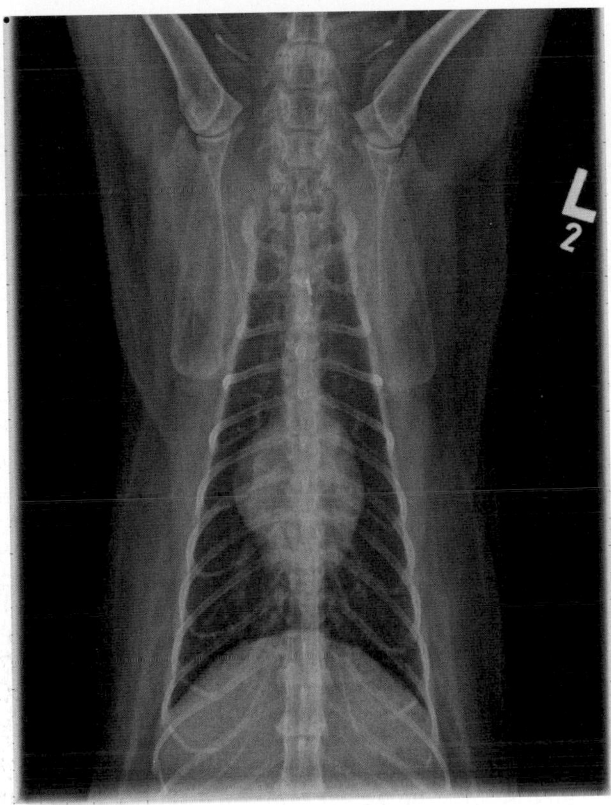

Fig. 118.3. Ventrodorsal thoracic radiograph of a cat exposed to smoke in a house fire. Radiograph shows a generalized diffuse bronchointerstitial pattern. Photo courtesy of Dana L. Clarke.

- Bronchoscopy and bronchoalveolar lavage can help diagnose smoke inhalation, bronchial obstruction, and disease localized to a single lung lobe.

Pathological Findings

- The gross and histopathological findings are determined by individual inhaled toxins, degree of injury to the respiratory tract and CNS, and extent of burns and ocular injury.
- On gross examination, there may be burns of varying severity and ocular injury such as corneal edema and ulcers, hyperemia, and foreign material in the conjunctival fornix.
- Nasopharyngeal, oropharyngeal, and laryngeal burns, erosions, ulcerations, inflammation, and edema may be present.
- Tracheal inflammation, edema, and particulate matter deposition may be present. Mucosal edema, mucosal sloughing, and pseudomembranous casts may also be seen.
- Histological evaluation of the pulmonary parenchyma may show particulate matter, edema, hyaline casts, intraalveolar hemorrhage, purulent material consistent with pneumonia, and atelectasis.
- Other than carbon particulate matter along the airway and within the alveoli, there are no characteristic histopathological changes associated with smoke inhalation.

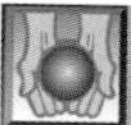

THERAPEUTICS

- The goals of treatment include supplemental oxygen, administration of toxin-specific antidotes (if possible), maintaining patency of the airway (especially the upper airway), preserving hydration, and supportive and nursing care.
- Supplemental oxygen therapy is vital. Methods of administering supplemental oxygen include flow-by, mask, nasal oxygen, oxygen cage, and intubation.
- Treatment of carbon monoxide toxicosis is discussed in chapter 117. Specific treatment of cyanide toxicosis is discussed below.
- Patients should be intensely monitored for signs of progressive upper airway inflammation, and obstruction. If upper airway obstruction is present, intubation and/or tracheostomy may be necessary.
- Mechanical ventilation may be necessary for patients with hypoxemia, hypoventilation, or continued respiratory distress despite therapy.
- If hypovolemic shock is present, patients should be treated with crystalloid and/or colloid therapy to correct their intravascular volume deficit. Once euvolemic, fluid therapy in smoke inhalation patients should be judicious due to the concern for pulmonary capillary leak and secondary pulmonary edema, especially in cats.

Appropriate Health Care

- Patients should be carefully monitored for vomiting, regurgitation, and inability to protect their airway. Aspiration pneumonia in addition to the pulmonary compromise from smoke inhalation can be a serious, if not fatal, complication.

- Smoke inhalation patients, especially those with significant dermal burns, are at increased risk for sepsis, therefore measures to prevent hospital-acquired infections, such as wearing gloves and gowns and hand washing, should be adhered to strictly.

Drugs and Antidotes of Choice

- Bronchodilators may be considered, especially in patients with concern about bronchoconstriction and wheezing.
    - Albuterol 2–3 puffs q 2–4 hours PRN.
    - Terbutaline 0.01 mg/kg IV, IM, SQ q 8 hours.
- Cough suppressants should be avoided. Opioids should be used judiciously as an analgesic due to their suppression of the cough reflex.
- Antiemetic therapy in vomiting or nauseated patients.
    - Maropitant 1 mg/kg SQ q 24 hours.
    - Ondansetron 0.1–0.5 mg/kg IV q 8–12 hours.
- Sodium thiosulfate (25%) can be used to treat cyanide toxicosis at a dose of 150–500 mg/kg IV as either a bolus or CRI.
- In people, inhalation therapies with heparin, N-acetylcysteine, and epinephrine are used for bronchodilation or free radical scavenging properties.

Precautions/Interactions

- Corticosteroids are not indicated for smoke inhalation patients as there is no evidence of clinical benefit and they may have unwanted side effects.
- Empiric antibiotic therapy is not recommended in victims of smoke exposure due to concerns for bacterial resistance. If bacterial pneumonia is documented via airway sampling, antibiotic selection should be based on culture and sensitivity testing.
- Sodium nitrate should not be used in smoke inhalation patients to treat cyanide toxicosis; may exacerbate decreased oxygen-carrying capacity via the formation of methemoglobinemia.

Nursing Care

- Supportive care for patients with smoke inhalation includes:
    - maintenance of oral and eye care for recumbent patients
    - saline nebulization for 15–20 minutes, every 4–6 hours as needed
    - wound care and pain management.

Follow-up

- Thoracic radiographs should be rechecked in 1–2 weeks from hospital discharge.

Diet

- For patients with any neurological compromise, vomiting, regurgitation, or those that are sedated, oral food and water should be withheld until the patient is neurologically appropriate and GI signs have resolved.

Activity

- Activity should be restricted until there is complete resolution of any pulmonary parenchymal disease.

Surgical Considerations

- Surgical tracheostomy could be necessary if there is upper airway obstruction impeding ventilation.
- For patients with significant dermal injuries requiring general anesthesia for debridement, sterile ETT and anesthetic tubing should be used. Other anesthetic considerations include avoidance of high airway pressures during ventilation and limiting the duration of anesthesia and number of anesthetic events as much as possible.

COMMENTS

Client Education

- Emergency first responders should be educated to provide all rescued smoke inhalation animals with oxygen supplementation prior to arrival to the hospital.

Patient Monitoring

- Pulse oximetry can be used several times per day to monitor for improvement in oxygenation; can be falsely elevated with carboxyhemoglobinemia and methemoglobinemia.
- Arterial or venous blood gas monitoring should be performed at least daily to assess oxygenation (arterial samples only), ventilation, and acid–base balance.

Possible Complications

- Limited information about long-term complications in veterinary patients.
- Concerns for long-term complications include pulmonary fibrosis, asthma, and chronic obstructive pulmonary disease.
- Patients with severe neurological dysfunction may have residual neurological deficits long term, though these would likely be mild in surviving patients.
- Patients may have a short-term increased risk of pulmonary and dermal infections, sepsis, and neurological dysfunction.

Expected Course and Prognosis

- In a retrospective study of 27 dogs with smoke exposure, four dogs died and four were euthanized. Dogs that were clinically worse by the second day of hospitalization were more likely to die, be euthanized, or have a prolonged course of hospitalization. Less complicated canine smoke exposure patients had improvement in their clinical signs after their first 24 hours of hospitalization.

- Dogs with acute neurological signs following smoke inhalation were found to have a mortality rate of 46% in one study.
- In a retrospective study of 22 cats with smoke exposure, two cats were euthanized because of severe respiratory or neurological signs but none died. There were similar findings compared with dogs in terms of clinical course over hospitalization depending on the severity of their signs at presentation.
- A more guarded prognosis is warranted in patients with significant dermal burns.
- Delayed neurological signs have been documented in canine patients after initial improvement from acute smoke inhalation injury. In dogs with a history of smoke inhalation and acute neurological signs at presentation, approximately half developed delayed neurological signs after a period of improvement and there was a 60% mortality rate in these dogs.

Synonyms

Smoke exposure

See Also

Carbon Monoxide

Suggested Reading

Ashbaugh EA, Mazzaferro EM, McKiernan BC, et al. The association of physical examination abnormalities and carboxyhemoglobin in 21 dogs trapped in a kennel fire. J Vet Emerg Crit Care 2012; 22(3):361–367.

Drobatz KJ, Walker LM, Hendricks JC. Smoke exposure in cats: 22 cases (1986–1997). J Am Vet Med Assoc 1999; 215(9):1312–1316.

Drobatz KJ, Walker LM, Hendricks JC. Smoke exposure in dogs: 27 cases (1988–1997). J Am Vet Med Assoc 1999; 215(9):1306–1311.

Fitzgerald KT, Flood AA. Smoke inhalation. Clin Tech Small Anim Pract 2006; 21:205–214.

Guillaumin J, Hopper K. Successful outcome in a dog with neurologic and respiratory signs following smoke inhalation. J Vet Emerg Crit Care 2013; 23(3):328–334.

Jasani S. Smoke inhalation. In: Silverstein DC, Hopper K, eds. Small Animal Critical Care Medicine, 2nd edn. St Louis, MO: Saunders, 2015; pp. 785–788.

Acknowledgment: The authors and editors acknowledge the prior contributions of Kenneth J. Drobatz, DVM, MSCE, DACVIM, DACVECC, who co-authored this topic in the previous edition.

Author: Dana L. Clarke, VMD, DACVECC

Consulting Editor: Katherine L. Peterson, DVM, DACVECC

section III

Reference Information

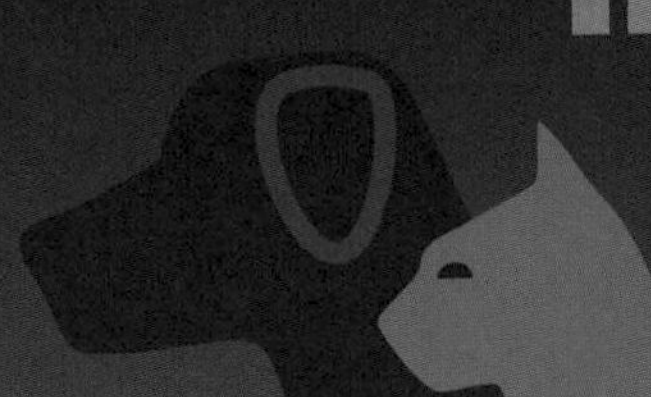

appendix 1

Abbreviations

2-PAM	pralidoxime
2,4-D	2,4-dichlorophenoxyacetic acid
4-MP	4-methylpyrazole
5-FU	5-fluorouracil
5-HT	5-hydroxytryptamine
5-HTP	5-hydroxytryptophan
AAFCO	Association of American Feed Control Officials
ABCB-1	ATP binding cassette
ABG	arterial blood gas
AC	activated charcoal
ACE	angiotensin converting enzyme
ACEi	angiotensin converting enzyme inhibitor
ACT	activated clotting time
ADH	alcohol dehydrogenase; antidiuretic hormone
ADHD	attention deficit hyperactivity disorder
ADP	adenosine diphosphate
ADWD	automatic dishwashing detergents
AKI	acute kidney injury
ALI	acute lung injury
ALP	alkaline phosphatase
ALT	alanine aminotransferase
ANS	autonomic nervous system
APAP	N-acetyl-p-aminophenol
ARDS	acute respiratory distress syndrome
ARF	acute renal failure
APCC	Animal Poison Control Center
ASA	aspirin
AST	aspartate aminotransferase/transaminase
ATN	acute tubular necrosis
ATP	adenosine triphosphate

Blackwell's Five-Minute Veterinary Consult Clinical Companion: Small Animal Toxicology, Second Edition.
Lynn R. Hovda, Ahna G. Brutlag, Robert H. Poppenga, and Katherine L. Peterson.

Companion website: www.fiveminutevet.com/toxicology

AV	atrioventricular
BAL	British anti-Lewisite
BBB	blood–brain barrier
BE	base excess
BG	blood glucose
BID	twice a day (*bis in die*)
BMBT	buccal mucosal bleeding time
BP	blood pressure
bpm	breaths per minute; beats per minute
BUN	blood urea nitrogen
BW	body weight
cAMP	cyclic adenosine monophosphate
CaNa2 EDTA	calcium disodium ethylene diamine tetra-acetate
CBC	complete blood count
CCB	calcium channel blocker
cECG	continuous ECG
CHF	congestive heart failure
CK	creatine kinase
CNS	central nervous system
CO	carbon monoxide
CO_2	carbon dioxide
COHb	carboxyhemoglobin
COP	colloidal osmotic pressure
COX	cyclooxygenase
CPK	creatine phosphokinase
cPL	canine pancreatic-specific lipase
CR	controlled release
CRI	continuous rate infusion
CRT	capillary refill time
CSF	cerebral spinal fluid
CT	computed tomography
CTZ	chemoreceptor trigger zone
CV	cardiovascular
CVP	central venous pressure
D5W	5% dextrose in water
DCM	dilated cardiomyopathy
DEA	Drug Enforcement Agency
DEET	diethyltoluamide
DIC	disseminated intravascular coagulation
DKA	diabetic ketoacidosis
DMSO	dimethyl sulfoxide
DMX	dextromethorphan
DNA	deoxyribonucleic acid

ECF	extracellular fluid
ECG	electrocardiogram
EDTA	ethylenediaminetetraacetic acid
EG	ethylene glycol
ELISA	enzyme-linked immunosorbent assay
EPS	extrapyramidal syndrome
ERG	electroretinogram
$ETCO_2$	end-tidal CO_2
ETT	endotracheal tube
Fab	fragment antigen binding
FBO	foreign body obstruction
FCE	fibrocartilaginous emboli
FDA	Food and Drug Administration
FDP	fibrin degradation products
FFP	fresh frozen plasma
Fib	fibrinogen
FiO_2	fraction of inspired oxygen concentration
FP	frozen plasma
GABA	gamma-aminobutyric acid
GC-MS	gas chromatography-mass spectrometry
GDV	gastric dilatation volvulus
GFR	glomerular filtration rate
GGT	gamma-glutamyl transferase
GHB	gamma hydroxybutyric acid
GI	gastrointestinal
GIT	gastrointestinal tract
GSH	glutathione
Hb	hemoglobin
HbO2	oxyhemoglobin
HCM	hypertrophic cardiomyopathy
HCO_3	bicarbonate
HDI	high-dose insulin
HF	hydrofluoric acid
Hg	mercury
Hgb	hemoglobin
HGE	hemorrhagic gastroenteritis
HPLC	high pressure/performance liquid chromatography
HR	heart rate
IBD	inflammatory bowel disease
ICF	intracellular fluid
ICP	intracranial pressure
IFE	intravenous fat emulsion
ILE	intravenous lipid emulsion

IgG	immuoglobulin G
IM	intramuscular
IMHA	immune-mediated hemolytic anemia
IMT	immune-mediated thrombocytopenia
INR	international normalized ratio
IOP	intraocular pressure
IP	intraperitoneal
IU	international units
IV	intravenous
IVDD	intervertebral disk disease
K	potassium
LAAC	long-acting anticoagulant
LC_{50}	median lethal concentration
LC-MS	liquid chromatography-mass spectrometry
LD	lethal dose
LD_{50}	median lethal dose
L	lowest observed lethal dose
LDH	lactate dehydrogenase
LOX	lipoxygenase
LRS	lactated Ringer's solution
LSAs	lysergic acid amide substances
LSD	lysergic acid diethylamide
MAO	monoamine oxidase; mechanism of action
MAOI	monoamine oxidase inhibitor
MAP	mean arterial pressure
MCPA	2-methyl-4-chlorophenoxyacetic acid
MCPP	2-(4-chloro-methylphenoxy) propionic acid
MDMA	3,4-methylene-2-dioxymethamphetamine
MDR	multidrug resistance
meth	methamphetamine
MetHb	methemoglobinemia
Mg	magnesium
MI	myocardial infarction
MRI	magnetic resonance imaging
NAC	N-acetylcysteine
NaCl	sodium chloride
NADPH	nicotinamide adenine dinucleotide phosphate
Na-K ATPase	sodium-potassium adenosine triphosphatase
NAPQI	N-acetyl-para-benzoquinone imine
NE	nasoesophageal/norepinephrine
NG	nasogastric
NMDA	N-methyl-D-aspartic acid
NPN	nonprotein nitrogen

NPO	nothing by mouth (*nil per os*)
NSAIDs	nonsteroidal antiinflammatory drugs
O_2	oxygen
OP	organophosphate
OTC	over-the-counter
PaO_2	partial pressure of arterial oxygen
PCO_2	partial pressure of carbon dioxide
PCP	phencyclidine
PCR	polymerase chain reaction
PCV	packed cell volume
PD	polydipsia
PDB	paradichlorobenzene
PE	physical exam
PEG	percutaneous endoscopic gastrotomy; polyethylene glycol
PEG-ES	polyethylene glycol electrolyte solution
PG	propylene glycol
PGE_2	prostaglandin E_2
PIVKA	proteins induced by vitamin K antagonism
PLR	pupillary light reflex/response
plt	platelet
PO	by mouth (*per os*)
PPA	phenylpropanolamine
ppb	parts per billion
ppm	parts per million
PPV	positive pressure ventilation
pRBC	packed red blood cells
PRN	as needed (*pro re nata*)
PSE	pseudoephedrine
PT	prothrombin
PTT	partial thromboplastin time
PU	polyuria
q	every
QID	four times a day (*quater in die*)
RBC	red blood cell
RNA	ribonucleic acid
ROS	reactive oxygen species
RR	respiratory rate
RTA	renal tubular acidosis
RTU	ready to use
Rx	prescription
SA	sinoatrial
SAMe	S-adenosyl-methionine
SaO_2	arterial oxyhemoglobin saturation

SE	serotonin
SI	small intestine
SLUDGE	salivation, lacrimation, urination, defecation, gastroenteritis
SNRI	serotonin and norepinephrine reuptake inhibitor
SpO_2	blood oxygen saturation
SQ	subcutaneous
SR	sustained release
SSRI	selective serotonin reuptake inhibitor
SVR	systemic vascular resistance
SVT	supraventricular tachycardia
T½	half-life
TCA	tricyclic antidepressant; tricarboxylic acid
tCO_2	total carbon dioxide
TEG	thromboelastography
TEPP	tetraethyl pyrophosphate
TIBC	total iron-binding capacity
TID	three times a day (*ter in die*)
TLC	thin-layer chromatography
TP	total protein
TPN	total parenteral nutrition
TPR	temperature, pulse, respiration
TS	total solids
UA	urinalysis
UOP	urine output
USG	urine specific gravity
VBP	venous blood gas
VPC	ventricular premature complex/contraction
WB	whole blood
WBC	white blood cell
WBI	whole bowel irrigation
XR	extended release
Zn	zinc

appendix 2

Information Resources for Toxicology

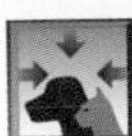

DEFINITION/OVERVIEW

- The tens of thousands of metals, minerals, natural products, and synthetic chemicals used in modern civilization provide numerous opportunities for exposure of small companion animals to dangerous or toxic materials.
- Of the hundreds of drugs and products used in a veterinary practice, many can interact with one another to either increase or mitigate the desired effects.
- Veterinarians receive questions and calls daily about the safety of a variety of products to which pets are exposed.
- Beyond the personal experience and knowledge gained from frequent encounters with the most familiar products, veterinarians need resources to bolster their personal knowledge when less frequently known chemical exposures or questions occur.
- This appendix presents several sources of information that can help veterinarians extend their service to clients by effectively using information resources in toxicology.
- Principal categories of assistance include the following.
    - Persons with in-depth experience relevant to specific toxicants or circumstances. Examples are agronomists, botanists, chemists, limnologists, mycologists, pest control specialists, pharmacists, pharmacologists, pathologists, veterinary extension faculty, wildlife specialists, state and federal regulatory professionals, and many others. Often, veterinary toxicologists are the initial experts consulted and many have developed a network of additional experts to consult if needed.
    - Textbooks and reference books prepared by knowledgeable experts and provided by reliable publishers.
    - Selected peer-reviewed, scientific veterinary journals that routinely accept original reports of toxicology clinical cases or toxicology research.
    - Animal poison control centers that maintain a staff of skilled and knowledgeable veterinary specialists for consultation when veterinary toxicology questions arise. Occasionally, human poison control centers can provide valuable information regarding a product's formulation or a chemical's general toxicity.
    - Government agencies with emphasis on toxicology scientific, regulatory, or educational services.

Blackwell's Five-Minute Veterinary Consult Clinical Companion: Small Animal Toxicology, Second Edition.
Lynn R. Hovda, Ahna G. Brutlag, Robert H. Poppenga, and Katherine L. Peterson.

Companion website: www.fiveminutevet.com/toxicology

- Reliable internet resources for quick and easy access to useful toxicology information on a 24/7 basis. The key to using internet resources is whether the information is reliable and based upon the best available evidence.

VETERINARY AND TOXICOLOGY INFORMATION RESOURCES

- As with all professional services, critical evaluation of resources available is essential to gathering reliable information for toxicology support.
- Sources that are well documented and subject to some form of peer review are usually most reliable.
- If regulatory or legal aspects of toxicology are important for a given situation, official government sources often provide that aspect of information.
- As with all critical information for patient care, the veterinarian must carefully and critically determine how the information applies to their individual practice needs.

Specialists with In-Depth Expertise Relevant to Veterinary Toxicology

- Examples are agronomists, botanists, chemists, limnologists, mycologists, pest control specialists, pharmacists, pharmacologists, pathologists, veterinary extension faculty, veterinary toxicologists, wildlife specialists, state and federal regulatory professionals and many others.
- Knowing about these highly skilled and focused individuals can be invaluable when an infrequently encountered question or exposure demands special knowledge at short notice.
- Prior contact or arrangements with experts that one already knows are often invaluable when a quick and thorough response is required to support a toxicology incident in small animals.

Principal Reference Books and Textbooks

- Many popular textbooks are updated on a regular basis and new information is incorporated for many toxicological topics. The use of the most current textbook is recommended for this reason, although for many toxicants little new information is available.
- While many textbooks are devoted exclusively to toxicology, other textbooks devoted to other topics such as pharmacology or internal medicine also contain useful information related to toxicology.
- The following textbooks or series of textbooks are useful for veterinarians.
  - Burrows GE, Tyrl RJ, eds. Handbook of Toxic Plants of North America, 2nd edn. Wiley–Blackwell, 2013.
  - Campbell A, Chapman MJ, eds. Handbook of Poisoning in Dogs and Cats. Wiley–Blackwell, 2000.

- Gfeller RW, Messonnier SP, eds. Handbook of Small Animal Toxicology. Mosby, 2004.
- Kirk's Current Veterinary Therapy Series (XV edition the most recent). The range of topics varies from edition to edition and relevant older topics are updated with new information. Older editions still contain valuable information.
- Knight AP, ed. A Guide to Poisonous House and Garden Plants. Teton New Media, 2006.
- Morgan RV, ed. Handbook of Small Animal Practice, 5th edn. Saunders, 2008.
- Peterson ME, Talcott PA, eds. Small Animal Toxicology, 3rd edn. Elsevier, 2013.
- Plumlee KH, ed. Clinical Veterinary Toxicology. Mosby, 2004.
- Poppenga RH, Gwaltney-Brant SM, eds. Small Animal Toxicology Essentials, Wiley–Blackwell, 2011.
- Tilley LP, Smith FWK, eds. Blackwell's 5-Minute Veterinary Consult, 5th edn. Wiley–Blackwell, 2011.
- Veterinary Clinics of North America Small Animal Practice. Periodic issues related to small animal toxicology, the most recent published in 2012.

Supportive Reference Books and Textbooks

- Macintire DK, Drobatz KJ, Haskins SC, Saxson WD, eds. Manual of Small Animal Emergency and Critical Care Medicine. Wiley–Blackwell, 2012.
- Papich MG, ed. Saunders Handbook of Veterinary Drugs, 3rd edn. Saunders, 2011.
- Plumb DC, ed. Plumb's Veterinary Drug Handbook, 8th edn. Wiley–Blackwell, 2015.
- Plunkett SJ, ed. Emergency Procedures for the Small Animal Veterinarian, 3rd edn. Saunders, 2011.
- Riviere JE, Papich MG, eds. Veterinary Pharmacology and Therapeutics, 9th edn. Wiley–Blackwell, 2009.

Selected Veterinary Journals as References in Toxicology

Advances in Veterinary Medicine
American Journal of Veterinary Research
Australian Veterinary Journal
Canadian Journal of Veterinary Research
Journal of the American Animal Hospital Association
Journal of the American Veterinary Medical Association
Journal of Medical Toxicology
Journal of Small Animal Practice
Journal of Veterinary Diagnostic Investigation
Journal of Veterinary Emergency and Critical Care
Journal of Veterinary Internal Medicine
Journal of Veterinary Pharmacology and Therapeutics
Research in Veterinary Science

Veterinary Clinics of North America Small Animal Practice
Veterinary Journal
Veterinary Quarterly
Veterinary Record

Animal Poison Control Centers

- ASPCA Animal Poison Control Center
  - www.aspca.org/pet-care/poison-control/
  - (888) 426-4435
  - $65 fee
- Pet Poison Helpline (animal poison control hotline)
  - www.petpoisonhelpline.com/
  - (855) 764-7661
  - $45 fee

Internet-Based Toxicology Resources

- Agency for Toxic Substances and Disease Registry (ATSDR)
  - www.atsdr.cdc.gov/
  - www.atsdr.cdc.gov/toxfaqs/index.asp
- American Association of Poison Control Centers (AAPCC)
  - www.aapcc.org/
  - American Association of Poison Control Centers assists 55 poison centers in the United States on a 24/7 basis.
  - Poison Help hotline at 1-800-222-1222 can be dialed from anywhere in the United States and will be automatically routed to an appropriate center.
  - Certifies poison control center personnel and owns and maintains the National Poison Data System (NPDS).
- Consultant
  - www.vet.cornell.edu/consultant/consult.asp
  - Consultant is a diagnostic support system to assist in possible differential diagnoses or causes based on clinical signs entered. When clinical signs are entered, it enables a wide selection of potential differential toxicology diagnoses.
  - Consultant is free of charge, but monetary support is welcome to help defray expenses. It is species specific, provides a brief synopsis of a selected diagnosis/cause, and is supported by 3–6 recent references pertinent to the diagnosis selected.
  - Supported by a database of approximately 500 signs/symptoms, 7000 diagnoses/causes, and 18,000 literature references, of which 3000 are web sources.
- Cornell University Poisonous Plants
  - www.ansci.cornell.edu/plants/
  - Maintained by the Animal Science Department at Cornell University as a reference only.

- Includes plant images, pictures of affected animals, and presentations concerning botany, chemistry, toxicology, diagnosis, and prevention of poisoning of animals by plants and other natural flora.
- The images are copyrighted but may be printed, downloaded, or copied, provided it is in an educational setting and proper attribution is provided.

■ Drug Compounding – FDA
- www.fda.gov/Drugs/GuidanceComplianceRegulatoryInformation/PharmacyCompounding/ucm339764.htm

■ FDA-Approved Animal Drugs
- FDA Approved Animal Drug Products (Green Book)
- www.fda.gov/AnimalVeterinary/Products/ApprovedAnimalDrugProducts/default.htm

■ FDA Center for Veterinary Medicine (FDA-CVM)
- www.fda.gov/animalveterinary/default.htm
- Official website for the Center for Veterinary Medicine
- Provides current information on pet food regulations, labeling, and food safety for pets.
- Monitors and investigates outbreaks of suspected toxicosis related to pet foods.
  - □ Provides a reporting portal for pet food complaints.
- Examples have included aflatoxins in dogs, melamine/cyanuric acid nephrosis in dogs and cats, and safety of imported pet jerky treats.

■ Household Products Database
- http://householdproducts.nlm.nih.gov/
- Provides a wealth of information about household products including ingredients, potential health risks, and appropriate safety and handling information.
- This database links over 14,000 consumer brands to health effects from Material Safety Data Sheets (MSDS) provided by manufacturers and allows scientists and consumers to research products based on chemical ingredients. The database is designed to help answer the following typical questions.
  - □ What are the chemical ingredients and their percentage in specific brands?
  - □ Which products contain specific chemical ingredients?
  - □ Who manufactures a specific brand? How can the manufacturer be contacted?
  - □ What are the acute and chronic effects of chemical ingredients in a specific brand?
  - □ What other information is available about chemicals in the toxicology-related databases of the National Library of Medicine?

■ InChem (International Programme on Chemical Safety)
- www.inchem.org
- Rapid access to internationally peer-reviewed information on chemicals, including contaminants in the environment and food.
- Primarily human and environment oriented.
- Consolidates information from a number of intergovernmental organizations to assist in sound management of chemicals.

    - Includes environmental health criteria as well as health and safety guidelines.
    - Provides poison information monographs.
- International Veterinary Information Service (IVIS)
    - www.ivis.org/home.asp
    - Free service to veterinarians, veterinary students, and animal health professionals.
    - Provides online peer-reviewed references.
    - Access to three veterinary toxicology textbooks and the IVIS Drug Database.
    - The Drug Database provides rapid access to listings of veterinary drugs by generic name, drug category, biological activity, and manufacturer/distributor.
    - The drug database is under continuing development, and the management advises that some information may be incomplete or contain omissions.
- Merck Veterinary Manual
    - www.merckvetmanual.com/mvm/index.html
- Medline
    - www.nlm.nih.gov/medlineplus/
    - Service provided by the National Library of Medicine and National Institutes of Health.
    - Updated daily.
    - Human focused, but can be a good source of information about human drugs encountered by animals.
    - Also a source of information about human antidotes useful in veterinary medicine.
    - Public access is allowed, as information is supported by two well-known federal agencies.
- MSDS Search
    - www.msdssearch.com/
    - A database service specializing in providing a digital source of MSDS (Material Safety Data Sheets) required by many commercial, business, and manufacturing companies.
    - MSDS sheets contain information about the characteristics and nature of thousands of chemicals to which animals could be exposed.
    - The information is often not assembled consistently in standard references.
    - The MSDS provides a relatively consistent and detailed documentation of composition, use, and potential adverse effects.
    - In many cases, MSDS information for a given product can be located through a search on the product.
- National Institute for Environmental Health Sciences (NIEHS)
    - www.niehs.nih.gov/
    - The NIEHS mission is to reduce the burden of human illness and disability by understanding how the environment influences the development and progression of human disease. Some of the NIEHS activities include:
        - rigorous research in environmental health sciences, and communicating the results of this research to the public

        - alphabetical listing of major health topics that are related to or affected by environmental exposures.
    - Access to materials and guidance for use by health professionals in educating, diagnosing, and treating patients with conditions and diseases influenced by environmental agents.
- National Pesticide Information Center (NPIC)
    - www.npic.orst.edu/
    - (800)-858-7378
    - NPIC provides objective, science-based information about pesticides and pesticide-related topics to enable people to make informed decisions about pesticides and their use. NPIC is a cooperative agreement between Oregon State University and the US Environmental Protection Agency.
- PubMed
    - www.ncbi.nlm.nih.gov/pubmed
    - PubMed is a search service of the United States National Library of Medicine.
    - It comprises more than 19 million citations for biomedical articles from Medline and life science journals.
    - Citations include links to full-text articles from PubMed Central or publisher websites.
    - Numerous major scientific and applied veterinary journals can be reliably accessed through PubMed.
- TOXNET (National Library of Medicine Toxicology Information)
    - http://toxnet.nlm.nih.gov
    - TOXNET is a collection of toxicology and environmental health databases.
        - Hazardous Substances Data Bank (HSDB) is a database of potentially hazardous chemicals. (http://toxnet.nlm.nih.gov/cgi-bin/sis/htmlgen? HSDB).
        - TOXLINE is a database of references to the world's toxicology literature (http://toxnet.nlm.nih.gov/cgi-bin/sis/htmlgen?TOXLINE).
    - ChemIDplus is a chemical dictionary and structure database (http://chem.sis.nlm.nih.gov/chemidplus/).
- USP Veterinary Drug Information
    - www.usp.org/
    - The US Pharmacopeial Convention (USP) is a scientific nonprofit organization that sets standards for the identity, strength, quality, and purity of medicines, food ingredients, and dietary supplements manufactured, distributed and consumed worldwide.
- Veterinary Information Network
    - www.vin.com
    - A veterinary organization and system of education and databases to help busy veterinary professionals be the best clinicians they can be, providing features to include the following.
        - Bringing veterinarians together worldwide as colleagues.
        - Bringing instant access to vast amounts of up-to-date veterinary information to colleagues.

- □ Bringing instant access to "breaking news" that affects veterinarians, their patients, and their practice.
- □ Bringing easy access to colleagues who have specialized knowledge and skills.
- □ Making continuing education available every day.

- ▪ Veterinary Toxicology Diplomate
  - www.abvt.org/public/index.html

Authors: Gary D. Osweiler, DVM, PhD,DABVT; Robert H. Poppenga, DVM, PhD, DABVT
Consulting Editor: Robert H. Poppenga, DVM, PhD, DABVT

appendix 3

Metallic Toxicants

For information on more frequent and serious metallic toxicants for small animals, see individual chapters on iron, lead, and zinc.

Metal & Sources	Toxicity	Clinical Effects	Diagnostics	Therapy/Prevention
Arsenic (As): Trivalent (+3) and pentavalent (+5) sources are of concern. Natural +5 sources are found in soil, coal, mine tailings, and seafoods (2–22 ppm). Both +3 and +5 valence in pesticides. Other: Pre-2004 treated wood (CCA). Well water ≤21 ppm. Weed and insect killers. Medical: immiticide (melarsomine) adult heartworm treatment (thiacetarsamide).	Absorbed via GIT, intact skin, inhalation. +3 is 3–10 times more toxic than +5 valence. Storage in liver, kidney, GIT, spleen, skin, hair. Excreted 50% in urine within 48 hours. Lethal dosage range 1–25 mg/kg. More toxic to cats than dogs. Toxicity order is As^{+3}(arsenite) > As^{+5} (arsenate) > trivalent organics. Melarsomine = severe toxicosis at 7.5 mg/kg.	Immediately postabsorption – oral irritation, dysphagia. Acute toxicosis 1–3 hours – GIT pain, vomiting, hematachezia, melena, rice-water stools, hypovolemia from capillary dilation and vascular transudation. Salivation, oral erosion, and ulceration. Subacute – tubular nephrosis, renal failure, azotemia.	Arsenical analysis of: Liver, kidney: >10 ppm is toxic. Urine: current exposure = 2–100 ppm. Hair: chronic levels ≥25 ppm. Blood: unreliable for arsenic concentration. CBC: hemoconcentration secondary to dehydration, hemolysis, anemia, ± basophilic stippling, possible pancytopenia, leukopenia, or thrombocytopenia. Urinalysis: monitor for whole cells, casts, protein, evidence of hemolysis, hematuria.	No emetics or gastric lavage unless very early and asymptomatic. Charcoal is *not* an effective adsorbent. Intensive care with IV fluids, demulcents, treat for shock, maintain body temp, dialysis for renal failure. Sucralfate, H_2 blockers, antiemetics, antidiarrheals. Monitor renal function. Acute prognosis guarded. Best antidote is succimer (DMSA), a metal chelator. Less toxic, more expensive, more effective than dimercaprol (BAL). *See dosages at end of table.*

(Continued)

Blackwell's Five-Minute Veterinary Consult Clinical Companion: Small Animal Toxicology, Second Edition.
Lynn R. Hovda, Ahna G. Brutlag, Robert H. Poppenga, and Katherine L. Peterson.

Companion website: www.fiveminutevet.com/toxicology

Metal & Sources	Toxicity	Clinical Effects	Diagnostics	Therapy/Prevention
Barium (Ba): Rodenticide (obsolete), welding fluxes, depilatories, dyes, glass manufacture, explosive detonators	Acid- or water-soluble barium salts act as strong cardiosuppressants and cause severe hypokalemia by blocking exit channels for K in muscle cells. Barium also stimulates skeletal, smooth, and cardiac muscle. Toxic dose, canine: 50 mg/kg BW.	Acute – vomiting, colic, salivation, diarrhea, ventricular tachycardia/ fibrillation, dyspnea, weakness. Violent peristalsis, arterial hypertension, and arrhythmias. Additional signs may include seizures, tremors, mydriasis.	Hypokalemia, from blocking cellular K+ exit. ECG changes from hypokalemia (ECG: QRS or QTc interval changes). Tissue levels – primarily in bones (replacing Ca^{++}). Soft tissue normal values generally less than 1 ppm. Blood values from acute poisoning expected at 2–10 ppm. ECG: QRS or QTc interval changes.	Emesis and activated charcoal not recommended. Saline diuresis, intravenous K^{+} to control hypokalemia and tachycardia is critical. Consider gastric lavage if patient is stabilized and airway protected. Magnesium sulfate (250 mL/kg PO) to form insoluble $BaSO_4$ and reduce absorption. Lidocaine recommended in humans if refractory to potassium.
Cadmium (Cd): Ores, mine tailings, smelters. Also in foods (shellfish), cigarettes, fertilizers, solders, batteries, art pigments, automotive paints, semiconductors, solar cells.	Multisystem effects. Accumulates in kidneys and very slowly excreted – oxidative damage and lysosomal release → renal damage. Competes with Ca and Zn. Dogs tolerate 10 ppm in diet; chronic toxicity occurs at 50 mg/kg.	Acute – dyspnea, vomiting, colic, diarrhea (mucosal damage), weakness, renal failure. Chronic – rhinitis, anorexia, renal tubular dysfunction, sodium retention, osteomalacia/ osteoporosis enlarges joints, testicular damage, potential copper deficiency.	Blood levels ≥100 µg/ dL reflect acute exposure; urine levels represent chronic exposure, but blood or urine values for small animals are poorly defined. Liver accumulates 1–2 ppm and kidney from 3–10 ppm. Diagnosis depends on history of exposure, typical clinical signs, and elevated cadmium in blood, urine, or tissue.	Treat symptomatically and supportive therapy for gastroenteritis and renal insufficiency. Zinc supplementation may reduce accumulation or persistence of Cd residues. $CaNa_2EDTA$ or d-penicillamine. *See dosages at end of table.*
Copper (Cu): Liver accumulation in dogs enhanced by autosomal recessive trait in Bedlington Terrier; also high risk	Absorbed readily from GIT, stored mainly in liver cell lysosomes, excreted in bile complexed with molybdenum.	Acute exposure to concentrated copper salts – moderate to severe gastroenteritis.	Samples for diagnosis:	Treat acute signs of liver disease and anemia symptomatically.

Metal & Sources	Toxicity	Clinical Effects	Diagnostics	Therapy/Prevention
in West Highland, Skye, Dalmatian, Doberman, and Labrador. Sources include coins, wiring, garden sprays, feeds, copper oxide capsules.	Excess accumulation causes hepatic cell necrosis. Hereditary copper accumulation is a liver disease. Acute release from liver may cause hemolytic crisis.	Chronic accumulations – hepatic insufficiency, possible encephalophathy, and occasional acute hemolytic crisis with icterus and hemoglobinuria.	Chemistry panel – elevated LDH, ALT, AST, bilirubin, bile acids. CBC – anemia, hemoglobinemia, hypoproteinemia. Urine – hemoglobinuria. Liver biopsy for histopathology and copper analysis may be diagnostic. Liver normal <400 ppm dry weight. Secondary Cu accumulation 400–800 ppm. Toxicosis >800 ppm.	If chronic toxicity – chelation of copper with d–penicillamine. *See dosages at end of table.* Continue therapy with monitoring up to 1 year. Biopsy for liver status again after 1 year of therapy.
Chromium (Cr): Occurs in nature in 4 oxidation states. Cr+6 is made and used by industrial processes. Cr+3 is used in leather tanning, pigments, and wood preservation. Few sources are generally available to small animals.	Cats tolerate 100 μg/day or 16 μg/kg/day. Dogs tolerate 50 μg/kg/day. Cr supports glucose tolerance and modulates serum triglycerides and cholesterol.	Reports of poisoning in small animals are rare. Signs in other species include vomiting, profuse diarrhea with mucosal sloughing, and dermatitis.	Cr is widely distributed in mammalian species at very low (ng/g) concentrations. Normal values in rats are 6 ppm (liver) and 8 ppm (kidney). Dosage of 100 mg/kg raises Cr values to 90 and 700 ppm in liver and kidney, respectively. Excreted mainly in urine.	Minimal toxicity is expected after ingestion. Some sources suggest activated charcoal, others do not. Overdose, if it occurs, is treated with general detoxification, fluids, and GIT therapy to manage potential or real gastroenteritis and dermatitis.
Gold: Gold-containing drugs are used primarily to manage rheumatoid arthritis. Forms include gold sodium thioglucose, gold sodium thiomalate, gold thiosulfate.	Rat IM LD_{50} = 35–440 mg/kg. Gold drugs are generally not available in a way that would expose small animals unless by malicious intent or extreme carelessness.	Most data are for parenteral exposure. Signs include ventricular tachycardia, vasodilation, hypotension, stomatitis, glossitis, ocular inflammation, pneumonitis, toxic encephalopathy, and polyneuropathy.	Urine assay for gold would establish exposure, but diagnostic values are not established. Human therapeutic use produces approximately 1 μg/mL blood levels.	Gold toxicosis has been treated in humans with steroids, BAL and N-acetylcysteine (NAC). *See dosages at end of table.* Animal treatment regimens are not established.

(Continued)

Metal & Sources	Toxicity	Clinical Effects	Diagnostics	Therapy/Prevention
Lithium (Li): Used in human medicine to treat manic depressive illness. Standard and sustained-release products available. Adult therapy range is 300–1800 mg/day. Tablet strength typically is 300 mg. Lithium batteries low risk: pass through GIT and contain limited lithium.	Rat oral LD_{50} = 525 mg/kg. Feline: Toxic dose >85 mg/kg. Animals with renal disease, dehydration, sodium depletion, cardiovascular disease, severe debilitation, or receiving diuretics are at higher risk. Crosses the placenta, concentrates in fetus, may be teratogen.	CNS – drowsiness, tremors, weakness, confusion, ataxia, seizures, or coma. GIT – vomiting, diarrhea, nausea, anorexia. Other –blurred vision, PU/PD, T-wave ECG changes. Signs prolonged if sustained-release product ingested.	History: excessive and/or sustained high dosages. Human serum values: Moderate toxicity = 1.5–2.5 mEq/L. Severe toxicity = 2.5–3 mEq/L. Fatal = >3 mEq/L. Recheck serum Li as needed. Follow clinical course with baseline labs, electrolytes, BUN, and creatinine.	Activated charcoal not effective. Decontaminate – gastric lavage if <1 hr post ingestion. Whole bowel irrigation if >1 hr post ingestion, using PEG @ 25–50 mg/kg followed by 0.5 mg/kg/hr oral infusion until effluent is clear. IV fluids @ 1.5–2× maintenance with 0.9% NaCl to aid renal excretion. Acetazolamide (10 mg/kg q 6 hrs) and aminophylline to enhance renal excretion. Hemodialysis may be option in some cases.
Mercury (Hg): Current sources are limited. Ointments, leather preservatives, thermometers, fungicides, barometers, anti-mildew paints, fluorescent bulbs, mercury vapor lamps. Fish-based diets potentially contain methyl mercury which has a long half-life and can potentially bioaccumulate.	Vapors and organic mercurials absorbed by inhalation and from GIT. Metallic mercury concentrates in GIT and kidney. Organic mercury concentrates in brain. All forms pass the placenta. Cats are highly susceptible.	Organic mercurials cause erythema, conjunctivitis, stomatitis, depression, ataxia, incoordination, proprioceptive deficits, abnormal postures, paresis, and blindness. Hypoproteinemia, proteinuria, and azotemia typical in inorganic Hg poisoning.	Blood (>6.0 ppm) and urine (>1.5 ppm) are good samples for acute to subacute exposure. Hair (>45 ppm) for chronic exposure. Liver (>30 ppm) and kidney (>20 ppm) associated with toxicosis in cats.	Acute inorganic mercury – egg white to inactivate mercury; activated charcoal results variable. Whole bowel irrigation with PEG recommended. Oral sodium thiosulfate (0.5–1.0 g/kg BW) may bind mercury. Antidote: oral d-penicillamine or succimer may bind Hg. *See dosages at end of table.*

Metal & Sources	Toxicity	Clinical Effects	Diagnostics	Therapy/Prevention
Selenium (Se): Selenium dietary supplements, gun bluing compound, pigments, photocells, photography developing products.	Canine lethal dosage is 1.5–3 mg/kg both oral and parenteral. Dietary levels of 10–20 ppm are toxic. Selenium causes glutathione depletion, lipid peroxidation, and replaces sulfur in amino acids. May also depress ATP formation.	Acute – vomiting, diarrhea, dyspnea, ataxia, hypovolemia and collapse result from acute exposure. Signs are similar to acute arsenic or iron toxicosis. Chronic – exposure may cause rough, dull haircoat, alopecia, weight loss, and infertility.	A normal blood Se value in dogs is approximately 0.220 ppm. Blood Se >1–2 ppm is suggestive of toxicosis. Kidney and liver values >12 ppm are considered toxic. Chronic exposure is detected with hair analysis.	Life support includes acute therapy for gastroenteritis and shock. Activated charcoal is recommended by some, not by others. Alternatively, gastric lavage with sodium thiosulfate 20% solution may be helpful. Treatment: NAC. *See dosages at end of table.*
Tin: Food preparation, toothpaste, pigments for ceramics and textiles. Organotins (alkyl tins) used as fungicides, insecticides, wood, leather, textile, preservatives.	Two valence forms (+2 and +4). Prior use of trimethyl/ triethyl tin as a fungicide. Organic tins are toxic and well absorbed from GIT, but inorganic forms are highly tolerated.	Organotin target organs are brain, liver, immune system, and skin. Cause skin and eye irritation, colic, diarrhea, hepatotoxicity and neurotoxicity (hyperactivity), seizures, ataxia.	Myelin edema (status spongiosis) and demyelization in CNS. Blood levels >0.3 ppm and liver levels of 0.6 ppm have been associated with organotin toxicosis.	Acute exposures not likely. If occurs, activated charcoal is recommended. BAL for 4 days effective in experimental animals. Sodium thiosulfate may improve response. Control fever and hypotension. *See dosages at end of table.*

Antidotes and dosages

For more details, consult Plumb DC. Plumb's Veterinary Drug Handbook, 8th edn. Wiley–Blackwell, 2015.

- $CaNa_2EDTA$: 100 mg/kg/day SQ in 4 divided doses diluted in D5W. Treat for 5 days and reevaluate metal concentration in 5–14 days to determine if additional course of therapy is necessary.
- BAL (dimercaprol): dogs/cats: 2.5–5 mg/kg IM q 4 for first 2 days of treatment then q 12 hours until recovery. Evidence is lacking to support any particular dosage regimen.
- Succimer: 10 mg/kg PO q 8 hours for 10 days and reevaluate metal concentration several days after course of therapy to determine if additional course of therapy is necessary.

- d-Penicillamine: for copper-associated hepatopathy, 7–15 mg/kg PO q 12 hours. Drug may cause vomiting. Give 1 hour prefeeding. Lower dosage of 7 mg/kg PO might be efficacious while reducing drug cost and incidence of vomiting.
- NAC: 140–180 mg/kg IV (5% solution) or 280 mg/kg PO initially, then 70 mg/kg q 6 hours PO or IV for a minimum of 7 treatments.
- Sodium thiosulfate: 40–50 mg/kg IV as 20% solution q 8–12 hours.

Abbreviations

ATP = adenosine triphosphate
BAL = British anti-Lewisite (dimercaprol)
$CaNa_2EDTA$ = calcium disodium ethylene diamine tetraacetate
CCA = chromated copper arsenate
LD_{50} = median lethal dose
NAC = N-acetylcysteine
PEG = polyethylene glycol

Authors: Gary D. Osweiler, DVM, PhD, DABVT; Ahna G. Brutlag, DVM, MS, DABT, DABVT
Consulting Editor: Robert H. Poppenga, DVM, PhD, DABVT

Toxic Plants and Their Clinical Signs: Antidotes and Treatment

appendix 4

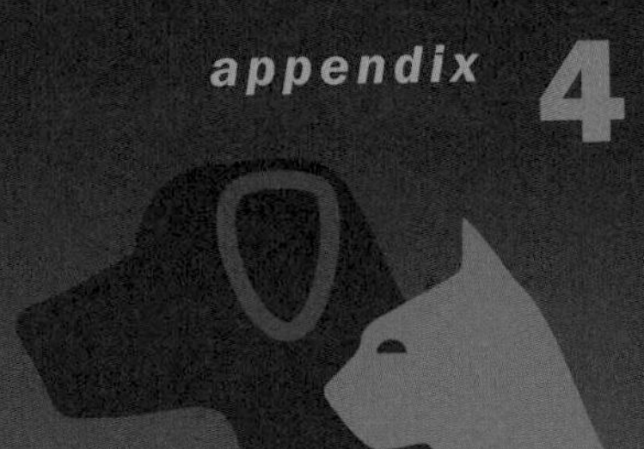

Plant and Characteristics	Clinical Signs	Antidotes and/or Treatment
Air plant, Cathedral bells (*Kalanchoe* spp.) Bright red-orange to pink blooms; umbel flower pattern. Plant contains cardiotoxins similar to azalea and rhododendrons, concentrated mainly in flowers.	Cardiac glycoside causes acute signs 1–3 hours after ingestion. Signs include depression, salivation, diarrhea, bradycardia, tachypnea, ataxia, tremors, and paralysis.	Emesis and/or activated charcoal early after ingestion. Treat as a cardiac glycoside. (see chapter 102).
Aloe, Octopus plant, Candelabra plant (*Aloe* spp.) Succulent plant, used in folk and herbal medicine. Toxic fraction is anthraquinone glycoside; disrupts water and electrolyte balance in large intestine.	Anorexia, depression, vomiting, colic, diarrhea, tremors (uncommon), and change in urine color. Generally mild in nature.	Drugs for abdominal pain/ diarrhea. Protect airway, treat locally for pharyngitis associated with oxalate crystals (rare).
Autumn crocus (Colchicum autumnale) Houseplant, garden plant. Typically blooms in fall, different from most other bulbs. Dosages above 6 g/kg BW considered lethal. Although the whole plant is toxic, the toxin (colchicine) is highest in bulbs.	Acute onset 2–12 hours post ingestion. Initial signs are nausea, salivation, vomiting, colic, diarrhea, incoordination, and weakness. Multiple organ systems (heart, lungs, and kidneys) also may be involved. Potential for coagulopathy and elevated serum enzymes.	Induce emesis if not vomiting. Activated charcoal if early. Evaluate CBC and serum chemistries, including prothrombin, LDH, CK. IV fluids, analgesics, anticonvulsants as needed.
Baneberry, Doll's eye, Cohosh (*Actea* spp.) Toxic principle is protoanemonin glycoside, as well as irritant essential oils.	Clinical response ranges from dermatitis and blistering of skin to oral irritation, drooling, pawing at face or mouth, emesis, diarrhea, and hematuria. Neurological and cardiovascular signs are occasionally reported.	Cleanse mouth thoroughly with water; apply appropriate local demulcents; control emesis and diarrhea as necessary; monitor for organ dysfunction, especially renal damage.

Blackwell's Five-Minute Veterinary Consult Clinical Companion: Small Animal Toxicology, Second Edition.
Lynn R. Hovda, Ahna G. Brutlag, Robert H. Poppenga, and Katherine L. Peterson.

Companion website: www.fiveminutevet.com/toxicology

Plant and Characteristics	Clinical Signs	Antidotes and/or Treatment
Belladonna lily (*Amaryllis* spp.) Potted plant, Bulbs are most toxic. Contains both lycorine alkaloid (systemic effects) and insoluble oxalates (local pharyngitis).	Nausea, vomiting, diarrhea, hypotension, depression. Oxalate crystals can cause direct pharyngeal irritation.	Gastric lavage, activated charcoal, fluids, and supportive treatment.
Bittersweet (*Celastrus* spp.) Weed, vine with red berries. Immature fruits are toxic. Toxins are sesquiterpene alkaloids (celapanine, celastrine, paniculatine).	Gastric irritation, vomiting, diarrhea.	Fluids, supportive care as needed.
Bleeding heart (*Dicentra* spp.) Garden, woods, potted plant. Roots more toxic than leaves. Toxins are isoquinoline alkaloids (apomorphine, cularine, protoberberine).	Vomiting, diarrhea, muscle tremors, convulsions or paralysis.	Fluids and seizure control.
Castor bean (Ricinus communis) Garden shrub or ornamental grows to 2 meters. Seeds are 1 cm, dark and light mottled, and highly toxic. Chewing the seed greatly increases toxicity. Toxin is ricin.	Severe, dangerous if seeds chewed before swallowing. Latent period 6–48 hours. Emesis, severe and hemorrhagic diarrhea, colic, muscle tremors, sudden collapse. Dehydration, hypotension, hemolysis and/or hemoglobinuria.	Emesis for recent exposure: sorbitol if diarrhea not present; charcoal, fluids, and electrolytes. Monitor electrolytes, liver, kidney, adrenal function up to 6 days; H_2 blockers for GI signs; diazepam for seizures. Antibiotics, lactulose, SAMe for liver damage.
Chinaberry tree (*Melia azedarach*) Other common names are Persian lilac, white cedar, Texas umbrella tree. Ornamental tree in temperate to subtropical areas: southern coastal states, Mexican border. Berry is most toxic. Toxins are meliatoxins.	Salivation, anorexia, vomiting, diarrhea. May be followed by weakness, ataxia, excitement or seizures. Fatalities have occurred, generally within 2 days post ingestion.	Early emesis, GI lavage and charcoal are considered beneficial. Fluid and electrolyte replacement, anticonvulsants and supportive care.
Christmas rose (*Helleborus niger*) House and garden plant. Entire plant is toxic, but fruits are most dangerous. Small amounts considered dangerous. Contains several toxins including ranunculin that is converted to protoanemonin when chewed, cardenolides, and bufadienolides.	Hypersalivation, vomiting, anorexia, diarrhea followed by cardiac arrhythmias, heart block with premature beats, premature beats, slow irregular pulse. Potent cardenolide action is greatest risk.	Gastric lavage or emesis; activated charcoal or saline cathartics to decontaminate the GI tract. Atropine may be helpful as for other cardenolide plants such as *Digitalis* spp.

Plant and Characteristics	Clinical Signs	Antidotes and/or Treatment
Daphne (*Daphne mezereum*) Landscape shrub; evergreen or deciduous. Entire plant is toxic. Bitter or acid taste discourages consumption, may reduce toxic effects. Toxins are tricyclic daphnane and diterpenes.	Vesication and edema of the lips and oral cavity associated with ingestion. Signs progress to salivation, thirst, abdominal pain, emesis, hemorrhagic diarrhea.	Analgesics to control pain. General GI detoxification, medical treatment for vomiting and diarrhea. Fluid and electrolyte replacement as needed. Monitor body fluids and electrolytes.
Delphinium/larkspur (*Delphinium* spp.) and/or pheasant's eye, yellow oxeye (*Adonis* spp.) Outdoor perennial: gardens, mountains; tall with blue, purple, or pinkish flowers. Seeds more toxic than leaves. Toxin is a diterpenoid alkaloid.	Small animal poisoning unlikely unless by access to seeds. Early signs are vomiting, colic, and diarrhea. May progress to trembling, ataxia, weakness, lateral recumbency.	GI detoxification; demulcents and antidiarrheal for GI signs; physostigmine to treat muscarinic signs.
English holly (*Ilex* spp.) Landscape plant; glossy green leaves with marginal spicules. Fruit (drupe) white, yellow, black, red, orange. Occurs in forested areas of eastern N. America; elsewhere as an ornamental. Fruit is most likely portion consumed. Fruit and leaves contain potentially toxic saponins.	Nausea, vomiting, diarrhea most common from consumption of berries. Some animals may be depressed. Clinical response most often mild/moderate and transient.	Relief of digestive distress; activated charcoal may be helpful. Fluid and electrolyte replacement as needed.
English ivy (*Hedera helix*), also known as Atlantic ivy, Irish ivy, common ivy. Houseplant, or in mild climates used as a ground cover. Occurs as a woody, climbing or creeping vine. Commonly grown throughout North America. Toxins are triterpenoid saponins.	Salivation, thirst, emesis, gastroenteritis, diarrhea, dermatitis. Relatively few reported cases, most are moderate GI irritation. Often moderate or mild.	Symptomatic relief of GI distress; supportive care for vomiting and diarrhea.
Golden angel's trumpet (*Brugmansia* spp.) Nonnative ornamental, similar to jimsonweed. Large pendulous flowers, similar to angel's trumpet. Toxin similar to jimsonweed (tropane alkaloid scopolamine) causes anticholinergic effects.	Typical anticholinergic effects are restlessness, dilated pupils, tachycardia, dyspnea, dry mouth, GI atony, rarely seizures. Rarely lethal.	Treat similar to *Datura* spp. (see Thornapple below).

(Continued)

Plant and Characteristics	Clinical Signs	Antidotes and/or Treatment
Horse chestnut or Ohio buckeye (*Aesculus* spp.) Landscape or forest tree; palmate leaves. Native range is Midwest, east to Appalachian Mountains, south into Texas. Planted as ornamental/landscape tree as well. Nuts and twigs most toxic; very early green foliage in spring. Horse chestnut highly toxic; Ohio buckeye very low toxicity. Contain several toxins including saponins, anthraquinones, and a coumarin glycoside.	Gastroenteritis, diarrhea, dehydration, electrolyte imbalance. Neurological signs possible, including incoordination, hypermetria, staggering. Usually transient, rarely fatal. Recovery usual within 24–48 hours.	Fluid and electrolyte replacement, demulcents, and therapy for gastroenteritis. Confine animals during neurological phase.
Iris or flag (*Iris* spp.) Perennial garden flower – very commonly available. Rootstock (rhizome) most toxic; most risk at transplantation. Close to soil surface, may be dug up by dogs. Advise clients of potential risk. Rootstock contains purgative toxin known as irisin.	Hypersalivation, vomiting, colic, diarrhea which may be hemorrhagic. Occasionally irritation of the lips and muzzle.	GI decontamination early. Fluid and electrolyte therapy as needed.
Irish potato (*Solanum tuberosum*) Vegetable garden plant. Vines, green skin, and sprouts are toxic. Toxins vary but are solanine and other glycoalkaloids.	Vomiting, diarrhea, depression, rapid heart rate, mydriasis, muscle tremors. Signs may vary from atropine-like to cholinesterase inhibition. Use antidotes accordingly and with caution.	GI decontamination. If atropine-like signs predominate, use physostigmine. If salivation and diarrhea are present, use atropine cautiously.
Jerusalem cherry, winter cherry (*Solanum pseudocapsicum*) Common ornamental houseplant. Toxin is the glycoalkaloid solanine similar to other plants of the nightshade (Solanaceae) family.	Severe GI irritation characterized by drooling, vomiting, diarrhea, ulceration, depression, and sometimes seizures.	GI decontamination if exposure is recent. If salivation and diarrhea are present and severe, use atropine cautiously. Provide fluid therapy based on condition of patient and results of laboratory tests.

Plant and Characteristics	Clinical Signs	Antidotes and/or Treatment
Lantana (*Lantana camara*) Occurs wild and in gardens in mild temperate to tropical areas. Naturalized in southeastern coastal states of the USA. Bright orange, yellow, red, purple, or pink flowers. Foliage and immature berries are most toxic. Toxins are pentacyclic triterpenoid lantadenes A,B, and C.	Weakness, lethargy, vomiting, diarrhea, mydriasis, dyspnea. Continued ingestion can lead to chronic disease. Advanced signs: cholestasis, hyperbilirubinemia. Liver changes predispose to photosensitization.	GI decontamination, activated charcoal for acute exposures. Provide fluids and respiratory support. Protect from sunlight and treat for hepatic insufficiency.
Lily of the valley (*Convallaria majalis*) Ornamental garden plant. Prefers moist, shaded areas. Blossoms nodding/drooping on stem. Toxic principle (cardenolides) persists in dried plants; highest concentration in roots.	Multiorgan failure. Tremors, thirst, vomiting, diarrhea, cardiac arrhythmia/bradycardia, weakness, shock. Monitor for cardiac arrhythmias, shock and hyperkalemia.	Emesis or gastric lavage. Control dehydration, maintain electrolytes; control diarrhea; monitor ECG and serum potassium.
Lupine, bluebonnet (*Lupinus* spp.) Common garden ornamental throughout USA; wild plants abundant in some regions, primarily western USA. Seeds more toxic than leaves, but plant, seeds and pods are toxic. Toxin is lupine.	Signs begin 1–24 hours post exposure. Salivation, ataxia, mydriasis, depression or seizures, disorientation, dyspnea. Liver and kidney damage may develop from continued ingestion. Lupines are teratogenic in ruminants. Risk in small animals is not well known.	GI decontamination with activated charcoal for acute exposure. Anticonvulsants may be needed if neurological signs are severe.
Mexican breadfruit, Swiss cheese plant, hurricane plant (*Monstera deliciosa*) Stems and leaves contain insoluble calcium oxalate spicules (raphides).	Chewing on the plant releases oxalate spicules into mouth, tongue and lips. Response is immediate irritation, pain, salivation, and inflammation. Signs include pawing at face, drooling, and vomiting; potential interference with upper airway.	Cleanse mouth thoroughly with water. Apply local and/or systemic antiinflammatory agents based on clinical condition of patient.
Mistletoe (*Phoradendron* spp.) Access to pets in homes at holiday time. Oval evergreen leaves with white berries. Leaves, stems, and berries are moderately toxic – contain toxic amines and proteins.	Vomiting, GI pain, diarrhea; ataxia, hypotension, occasional seizures, cardiovascular failure. Principal risk may be from use during holiday season.	Fluid and electrolyte replacement; demulcents for gastroenteritis.

(Continued)

Plant and Characteristics	Clinical Signs	Antidotes and/or Treatment
Monkshood (*Aconitum* spp.) Perennial garden ornamental. Entire plant is toxic, contains diterpene alkaloids that are primarily neurotoxic.	Interferes with inactivation of Na+ channels in nerves. Salivation, vomiting, diarrhea. Muscle tremors, weakness, cardiac arrhythmia and/or heart failure; respiratory depression.	GI decontamination, fluid and electrolyte replacement. Manage similar to digitalis glycoside overdose, with caution for potassium administration.
Morning glory (*Ipomoea purpurea* and *Ipomoea tricolor*) Garden annual, potted plant. Seeds most toxic. Increased risk when seeds are presoaked, consumed by dogs. Indole alkaloid toxin similar to ergot alkaloids; abused as hallucinogen.	Nausea, mydriasis, ataxia, muscle tremors, hallucinations, decreased reflexes, diarrhea, hypotension.	Dark, quiet surroundings; tranquilization as needed. GI decontamination is not routinely recommended.
Mountain laurel (*Kalmia* spp.) Native of eastern and southeastern woods, mountains. Both leaves and flowers are toxic. Honey from nectar also toxic. Toxins are diterpenoids, in particular grayanotoxins I and II.	Oral irritation, salivation, projectile vomiting, diarrhea, weakness, impaired vision, bradycardia, hypotension, AV block.	Activated charcoal, fluid replacement, and respiratory support as needed.
Narcissus, daffodil, jonquil (*Narcissus* spp.) Garden ornamental bulb. Bulb is most toxic. Contains lycorine alkaloid.	Nausea, vomiting, salivation, hypotension, diarrhea. Prolonged signs may cause dehydration.	Gastric lavage, activated charcoal, fluid replacement, supportive treatment for gastroenteritis.
Nettle (*Urtica spp.*) Garden or waste area weed. Hairs on leaves contain toxin that enters skin on contact. Most common in hunting or outdoor free-roaming dogs. Toxins are biogenic amines (acetylcholine, histamine, etc.).	Oral irritation and pain, hypersalivation, swelling and edema of nose and periocular areas or other areas of skin contact.	Antihistamines and analgesics. Local or systemic antiinflammatory supportive therapy to treat affected contact areas.
Persian violet, sowbread (*Cyclamen persicum*) Popular florist's plant; widely available. Irritant saponins in all parts of the plant, especially tubers or roots.	Chewing plant parts causes oral irritation with drooling, vomiting and diarrhea. Occasional hemoglobinuria may color urine red-brown. Large amounts may cause cardiac arrhythmias, seizures and rarely mortality.	Control vomiting and diarrhea if severe; administer fluids as needed. Monitor urine for color and/or hemoglobin. Control seizures and cardiac arrhythmias as needed.

Plant and Characteristics	Clinical Signs	Antidotes and/or Treatment
***Philodendron* spp.** Very common indoor ornamental vine. Toxic principle is insoluble oxalate.	Chewing on the plant releases oxalate spicules into mouth, tongue and lips. Response is immediate irritation, pain, salivation, and inflammation. Signs include pawing at face, drooling, and vomiting; also potential interference with upper airway.	Cleanse mouth thoroughly with water. Apply local and/or systemic antiinflammatory agents based on clinical condition of patient.
Poinsettia (Euphorbia pulcherrima) Garden or potted plant, especially during the Holiday season. Sap of stem and leaves mild irritant. Contains a variety of diterpenoid euphorbol esters.	Irritation of mouth: may cause vomiting, diarrhea, and dermatitis. Usually transient and not life-threatening.	Demulcents for local lesions; fluids to prevent dehydration.
Rosary pea, precatory bean (*Abrus precatorius*) Native of Caribbean islands. Seeds (when broken or chewed) are highly toxic. Seeds used in ornamental jewelry in some countries. Illegal to import into USA. Toxin is abrin.	Signs may be delayed up to 2 days after ingestion. Early signs are nausea, vomiting, diarrhea (often hemorrhagic) followed by weakness, tachycardia, possible renal failure, coma, death.	Emesis or lavage followed by activated charcoal, demulcents, fluids, and electrolytes. Early and thorough detoxication is important for survival.
Thorn apple, jimsonweed (*Datura stramonium*) Annual weed, some species are ornamental *(Datura metel)*. Entire plant is toxic, but seeds are most toxic and available. Toxins are tropane alkaloids (hyoscyamine and scopolamine) with effects similar to atropine.	Thirst, disturbances of vision, delirium, mydriasis, thirst, tachycardia, hyperthermia, GI atony/constipation. Commonly described as "Hot as a pistol, blind as a bat, red as a beet, mad as a hatter."	GI decontamination if early after ingestion. Parasympathomimetic drug (e.g., physostigmine).
Tulips (*Tulipa* spp.) and hyacinths (*Hyacinthus* spp.) Poisoning usually occurs when dogs consume available bulbs or dig up freshly planted bulbs. Toxic principle includes allergenic lactones and similar alkaloids.	Signs reflect direct irritation and include drooling, nausea, vomiting, diarrhea, dyspnea, tachycardia and dyspnea and hyperpnea.	GI decontamination if early after ingestion. Apply local and/or systemic antiinflammatory agents based on clinical condition of patient. Monitor and control gastrointestinal effects; medicate as needed for tachycardia and dyspnea.

(Continued)

Plant and Characteristics	Clinical Signs	Antidotes and/or Treatment
Tobacco (*Nicotiana tabacum*) Garden plant, weed, cigarettes. Entire plant toxic. Nicotine alkaloid is toxic principle.	Rapid onset of salivation, nausea, emesis, tremors, incoordination, ataxia, collapse and respiratory failure.	Assist ventilation, provide vascular support. Gastric lavage with activated charcoal.
Wisteria (*Wisteria* spp.) Woody vine or shrub with bluish purple to white legume flowers. Entire plant is toxic. Toxin is a glycoprotein lectin	Nausea, abdominal pain, prolonged vomiting; diarrhea. Signs may persist 2–3 days.	Antiemetics and fluid replacement therapy.
Yellow jessamine (*Gelsemium sempervirens*) Mild temperate to subtropical climates; mainly SE United States. Yellow trumpet-shaped flowers grow on evergreen vines. Neurotoxic alkaloids and semipervirine, and indole, are toxins.	Weakness, ataxia, clonic/tonic seizures, paralysis, respiratory failure.	GI decontamination early in course of toxicosis. Symptomatic and supportive therapy for respiration. Fluid replacement therapy as needed.

Supplemental Resources

- Barr AC. Household and garden plants. In: Peterson ME, Talcott PA, eds. Small Animal Toxicology, 3rd edn. Elsevier, 2013; pp. 357–400.
- Burrows GE, Tyrl RJ. Toxic Plants of North America. Iowa State University Press, 2001.
- Frohne D, Pfander HJ. Poisonous Plants, 2nd edn. Timber Press. 2005.
- Williams MC, Olsen JD. Horse chestnut: a multidisciplinary clinical review. Am J Vet Res 1984; 45(3):539–542.

Authors: Gary D. Osweiler, DVM, PhD, DABVT; Lynn R. Hovda, RPh, DVM, MS, DACVIM

Topical Toxins: Common Human OTC Dermatological Preparations

appendix 5

For information on topical preparations with a greater potential for toxicity, including 5-fluoruracil (5-FU), calcipotriene (vitamin D), imidazoline decongestants, nicotine or fentanyl transdermal patches, NSAIDs, pyrethrin/pyrethroid insecticides, salicylate (aspirin) creams, and tea tree oil (melaleuca oil), see the individual chapter.

Blackwell's Five-Minute Veterinary Consult Clinical Companion: Small Animal Toxicology, Second Edition.
Lynn R. Hovda, Ahna G. Brutlag, Robert H. Poppenga, and Katherine L. Peterson.

Companion website: www.fiveminutevet.com/toxicology

Product Category and Trade Name	Active Ingredients	Toxicity	Clinical Signs	Treatment	Prognosis
Analgesics (camphor): Campho-Phenique Carmex Tiger Balm Arthritis Rub; White; Red Vicks VapoRub	Camphor, up to 11%.	Toxicity is not well established in cats/dogs. <1 g of camphor has caused death in children. Mouse LD_{50} (oral) = 1310 mg/kg. Camphor is readily absorbed across the skin.	Onset of signs is 5–20 minutes. Dermal application can cause local irritation. Any ingestion can cause GI distress. Large ingestion can cause CNS depression and seizures (humans). Death from respiratory depression/seizures.	No antidote. GI protectants if needed. Benzodiazepines or barbiturates for seizures. Respiratory support. Monitor blood pressure and vitals.	Good with treatment/ mild signs. Severe signs without treatment have a poorer prognosis. If no signs by 60 min, toxicosis unlikely.
Antibiotics: Duospore Polysporin Lanabiotic Medi-Quik Neosporin Triple Antibiotic	Bacitracin Neomycin Polymyxin B	Not established. Severe toxicity is not expected from acute ingestion/application.	Self-limiting vomiting and diarrhea (partly from the petroleum-based carrier). Anaphylaxis in cats with ocular administration (very rare).	Supportive GI care. Treat for anaphylaxis with O_2, epinephrine, fluids, diphenhydramine, possible steroids.	Excellent with acute ingestions and appropriate treatment for anaphylaxis if needed.
Antifungals: Femstat Lamisil AT Lotrimin AF Monistat Neosporin AF Nizoral A-D Spectazole Vagistat	Butoconazole, 2% Clotrimazole, 1–2% Econazole, 1% Ketoconazole, 1–2% Miconazole, 2–4% Terbinafine, 1% Tioconazole, 1–6.5% Tolnaftate, 1%	Generally, all OTC antifungal preparations have a wide margin of safety, especially in acute ingestions.	Self-limiting vomiting and diarrhea (partly from the carriers).	Supportive GI care.	Excellent with acute ingestions.

Product Category and Trade Name	Active Ingredients	Toxicity	Clinical Signs	Treatment	Prognosis
Antihistamines: Benadryl Caladryl Dermamycin Ziradryl	Diphenhydramine (DPH), 1–2%	Toxicity unlikely with ingestion of topical DPH or significant topical application (poor dermal absorption). Oral: 2–4 mg/kg (therapeutic dose), mild CNS depression and anticholinergic effects. Large oral overdoses may cause severe CNS stimulation.	Following ingestion: Common – vomiting and diarrhea, especially from carriers. Lethargy, dry mouth, urinary retention. Uncommon – CNS stimulation, agitation, and tachycardia from large oral overdoses.	Emesis and activated charcoal (large ingestions only). Sedation and GI support as needed.	Excellent following ingestion of topical preparations.
Antiseptics (benzoyl peroxide): Clean & Clear PERSA Gel-10 Clearasil Acne Treatment PanOxyl Acne Face Wash Proactiv Acne Cleanser	Benzoyl peroxide, 2.5–10%	Minimal systemic absorption may occur from topica administration. Severe toxicity is not expected from small, acute ingestions/ applications. Large ingestions may cause tissue irritation. Mouse oral LD_{50} = 5700 mg/kg.	Dermal and ocular irritation, including hyperemia and blistering or ulceration (rare) following topical exposure. GI irritation (vomiting, pain, gas, diarrhea) likely with small ingestions. Erosion/ulceration possible with massive ingestions.	Dermal or ocular decontamination. Dilution or gas decompression if ingested. Supportive GI care and GI protectants.	Good with acute ingestions or topical reactions.
Corticosteroids: Cortaid Penecort Procort Scalpicin	Hydrocortisone, 0.5–1%	Ingestion, even in massive doses, is unlikely to cause harmful effects. Therapeutic dose = 5 mg/kg PC.	Self-limiting vomiting, diarrhea (partly from carriers) with possible PU/ PD.	Supportive GI care. Access to water.	Excellent with acute ingestions.

(Continued)

Product Category and Trade Name	Active Ingredients	Toxicity	Clinical Signs	Treatment	Prognosis
Local anesthetics: Cetacaine Chigger X Plus Goodwinol Solarcaine	Benzocaine, 5–20% Dibucaine, 1% Lidocaine, 0.5–2.5% Prilocaine, 2.5%	Oral toxic dose is not established. 1–2 licks are unlikely to cause toxicity. Larger ingestions pose greater risk. Dibucaine is more toxic than lidocaine. Topical lidocaine is systemically absorbed; toxicity unlikely unless used chronically. High first-pass effect makes oral toxicity less likely.	Anesthetization of the pharynx can lead to aspiration. Methemoglobinemia and Heinz bodies can occur with ingestion. Cats are more sensitive and can develop methemoglobinemia or seizures more readily than dogs. Dibucaine can cause seizures, arrhythmias, hypotension, death.	Emesis of questionable efficacy. Charcoal if no risk of aspiration (stomach tube). Treat for methemoglobinemia if present. More aggressive treatment needed for some exposures and species.	Good with appropriate care.

Abbreviations

See Appendix 1 for a complete list.

AC = activated charcoal

Suggested Reading

Welch S. Local anesthetic toxicosis. Vet Med 2000; 95(9):670–673.
Welch S. Oral toxicity of topical preparations. Vet Clin Small Anim Pract 2002; 32:443–453.

Acknowledgment: The authors and editors acknowledge the prior contributions of Catherine M. Adams, DVM, who co-authored this appendix in the previous edition.
Author: Ahna G. Brutlag, DVM, MS, DABT, DABVT

Index by Toxins and Toxicants

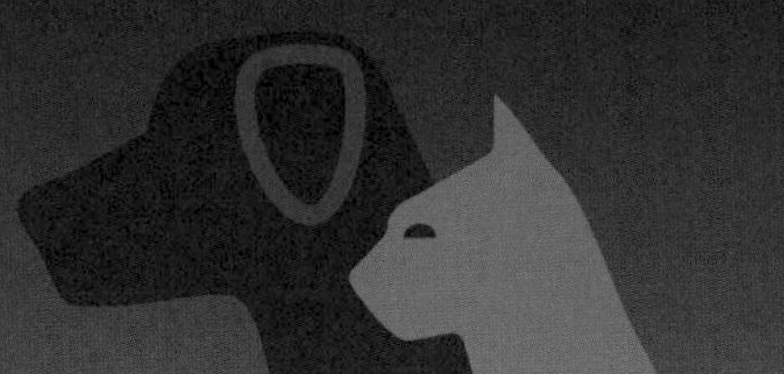

Note: Chapter titles are bolded and chapter paging shows inclusive pages. Page numbers followed by "t" refer to tables; page numbers followed by "f" are figures.

Index by Clinical Signs

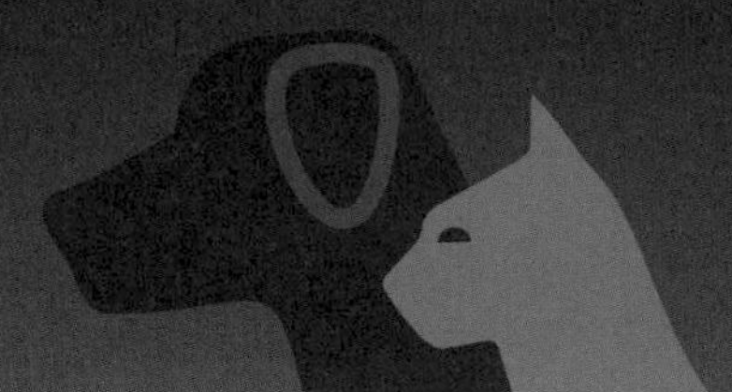

This index is intended to assist clinicians with differential diagnoses of the specific toxins and toxicants documented in this book by providing a quick review of associated clinical signs or physiological conditions.

Acidosis
- Alcohols/glycol ethers
- Amphetamines
- Aspirin
- Azaleas and rhododendrons
- Beta receptor antagonists (beta-blockers)
- Bread dough (with yeast)
- Cardiac glycosides
- Chlorine bleach (large ingestions only)
- Cholecalciferol
- Colchicine
- Ethylene glycol
- Hops
- Methionine
- Hydrofluoric acid
- Iron
- Metaldehyde
- Methamphetamine
- Organophosphates/carbamates
- PCP
- Phenols
- Phosphides
- Pine oil
- Propylene glycol
- Smoke inhalation
- SSRIs and SNRIs
- Strychnine

Agitation – see CNS stimulation/agitation

Alkalosis
- Aspirin (respiratory)
- Calcium supplements
- Diuretics (rare)
- Foreign objects
- Phenols and pine oils

Anemia (also see Heinz body anemia)
- 5-Fluorouracil (5-FU)
- Anticoagulant rodenticides
- Arsenic
- Aspirin
- Batteries (secondary to zinc intoxication)
- Brown recluse spider (*Loxosceles reclusa*)
- Copper
- Elapids (coral snakes)
- Grapes and raisins
- Lead
- Methionine
- Mothballs
- Naphthalene (see Mothballs)
- NSAIDs
- Onions/garlic
- Pine oil
- Propylene glycol
- Sago palm
- Vitamin A
- Wasps, hornets, and bees
- Zinc

Arrhythmias
- 5-Fluorouracil (5-FU)
- Amaryllis (*Hippeastrum* spp.) and daffodils (*Narcissus* spp.)
- Amphetamines
- Antipsychotics, atypical
- Azaleas and rhododendrons
- Baclofen
- Barium (fireworks; see Chapter 84)
- Bath salts
- Beta$_2$ receptor agonists
- Bread dough (with yeast)
- Bufo toads
- Calcipotriene/calcipotriol
- Calcium channel blockers
- Calcium supplements
- Cardiac glycosides
- Chocolate/caffeine
- Cholecalciferol
- Cocaine
- Colchicine
- Crotalids (pit vipers)
- Deferoxamine chelation therapy
- Diuretics
- Fireworks (barium)
- Hydrofluoric acid
- Lily-of-the-valley (*Convallaria* spp.)
- Local anesthetics
- MDMA
- Methamphetamine

Arrhythmias (*continued*)
Minoxidil
Opiates and opioids (cats)
PCP
Phosphides
Pimobendan (massive overdose)
Propylene glycol
Thyroid hormones
Venomous lizards
Yew (*Taxus* spp.)
Ataxia/incoordination
5-Fluorouracil (5-FU)
Alcohols/glycol ethers
Amitraz
Anticoagulant rodenticides
Antipsychotics, atypical
Baclofen
Benzodiazepines
Bread dough (with yeast)
Bromethalin
Bufo toads
Chinaberry (*Melia* spp.)
Cocaine
Dextromethorphan
Elapids (coral snakes)
Essential oil
Larkspur (*Delphinum* spp.)
Lilies (*Lilium* spp.)
Lithium
Lupin (*Lupinus* spp.)
Macadamia nuts
Macrocyclic lactones (e.g., ivermectin)
Marijuana
Melaleuca/tea tree oil
Mercury
Neonicotinoids
Nicotine
Nonbenzodiazepine sleep aids
Paintballs (hypernatremia)
Phenols
Phosphides
Pine oil
Propylene glycol
Pyrethrins/pyrethroids
Scorpions
Selenium
Synthetic cannabinoids
Table salt
Tea tree /melaleuca oil
Tobacco (*Nicotiana* spp.)
Vitamin B_6 (pyridoxine)
Xylitol
Yesterday, today, and tomorrow plant (*Brunfelsia* spp.)
Yew (*Taxus* spp.)
AV block
Alpha$_2$-adrenergic agonists
Azaleas and rhododendrons
Bufo toads
Calcium channel blockers
Cardiac glycosides
MDMA
Mountain laurel (*Kalmia* spp.)
Opiates and opioids
Yew (*Taxus* spp.)

Blindness
Alcohols/glycol ethers
Anticoagulant rodenticides
Azaleas and rhododendrons
Bread dough (with yeast)
Lead
Macrocyclic lactones (e.g., ivermectin)
Mercury
Metaldehyde
Paintballs
Bloat
Alcohols/glycol ethers
Amitraz
Bread dough (with yeast)
Glue, diisocyanate (e.g., Gorilla Glue)
Phosphides
Bone marrow suppression
5-Fluorouracil
Aspirin (rare)
Colchicine
Bradycardia
Alpha$_2$-adrenergic agonists
Amitraz
Azaleas and rhododendrons
Baclofen
Barium (fireworks; see Chapter 84)
Benzodiazepines
Beta receptor antagonists (beta-blockers)
Bread dough (with yeast)
Bufo toads
Calcipotriene/calcipotriol
Calcium channel blockers
Cardiac glycosides
Cholecalciferol
Fireworks (barium)
Foxglove (*Digitalis* spp.)
Imidazoline decongestants
Lily-of-the-valley (*Convallaria* spp.)
Marijuana
Monkshood (*Aconitum* spp.)
Mountain laurel (*Kalmia* spp.)
Mushrooms
Oleander (*Nerium* spp.)
Opiates and opioids
Organophosphorus/carbamate insecticides
Oxalates, soluble
PCP
Phenylephrine (reflex)
Phenylpropanolamine (reflex)

Hypercalcemia
- Calcipotriene/calcipotriol
- Calcium supplements
- Cholecalciferol
- Grapes/raisins
- Vitamin D

Hyperchloremia
- Paintballs

Hyperkalemia
- Beta receptor antagonists (beta-blockers)
- Cardiac glycosides
- Chlorates (fireworks, matches)
- Diuretics
- Ethylene glycol
- Fireworks (chlorates)
- Fluoride
- Foxglove (*Digitalis* spp.)
- Grapes/raisins
- Hops
- Hydrofluoric acid
- Lily-of-the-valley (*Convallaria* spp.)
- Matches (chlorates)
- Oleander (*Nerium* spp.)

Hypernatremia
- Chlorine bleach (large ingestions only)
- Cocaine
- Paintballs
- Table salt

Hypersalivation
- Amphetamines
- Antipsychotics, atypical
- Azaleas and rhododendrons
- Baclofen
- Batteries
- Black widow spider (*Latrodectus* spp.)
- Blue-green algae
- Bufo toads
- Calcipotriene/calcipotriol
- Cardiac glycosides
- Citrus oil
- Cocaine
- Crotalids (pit vipers)
- Essential oils
- Glow jewelry
- Lilies (*Lilium* spp.)
- Macrocyclic lactones (e.g., ivermectin)
- Matches and fireworks
- Minoxidil
- Mycotoxins, tremorgenic
- Nicotine
- Oxalates, insoluble
- Phenols
- Pine oil
- Pyrethrins/pyrethroids
- Scorpions
- Smoke inhalation
- Spring-blooming crocus (*Crocus* spp.)
- Strong acids/alkalis
- Yesterday, today, and tomorrow plant (*Brunfelsia* spp.)

Hypertension
- Amphetamines
- Baclofen
- Barium (fireworks; see Chapter 84)
- Beta$_2$ receptor agonists
- Black widow spider (*Latrodectus* spp.)
- Chocolate/caffeine
- Cocaine
- Ephedra
- Fireworks (barium)
- Imidazoline decongestants (initially)
- Ma huang
- MDMA
- Methamphetamine
- Nicotine
- PCP
- Phenylephrine
- Phenylpropanolamine
- Pimobendan (rare)
- Pseudoephedrine
- Scorpions
- SSRIs and SNRIs
- Thyroid hormones

Hyperthermia
- Amphetamines
- Bath salts
- Bittersweet (*Celastrus* spp.)
- Bufo toads
- Cationic surfactants
- Cocaine
- Ephedra
- Hops
- Ma huang
- Macadamia nuts
- MDMA
- Metaldehyde
- Methamphetamine
- Mycotoxins, tremorgenic
- PCP
- Phenylephrine
- Phenylpropanolamine
- Pseudoephedrine
- SSRIs and SNRIs
- Thyroid hormones
- Tin
- Yew (*Taxus* spp.)

Hypocalcemia
- Builders and cleaners (soaps, detergents, etc.; see Chapter 88)
- Colchicine
- Ethylene glycol
- Fluoride
- Hydrofluoric acid
- Oxalates, soluble
- Strychnine

Pine oil
Pseudoephedrine
Scorpions
SSRIs and SNRIs
Synthetic cannabinoids
Yew (*Taxus* spp.)

Pain
5-Fluorouracil (5-FU) (GI pain)
Antiseptics
Arsenic (GI pain)
Batteries (corrosive injury)
Black widow spider (*Latrodectus* spp.)
Bufo toads
Calcipotriene/calcipotriol
Cationic surfactants
Colchicine
Diquat/paraquat
Fluoride
Foreign objects
Glue, diisocyanate (e.g., Gorilla Glue) (GI pain)
Hops
Hydrofluoric acid
Iron (GI pain)
Lead (GI pain)
Macadamia nuts
Mushrooms
NSAIDs, veterinary and human (GI pain)
Onions/garlic (GI pain)
Oxalates, insoluble
Phosphides (GI pain)
Scorpions
Smoke inhalation
Strong acids/alkalis
Tacrolimus
Venomous lizards
Wasps, hornets, and bees

Pancreatitis
Angiotensin converting enzyme inhibitors (rare)
Bone and blood meal
Fertilizers
Foreign objects
Lilies (*Lilium* spp.) (rare)
Macadamia nuts
Organophosphorus/carbamate insecticides
Pennyroyal oil
Zinc

Paralysis
Azaleas and rhododendrons
Baclofen (flaccid)
Black widow spider (*Latrodectus* spp.) (cats)
Blue-green algae
Elapids (coral snakes)
Magnesium (flaccid paralysis)
Nicotine
Quaternary ammonium compounds (soaps, detergents, etc.; see Chapter 88)
Vitamin A
Yesterday, today, and tomorrow plant (*Brunfelsia* spp.)

Paresis
Albuterol
Anticoagulant rodenticides
Bromethalin
Elapids (coral snakes)
Macadamia nuts
Mercury
Organophosphorus/carbamate insecticides

Pharyngitis
Oxalates, insoluble

Pigmenturia – see Hemoglobinuria/pigmenturia

Piloerection
Phenylpropanolamine

Pruritus
Blue-green algae
Brown recluse spider (*Loxosceles reclusa*)
Cyclosporine A
Glow jewelry
Miscellaneous insecticides
Neonicotinoids
Scorpions
Wasps, hornets, and bees

Pulmonary edema
5-Fluorouracil (5-FU)
Aspirin (rare)
Compound 1080
Diquat/paraquat
Hydrocarbons
Hydrofluoric acid
Metaldehyde
Minoxidil
Organophosphorus/carbamate insecticides
Phenols
Phenols/pine oils
Phosphides
Pine oil
Scorpions (rare)
Smoke inhalation
Table salt
Tacrolimus (rabbits)

Respiratory depression
Alcohols
Alpha$_2$-adrenergic agonists
Amitraz
Baclofen
Benzodiazepines (rare)
Bread dough (ethanol)
Bromethalin
Camphor
Club drugs

Sago palm
Strychnine
Table salt
Xylitol
Yew (*Taxus* spp.)

Tachycardia
Amphetamines
Anticoagulant rodenticides (due to hypovolemia)
Antipsychotics, atypical
Azaleas and rhododendrons
Baclofen
Barium
Bath salts
Beta$_2$ receptor agonists
Black widow spider (*Latrodectus* spp.)
Bread dough
Brown recluse spider (*Loxosceles reclusa*)
Bufo toads
Carbon monoxide
Cardiac glycosides
Chocolate/caffeine
Cocaine
Elapids (coral snakes)
Ephedra
Ethylene glycol
Gold
Golden angel's trumpet (*Brugmansia* spp.)
LSD
Ma huang
Marijuana
MDMA
Metaldehyde
Methamphetamine
Minoxidil
Mycotoxins, tremorgenic
Nicotine
Organophosphorus/carbamate insecticides
PCP
Phenylephrine
Phenylpropanolamine
Pimobendan (reflex)
Pseudoephedrine
Rosary pea (*Abrus precatorius*)
Scorpions
Smoke inhalation
SSRIs and SNRIs
Strychnine
Thyroid hormones
Tulips (*Tulipa* spp.)
Venomous lizards
Wasps, hornets, and bees
Yew (*Taxus* spp.)

Tachypnea
Amphetamines
Anticoagulant rodenticides
Beta$_2$ receptor agonists
Bread dough (with yeast)
Bufo toads
Carbon monoxide
Diquat/paraquat
Elapids (coral snakes)
Ethylene glycol
Hops
MDMA
Methamphetamine
Phosphides
Smoke inhalation

Tremors
Amphetamines
Antipsychotics, atypical
Azaleas and rhododendrons
Blue-green algae
Chocolate/caffeine
Cocaine
Compound 1080
Dextromethorphan
Ephedra
GHB
Lilies (*Lilium* spp.) (rare)
Ma huang
Macadamia nuts
Macrocyclic lactones (e.g., ivermectin)
Marijuana
Melaleuca/tea tree oil
Methamphetamine
Mycotoxins, tremorgenic
Neonicotinoids
Nicotine
Paintballs (hypernatremia)
Phenylpropanolamine
Pyrethrins/pyrethroids
Scorpions
Synthetic cannabinoids
Table salt
Tea tree/melaleuca oil
Thyroid hormones
Vitamin A
Vitamin B$_3$ (niacin)
Xylitol
Yesterday, today, and tomorrow plant (*Brunfelsia* spp.)

Uroliths
Calcium supplements
Magnesium
Phosphorus
Vitamin C

Vocalization
- Alcohols
- Baclofen
- Black widow spider (*Latrodectus* spp.)
- Bread dough (ethanol)
- Bufo toads
- Hallucinogens
- LSD
- Marijuana (rare)
- Mushrooms
- Oxalates, insoluble
- SSRIs and SNRIs
- Yesterday, today, and tomorrow plant (*Brunfelsia* spp.)

Vomiting
- 5-Fluorouracil (5-FU)
- Alpha$_2$-adrenergic agonists
- Amaryllis (*Hippeastrum* spp.), hyacinths (*Hyacinthus* spp.), and daffodils (*Narcissus* spp.)
- Amphetamines
- Angiotensin converting enzyme inhibitors
- Antipsychotics, atypical
- Aspirin
- Azaleas and rhododendrons
- Baclofen
- Black widow spider (*Latrodectus* spp.)
- Blood and bone meal
- Brown recluse spider (*Loxosceles reclusa*)
- Bufo toads
- Calcipotriene/calcipotriol
- Calcium channel blockers
- Calcium supplements
- Cardiac glycosides
- Chlorates (fireworks, matches)
- Chocolate/caffeine
- Cocaine
- Colchicine
- Crotalids (pit vipers)
- Cyclosporine A
- Fertilizers
- Fireworks (chlorates)
- Fluoride
- Foreign objects
- Glues/adhesives
- Grapes and raisins
- Herbicides
- Hops
- Hydrofluoric acid (with corrosive burns)
- Iron
- Lilies (*Lilium* spp.)
- Marijuana
- Matches (chlorates)
- Methionine
- Minoxidil
- Mothballs
- Mushrooms
- Mycotoxins, aflatoxins
- Mycotoxins, tremorgenic
- Nicotine
- NSAIDs, veterinary and human
- Oil of wintergreen
- Oxalates, insoluble
- Paintballs
- Peppermint oil
- Phenols
- Phenylephrine
- Phenylpropanolamine
- Pine oil
- Pseudoephedrine
- Sago palm
- Soaps, detergents, cleaners, etc.
- Spring-blooming crocus (*Crocus* spp.)
- SSRIs and SNRIs
- Synthetic cannabinoids
- Table salt
- Tacrolimus
- Thyroid hormones
- Venomous lizards
- Xylitol
- Yesterday, today, and tomorrow plant (*Brunfelsia* spp.)

Weakness
- Azaleas and rhododendrons
- Blue-green algae
- Calcium channel blockers
- Crotalids (pit vipers)
- Diuretics
- Melaleuca/tea tree oil
- Minoxidil
- Nicotine
- Paintballs
- Quaternary ammonium compounds (soaps, detergents, etc.; see Chapter 88)
- Tea tree/melaleuca oil
- Venomous lizards